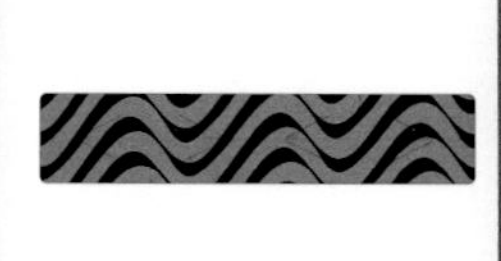

CARDIAC SURGERY
Operative Technique

CARDIAC SURGERY
Operative Technique

2nd EDITION

Donald B. Doty, M.D.
John R. Doty, M.D.
Division of Cardiovascular and Thoracic Surgery
Intermountain Medical Center
Salt Lake City, Utah

with illustrations by
Jill Rhead, MA, CMI, FAMI
Salt Lake City, Utah
Christy Krames, MA, CMI, FAMI
Austin, Texas

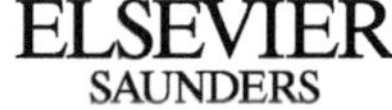

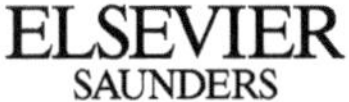

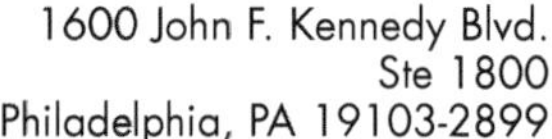

1600 John F. Kennedy Blvd.
Ste 1800
Philadelphia, PA 19103-2899

CARDIAC SURGERY: OPERATIVE TECHNIQUE, 2ND EDITION ISBN: 978-1-4160-3653-1

Notices

Knowledge and best practice in this field are constantly changing. As new research and experience broaden our understanding, changes in research methods, professional practices, or medical treatment may become necessary.

Practitioners and researchers must always rely on their own experience and knowledge in evaluating and using any information, methods, compounds, or experiments described herein. In using such information or methods they should be mindful of their own safety and the safety of others, including parties for whom they have a professional responsibility.

With respect to any drug or pharmaceutical products identified, readers are advised to check the most current information provided (i) on procedures featured or (ii) by the manufacturer of each product to be administered, to verify the recommended dose or formula, the method and duration of administration, and contraindications. It is the responsibility of practitioners, relying on their own experience and knowledge of their patients, to make diagnoses, to determine dosages and the best treatment for each individual patient, and to take all appropriate safety precautions.

To the fullest extent of the law, neither the Publisher nor the authors, contributors, or editors, assume any liability for any injury and/or damage to persons or property as a matter of products liability, negligence or otherwise, or from any use or operation of any methods, products, instructions, or ideas contained in the material herein.

Library of Congress Cataloging-in-Publication Data

Doty, Donald B.
Cardiac surgery: operative technique / Donald B. Doty, John R. Doty ; with illustrations by Jill Rhead, Christy Krames. – 2nd ed.
p. ; cm.
Includes index.
ISBN 978-1-4160-3653-1 (hardcover : alk. paper)
I. Doty, John R. II. Title.
[DNLM: 1. Heart Diseases–surgery–Atlases. 2. Cardiac Surgical Procedures–methods–Atlases. WG 17]
617.4'12–dc23

2012001906

Content Strategist: Michael Houston
Content Development Specialist: Rachel Miller
Publishing Services Manager: Julie Eddy
Project Manager: Jan Waters
Design Direction: Steven Stave

Last digit is the print number: 9 8 7 6 5 4 3 2 1

To those who have shaped our lives, Our family,
Our wives and children – Cheryl, Kristy, Grant, Madeline, and Ainsley,
Teachers, Mentors in cardiac surgery, Leaders of our Faith. They have
shown us that Knowledge of the Science of Medicine and Ability to
understand and perform the operations must be in addition to Honesty,
integrity, caring, compassion, and respect for God and fellow man
(our patients) to be competent and successful as a Cardiac Surgeon.

PREFACE

Cardiac Surgery: A Looseleaf Workbook and Update Service, published in 1985, consisted of a core set of chapters including an atlas section demonstrating operations, followed by a collection of abstracts of important articles from the literature. Additional complete chapters and abstracts were added at six month intervals for five years, keeping the book up to date through 1990. This service was discontinued and the book went out of print in 1991. The atlas portions of the chapters were revised to include all of the original illustrations extensively supplemented by new illustrations and published in 1997 as *Cardiac Surgery: Operative Technique*. The operations were presented with illustrations supported by text in sufficient detail to demonstrate exactly how to perform the steps of the procedure. The book was comprehensive including nearly all operations that were performed in cardiac surgical practice. The unique talent of Christy Krames is acknowledged. She spent countless hours over a 15 year period to produce the original 916 illustrations of operative technique. The illustrations were presented from the surgeon's perspective to reproduce what was actually seen at the operation.

The second edition of *Cardiac Surgery* has required more than seven years of work. Jill Rhead added color to the original illustrations with some modifications to reflect current practice. This method produced a wonderful blend of the work of two illustrators and preserved the legacy contributed by Christy Krames to the original edition of this book. Jill Rhead has independently created many new illustrations to be representative and inclusive of the operations presently performed in cardiac and great vessel surgery. As this illustration process has gone forward, we have been pleased with the added dimension that color has contributed. In addition to the hours she spent producing beautiful illustrations, she also did the tedious and time consuming process of page layout and labeling.

Photographs have been added to demonstrate cardiac anatomy, the morphology of the cardiac defects, or elements of the corrective operations. High quality color corrected digital images were taken in the operating room by the authors. We also photographed hundreds of anatomic cardiac specimens at the University of Iowa School of Medicine, Division of Pediatric Cardiology during August 2006, when Larry T. Mahoney, M.D. was Director of the unit, and, in February 2007 at the Jesse E. Edwards Registry of Cardiovascular Disease, Shannon M. Mackey-Bojack, M.D. Medical Director. We express sincere appreciation to these helpful, dedicated medical doctors for allowing us to produce photographs that would not be available to most cardiac surgeons.

We gratefully acknowledge guidance, encouragement, respectful cajoling, and patience of Judith Fletcher, Content Strategist, Rachel Miller, Content Development Specialist, and Jan Waters, Project Manager, as well as the design and production staff and all others at Elsevier who helped on this project. It is our hope that these collective efforts have resulted in a book that will be helpful to those who read and use it.

Donald B. Doty, M.D.
John R. Doty, M.D.

CONTENTS

part I

Basic Considerations

chapter 1 CARDIAC ANATOMY

Understanding cardiac anatomy is fundamental to success in cardiac surgery. The following drawings show the cardiac surgeon's view of the heart from the right side of a supine patient through a midsternal incision. Photographs illustrate the anatomic position as if looking at an upright patient, unless otherwise noted.

Figure 1-1

A The cardiac structures most accessible to view are the superior vena cava, right atrium, right ventricle, main pulmonary artery, and aorta. Only a small portion of the anterior wall of the left ventricle is visible. Medial displacement of the right atrium exposes the left atrium and right pulmonary veins.

B The right coronary artery is partly visible in the fat of the atrioventricular groove, with the ventricular branches and the acute marginal branch in full view. The posterior descending artery originates from the right coronary artery near the crux of the heart. The crux is defined as the cross point or junction of the atrioventricular septum and the atrioventricular groove. In its course in the atrioventricular groove, the right coronary artery is in close relation to the anterior portion of the annulus of the tricuspid valve. The distal portion of the right coronary artery supplies blood to the atrioventricular node and is in close proximity to the annulus of the mitral valve. The left coronary artery originates posteriorly from the aorta and, after a short distance, divides into the anterior descending and circumflex branches. The anterior descending coronary artery deviates from the atrioventricular groove onto the left ventricle, lateral to the pulmonary artery. Once it is on the anterior wall of the heart over the ventricular septum, the left anterior descending coronary artery becomes visible. The circumflex coronary artery lies in the atrioventricular groove posteriorly, in close relation to the annulus of the mitral valve. Marginal branches of the circumflex coronary artery supply the posterolateral surface of the left ventricle.

C Visualization of the distal portion of the right coronary artery requires displacement of the acute margin of the heart to expose the diaphragmatic surface. The posterior descending coronary artery takes a course over the ventricular septum on the diaphragmatic surface of the heart. An exception to this anatomic configuration occurs when the posterior descending coronary artery originates from the left dominant coronary artery. The distal right coronary artery generally continues in the atrioventricular groove to supply one or more branches in the posterior wall of the left ventricle.

D Exposure of the branches of the left coronary artery requires displacement of the heart superiorly and to the right. The circumflex branch of the left coronary artery is in the atrioventricular groove, giving off marginal branches to supply blood to the posterolateral surfaces of the left ventricle. The obtuse marginal branch is usually near the base of the left atrial appendage. The obtuse marginal branch may not be visible on the surface of the heart when it lies within the myocardium. In this situation it can usually be identified as a slightly yellowish discoloration of the otherwise red-brown myocardium. The anterior descending coronary artery takes a course along the ventricular septum anteriorly, providing one or more diagonal branches to supply blood to the anterolateral surfaces of the left ventricle. The size of the diagonal branches depends on the relative size of the circumflex marginal branches because the blood supply to the lateral wall of the ventricle is shared.

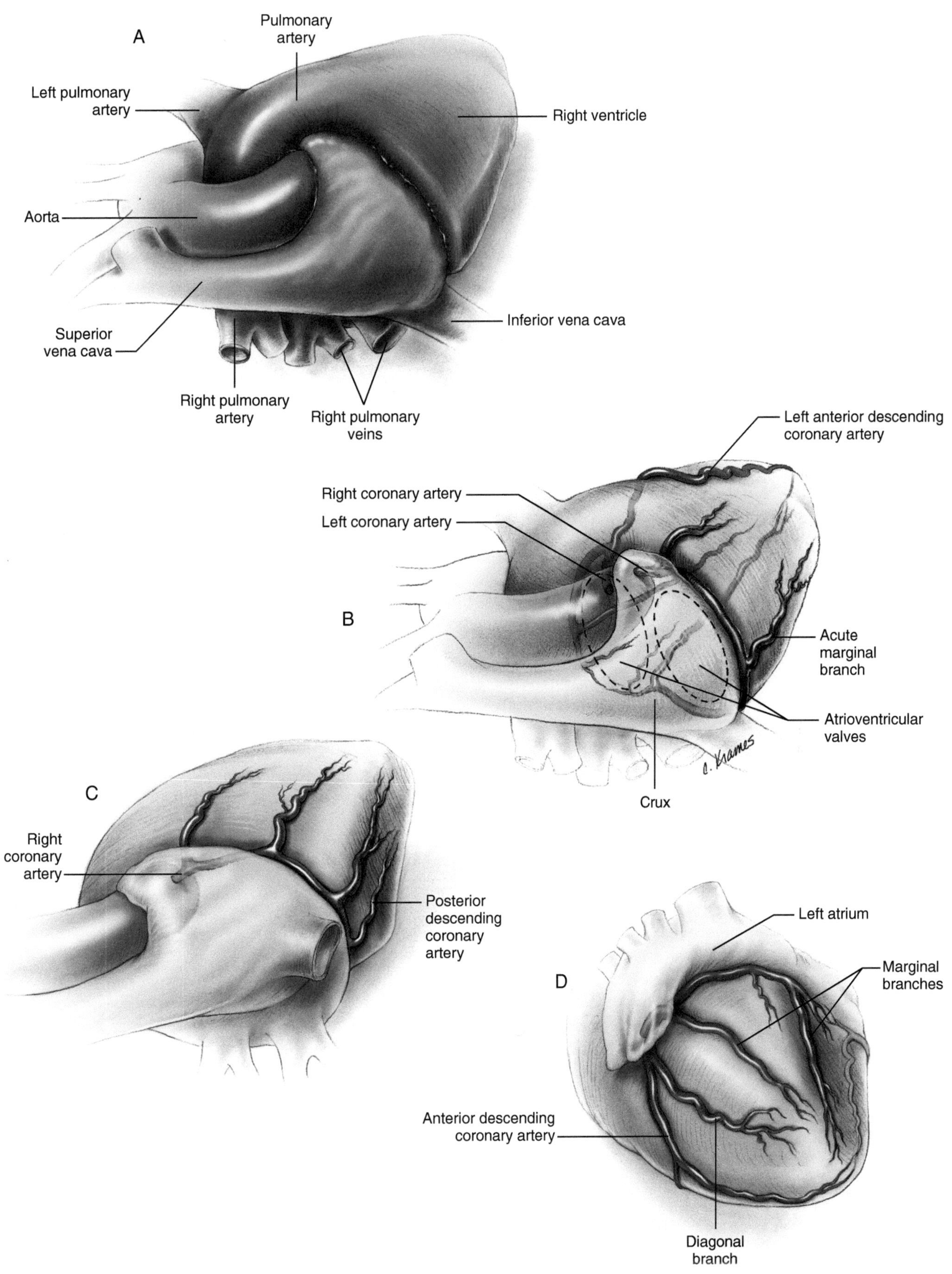
A
Pulmonary artery
Left pulmonary artery
Right ventricle
Aorta
Superior vena cava
Inferior vena cava
Right pulmonary artery
Right pulmonary veins
B
Left anterior descending coronary artery
Right coronary artery
Left coronary artery
Acute marginal branch
Atrioventricular valves
Crux
C. Krames
C
Right coronary artery
Posterior descending coronary artery
D
Left atrium
Marginal branches
Anterior descending coronary artery
Diagonal branch

Figure 1-2

A Coronary veins of the right ventricle drain directly to the right atrium or through thebesian veins to the right ventricle. Most of the venous return of the left ventricle is via the coronary sinus. Large cardiac veins located on the posterior surface of the heart collect through a common venous channel in the atrioventricular groove, which is anatomically related to the posterior portion of the annulus of the mitral valve. These veins drain into the right atrium at the coronary sinus. The orifice of the coronary sinus is located in close proximity to the septal portion of the annulus of the tricuspid valve. The sinoatrial node is located on the lateral surface of the right atrium at the junction with the superior vena cava at the origin of the crista terminalis. It occupies a considerable area, often greater than 1 cm in diameter, of the lateral wall of the right atrium.

B Three interatrial conduction pathways are thought to arise from the sinoatrial node. The anterior and medial interatrial conduction pathways course anterior and posterior to the orifice of the superior vena cava and through the atrial septum, anterior to the foramen ovale. The posterior interatrial conduction pathway follows the crista terminalis and crosses the atrial septum caudal to the foramen ovale on the superior rim of the coronary sinus. The atrioventricular node is located in the floor of the right atrium at a point approximately one-third the distance along a line from the coronary sinus to the commissure of the anterior and septal leaflet of the tricuspid valve. The bundle of His generally follows this line to penetrate the annulus of the tricuspid valve and enter the ventricular septum just below the membranous portion. The triangle of Koch is bounded by the coronary sinus, the septal attachment of the tricuspid valve, and (laterally) a ridge of tissue referred to as the tendon of Todaro. The commissure of the septal and anterior leaflet of the tricuspid valve is usually well defined. The commissure of the septal and posterior leaflet of the tricuspid valve may be less obvious. This commissural cleft can generally be identified by the relationships of the chordae tendineae of the papillary muscle attached to the leaflets. The commissure of the anterior and posterior leaflets may also be poorly defined, but this is not of great anatomic importance because these leaflets function as a unit to approximate the septal leaflet.

C A magnified view of the tricuspid valve shows the details of the septal leaflet, with the delicate chordae tendineae and papillary muscle attached. A portion of the posterior leaflet is seen, with the commissure between the posterior and septal leaflets. The coronary sinus is in the lower right corner of the image.

D With the atrial septum removed, the anatomic relations of the right and left atrioventricular valves and the aortic valve are delineated at the fibrous body of the heart. Anatomically, the commissure of the septal and anterior leaflet of the tricuspid valve is closely related to the aortic annulus and the right atrium. Similarly, the noncoronary portions of the annulus of the aortic valve are closely related to the superior wall of the left atrium and the anterior leaflet and annulus of the mitral valve.

E With the anterior wall of the right ventricle opened, the crista supraventricularis, with its septal and parietal bands, separates the tricuspid valve annulus from the annulus of the pulmonary valve. Space between the crista supraventricularis and the pulmonary annulus forms the infundibular chamber. The papillary muscle of the conus is attached to the ventricular septum caudal to the crista supraventricularis and marks the most distal portion of the bundle of His on the ventricular septum. The surface of the right ventricle is trabecular, making identification of small defects of the muscular portion of the ventricular septum extremely difficult.

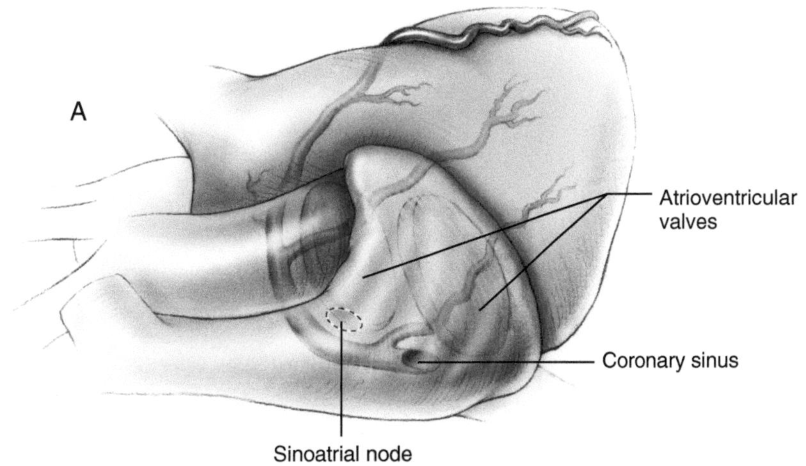
A
Atrioventricular valves
Coronary sinus
Sinoatrial node

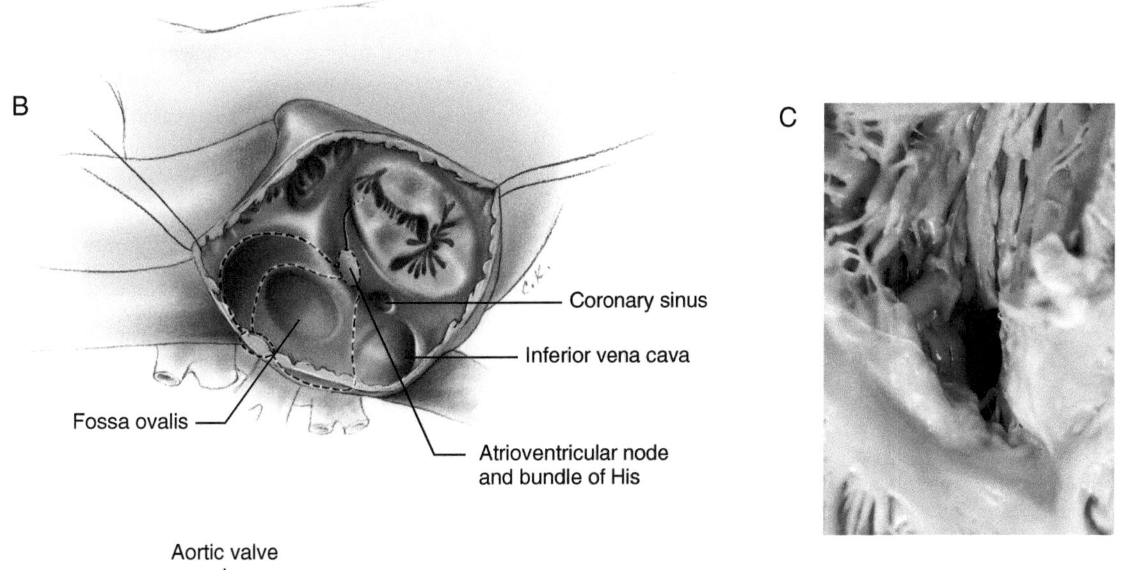
B
Coronary sinus
Inferior vena cava
Fossa ovalis
Atrioventricular node and bundle of His
C

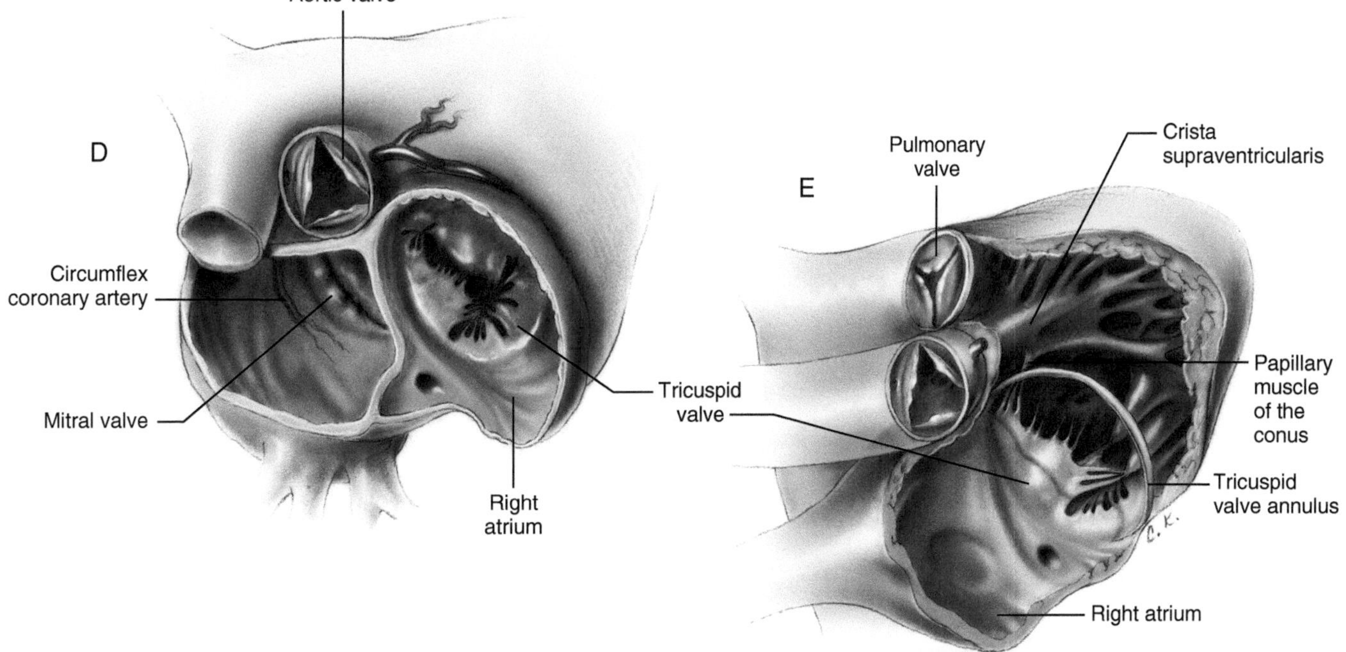
Aortic valve
D
Circumflex coronary artery
Mitral valve
Tricuspid valve
Right atrium
Pulmonary valve
E
Crista supraventricularis
Papillary muscle of the conus
Tricuspid valve
Tricuspid valve annulus
Right atrium

Figure 1-2 (continued)

F Right ventricle, normal. The thin wall of the right ventricle is compared with the thick wall of the left ventricle (behind and to the left of the image). Trabeculations are coarse in the right ventricle. The tricuspid valve septal leaflet is barely visible, attached by chordae to the papillary muscle of the conus on the ventricular septum. The pulmonary valve is separated from the tricuspid valve by the infundibular (conus) portion of the right ventricle. The pulmonary valve is attached directly to the right ventricular outflow tract, with myocardium completely surrounding it.

G Right ventricle, normal. This specimen shows the three segments of the right ventricle. The smooth wall of the right ventricle directly below the tricuspid valve is the inflow segment. This gives way almost immediately to the coarsely trabeculated body of the right ventricle, constituting most of the pumping chamber. The free wall portion is reflected to the left of the image, and the septal wall of the body of the right ventricle is on the right. The infundibular or conal segment of the right ventricle is smooth and is delineated by the ventricular-infundibular fold on the left and the trabecula septomarginalis on the right. These myocardial muscle bundles are minimally defined in the normal right ventricle but become prominent when the right ventricle is hypertrophied. These muscle bundles are also called the parietal and septal bands when they are sufficiently hypertrophied to obstruct the right ventricular outflow tract. In this state, a ridge forms on the infundibular septum, separating the body of the right ventricle from the conus portion, called the crista supraventricularis.

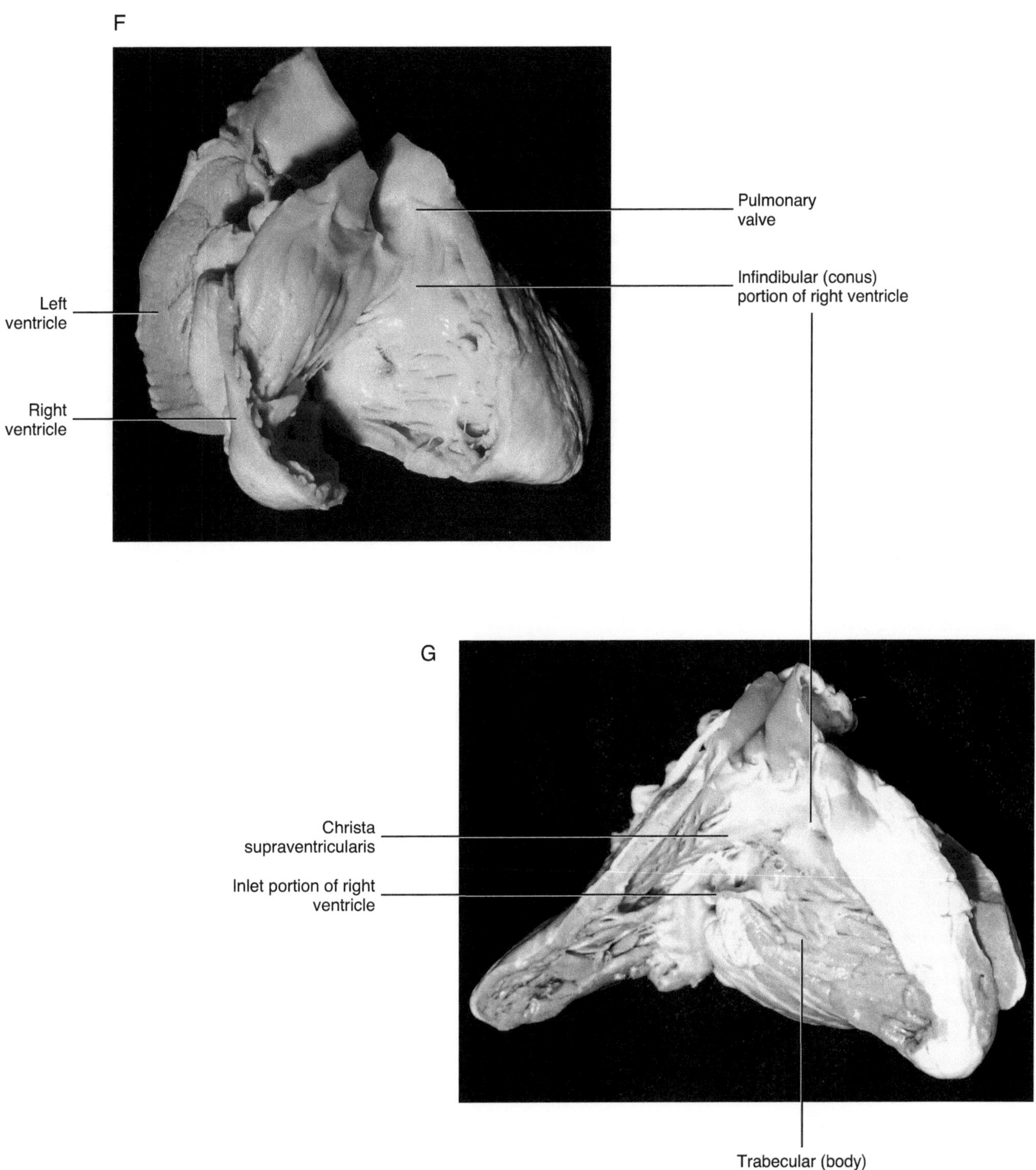
F
Left ventricle
Right ventricle
Pulmonary valve
Infindibular (conus) portion of right ventricle
G
Christa supraventricularis
Inlet portion of right ventricle
Trabecular (body) of right ventricle

Figure 1-3

A The aorta (Ao) and pulmonary artery trunk (PA) are closely related anteriorly. The plane of the semilunar valves is different owing to the presence of the infundibular or conal portion of the right ventricle. This extension of the right ventricular outflow tract carries the plane of the pulmonary valve higher than the aortic valve and directs the pulmonary trunk more posteriorly. The interleaflet triangle is the space between the fibrous attachments of the semilunar leaflets to the aorta or pulmonary artery. The fibrous connective tissue of the interleaflet triangle is looser and more flexible than other portions of the aortic root. The interleaflet triangle between the right and left cusp of the aortic valve is closely related to the pulmonary trunk and the outflow tract of the right ventricle. The anterior interleaflet triangle of the aortic valve, located between the right (R) and posterior (P) or noncoronary cusps, extends to the membranous septum.

B The anterior relationships of the aortic root are best appreciated and illustrated by removing the entire anterior wall of the right ventricle, leaving only the fibrous attachment structure of the pulmonary valve. The aortoventricular junction is on the sinus portion of the aorta, leaving the lowest portion of the aortic valve attached to the ventricle and the commissures above in the aorta. The right (R) coronary sinus of the aorta is related to the right ventricular outflow tract. The left anterior descending branch of the left coronary artery passes posterior to the pulmonary trunk, giving off the first septal branch near the medial posterior commissure of the pulmonary valve. The first septal branch courses toward the papillary muscle of the conus (medial papillary muscle).

C The course of the left anterior descending coronary artery posterior to the pulmonary trunk is appreciated when viewed from above. The relationship of the medial posterior commissure of the pulmonary valve to the origin of the first septal branch is demonstrated.

D Views of the superior aspect of the heart illustrate the central location of the aorta, with other valves displayed around it. IVC, inferior vena cava; LV, left ventricle; RV, right ventricle; SVC, superior vena cava.

E Posterior relations of the aortic valve demonstrate that the posterior interleaflet triangle between the left (L) and posterior (P) noncoronary cusps is exactly in the middle of the anterior leaflet of the mitral valve. The shape of the mitral annulus is not round; rather, it conforms to the primarily round shape of the aortic outflow tract.

F Views of the anterior leaflet of the mitral valve through the aortic root demonstrate the importance of the conformity of the mitral valve to the left ventricular outflow tract.

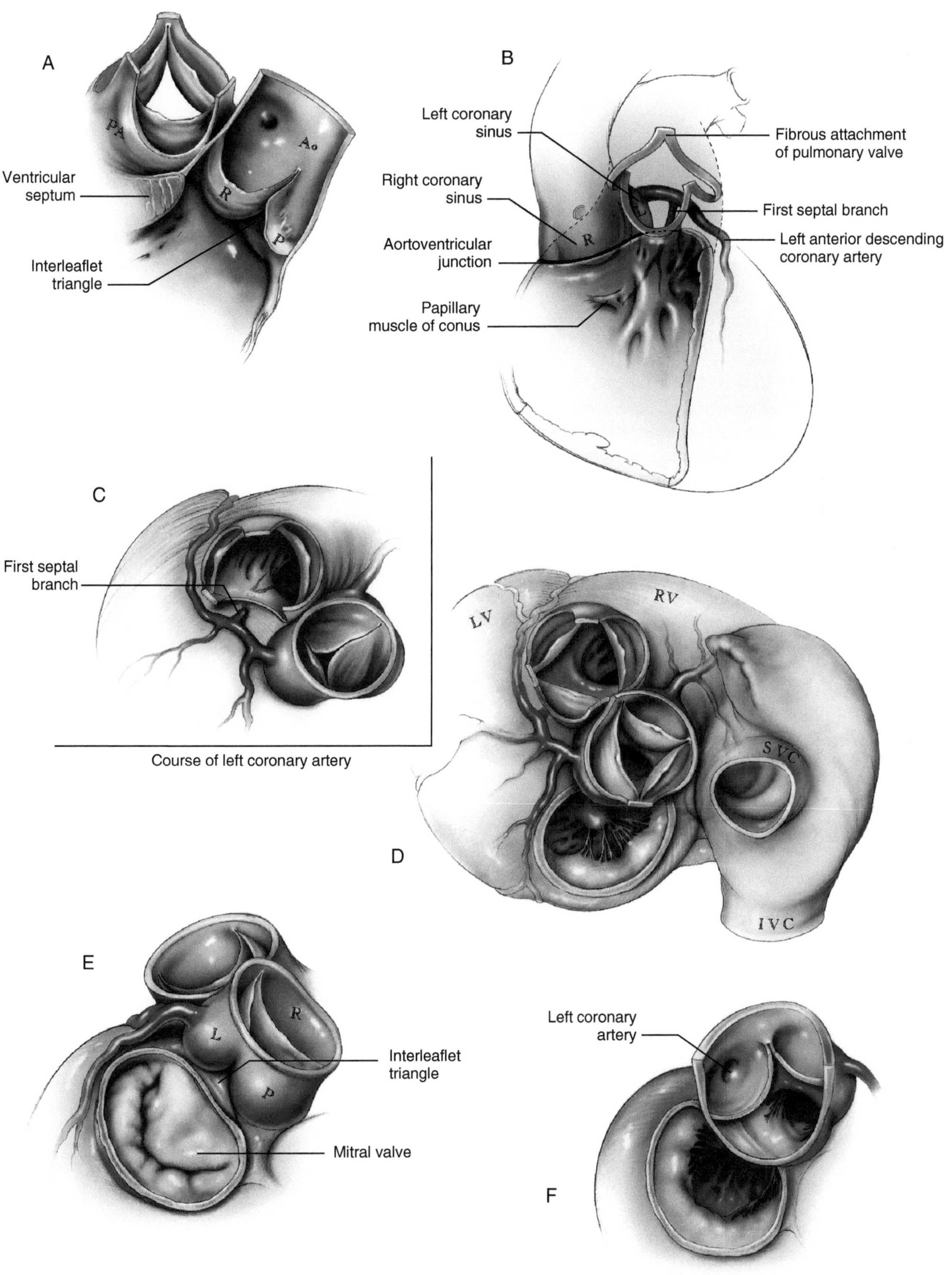
A
PA
Ao
R
P
Ventricular septum
Interleaflet triangle
B
Left coronary sinus
Right coronary sinus
Aortoventricular junction
Papillary muscle of conus
Fibrous attachment of pulmonary valve
First septal branch
Left anterior descending coronary artery
R
L
C
First septal branch
Course of left coronary artery
D
LV
RV
SVC
IVC
E
L
R
P
Interleaflet triangle
Mitral valve
F
Left coronary artery

Figure 1-4

A Aortic and mitral valves, anterior leaflet. The aortic valve is shown with typical thin, semilunar-shaped leaflets attached to the aorta by three commissures. The junction of the aorta and the left ventricular myocardium (aortoventricular junction) is partially bridged by the fibrous hinge point of the aortic valve at the lowest point of the aortic sinus. There is no "annulus," or circular fibrous ring, of the aortic valve; the valve is attached to the left ventricular outflow tract and aorta by the crown-shaped fibrous hinge point. For convenience, surgeons refer to the "annulus" of the aortic valve to describe the diameter of the left ventricular outflow tract at the level of the aortoventricular junction after excision of the aortic valve. There is continuity between the aortic valve fibrous structure and the anterior leaflet of the mitral valve. The midpoint of the anterior leaflet of the mitral valve is directly below the commissure, between the left coronary leaflet and the noncoronary leaflet of the aortic valve. Chordae tendineae attaching the mitral valve to the papillary muscle are demonstrated. The left ventricular outflow tract leading to the aortic valve and aorta is delineated by the anterior leaflet of the mitral valve and the wall of the left ventricle, shown here in cut section.

B Aortic valve, close-up view. Note the thin, translucent appearance of the aortic valve leaflets. The junction of the sinus aorta with the ascending aorta is called the sinotubular junction. This is an important anatomic structure in aortic reconstructive surgery. The ratio of the diameter of the sinotubular junction to the aortic "annulus" is normally 0.85 to 1.0. Although the aorta tends to enlarge somewhat with age, enlargement of the sinotubular junction due to aortic dilation resulting in a ratio greater than 1.0 is considered abnormal, regardless of the patient's age.

C Mitral valve. The anterior leaflet is to the left, the posterior leaflet is to the right, and the commissure is in between. Thin, translucent normal leaflets are attached to the posterior papillary muscle by delicate but remarkably strong chordae tendineae. The distribution of chordae from a single papillary muscle is to half the anterior leaflet and half the posterior leaflet. Note the chordae supporting the commissure.

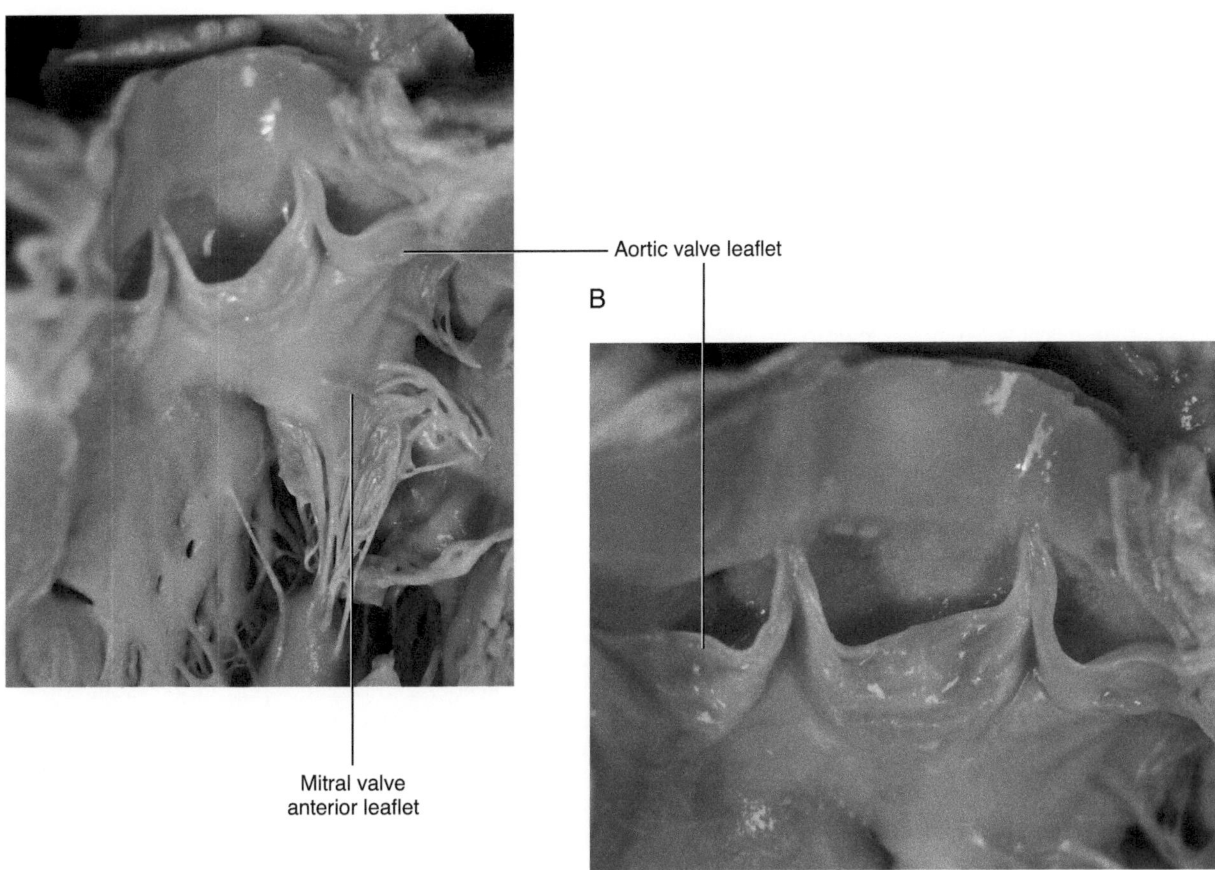
A
B
Aortic valve leaflet
Mitral valve
anterior leaflet

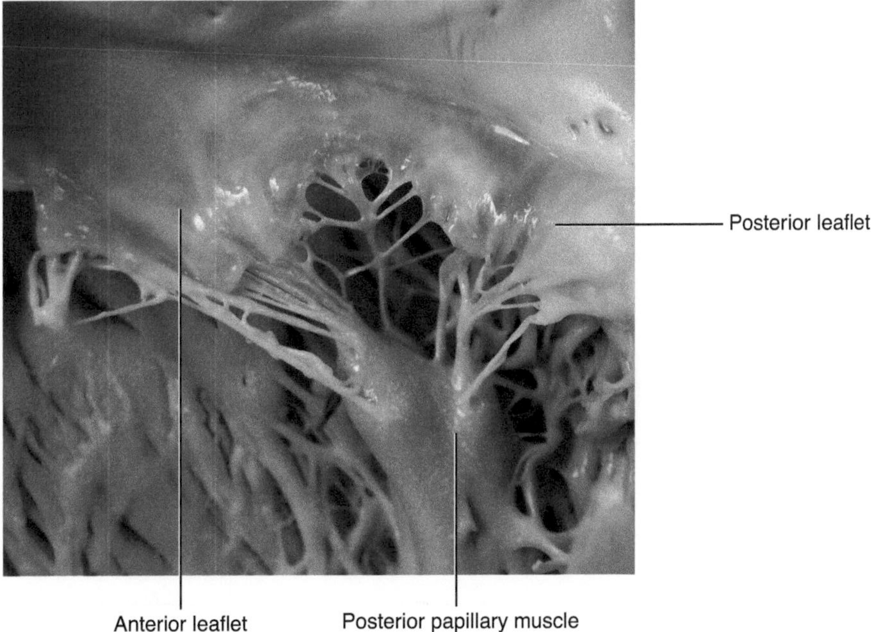
C
Posterior leaflet
Anterior leaflet
Posterior papillary muscle

Figure 1-5

A The heart is sectioned in the horizontal plane to demonstrate the left atrium, mitral valve, and left ventricular outflow tract during diastole. The anterior leaflet of the mitral valve moves toward the left ventricular outflow tract.

B During systole, the anterior leaflet of the mitral valve apposes the posterior leaflet, closing the atrioventricular orifice. At the same time, the left ventricular outflow tract is widely opened. Papillary muscles shorten to maintain the proper length as the ventricle moves inward during systole.

C The unique shape of the mitral valve is demonstrated during systole and diastole. The mitral valve conforms to adjacent structures to allow maximal area for flow at low pressure during diastole and to provide firm closure at high pressure during systole. Note that the anterior leaflet not only swings anteriorly into the subaortic left ventricle (left ventricular outflow tract) but also flexes to provide maximal opening.

D Left ventricular inflow tract, normal. The left ventricular inflow tract is shown with the left atrium above, separated from the left ventricle below by the mitral valve. The section is directly through the anterior papillary muscle so that some chordal attachments to the posterior leaflet of the mitral valve have been severed. The anterior leaflet is wider than the posterior leaflet. The anterior leaflet, however, constitutes one-third of the annular circumference, whereas the posterior leaflet is attached to two-thirds of the mitral valve annulus. Dual chordal attachment of the anterior leaflet to the anterior and posterior papillary muscles is present. The left ventricular wall is finely trabeculated, compared with the coarse trabeculation of the right ventricle (opening on the right side of the image). Note also the thick left ventricular myocardial muscle mass compared with that of the thin right ventricle.

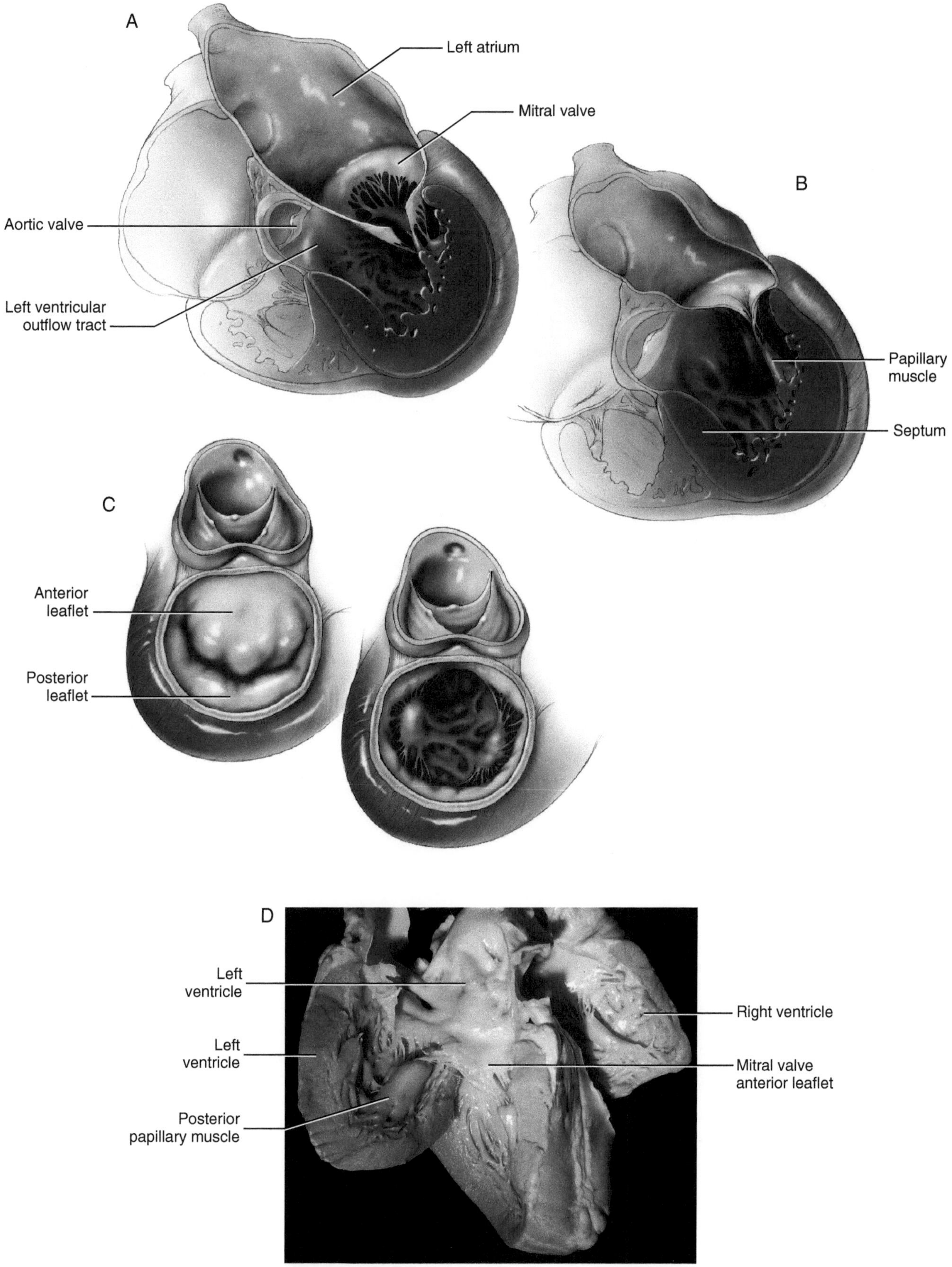

A
Left atrium
Mitral valve
Aortic valve
Left ventricular outflow tract
B
Papillary muscle
Septum
C
Anterior leaflet
Posterior leaflet
D
Left ventricle
Left ventricle
Posterior papillary muscle
Right ventricle
Mitral valve anterior leaflet

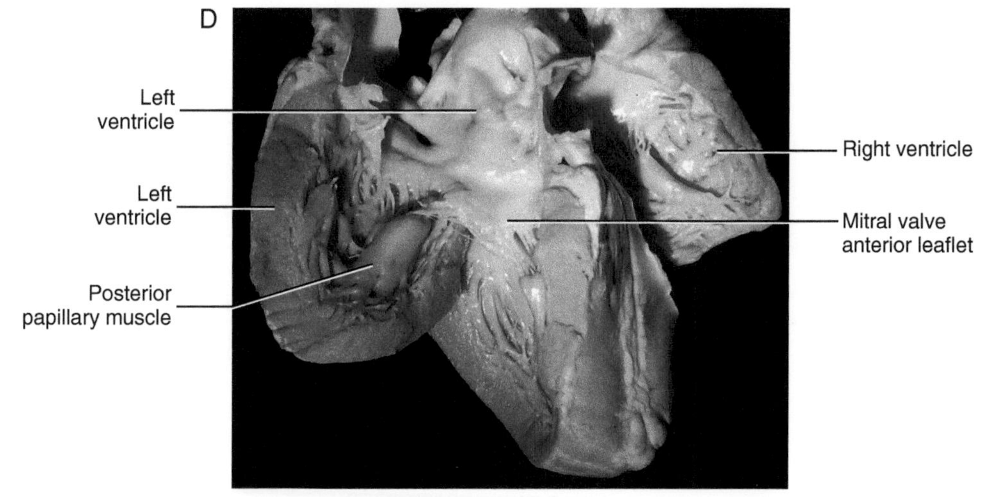

Figure 1-5 (continued)

E Left ventricular outflow tract, normal. The left ventricular outflow tract is delineated by the anterior leaflet and the free wall of the left ventricle. This passageway conducts blood from the left ventricle to the aortic valve and the aorta. The dual chordal attachment of the anterior leaflet of the mitral valve to the two papillary muscles is appreciated.

F This view of the pericardial reflections over the great vessels with the heart excised is not one usually seen by surgeons. Because this is not actually a surgical perspective, these relationships are shown in the anatomic position for clarity. As the aorta leaves the pericardial sac, it is located anterior and to the right of the bifurcation of the pulmonary artery. The superior and inferior venae cavae enter the pericardial sac on the right side. The pulmonary veins enter posteriorly on the right and left sides of the pericardial sac. The left atrium is attached at its superior aspect by two folds of the pericardium, with a narrow space between them. Thus, the left atrium is a midline structure with mostly free pericardial space behind it. The channel above the pericardial reflection over the left atrium and below the aorta and pulmonary artery is referred to as the transverse sinus. The vertical passageway between the pulmonary veins (through the left atrial pericardial reflection) is referred to as the oblique sinus. These sinuses have been used as pathways for coronary bypass grafts from the aorta to the posterior wall of the left ventricle.

G The posterior wall of the excised heart is shown to appreciate the pericardial reflections on the surface of the heart. The relatively narrow space between pericardial reflections over the inferior vena cava is shown. The back wall of the left atrium is mostly free pericardial space, and the distance between the superior and inferior pericardial reflections over the oblique sinus is demonstrated.

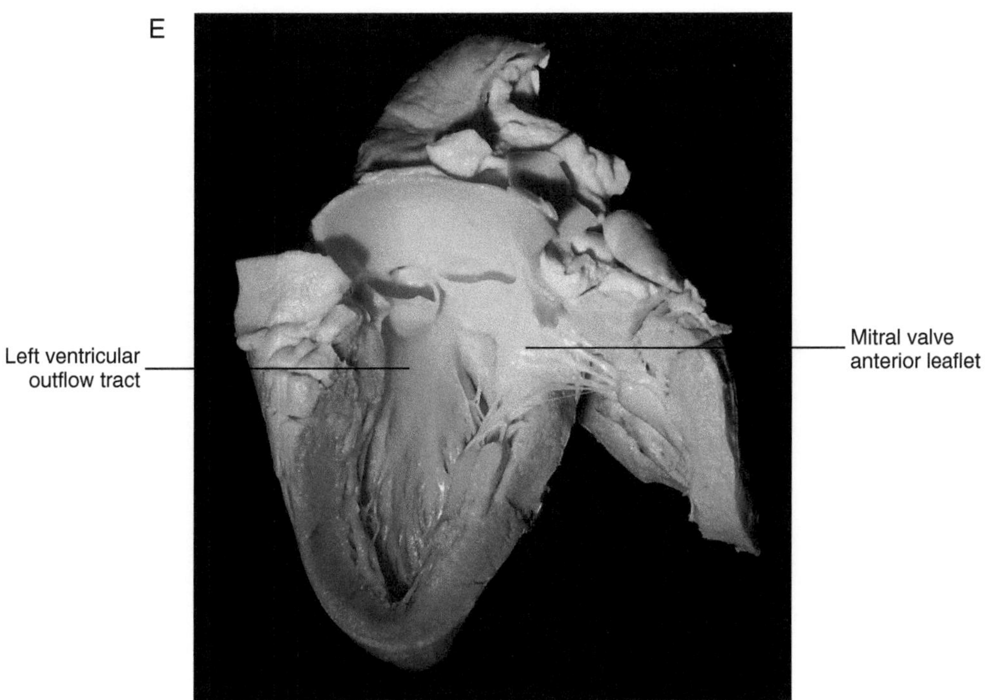
E
Left ventricular outflow tract
Mitral valve anterior leaflet

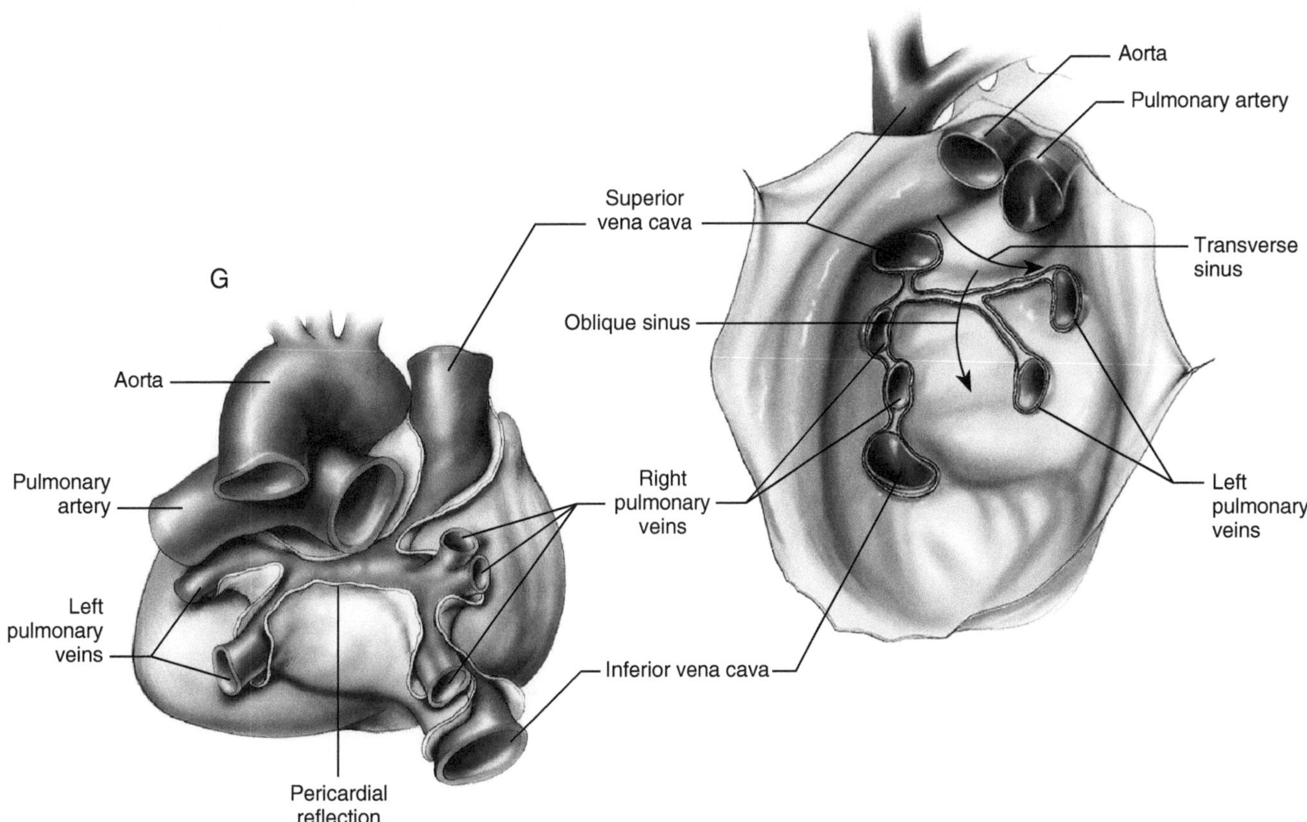
F
Aorta
Pulmonary artery
Superior vena cava
Transverse sinus
Oblique sinus
Right pulmonary veins
Left pulmonary veins
Inferior vena cava
G
Aorta
Pulmonary artery
Left pulmonary veins
Pericardial reflection

chapter 2 SETUP FOR CARDIAC SURGERY

Incision

Successful cardiac surgeons know that a standardized routine for cardiac operations is essential. An established routine makes every operation more efficient and, in the case of an emergency, allows one to proceed with speed and accuracy.

Figure 2-1

A A midsternal incision is made for nearly all cardiac operations. The exceptions are operations on the branch pulmonary arteries or the thoracic aorta, such as palliative procedures in which a thoracotomy is used. The midsternal incision begins below the sternal notch over the sternal manubrium and extends to the xiphoid process. Low, short incisions are preferred for cosmetic reasons and should be used unless they would limit exposure of the heart. The incision is taken through the periosteum of the anterior table of the sternum using electrocautery dissection. A thyroid retractor is inserted to gain exposure of the upper end of the sternum, and a right-angled clamp is used to open the mediastinum behind the sternum. The sternal saw is tested for proper operation before placing it against the upper end of the sternum. The sternal saw is grasped firmly with the thumb at the top and the fourth and fifth fingers at the back and bottom so that the saw blade can be held firmly against the sternum and the saw's protective "toe" guard is forced against the posterior table of the sternum. Ventilation of the patient is stopped momentarily to allow the lungs to deflate and retract away from the anterior chest wall as the sternum is divided with the saw. It is usually advisable to back up the saw once or twice during division of the sternum to release mediastinal tissue that may be caught up in the instrument; this permits the pleura to be left intact. The sternal edges are separated initially with a thyroid retractor, and hemostasis is obtained using electrocautery with a ball-tipped electrode and a thin layer of bone wax or Gelfoam reconstituted with antibiotic solution.

B The sternal retractor is used to separate the sternal edges for optimal exposure of the heart. The pericardium is opened in the midline, and retraction stitches are placed to gain access to the heart. The pericardium is cut back to the full extent of the reflection off the aorta superiorly and onto the diaphragm inferiorly. Extension of the pericardial incisions inferiorly to the right or left toward the pleural spaces may be required to expose the lower aspects of the right atrium or the apex of the heart. Retraction stitches of 2/0 silk are placed from the pericardium to the subcutaneous tissues or the retractor. The aorta, right ventricle, pulmonary artery, and right atrial appendage are clearly in view and freely accessible. The left ventricle, left atrium, and lower aspects of the right atrium must be exposed by retraction or displacement of the heart.

C Placement of a small vinyl catheter for monitoring the left atrial pressure is the initial step of the setup for cardiac surgery. The right atrium is retracted to expose the right superior pulmonary vein. A box stitch is placed in the pulmonary vein using 4/0 polypropylene suture. A needle with a catheter is used to enter the pulmonary vein within the box stitch, and the catheter is advanced precisely for a measured length so that the catheter tip is located just inside the left atrium. The needle is withdrawn, and the catheter is secured by tying the box stitch and making an additional stitch of 5/0 silk through the pericardium around the catheter. The catheter is brought out through the skin to the left of the skin incision.

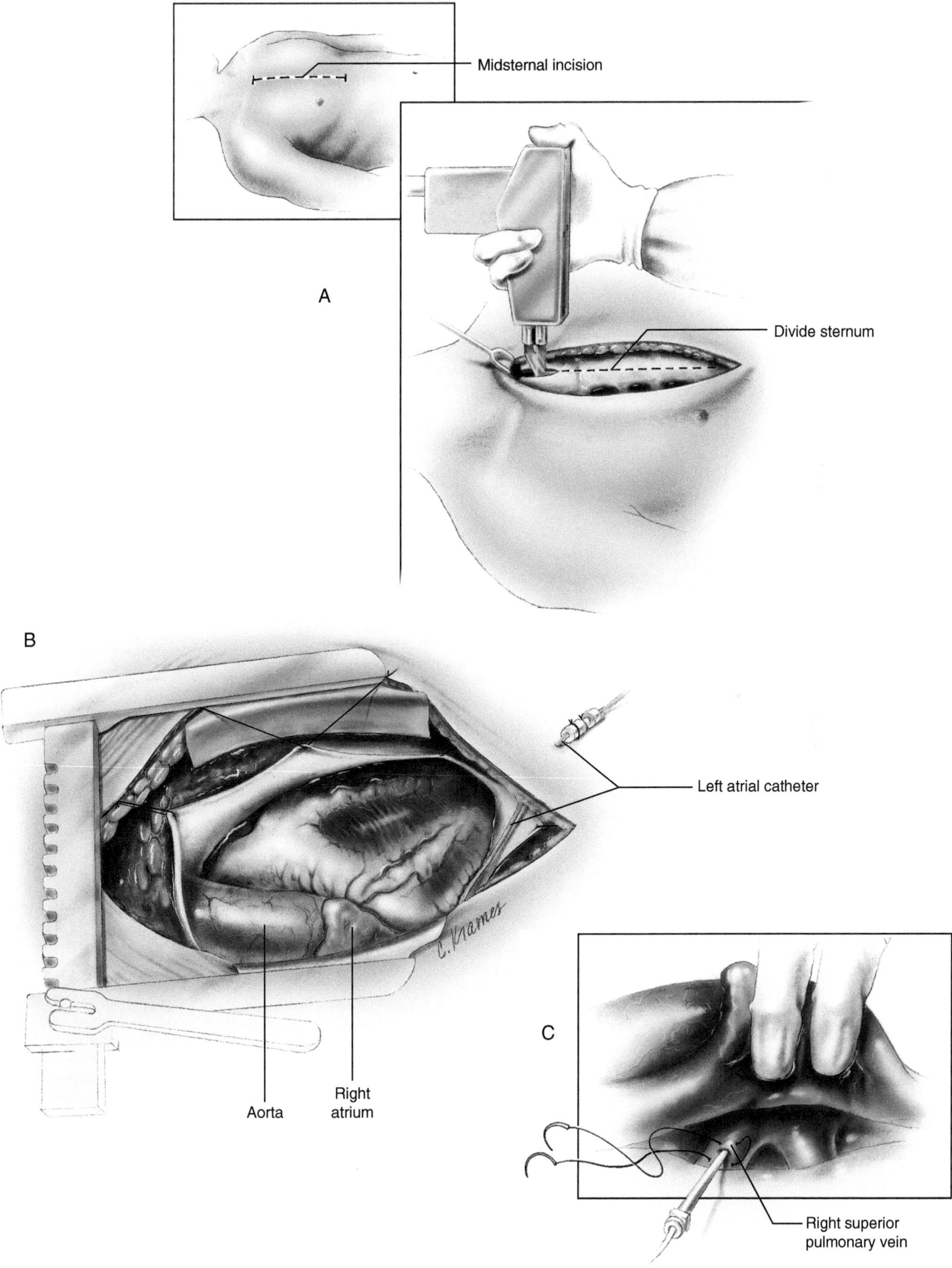

Midsternal incision
A
Divide sternum
B
Left atrial catheter
Aorta
Right atrium
C
Right superior pulmonary vein

Control of Venae Cavae

For most procedures to address congenital cardiac conditions, and for the surgical correction of some acquired conditions in which access to the right intracardiac structures is required, it is necessary to control the superior and inferior venae cavae with tourniquets, that can be drawn tightly around the venous uptake cannulae.

Figure 2-2

A The pericardium over the anterior aspect of the right pulmonary artery just medial to the superior vena cava is opened.

B Exposure of this area is enhanced by retraction of the aorta anteriorly and to the left. A right-angled clamp is passed behind the superior vena cava from its lateral aspect. The pericardial reflection lateral to the cava is usually thin and can be easily and safely perforated as it is invaginated toward the incision medially and anterior to the right pulmonary artery. Umbilical tape or heavy No. 3 silk suture is passed around the vena cava and through the polyethylene catheter tourniquet.

C Similar steps are used to control the inferior vena cava. The pericardium is incised in the space between the inferior pulmonary vein and the inferior vena cava. The pericardium may be quite thick in this area, so it is safer to use a sharp incision rather than forceful blunt dissection to obtain access to the delicate tissues posterior to the cava.

D A right-angled clamp is passed posterior to the inferior vena cava from the lateral aspect. The tip of the clamp can be seen as it emerges from behind the cava on the medial aspect by retracting the diaphragmatic surface of the heart superiorly. This maneuver usually upsets the hemodynamics considerably, so it should be performed efficiently but without compromising accurate exposure of the vena cava. The clamp is used to perforate the thin layer of pericardium medially and make an opening behind the vena cava large enough to draw the tourniquet tape safely around the vena cava.

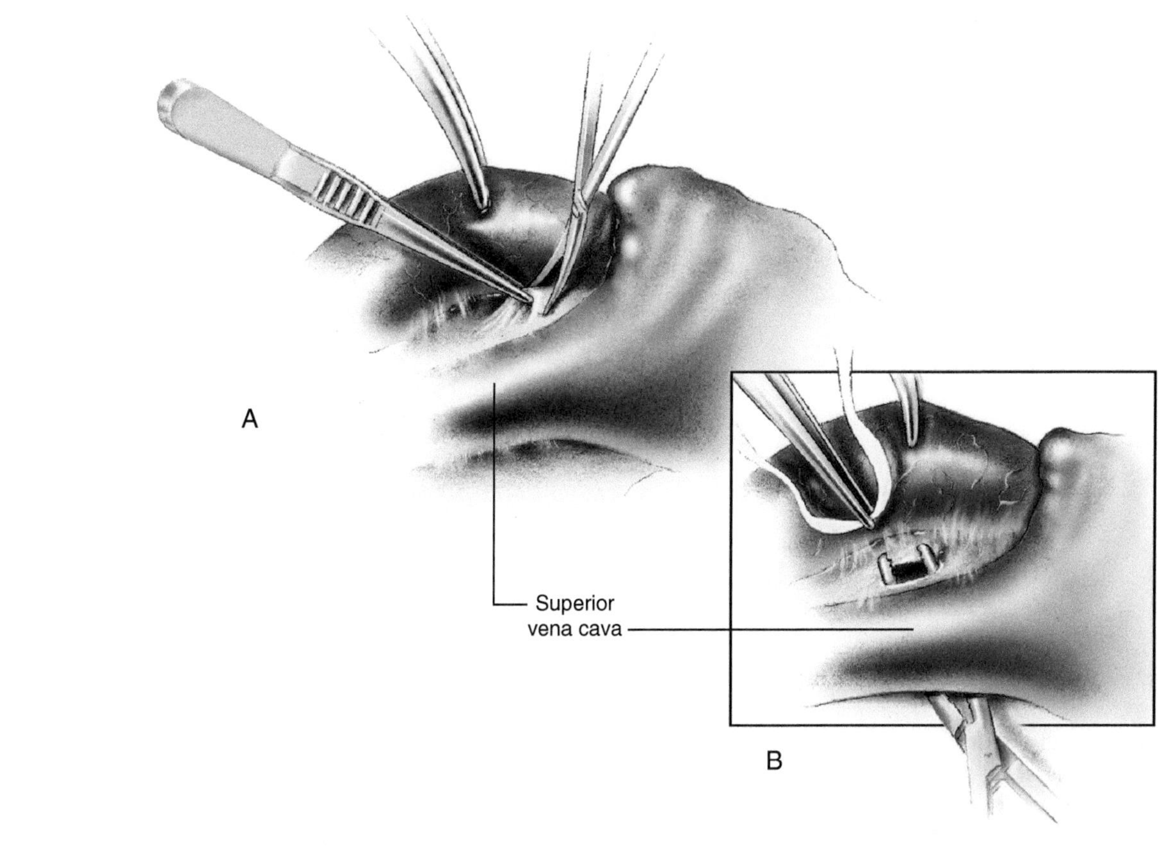
A
Superior
vena cava
B

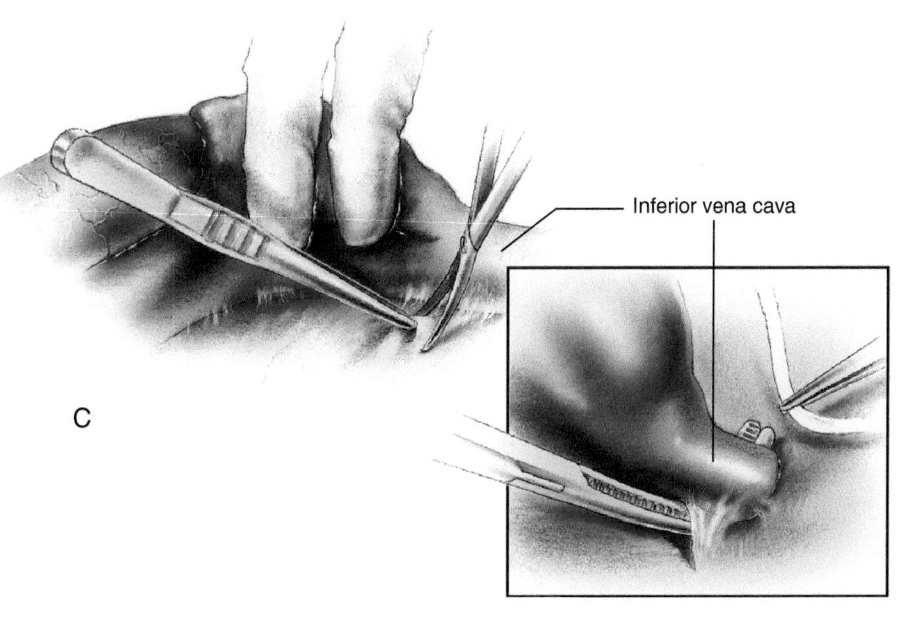
Inferior vena cava
C
D

Cannulation of the Ascending Aorta

The aorta is used in most operations for the return of oxygenated blood from the extracorporeal circuit.

Figure 2-3

A The aorta is prepared for cannulation by placing a purse-string stitch on the anterior aspect near the pericardial reflection. Polypropylene 3/0 suture material and a small needle are used exclusively for purse-string construction because the frequency of aortic perforation is reduced, bleeding around the cannula is less than with braided suture material, and closure of the aorta after removal of the cannula is more secure so that reinforcing pledget material is seldom required. The stitches are placed through the pericardial layer and into the adventitia of the aorta but should not penetrate the lumen of the aorta. Thus, the purse string is located in loose and mobile tissue that is nevertheless strong and will firmly hold the cannula in the aorta and close the aortic incision securely when the purse string is drawn up later. If the needle inadvertently penetrates the aorta, the entire suture should be removed and a new one placed. Stitches that are left in the fixed tissues of the aortic wall are likely to tear through when the purse string is drawn up, leaving an even larger hole in the aorta rather than sealing it. A tourniquet is placed on the purse-string stitch to secure the cannula after it is placed in the aorta. A second stitch is placed immediately outside the first one for added security, but a tourniquet is not necessary. An alternative cannulation site on the right lateral aspect of the aorta may be used if greater access to the anterior wall of the aorta is desired.

B The pericardium inside the purse string is removed to expose the aortic wall. This excision removes any loose tissue that could interfere with smooth passage of the aortic cannula into the lumen.

C Care must be taken not to mobilize or undermine tissue that is actually supporting the purse string. The area inside the purse string may be cleaned with a Kuettner sponge to remove blood or bits of loose tissue for accurate visualization of the cannulation site.

D The size of the cannulation site and the diameter of the surrounding purse string should be 4 to 5 mm larger than the diameter of the cannula to be introduced. A No. 11 blade is used to incise the aorta. The tip of the blade is placed inside the purse string, with the noncutting edge of the blade directed toward the outside. The blade is used to perforate the aorta to a depth sufficient to create an incision equal to the diameter of the cannula to be inserted. Not much blood escapes, provided that the blade is kept absolutely straight and is not allowed to twist.

E The thumb of the opposite hand is used to cover the aortic incision to control hemorrhage after the blade is removed from the aorta. Alternatively, the adventitia at the edge of the purse string can be grasped with forceps and pulled toward the aortotomy to control hemorrhage.

F The bevel of the aortic cannula is aligned with the aortic incision, the thumb is slid aside or the adventitia is pulled open with the forceps, and the cannula is inserted. Cannulae with removable, tapered point introducers aid the insertion process. Occasionally, the incision in the aorta is not adequate, or loose tissue has been drawn in that interferes with insertion of the cannula. Under these circumstances, the thumb is simply replaced to control hemorrhage while a tonsil clamp is passed beneath the thumb and into the aorta to dilate the opening. This dilation is usually sufficient to allow the cannula to be inserted. If this fails or the hemorrhage cannot be controlled, a partial-occlusion clamp can be placed for better control and assessment of the situation.

G The purse-string tourniquet is tightened to achieve hemostasis around the cannula. The cannula is secured to the aorta by simply tying the tourniquet to the cannula. The perfusion tubing is secured to the patient drapes.

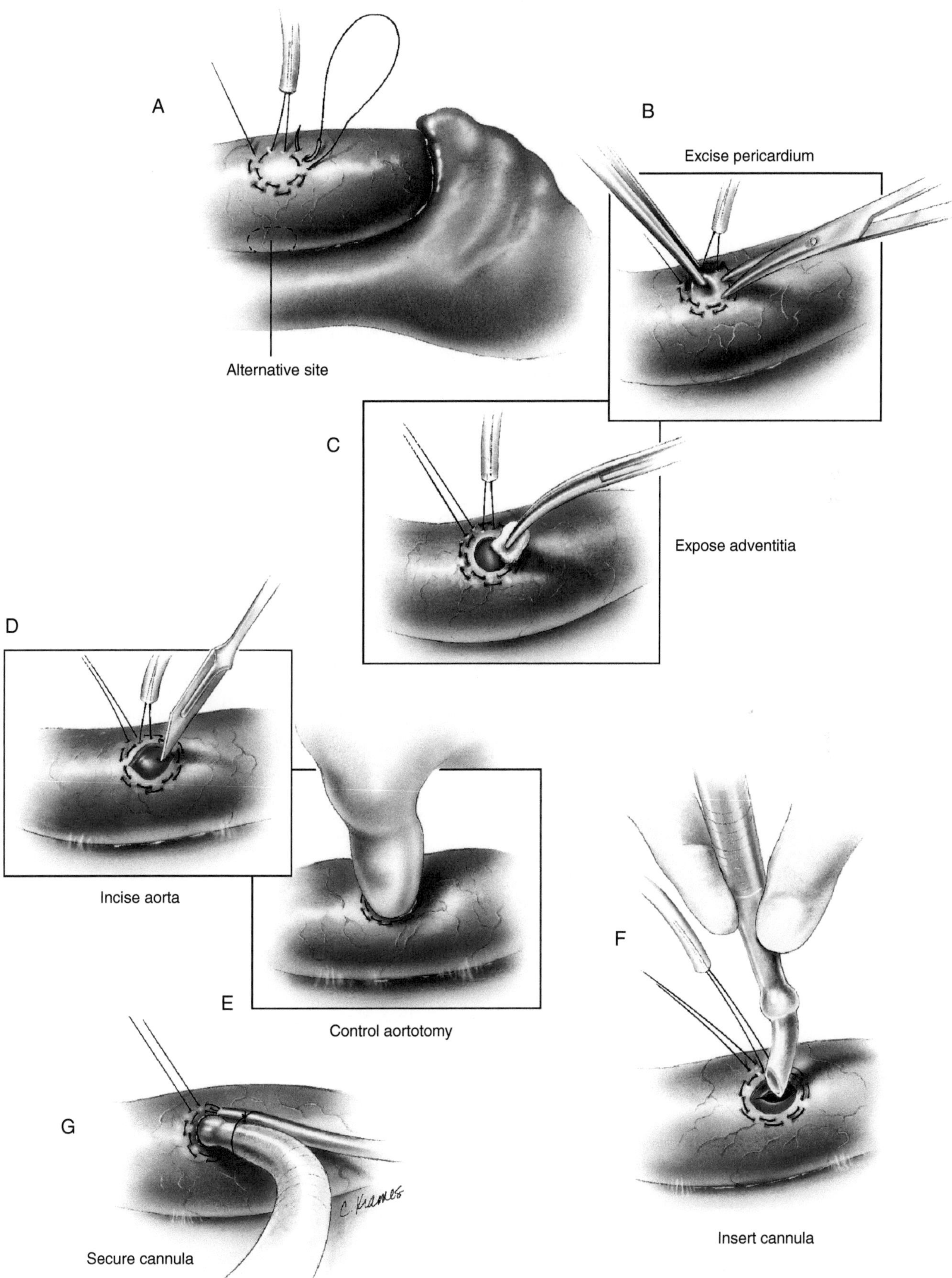
A
Alternative site
B
Excise pericardium
C
Expose adventitia
D
Incise aorta
E
Control aortotomy
F
Insert cannula
G
Secure cannula
C. Krames

Cannulation of the Femoral Artery

In some situations the femoral artery may be used for arterial return.

Figure 2-4

A When it is desirable to return blood from the pump oxygenator to a site other than the ascending aorta, the common femoral artery is the most convenient alternative. An incision is made in the groin over the femoral artery. Sufficient femoral artery is mobilized to identify the superficial and profunda branches so as to ensure that the point of cannulation will be the common femoral artery. A vinyl catheter or vessel loop is used to control the artery. Generally, 35-degree-angle vascular occlusion clamps are used, but they should be chosen carefully because the distal clamp will remain in place during cannulation and should lie conveniently out of the way. Scissors are used to incise the femoral artery through about half the circumference.

B A small curved hemostat is used to dilate the artery both proximally and distally. This is done to ease the passage of the cannula proximally and to ensure that the distal length of the femoral incision approximates the proximal length, allowing accurate repair of the femoral artery after the cannula is removed.

C The greatest hazard associated with cannulation of the femoral artery is dissection of the arterial wall, which could extend to the entire aorta after blood is perfused through the cannula. Absolute care during insertion of the cannula is essential to reduce the risk of arterial wall dissection. The intima of the artery must be accurately viewed, especially in cases of degenerative arterial disease. Smooth-tipped plastic cannulae that are slightly flexible may be somewhat safer than metal cannulae, but either type is acceptable as long as proper care is used during insertion. The cannula is introduced with the bevel directed toward the intact back wall of the artery up to the point of vascular clamp occlusion.

D The vascular clamp is removed, and the cannula is advanced into the femoral artery with a twisting motion that brings the bevel of the cannula anterior. Advancing the cannula against any resistance is extremely hazardous and should be avoided. Free flow of pulsatile blood into the cannula is a good sign that it has been introduced properly.

E The vessel loop is drawn up using a right-angled clamp to achieve a tight seal between the femoral artery and the cannula. The loop is simply tied below the clamp to secure the seal. The vessel loop is then tied to the perfusion cannula. Free flow of blood from the cannula and good pulsatile pressure in the cannula must be ensured before initiating infusion of the perfusate through the cannula. Perfusion pressures during femoral artery perfusion are usually higher than those observed during perfusion of the ascending aorta. Excessively high perfusion pressures are cause for alarm, indicating the possibility of dissection of the artery.

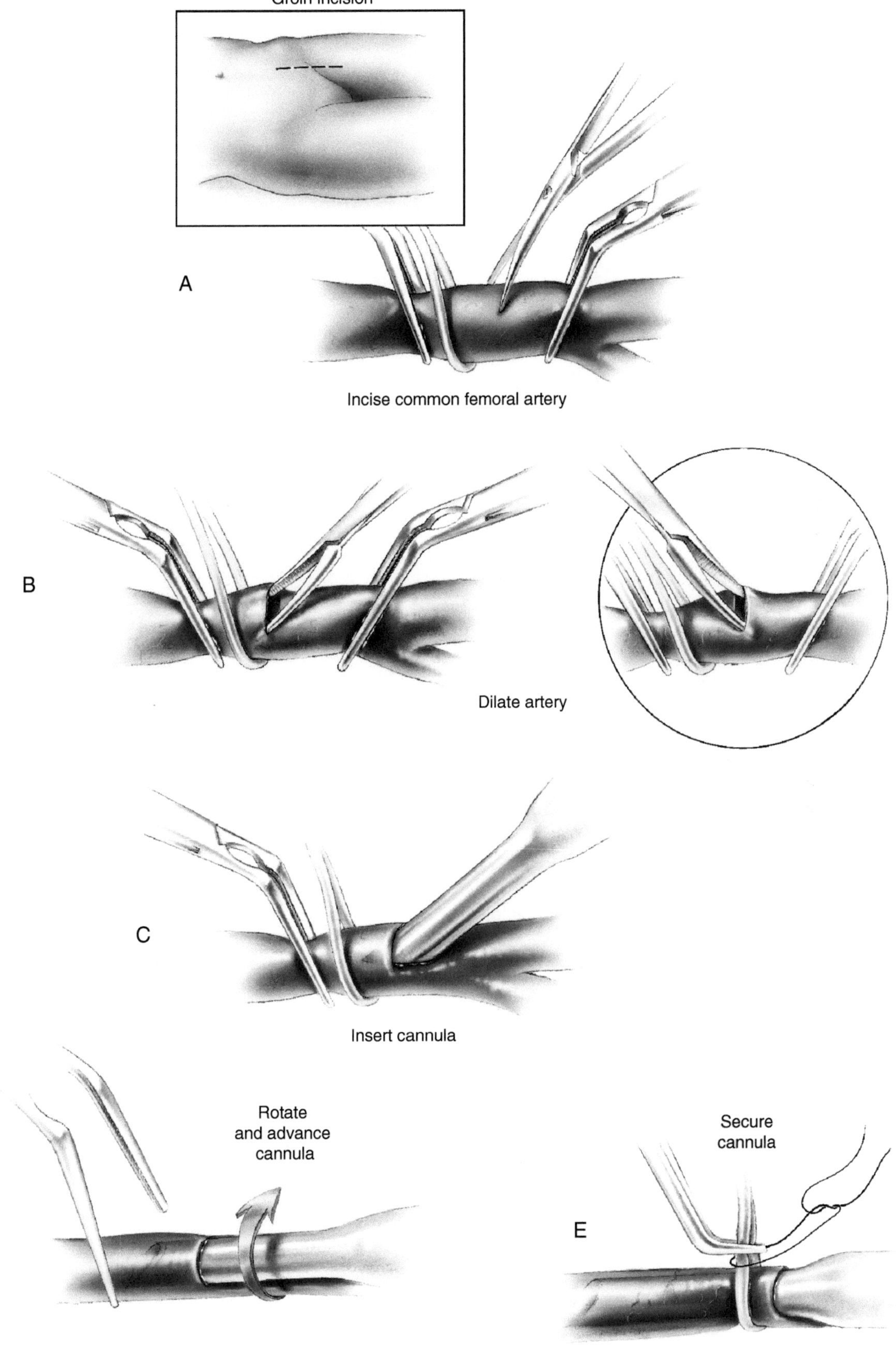
Groin incision
A
Incise common femoral artery
B
Dilate artery
C
Insert cannula
D
Rotate
and advance
cannula
E
Secure
cannula

Cannulation of the Veins

Cannulation of the right side of the heart for venous uptake is performed through the right atrium.

Figure 2-5

A The right atrial appendage is the site of cannula insertion for right atrium single-cannula techniques and for some superior vena cava cannulations. A 3/0 polypropylene suture is placed around the base of the right atrial appendage, using four or five very shallow bites into the atrial epicardium simply to hold the suture in place. Deep bites into the atrial lumen could tear through and cause hemorrhage. A side-biting vascular occlusion clamp is placed across the base of the atrial appendage so as to exclude the tip. An incision is made with scissors on the lateral aspect of the appendage near the tip. Tonsil clamps are placed on the edges of the incision to separate the edges and expose the inside. Crossing trabeculae are divided so that an unobstructed passageway to the right atrium is assured. The venous cannula is passed into the right atrium as the vascular clamp is removed. Alternatively, the appendage can be grasped with forceps, an incision made with scissors, and the cannula simply slipped into the atrium. Hemostasis is achieved by tightening the tourniquet catheter placed over the suture at the base of the appendage. For single venous cannula techniques, the tip of the cannula is placed near the coronary sinus at the opening of the inferior vena cava to the right atrium; alternatively, the large-stage port of a two-stage cannula is placed in a similar location, with the caval port advanced into the inferior vena cava. The position of the cannula is secured by tying it to the tourniquet occluder.

B In some instances, such as when better intraatrial exposure is required or when use of the right atrial appendage is an integral part of the operative repair, it is best to cannulate the superior vena cava directly. The pericardium is mobilized off the anterior wall of the superior vena cava above the pericardial reflection. A purse-string stitch of 3/0 polypropylene is placed superficially in the anterior wall of the vena cava. The suture can easily be removed upon completion to allow direct repair of the incision in the superior vena cava. The cannulation technique is similar to that used for the inferior vena cava.

C The inferior vena cava is cannulated through the inferior aspect of the lateral wall of the right atrium. A purse-string stitch of 3/0 polypropylene is placed in the epicardium of the right atrium just above the inferior vena cava junction. A tonsil hemostat is placed on the right atrium just inside the inferior portion of the purse string. A vascular forceps is used to grasp the atrium on the opposite side of the purse string. Using a No. 15 blade, an incision is made through the adventitia of the vena cava, long enough to accommodate the cannula. The scalpel is then passed into the caval lumen, and blood loss is controlled by approximating the forceps. A tonsil hemostat is used to dilate the incision up to the extent of the adventitial incision, again controlling hemorrhage by approximating the forceps. The forceps is then used to separate the edges of the incision as the cannula is introduced and advanced into the vena cava. Hemostasis is achieved by tightening the tourniquet occluder, which is tied to the cannula.

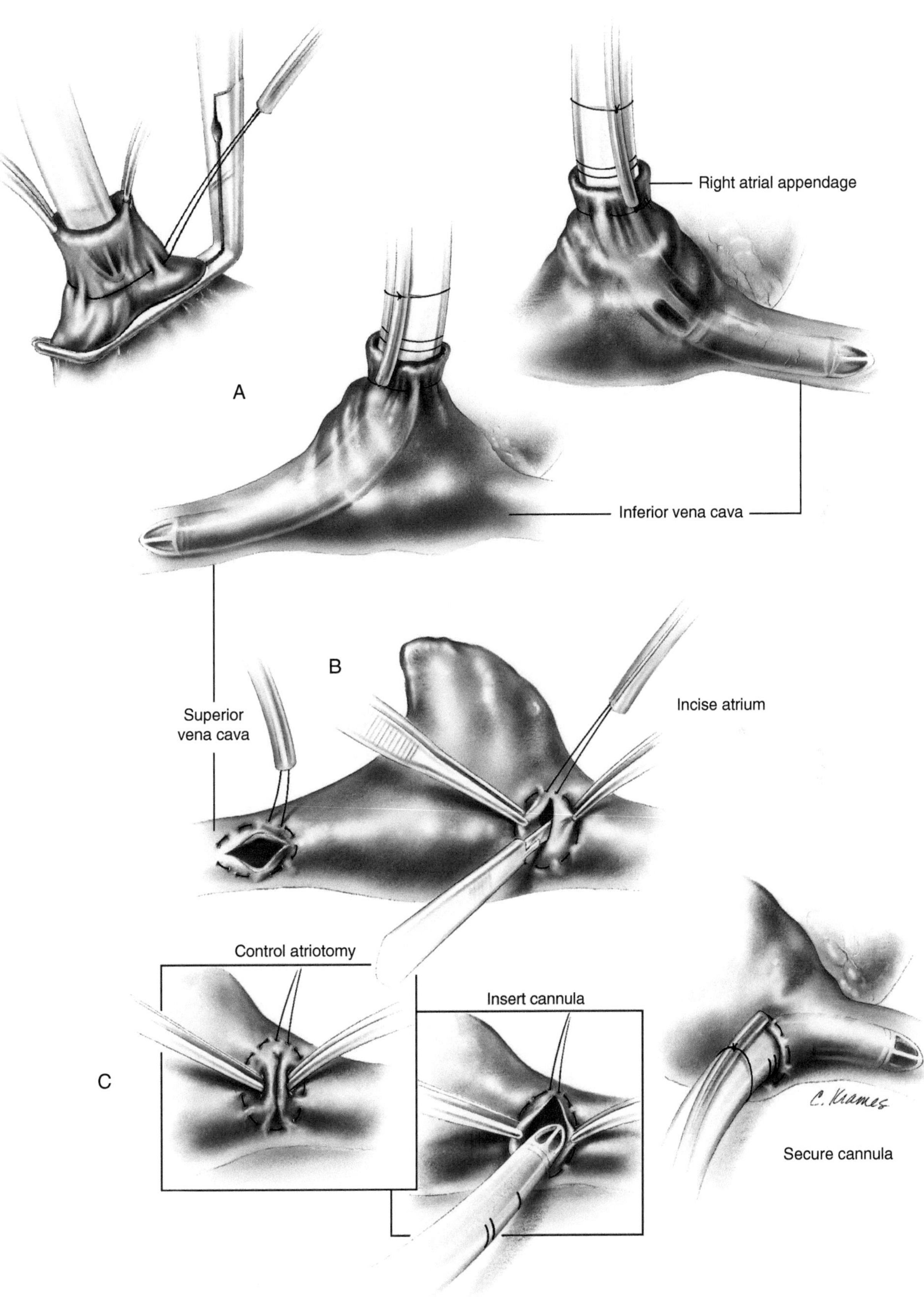
Right atrial appendage
A
Inferior vena cava
B
Superior vena cava
Incise atrium
Control atriotomy
Insert cannula
C
C. Krames
Secure cannula

Cervical Venous Cannulation and Left Heart Venting

There are some situations in which venous cannulation outside the thorax is desirable. The usual site for extrathoracic venous cannulation is the common femoral vein, but in some cases cannulation of the internal jugular vein may be useful. The left atrium is cannulated (vented) to remove blood that enters from the bronchial arterial circulation.

Figure 2-6

A A skin-line incision is made above the right clavicle. The sternal and clavicular heads of the sternocleidomastoid muscle are separated to expose the underlying internal jugular vein. The internal jugular vein is mobilized sufficiently to allow control and placement of a purse-string stitch of 4/0 polypropylene in the adventitia. A tourniquet is attached. Extensive mobilization is not required, and it is not necessary to completely surround the vein with tapes or sutures. The vein is incised longitudinally. The venotomy is controlled by approximating forceps placed at the edges of the purse-string stitch.

B The edges of the venotomy are retracted, and a venous cannula is inserted. The internal jugular vein easily accommodates a 32 F cannula, and often a 36 or 40 F can be passed through the vein into the right atrium. These cannulae are sufficient to achieve full bypass (2.2 L/min/m^2) in most adult patients by gravity drainage. Smaller cannulae (24 F) can be inserted by needle-guidewire technique, provided vacuum-assisted venous drainage is employed.

C The internal jugular venous cannula is placed so the tip lies within the right atrium. If desired, a second venous cannula can be passed through the wall of the right atrium into the inferior vena cava once the heart is exposed through the sternotomy.

D For procedures restricted to the left side of the heart, venting is accomplished using a vent catheter introduced through the right superior pulmonary vein. A triangular stitch of 3/0 suture is placed deep in the interatrial tissue to penetrate the anterior wall of the left atrium. The stitch should encompass an area medial and inferior to the site of the left atrial monitoring catheter. An incision is made in the center of the purse-string stitch using a No. 15 blade and is dilated using a tonsil hemostat. A right-angled atrial vent catheter is passed into the left atrium. In most instances the catheter is advanced across the mitral valve to vent the left ventricle. This maneuver is enhanced by using a stiff catheter guide or by soaking the catheter in iced water to maintain the stiffness and right-angled shape. A pediatric vent catheter (12 F with multiple holes) is usually adequate to drain the left heart using low-level suction. The position of the catheter is maintained by tightening the tourniquet on the purse-string stitch. It is not advisable to tie the catheter in place, since this can increase the risk of perforating the left ventricle during retraction of the heart.

E During operations in which the right side of the heart is to be opened, or when there is any possibility of a patent foramen ovale, the vent catheter can simply be introduced into the left atrium across the atrial septum and through the right atrium. If the foramen ovale is open, it is dilated with a tonsil hemostat to allow passage of a straight vent catheter. When the atrial septum is intact, an incision is made in the foramen ovale. The catheter insertion site is repaired at completion with 3/0 suture.

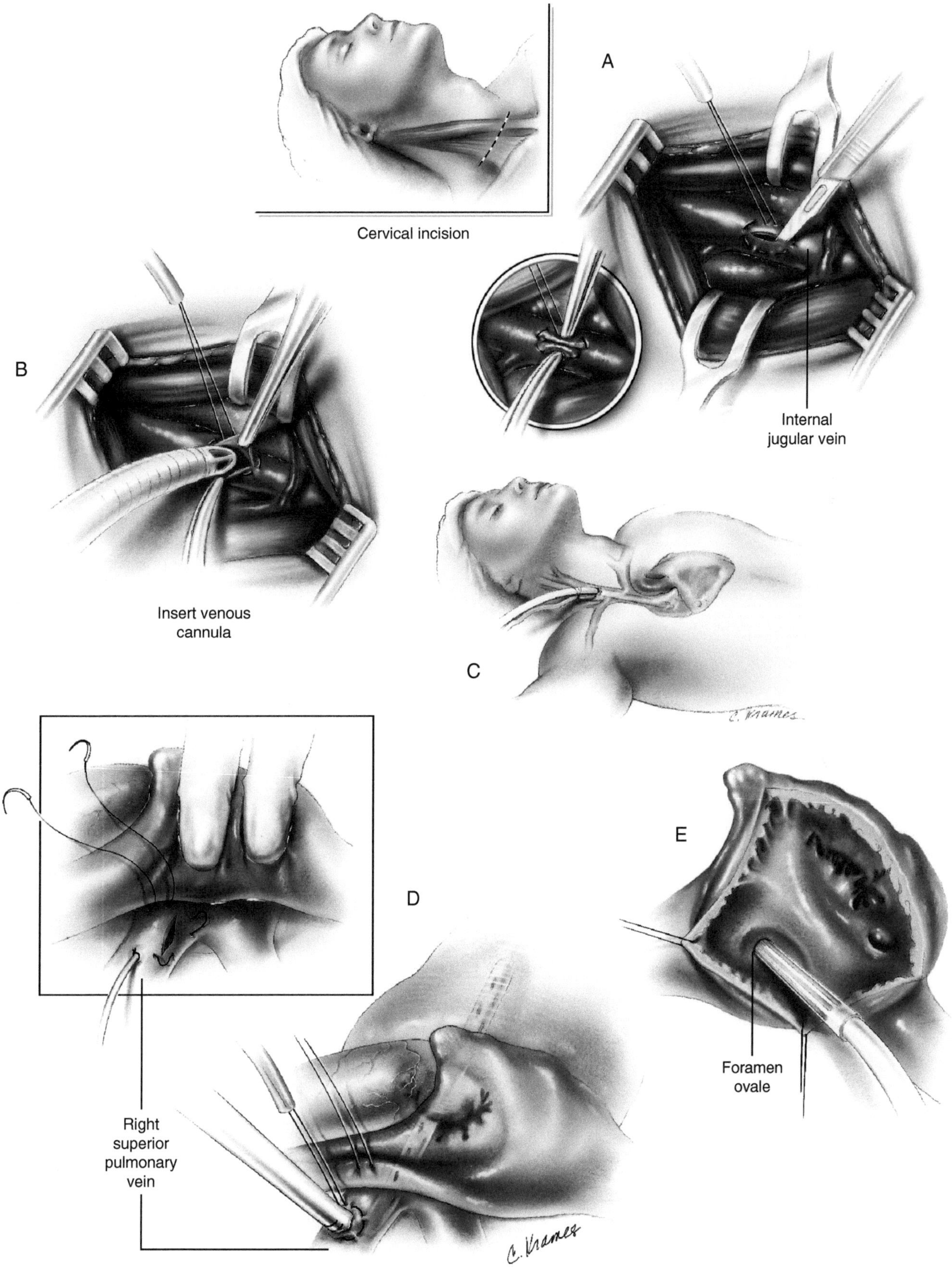
A
Cervical incision
Internal jugular vein
B
Insert venous cannula
C
C. Kramer
D
Right superior pulmonary vein
E
Foramen ovale
C. Kramer

Femoral Cannulation for Cardiopulmonary Bypass

There are situations in which arterial and venous access for the institution of cardiopulmonary bypass is achieved by the cannulation of peripheral vessels. Femoral cannulation for cardiopulmonary bypass is applicable in cases of reentry sternotomy, when there may be significant risk of cardiac or great vessel injury; for operations in which direct cannulation of the thoracic aorta is undesirable; and in some emergency situations. The preferred method of insertion of femoral perfusion cannulae is the needle–guidewire–cannula over guidewire technique.

Figure 2-7

A A skin-line incision is made in the groin over the femoral vessels.

B Short segments of the common femoral artery and vein are exposed and separated from the tissues in the femoral sheath.

C Rather than incising the wall of the artery, a purse-string stitch using 3/0 polypropylene is placed in the adventitia of the artery. A needle is inserted through the purse string, and a guidewire is passed into the artery, assuring that there is no resistance to advancing the wire proximally.

D A tapered dilator with a cannula is then passed into the artery over the guidewire and into the vessel lumen. A short incision of the vessel wall over the dilator enhances subsequent passage of the cannula and prevents tearing of the vessel wall.

E The cannula is inserted over the dilator and guidewire into the lumen of the vessel. No resistance should be encountered during this process.

F Active suction on the venous uptake is achieved by use of a centrifugal pump in the bypass circuit or by direct application of suction to a hard-shell oxygenator and reservoir. Blood on the arterial side of the circuit is returned, as usual, via a roller or centrifugal pump.

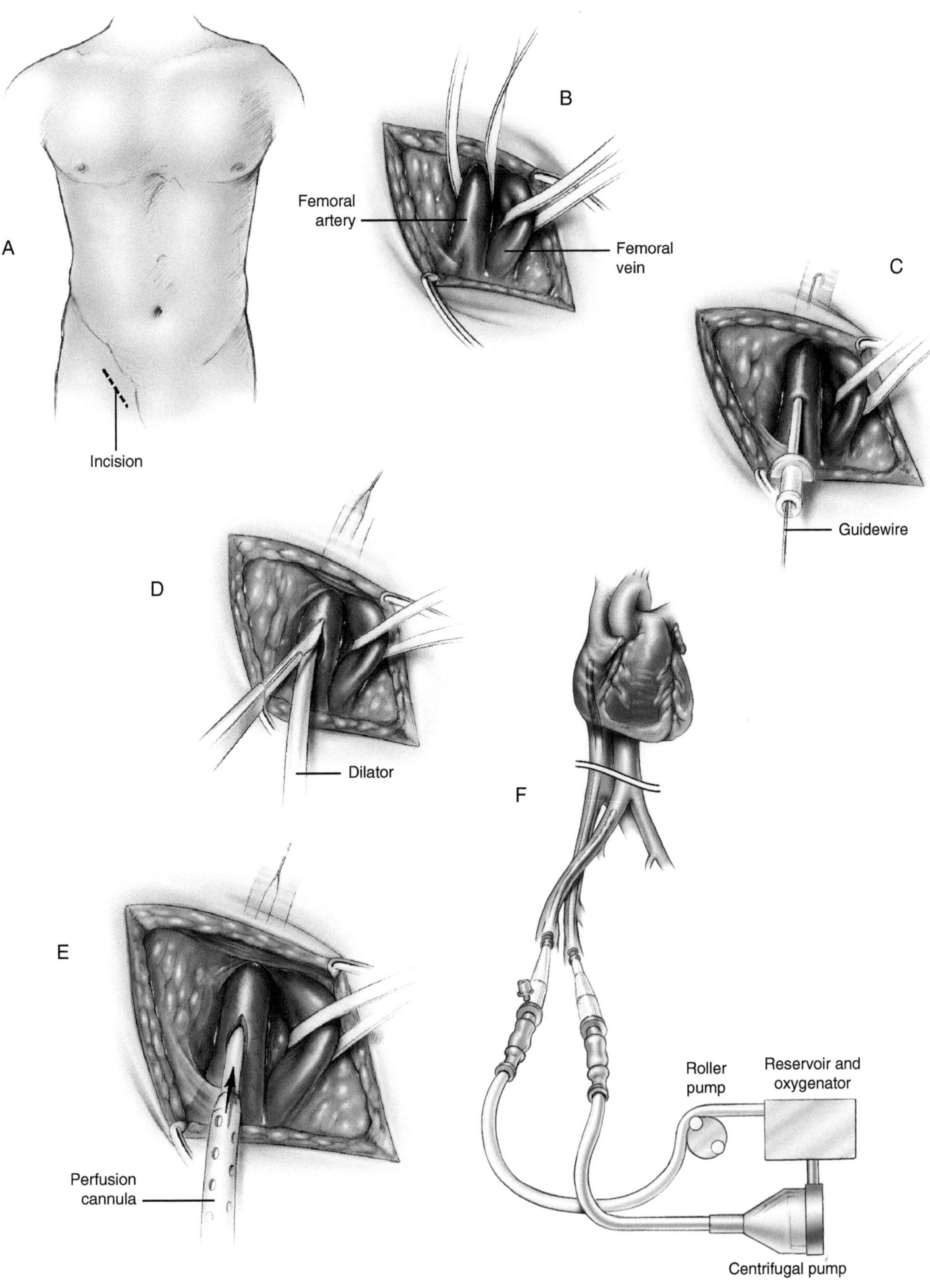
A
Incision
B
Femoral artery
Femoral vein
C
Guidewire
D
Dilator
E
Perfusion cannula
F
Roller pump
Reservoir and oxygenator
Centrifugal pump

Cannulation for Aortic Operations

Arterial cannulation for aortic disease, aneurysm, or dissection requires special considerations. The location of the disease in the ascending aorta, arch, or descending thoracic aorta dictates where the aortic perfusion cannula is best placed.

Figure 2-8

Aneurysmal disease of the ascending aorta extending into the proximal aortic arch can be treated by cannulation of the distal arch and the use of deep hypothermia and circulatory arrest.

A The pericardium is dissected away from the aorta at the pericardial reflection. A dissection plane is established on the anterior wall of the aortic arch, and a space in the mediastinum is opened to the distal portion of the arch. A purse-string stitch using 3/0 polypropylene is placed in the distal arch.

B A tapered dilator with a perfusion cannula is placed in the aortic lumen through a stab incision within the purse string. The cannula is advanced over the dilator into the upper portion of the descending thoracic aorta. A guidewire may be used for additional safety.

For disease of the descending aorta, it may be desirable to use left atrium–to–femoral artery or descending aorta bypass to assure visceral, spinal cord, and lower extremity blood flow.

C A left thoracotomy incision is made, entering the chest through the bed of the third or fourth rib. The pericardial sac is opened, and a purse-string stitch of 3/0 polypropylene is placed on the left inferior pulmonary vein. A 24 F cannula is placed in the left atrium. A roller or centrifugal pump takes blood from the left atrium and returns it to a cannula placed in the femoral artery. The lungs are ventilated so that no oxygenator is required.

D If there is sufficient normal aorta above the diaphragm and below the aneurysm or dissection, the uptake cannula can be placed in the distal arch, and the return cannula is placed in the descending thoracic aorta. Again, no oxygenator is required because the lungs are ventilated.

E When the disease in the descending thoracic aorta is extensive and complex, including thoracoabdominal aneurysm, it is best to use femoral vein–to–femoral artery perfusion, employing an oxygenator and heat exchanger in the perfusion circuit. Deep hypothermia and circulatory arrest are used for spinal cord and visceral protection.

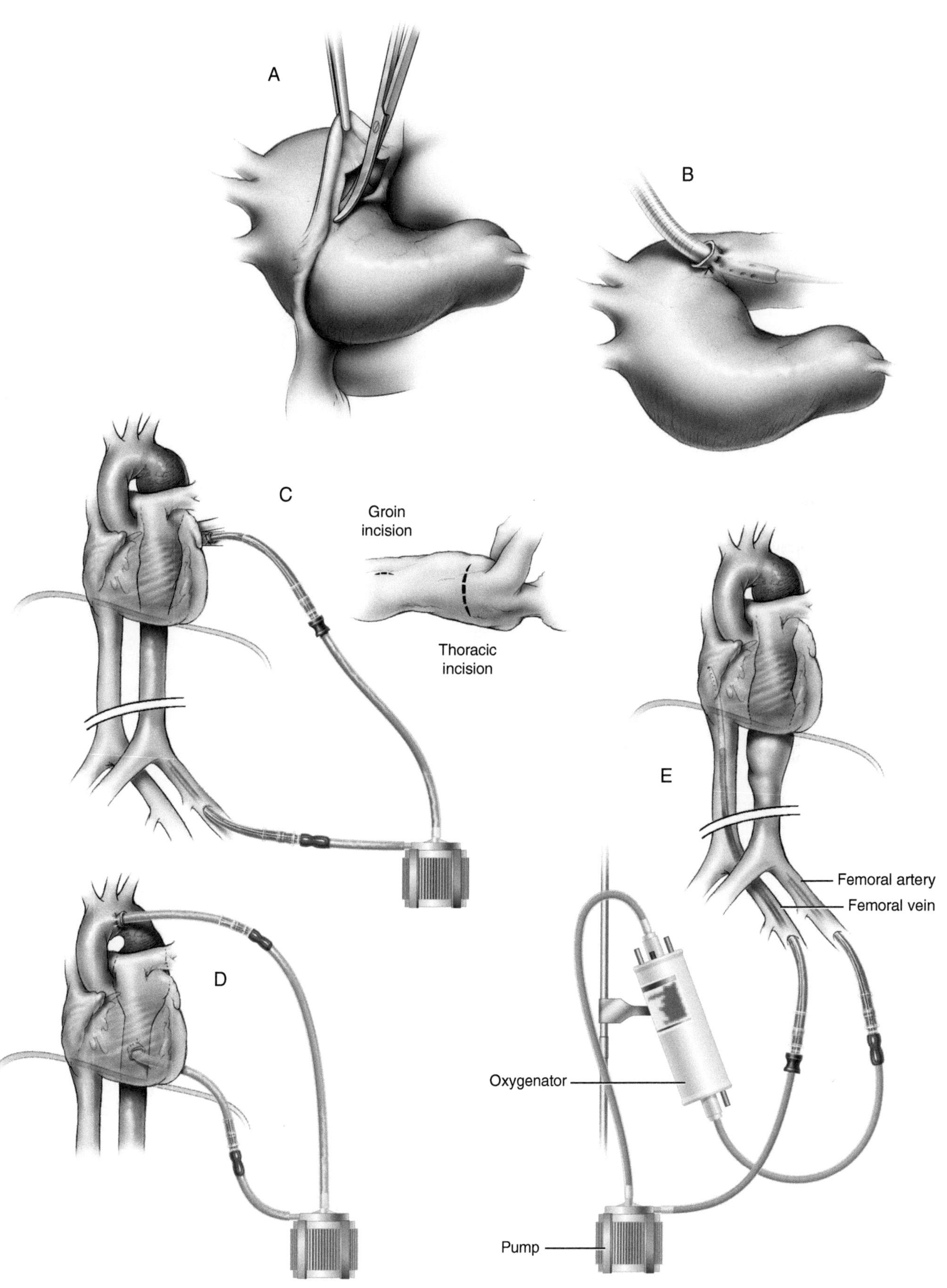
A
B
C
Groin incision
Thoracic incision
D
E
Femoral artery
Femoral vein
Oxygenator
Pump

Cannulation of the Axillary Artery

Cannulation of the right axillary artery has advantages in operations to repair an aortic arch aneurysm or acute aortic dissection. Arterial return can be established prior to sternotomy, thereby reducing risk. Perfusion of the right common carotid artery can be continued with the aortic arch open when the arch repair is complex and time-consuming.

Figure 2-9

A A transverse incision is made 2 cm below the lateral one-third of the clavicle. Fibers of the pectoralis major muscle are separated and retracted. The clavipectoral fascia is incised. Small arterial and venous branches are often encountered in the fatty tissue below the fascia and are divided as necessary. The axillary vein is located anterior to the axillary artery. The vein is mobilized to gain access to the artery. The artery is mobilized and separated from neural components of the brachial plexus. The artery is controlled by passing a vessel loop around it. Traction on the vessel loop aids dissection and mobilization of the artery.

B The axillary artery can be cannulated directly if it is free of atherosclerotic disease and if it is large enough to accept the cannula. The left radial or brachial artery should be used for arterial pressure monitoring because the axillary artery cannula will obstruct blood flow to the right arm. Small vascular clamps are used for proximal and distal control of the artery. Scissors are used to incise the axillary artery through half the circumference. A small curved hemostat is used to dilate the artery proximally and distally to allow easier passage of the cannula and to facilitate more accurate repair of the artery once the cannula is removed. The cannula is placed into the arteriotomy with the bevel toward the clearly visualized intima on the intact back wall.

C The occlusion clamp is opened to allow careful advancement of the cannula into the arterial lumen, while rotating the cannula to position the bevel anteriorly. The cannula should not be advanced against resistance. Free flow of pulsatile blood into the cannula is a good sign that it has been introduced properly. The vessel loop is drawn up tight under a small clamp to achieve hemostasis, and it can be tied to the cannula securely. Perfusion pressure in the axillary artery is always higher than pressure through cannulae placed directly in the aorta. Excessively high pressure suggests arterial dissection or other obstruction and is an indication to stop the flow through the cannula immediately.

D An alternative method for perfusion of the axillary artery is to place a prosthetic graft on the side of the artery and cannulate through the graft. This method has the advantages of avoiding dissection or damage to the artery, allowing the use of a larger perfusion cannula, and providing continuous distal perfusion of the arm during cardiopulmonary bypass. The axillary artery is approached, mobilized, and controlled in the same fashion as described earlier. A single side-biting clamp is used to control the artery proximally and distally. A longitudinal arteriotomy is made, long enough to accommodate an 8 mm woven polyester graft. The graft is beveled, and the tip of the graft is positioned toward the proximal end of the arteriotomy. Continuous stitches of 5/0 polypropylene are used to approximate the graft to the arteriotomy, beginning at the distal end and at the heel of the graft. The anastomosis is sealed with BioGlue. The vascular clamp is removed from the artery and placed on the graft to assure pulsatile flow into the graft and a secure anastomosis. The graft is shortened appropriately. A 24 F arterial perfusion cannula is inserted into the end of the graft and secured using 3 silk suture or umbilical tapes tied around the graft.

E After separation from cardiopulmonary bypass, the axillary artery is repaired with 5/0 or 6/0 polypropylene suture if direct cannulation has been used. When a side graft is used, the graft is clamped close to the artery, divided, oversewn with continuous stitches of 4/0 polypropylene suture, and sealed with BioGlue.

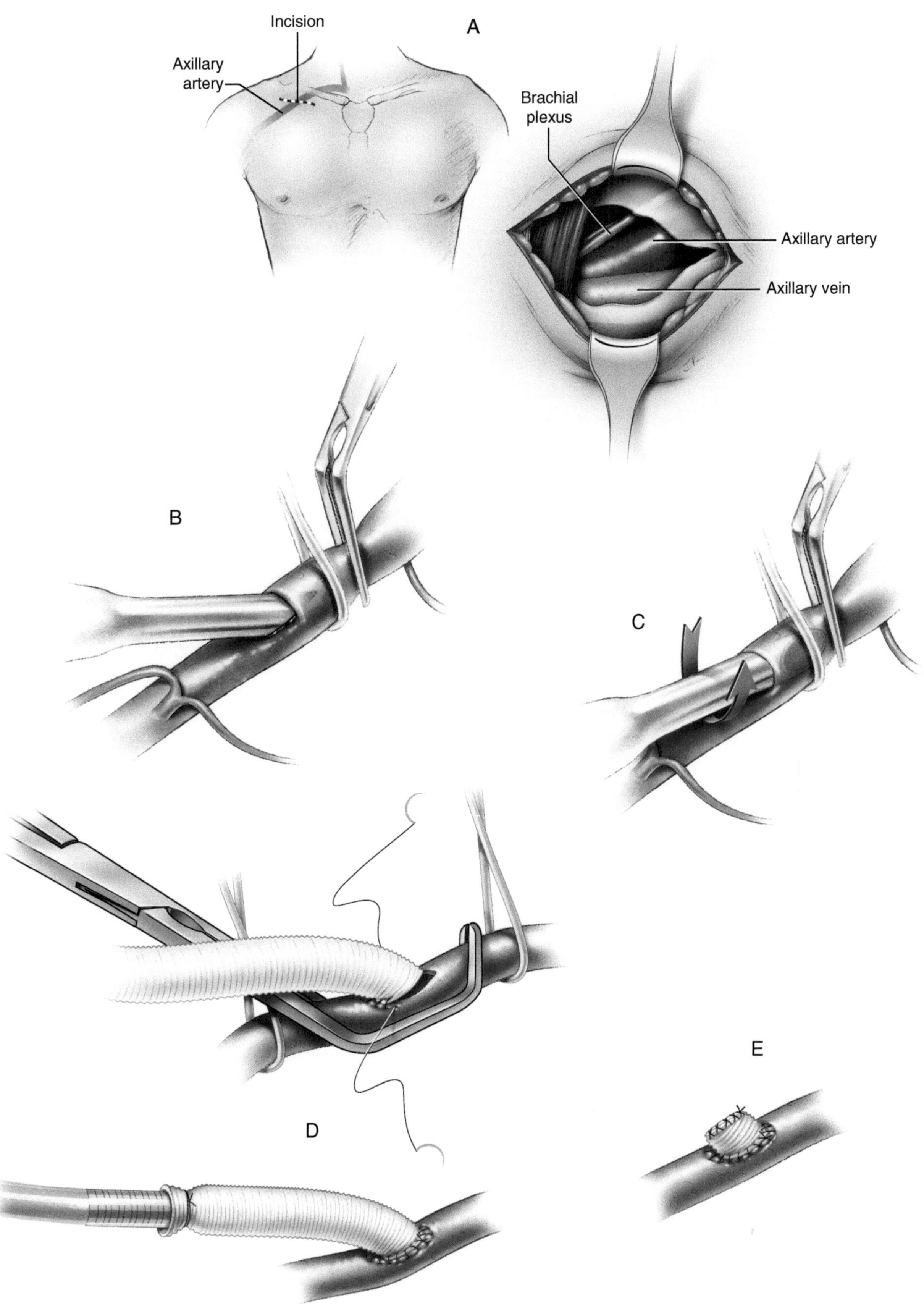
Incision
A
Axillary
artery
Brachial
plexus
Axillary artery
Axillary vein
B
C
D
E

Myocardial Protection

Myocardial protection by cardioplegic techniques has become standard procedure for most cardiac operations. The methods of delivery and the content of cardioplegic solutions in current use, however, are quite variable. In general, blood cardioplegia has become standard, with the use of various additives to reduce or buffer metabolic by-products. The addition of adenosine and lidocaine stabilizes the membrane potential of the myocardial sarcomere and allows the reduction of potassium to physiologic levels. Use of a "microplegia" delivery system provides precise control over the additives continuously infused into the blood cardioplegic solution.

The cardioplegic solution is initially delivered at normothermia until myocardial arrest is achieved. The temperature is then reduced in the microplegia system, and cold cardioplegic solution is given until the myocardial temperature reaches 10°C to 15°C. Doses of cardioplegic solution are administered at 20-minute intervals to maintain this myocardial temperature. At the conclusion of the operation, a second normothermic dose of cardioplegia is administered to provide controlled rewarming and reperfusion of the myocardium.

Figure 2-10

A Operations are performed during a single aortic occlusion period. Antegrade cardioplegia delivered through the aortic root is the preferred technique for coronary artery bypass and other operations in which the aortic valve remains competent. A pledget-reinforced mattress stitch of 3/0 polypropylene is placed in the anterior wall of the ascending aorta, and a tourniquet is attached.

B The cardioplegia delivery cannula is size 10 F, with a separate lumen for pressure monitoring. The cannula is introduced into the ascending aorta, and backflow from the aorta is assured. The cannula is held in place using the mattress stitch, and the pressure port is used to monitor aortic root pressure continuously. Infusion pressure should be in the range of 80 to 90 mm Hg (mean). The left ventricle is vented in all cases to prevent distension of the left heart.

C Retrograde cardioplegia is preferred when there is coronary artery disease with high-grade stenoses, aortic valve or aortic root disease, mitral valve disease, or during operations on the ascending aorta. This method has the advantage of providing uniform perfusion of the myocardium through the completely unobstructed venous system when there is coronary artery disease that may inhibit flow to some segments of the heart. A purse-string stitch is placed in the right atrium opposite the acute margin of the heart near the atrioventricular groove. An incision is made within the purse string, and a retrograde perfusion catheter is introduced into the right atrium and directed into the coronary sinus. The catheter can also be guided into the coronary sinus by placing the fingers of the right hand medial to the inferior vena cava near the posterior atrioventricular groove to monitor the catheter's position. As the catheter enters the coronary sinus anterior to the venous uptake cannula, it is directed more cephalad to follow the course of the coronary sinus along the atrioventricular groove. The tip of the catheter is positioned at about the midpoint of the coronary sinus. Catheters with manual or self-inflating balloons are available. The pressure port is attached to an appropriate pressure monitoring device, and retrograde cardioplegia is delivered with the coronary sinus pressure about 50 mm Hg.

D Attachment of a Y-connector to the cardioplegia system allows the tailored delivery of cardioplegic solution. In patients with high-grade coronary artery stenosis or acute occlusion of a major coronary artery with infarction, a combination of antegrade and retrograde cardioplegia delivers optimal protection of the myocardium. The second arm of the Y-connector can also be attached to a reversed saphenous vein graft, providing unobstructed perfusion of that area of the myocardium and the measurement of pressure and flow down the graft. In unusual situations in which retrograde cardioplegia is not possible, direct antegrade perfusion of the coronary ostia may be employed. Handheld cannulae are attached to the cardioplegia line and introduced just inside each main coronary ostium under direct vision. Care should be taken to avoid injuring the coronary ostium when placing these small cannulae.

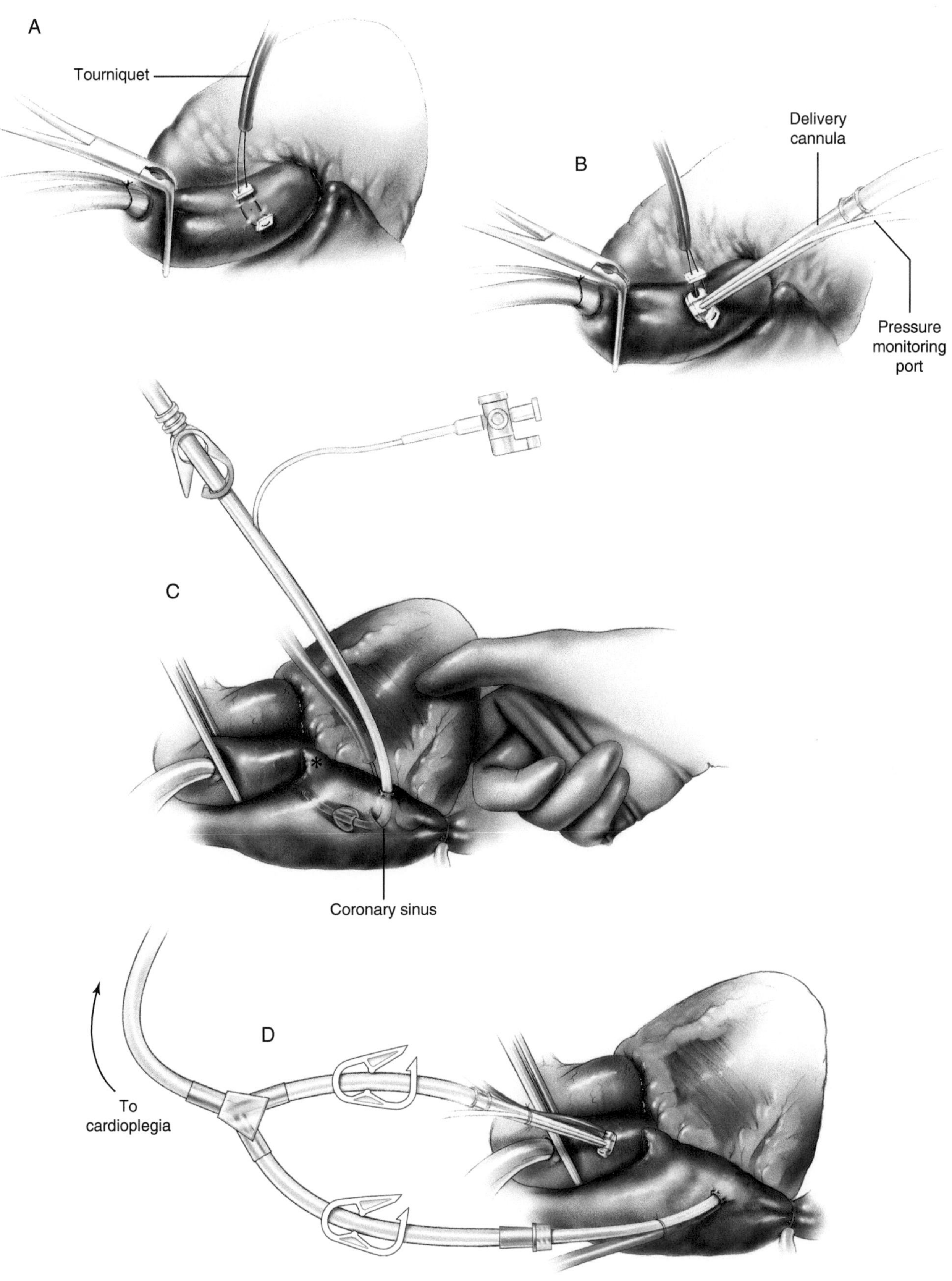
A
Tourniquet
B
Delivery cannula
Pressure monitoring port
C
*
Coronary sinus
D
To cardioplegia

Minimally Invasive Approaches in Cardiac Surgery

Numerous procedures have been developed to make cardiac surgery less invasive. In general, these smaller incisions limit visualization of and access to specific regions of the heart. Femoral cannulation is typically employed when cardiopulmonary bypass is required. Technical adaptations include partial sternotomy, small thoracotomy, cervical cannulation for retrograde cardioplegia, and percutaneous placement of retractors and clamps.

Figure 2-11

A Partial sternotomy requires division of the sternum in a transverse fashion in addition to a vertical incision. Care is taken to avoid injury to the internal mammary arteries. All cardiac operations can be performed through a lower-half partial sternotomy, and standard central cannulation can be utilized.

B A small thoracotomy avoids division of the sternum, but it must be located precisely for adequate exposure. The right third interspace is used for aortic valve operations. The right fourth interspace is used for tricuspid and mitral valve operations, as well as for surgical procedures to address atrial fibrillation and repair septal defects. The left third interspace is used for access to the left atrial appendage during atrial fibrillation operations. The left fourth interspace is used for beating heart coronary artery bypass grafting of the left anterior descending artery. MIDCAB, (minimally invasive direct coronary artery bypass).

C For minimally invasive operations that require cardioplegic arrest of the heart, retrograde cannulation of the coronary sinus can be performed through the jugular vein. This is accomplished under fluoroscopic or echocardiographic guidance. Alternatively, an extended antegrade cardioplegia cannula can be placed through an interspace directly into the ascending aorta.

D Adequate exposure of the heart and intracardiac structures is facilitated by retraction systems. Soft tissue retractors open the intercostal space and keep the tissues out of the visual field. Low-profile interatrial retractors and a flexible aortic cross-clamp can be inserted through separate stab wounds to prevent cluttering of the operative field.

E Beating heart, or "off-pump," coronary artery bypass operations require stabilization for a satisfactory technical result. Apical retraction devices allow displacement of the heart for exposure of the inferior and lateral walls. Once the heart is positioned, a localized stabilizer is used to reduce motion at the area of arterial grafting.

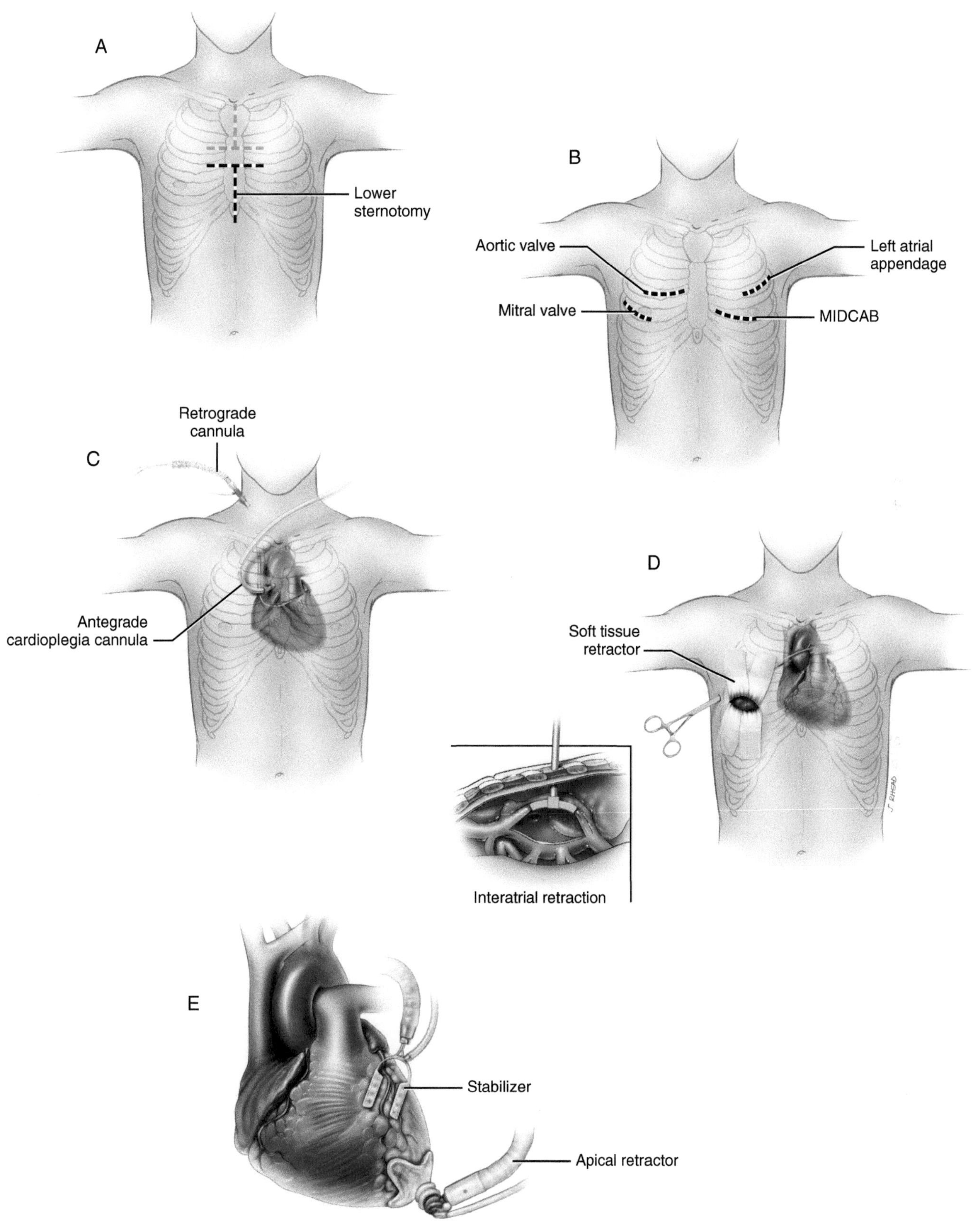

A
Lower sternotomy
B
Aortic valve
Left atrial appendage
Mitral valve
MIDCAB
C
Retrograde cannula
Antegrade cardioplegia cannula
D
Soft tissue retractor
Interatrial retraction
E
Stabilizer
Apical retractor

chapter 3 CIRCULATORY SUPPORT

Cannulation for Left and Right Heart Bypass

Left or right heart bypass is commonly employed to assist a patient's failing circulation. This method utilizes readily available cannulae and pumping devices. Pump circuits are extracorporeal, so this type of assisted circulation can be used for only a limited time (usually days).

Figure 3-1

A Left and right heart bypass may be instituted via a right anterior thoracotomy in patients in whom it is desirable not to violate the pericardial space. This may be important if cardiac transplantation is being considered and assisted circulation is being used as a bridge to the definitive procedure.

B Thin-walled, metal-tipped, right-angled cannulae (28 or 31 F) are introduced through purse-string stitches with tourniquets. One cannula is placed through the right superior pulmonary vein to the left atrium. The other cannula is placed in the right pulmonary artery. The cannulae are brought through intercostal spaces to the skin on the right side below the primary incision.

C Thin-walled percutaneous perfusion cannulae are introduced through the femoral vessels and advanced to the right atrium and the iliac artery. Right heart bypass is instituted by the uptake of blood from the right atrial percutaneous cannula and its return via centrifugal pump to the right pulmonary cannula. Left heart bypass is instituted by the uptake of blood from the left atrial cannula and its return via centrifugal pump to the iliac artery cannula.

D The cannulae for left and right heart bypass are more commonly introduced through a midline sternotomy during cardiac operations. When pharmacologic and intraaortic balloon counterpulsation support of the failing circulation is insufficient to sustain life, left or right heart bypass, or both, may be necessary.

E Cannulae are usually placed in the right atrium and the aorta during cardiac operations. These are utilized for left and right heart bypass. A thin-walled, metal-tipped, right-angled cannula is introduced into the left atrium via the right superior pulmonary vein through a purse-string stitch with a tourniquet. A 20-degree arterial perfusion cannula is placed in the main pulmonary artery.

F Left heart bypass is established by connecting the left atrial cannula to the aortic cannula through a centrifugal pump. Right heart bypass involves connecting the right atrial cannula to the pulmonary artery cannula through a centrifugal pump. The cannulae are brought through the fascia, muscle, and skin into the left and right upper quadrants of the abdomen. Teflon felt strips are placed tightly around the cannulae in the subcutaneous tissues to seal the exit tracts. The midline incision is closed primarily. In some cases the cannulae are brought out through the wound.

G The wound may be left open when the heart cannot tolerate the compression of wound closure. An Esmarch or Silastic membrane is attached to the skin edges using staples to seal the mediastinum.

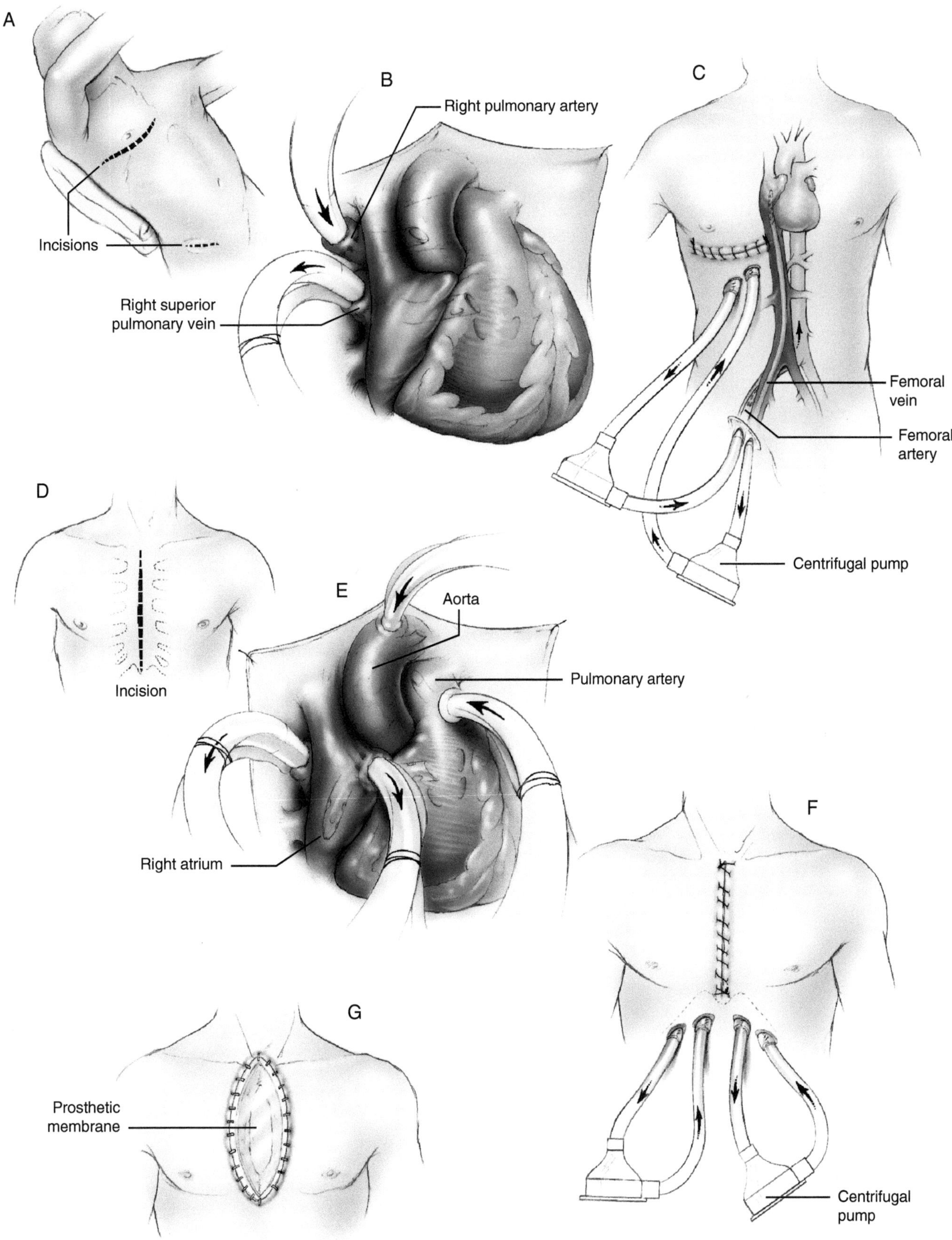
A
Incisions
B
Right pulmonary artery
Right superior
pulmonary vein
C
Femoral
vein
Femoral
artery
Centrifugal pump
D
Incision
E
Aorta
Pulmonary artery
Right atrium
F
Centrifugal
pump
G
Prosthetic
membrane

Percutaneous Ventricular Assist Device

Percutaneous ventricular assist devices (PVADs) are designed to be inserted in the operating room, the cardiac catheterization laboratory, the intensive care unit, or even regular hospital rooms. These devices provide short-term support for hours up to 14 days.

Figure 3-2

A The TandemHeart (CardiacAssist Inc., Pittsburgh, PA) is a left atrium–to–femoral artery bypass system. Cannulae are inserted by the percutaneous needle–catheter–over–guidewire technique. The femoral venous cannula is advanced through the atrial septum into the left atrium to receive oxygenated blood. An oxygenator is therefore not required. The femoral artery cannula is inserted by percutaneous technique. A second small cannula may be directed distally in the femoral artery to provide distal limb blood flow in case the primary cannula obstructs the artery. The pump is a continuous-flow centrifugal device capable of delivering blood flow at a rate up to 4 L/min. The pump has a fluid-infusion system for cooling and lubrication of the impeller. Local anticoagulation of the blood inside the pump is possible. The pump is placed outside the body (extracorporeal) on the patient's leg and is driven by a controller console. The cannulae are connected to the pump by appropriate wet-to-wet connections to prevent the entry of air into the bypass circuit. Cardiac-assist blood flow is established from the left atrium to the femoral artery.

B Cardiopulmonary support (CPS) is another form of PVAD system. The femoral vein is cannulated percutaneously, and the cannula is advanced to the right atrium for systemic venous uptake. The femoral artery is cannulated percutaneously for the return of blood to the body. Right atrium–to–femoral artery bypass is established using a magnetically driven centrifugal pump and a membrane oxygenator.

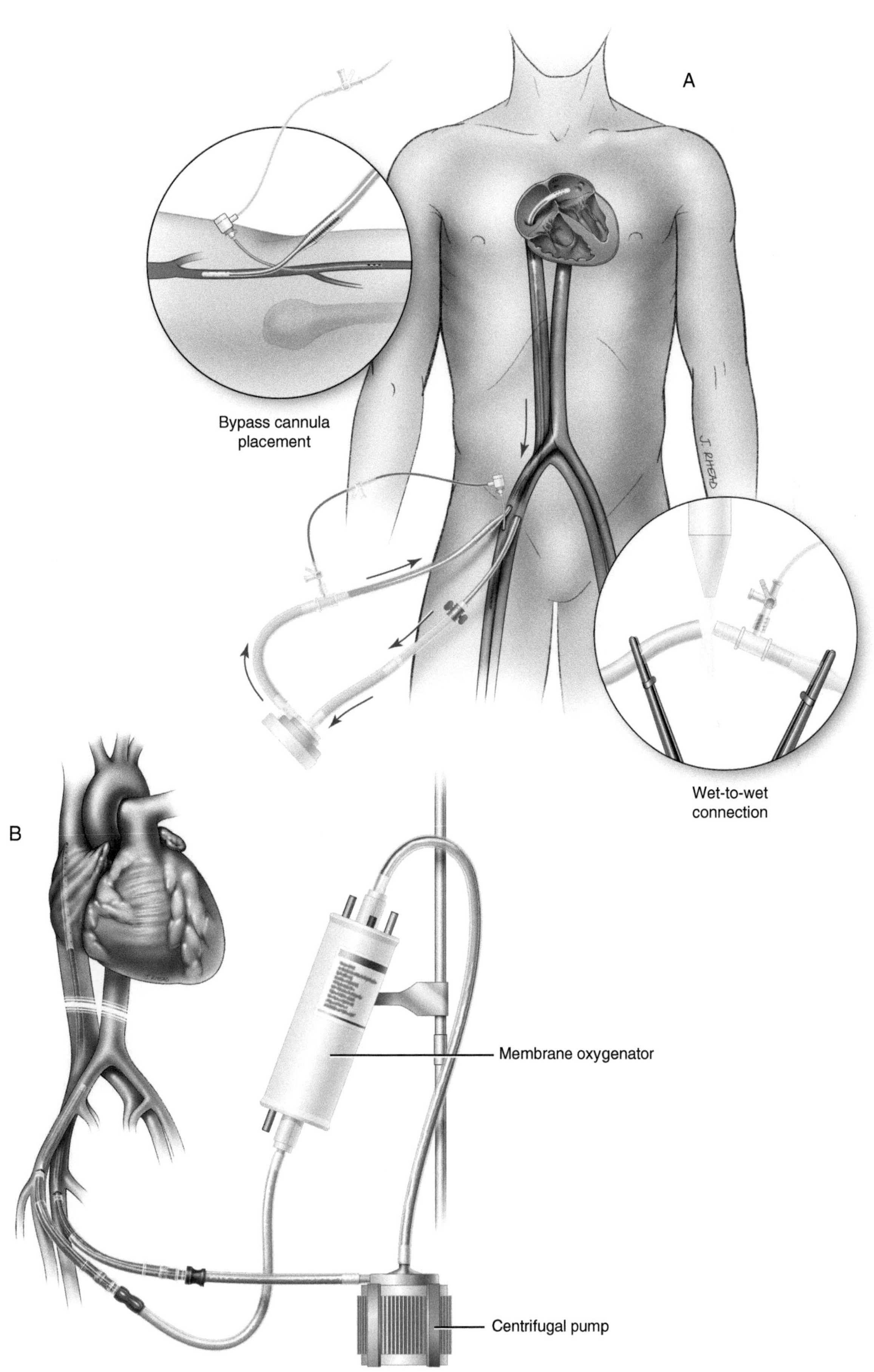
A
Bypass cannula placement
J. RHEAD
Wet-to-wet connection
B
Membrane oxygenator
Centrifugal pump

Left Ventricular Assist Device

Patients whose congestive cardiac failure is limited to the left ventricle may benefit from the implantation of a left ventricular assist device, which effectively supports the circulation provided that right ventricular function is normal. This device is generally used as a temporary measure to sustain the patient while awaiting a suitable donor for cardiac transplantation. Semipermanent or permanent implantation of a left ventricular assist device may also be performed.

Figure 3-3

A Implantation of the pneumatically driven HeartMate left ventricular assist device (Thoratec Inc., Pleasanton, CA) is shown. It was the first device approved for this purpose, and a large number of them were implanted successfully. This model of the HeartMate is now obsolete, but the insertion of all subsequent models uses the same operative principles. A midline sternotomy incision is made. The incision is extended to the umbilicus. The pump device is placed in a preperitoneal or intrarectus sheath pouch in the left upper quadrant of the abdomen. The peritoneum is mobilized from the anterior abdominal wall and off the inferior surface of the diaphragm.

B Cardiopulmonary bypass is established using two venous uptake cannulae, with the return of blood occurring through a cannula in the ascending aorta. Tourniquets are secured around the venae cavae. An incision is made in the right atrium parallel to the atrioventricular groove. A perfusion catheter is placed directly in the coronary sinus, and cold cardioplegic solution is administered through it. The atrial septum is inspected for defects, and appropriate repair is performed to prevent a shunt across the atrial septum following the institution of left heart bypass. A cross-clamp is placed on the ascending aorta. A longitudinal incision is made as low as possible in the ascending aorta to allow undistorted anastomosis of the return graft to the aorta. An end-to-side anastomosis of the Dacron graft to the aorta is performed using continuous stitches of 3/0 polypropylene. The anastomosis is started by placing several suture loops around the "heel" of the graft. The suture loops are pulled up, and the graft is approximated to the aorta. The anastomosis is completed by continuing the suture line around the "toe" of the graft. If the aorta is large, the anastomosis can be accomplished under a clamp that partially occludes the aorta and allows continued coronary artery perfusion.

C The point at which the left ventricular apex approximates the diaphragm is located. The apex is elevated from the pericardial sac. A core-cutting device is used to create an opening in the left ventricular apex.

D The apex connector is attached to the left ventricular myocardium using interrupted Teflon pledget-reinforced stitches of 2/0 braided suture. The stitches are placed through the epicardium and penetrate approximately three-fourths the thickness of the left ventricular wall.

E The sutures are tied to firmly approximate the apex connector to the apex of the left ventricle.

F In cases of acute myocardial infarction involving the apex of the left ventricle, it is necessary to reinforce the myocardium to prevent rupture around the apex connector. A sheet of Teflon felt is used to fashion a skirt to protect the left ventricle. A large circle of felt is formed, and a hole of the appropriate size is cut in the center of it. About one-fourth of the circle is removed. Removal of this segment allows the graft to be formed into a skirt, which can be used to reinforce the left ventricular apex. Pledget-reinforced mattress sutures are placed through the skirt and the myocardium to attach the apex connector to the heart.

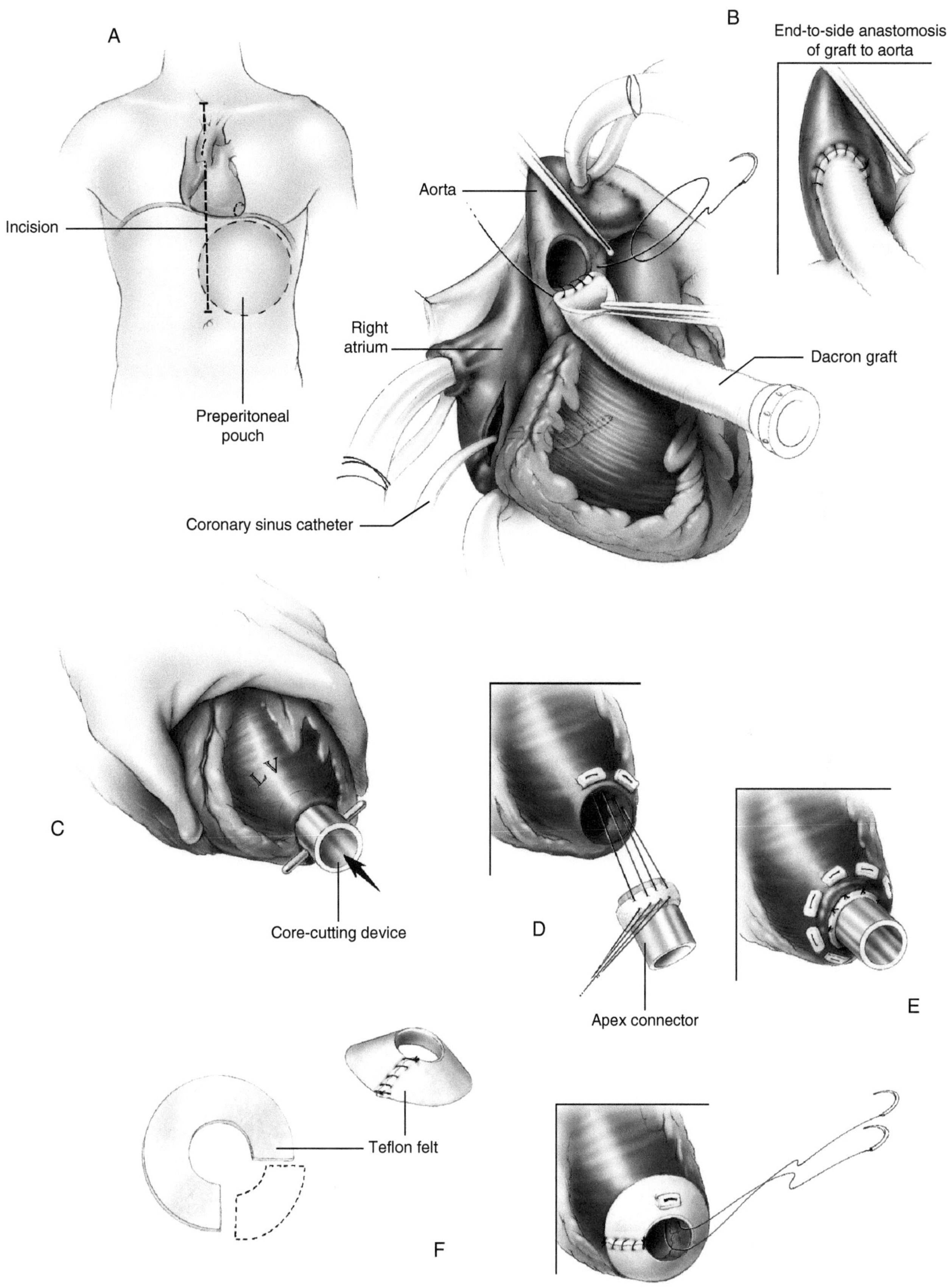
A
Incision
Preperitoneal
pouch
B
End-to-side anastomosis
of graft to aorta
Aorta
Right
atrium
Dacron graft
Coronary sinus catheter
C
LV
Core-cutting device
D
Apex connector
E
Teflon felt
F

Figure 3-3 (continued)

G The HeartMate left ventricular assist device is placed in the preperitoneal pouch in the left upper quadrant of the abdomen. An opening is made in the diaphragm directly opposite the apex connector. The inflow conduit is passed through the diaphragm.

H The inflow conduit is attached to the apex connector and tightly secured with suture and a conduit strap.

I The aortic graft is attached to the outflow conduit. The connection is secured by suture, which prevents the possibility of release.

J The drive line from the device exits from a tunnel in the left lower quadrant of the abdominal wall to complete the implant. It is connected to the drive console. Left ventricle–to–aorta bypass can then be established.

K The HeartMate XVE left ventricular assist system (Thoratec Inc., Pleasanton, CA) is the model currently in use and is approved for long-term permanent implantation (destination therapy). Improvements to this electrically driven device include a longer, smaller-diameter, and more flexible lead for patient comfort; enhanced controller software to reduce pressure and wear on moving parts; and a new inflow valve conduit with enhanced durability. The main difference in operative technique is that the exit point of the driver lead is from the right upper quadrant on the abdominal wall.

L HeartMate 2 (Thoratec Inc., Pleasanton, CA) is an axial-flow left ventricular assist device that is one-seventh the size and one-fourth the weight of the HeartMate XVE. The device employs a continuous-flow (i.e., pulseless) rotary pump that is virtually silent. The implantation technique is similar to that for the HeartMate pulsatile models, with placement of the device in a preperitoneal pouch in the left upper abdomen.

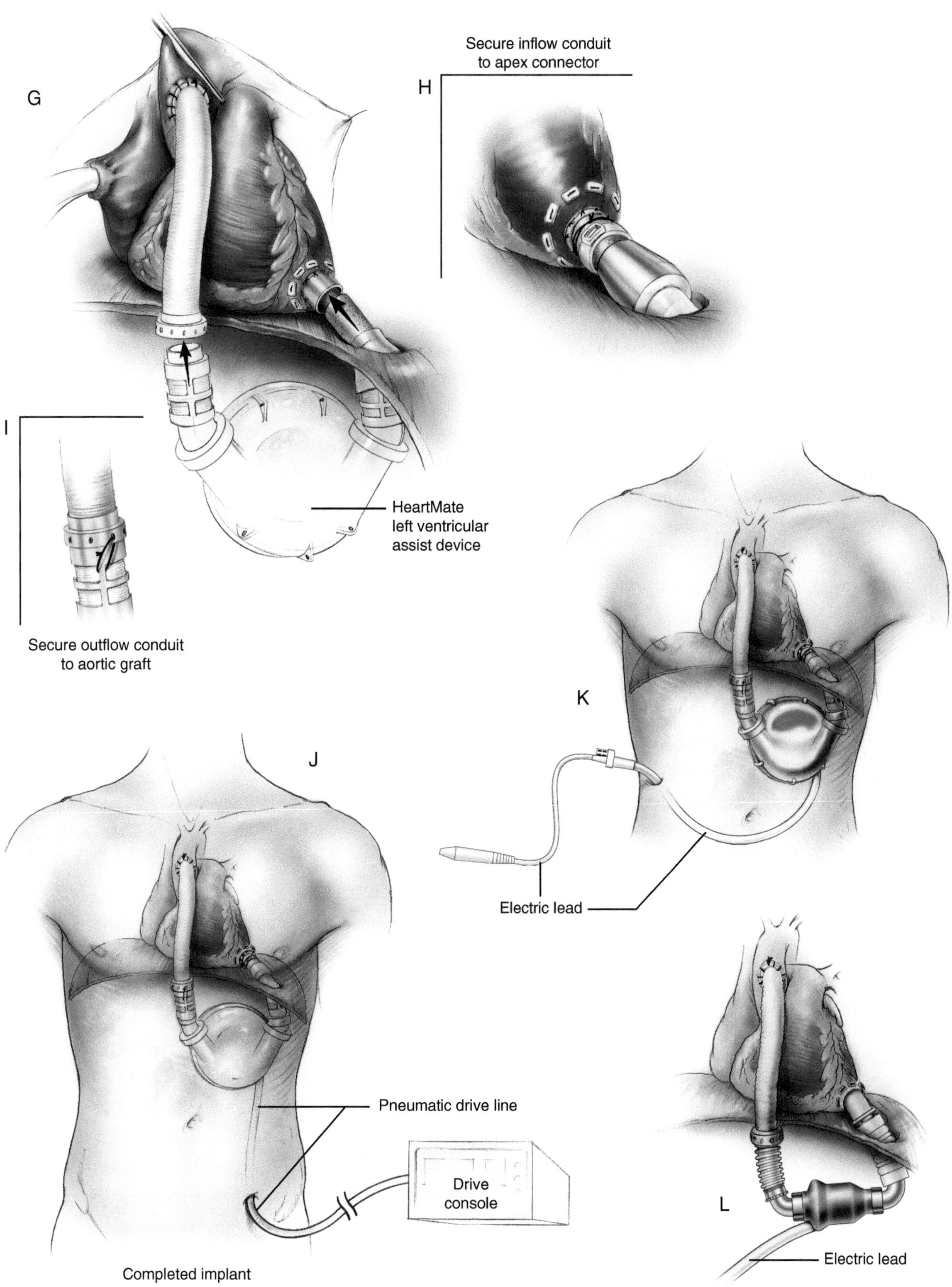

G
Secure inflow conduit
to apex connector
H
I
HeartMate
left ventricular
assist device
Secure outflow conduit
to aortic graft
K
J
Electric lead
Pneumatic drive line
Drive
console
L
Electric lead
Completed implant

Total Artificial Heart

The total artificial heart is implanted when there is irreversible heart failure and no chance of immediately locating a suitable donor for cardiac transplantation. The device is used as a bridge to support the circulation until it is possible to perform transplantation. The total artificial heart is used when there is both right and left heart failure, precluding support of only the left ventricle.

Figure 3-4

A Cardiopulmonary bypass is instituted using two venous uptake cannulae, with oxygenated blood returned to the ascending aorta. Tourniquets are secured around the caval cannulae. The aorta is occluded. The heart is excised through the ventricular mass below the atrioventricular groove. The aorta and pulmonary arteries are divided at the sinus rim. The ventricular mass is cut back to the atrioventricular groove, preserving the mitral and tricuspid valve annuli.

B The valve leaflets are nearly excised, retaining a rim of tissue on the annulus. The aortic valve's continuity with the mitral valve is preserved.

C Each atrioventricular connector of the artificial heart is supplied with a skirt of material to allow proper sizing of the device to match the atrioventricular orifice. The skirts of the connectors are cut down to the appropriate size in a circular fashion, except for the portion used to approximate the septum, which is cut straight. There is also a straight cut in the region of the aortic-mitral continuity.

D The connectors are inverted for easier approximation to the atrioventricular orifice. A continuous horizontal mattress stitch of 2/0 polypropylene is used to attach the right and left atrioventricular connectors to the septum. The stitch is started at the aortic-mitral continuity and continued to the crux posteriorly.

E The opposite end of the suture is used to oversew the septal suture line, continuing to the crux. A second suture is started at the 2 o'clock position on the left atrioventricular connector. Continuous stitches are used to approximate the connector to the left atrioventricular orifice, working counterclockwise across the aortic-mitral continuity. The opposite end of the suture is continued in a clockwise fashion to the crux, where it is tied off to the septal suture. A strip of Teflon felt may be worked into the suture line for better hemostasis.

F The septal suture is continued in a clockwise fashion to approximate the right atrioventricular connector to the right atrioventricular orifice. The suture line is completed by taking the anterior suture in a counterclockwise fashion to the 10 o'clock position to join the other suture. The connectors are everted to their proper position.

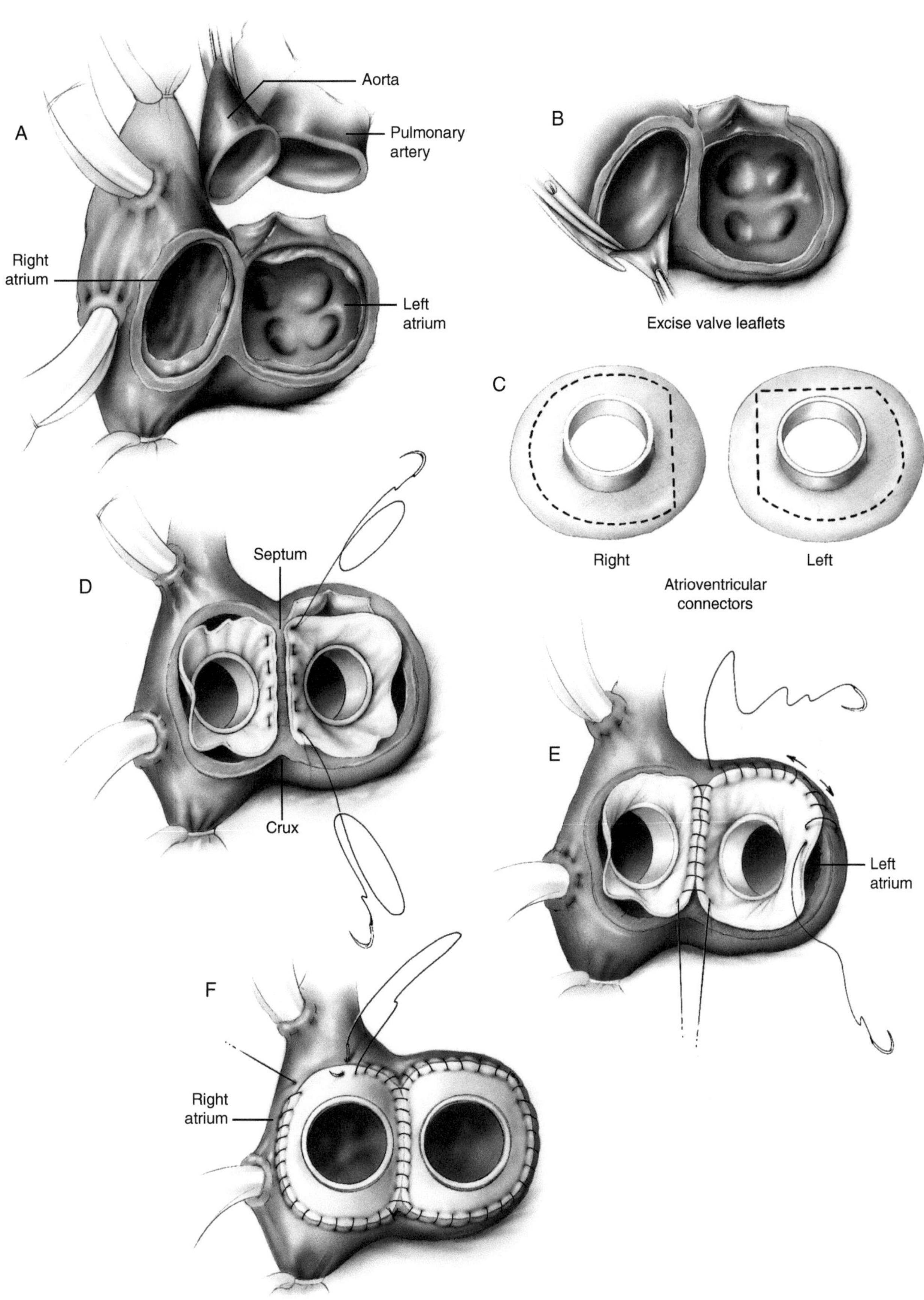
A
Aorta
Pulmonary artery
Right atrium
Left atrium
B
Excise valve leaflets
C
Right
Left
Atrioventricular connectors
D
Septum
Crux
E
Left atrium
F
Right atrium

Figure 3-4 (continued)

G The artificial heart is brought into position in the pericardial sac to allow measurement of the distance between the aorta and pulmonary artery and the device. The aortic connector and Dacron graft are usually 5 to 7 cm long, whereas the pulmonary connector and graft are usually 7 to 9 cm long. An end-to-end anastomosis of the aortic graft to the aorta is constructed using 4/0 polypropylene suture.

H An end-to-end anastomosis of the pulmonary graft to the pulmonary artery is constructed using continuous stitches of 4/0 polypropylene.

I The left ventricle of the artificial heart is connected first. The drive line is brought out through the pericardial sac to the left upper quadrant of the abdomen, a comfortable distance below the costal margin. The atrioventricular connectors are joined, with careful attention to the proper position of the artificial left ventricle so as not to obstruct the left atrium. The aortic connectors are joined, with careful attention to the proper orientation of the artificial left ventricle to prevent rotation of the aortic graft.

J The right ventricle of the artificial heart is placed in the pericardial sac, and the drive line is brought out below the left costal margin. The right atrioventricular connectors are joined, with careful attention to proper orientation to avoid a rotation defect of the right atrium. The artificial left ventricle is drawn to the left side of the pericardial sac, and the artificial ventricles are attached to each other. It is then possible to properly orient the pulmonary artery connectors anterior to the aortic graft.

K Implantation of the pneumatically driven total artificial heart is complete.

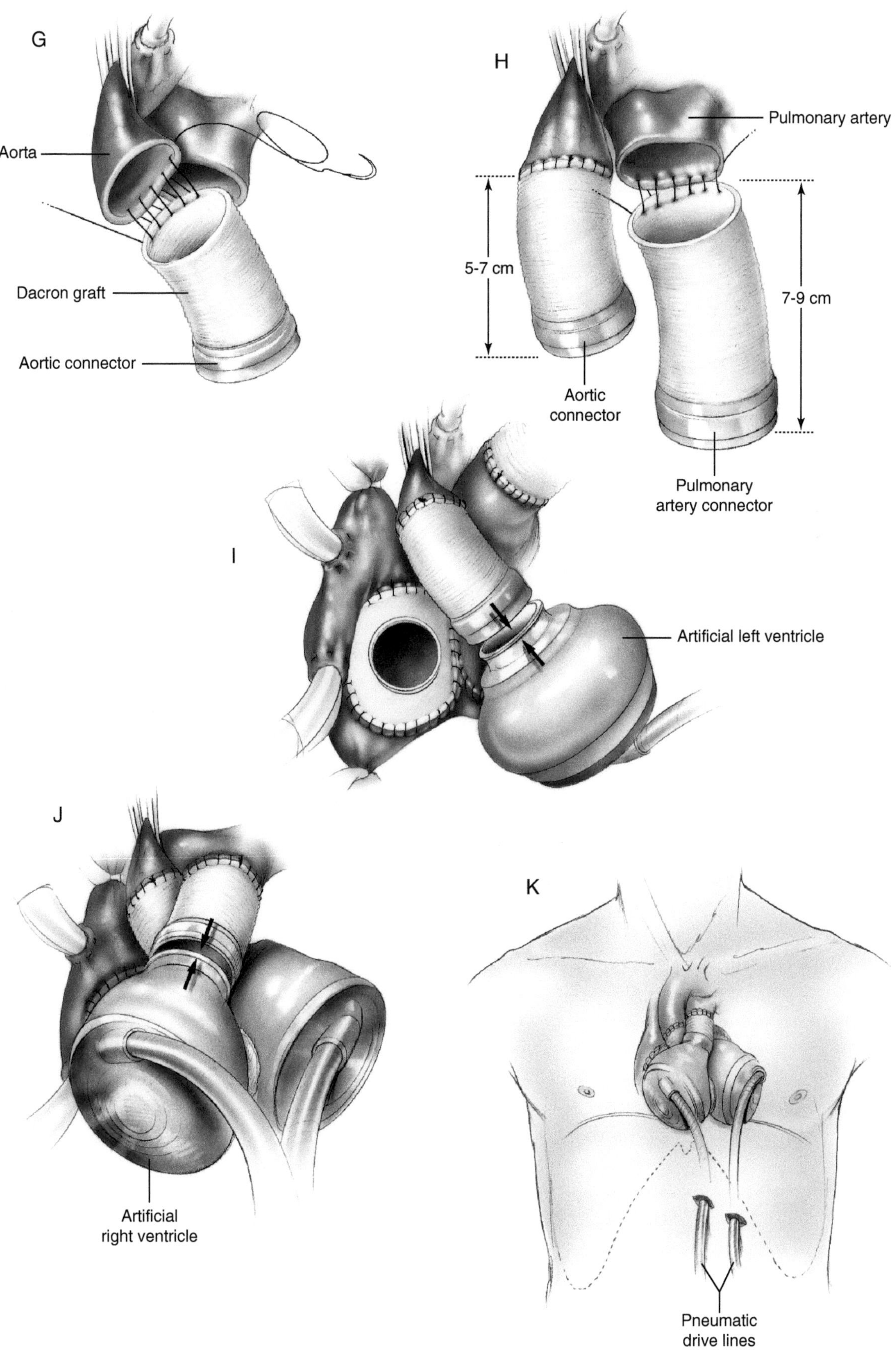
G
Aorta
Dacron graft
Aortic connector
H
Pulmonary artery
5-7 cm
7-9 cm
Aortic connector
Pulmonary artery connector
I
Artificial left ventricle
J
Artificial right ventricle
K
Pneumatic drive lines

part II

Septal Defects

chapter 4 ATRIAL AND ATRIOVENTRICULAR SEPTAL DEFECTS

Defects of the atrial septum are common cardiac anomalies. The surface cardiac anatomy is assessed for cardiac chamber and pulmonary artery enlargement, status of the mitral and tricuspid valves, location of the pulmonary veins (especially the right superior pulmonary vein), persistent left superior vena cava, and patent ductus arteriosus.

Morphology

Figure 4-1

A There are three main types of atrial septal defects. The most common is the secundum type, in which the defect occupies the location of the foramen ovale. The ostium primum type is actually a defect of the atrioventricular septum and is located low in the septum. The defect is crescent-shaped and is associated with atrioventricular valve abnormalities. The sinus venosus type of atrial septal defect is located high in the septum, near the superior vena cava orifice, and is often associated with an anomalous connection of the right superior pulmonary vein.

B Atrial septal defect, secundum type. The ostium secundum defect is an embryologic failure of atrial septation related to excessive fenestration of the septum primum during formation of the ostium secundum or inadequate coverage of the ostium secundum by the septum secundum as it descends from the roof of the atrium. This specimen shows some features of both mechanisms: there are fenestrations extending inferiorly to the limbus of the fossa ovalis, and the atrial septum is clearly thicker in the fossa above the fenestrations. There is also a patent foramen ovale due to failure of fusion after birth. Thus, there are two defects within the fossa ovalis, both some distance above the annulus of the tricuspid valve.

C Atrial septal defect, ostium primum type. The term *atrioventricular septal defect* has been proposed to describe the group of defects variously termed *endocardial cushion defects* and *atrioventricular canal defects*. The pathognomonic feature of this group of malformations, whatever the specific type, is a defect at the site of the atrioventricular septum. The normal atrioventricular septum is composed of the fibrous extension of the central fibrous body, located at the junction of the aortic root and the atrioventricular valve rings, and a muscular portion that is the cephalic segment of the inlet ventricular septum. These defects also have a virtually identical common atrioventricular junction guarded by a basically six-leaflet common atrioventricular valve. It is the anatomy of these leaflets bridging the ventricular septum that differentiates the partial and complete forms of the defect. In the partial form of the anomaly, the bridging leaflets of the atrioventricular valve are joined by a connecting tongue of valve tissue and are usually firmly adherent to the crest of the ventricular septum. This specimen demonstrates an intact fossa ovalis with a small rim of septum that extends to the coronary sinus. The septal rim borders a low-lying atrial septal defect extending to the atrioventricular valves. This defect is caused by the embryologic failure of the septum primum to fuse with the endocardial cushions. The left atrioventricular valve shows a prominent "cleft" in its septal portion, but the valve is fused to the ventricular septum.

D Atrioventricular septal defect, left ventricular outflow tract. The left ventricular outflow tract is abnormal in all patients with this defect. It is longer and narrower than normal because of the left atrioventricular valve's attachment to the ventricular septum at the edge of the septal deficiency, which may or may not be an open defect. The extent of narrowing is determined by how far the septal deficiency extends across the septum below the aortic valve. In this case, the narrowing of the left ventricular outflow tract is moderate, extending only halfway across the diameter of the aortic orifice.

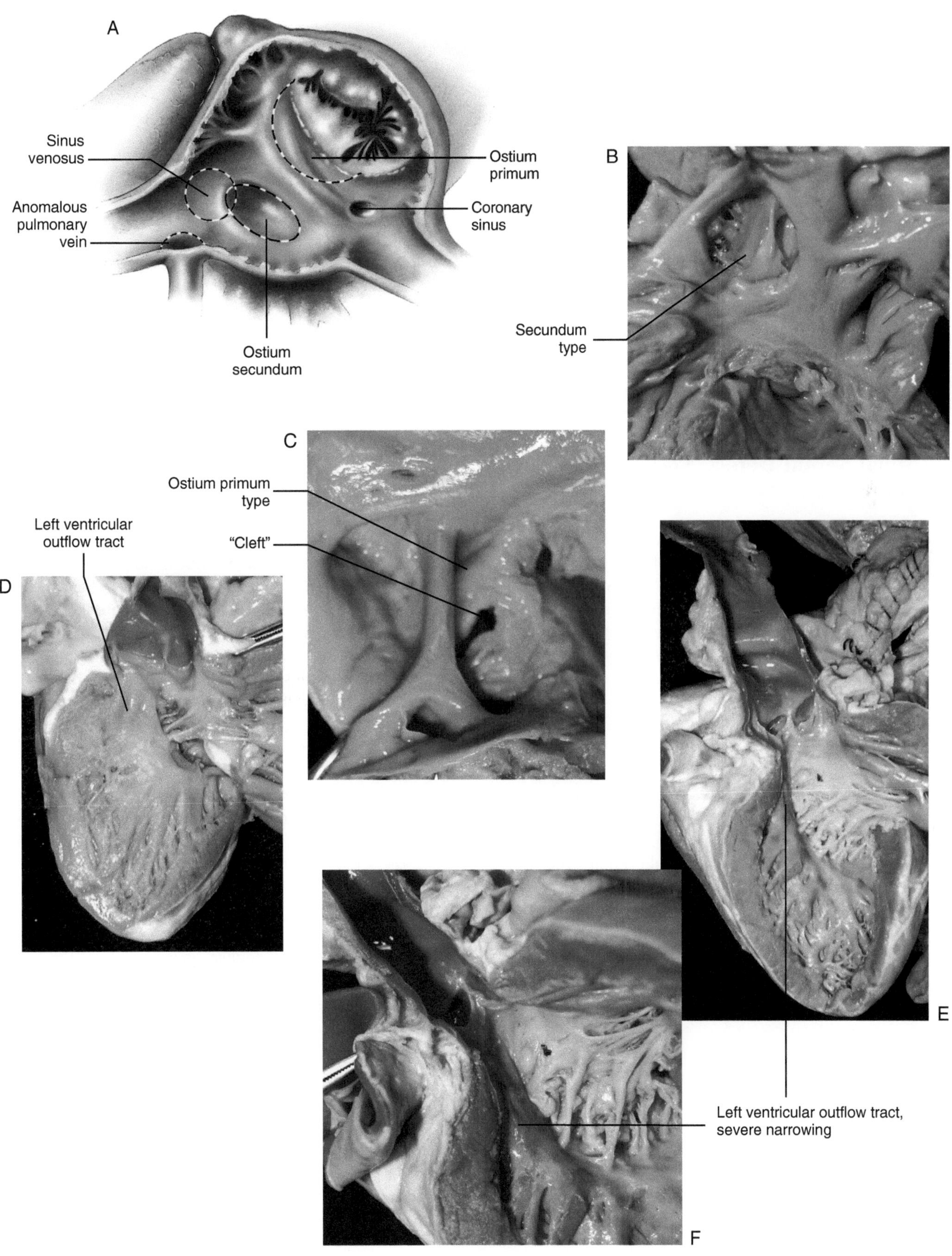
A
Sinus venosus
Anomalous pulmonary vein
Ostium primum
Coronary sinus
Ostium secundum
B
Secundum type
C
Ostium primum type
"Cleft"
Left ventricular outflow tract
D
E
F
Left ventricular outflow tract, severe narrowing

Figure 4-1 (continued)

E Atrioventricular septal defect, left ventricular outflow tract, severe narrowing. This specimen shows severe narrowing of the left ventricular outflow tract due to the left atrioventricular valve's attachment to a large ventricular septal deficiency that involves most of the septum below the aortic valve. Note that there is no opening in the ventricular septum due to dense atrioventricular valve tissue occluding the septum.

F Atrioventricular septal defect, left ventricular outflow tract, severe narrowing. This specimen illustrates a steeper angle than that in Figure 4-1, *E*, with severe narrowing of the left ventricular outflow tract.

Atrial Septal Defect, Secundum Type
Figure 4-2

A After the ascending aorta is occluded, the right atriotomy is made parallel and close to the atrioventricular groove. When an anomalous connection of the right superior pulmonary vein is encountered, an optional counterincision in the superior vena cava may provide better exposure of the superior margin of the anomalous venous connection.

B The secundum type of atrial septal defect is usually repaired without emptying the left heart. After the incision is made in the right atrium, the right heart is aspirated with the cardiotomy suction device in the coronary sinus so as not to empty the left atrium and to allow blood to continue overflowing the atrial septal defect into the right atrium. The amount of overflow is controlled by the flow rate of the pump-oxygenator. Exposure is obtained with the cardiotomy suction device acting as a retractor on the anterior rim of the atriotomy. A stitch is placed in the posterior rim of the atriotomy for lateral traction. A stitch of 3/0 silk is started on the medial side of the inferior rim of the atrial septal defect. The stitch should be placed in firm tissue but should not penetrate too far beyond the rim of the defect, so as to prevent injury to the atrioventricular node.

C The inferior rim of the defect is then reefed onto the needle by repeatedly penetrating the tissue at the rim. This maneuver is continued to a point on the lateral side of the rim exactly opposite the starting point. The knot of the plication suture is secured, and the circular defect is converted to a slit-like orifice. The defect is closed by continuous suture. The initial stitch should be inferior to or through the reefed up tissue to ensure that there is no crevice at the inferior rim of the defect. Positive pressure is held on the lungs to expel blood from the left atrium, along with any air that could have accumulated beneath the atrial septum on the left side. The final stitch is placed and tied to complete the closure of the atrial septal defect.

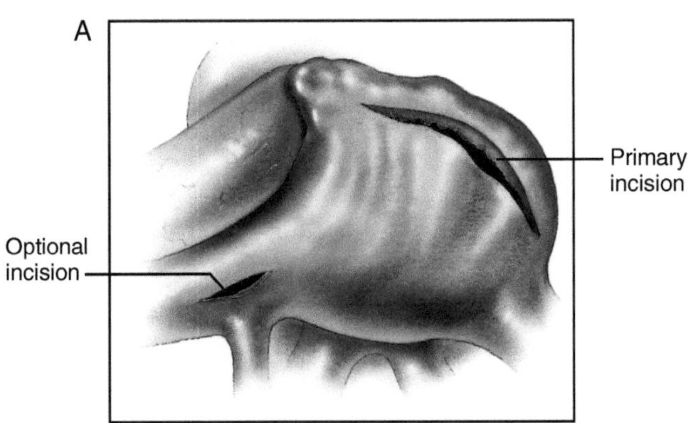
A
Primary
incision
Optional
incision

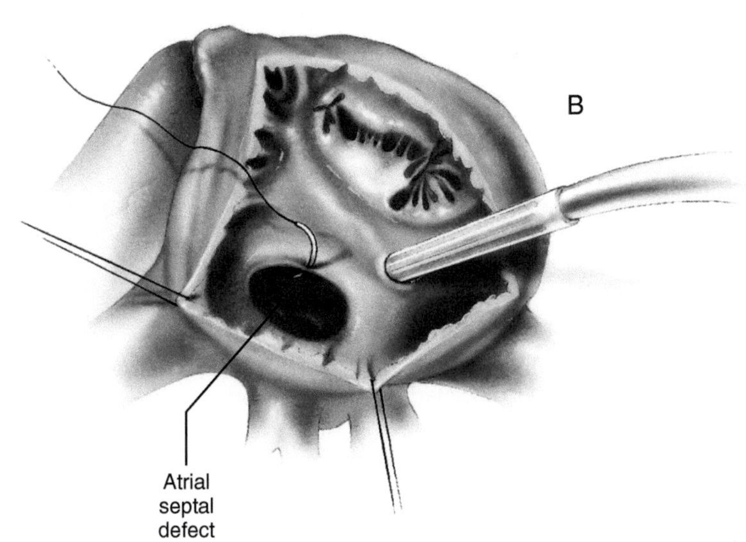
B
Atrial
septal
defect

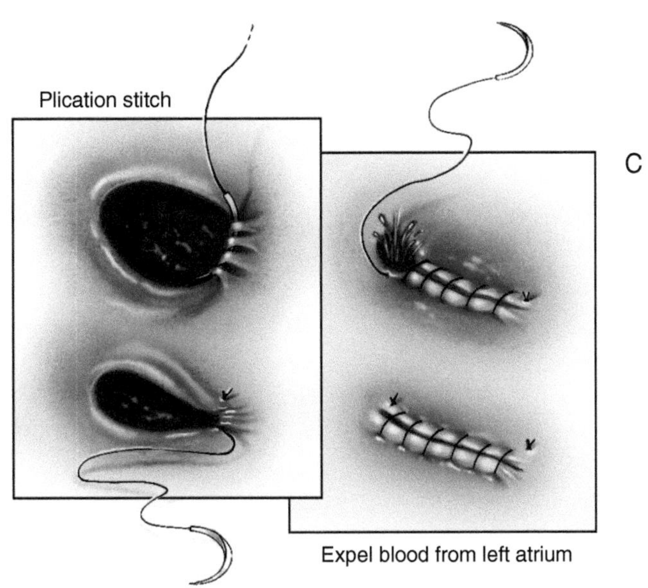
Plication stitch
C
Expel blood from left atrium

Figure 4-2 (continued)

D If the atrial septal defect is very large or if the inferior rim of the defect is absent, it may be desirable to close the defect using a pericardial patch. A rectangular patch is fashioned from the anterior portion of the pericardium. Traction sutures of 4/0 silk are passed through the tips of the rectangular pericardial patch and through the lateral rim of the atrial septal defect to keep the pericardial patch flat. Double-needle 4/0 polypropylene suture is started at the midportion of the pericardial patch and the medial rim of the atrial septal defect.

E The pericardium is sutured to the rim of the atrial septal defect by continuous suture beginning in a counterclockwise fashion. The suturing continues around the superior rim of the defect to the point of the upper lateral traction stitch, which can then be removed. The suture line is completed in a clockwise fashion around the rest of the rim of the atrial septal defect using the opposite needle. Stitches at the inferior rim of the defect should be placed into substantial tissue, but deep bites into the area of the atrioventricular node must be avoided. The stitches must also avoid obstructing the inferior vena cava orifice. The stitch is continued along the lateral rim of the defect to join the opposite end of the suture and complete the repair.

F A unidirectional patch may be used to close atrial or ventricular septal defects in patients with severe pulmonary hypertension. The patch is constructed from a piece of Dacron, and a 5 mm hole is placed eccentrically in the patch. A pericardial patch is attached to cover the hole. Only three sides of the pericardial patch are attached, leaving one side loose to act as a flap valve.

G The composite unidirectional patch is attached to the edges of the septal defect in the usual manner, placing the pericardial flap on the left (systemic) side.

H The valve patch permits one-way flow from right to left, allowing the right side to decompress during periods of extraordinarily high pulmonary pressure.

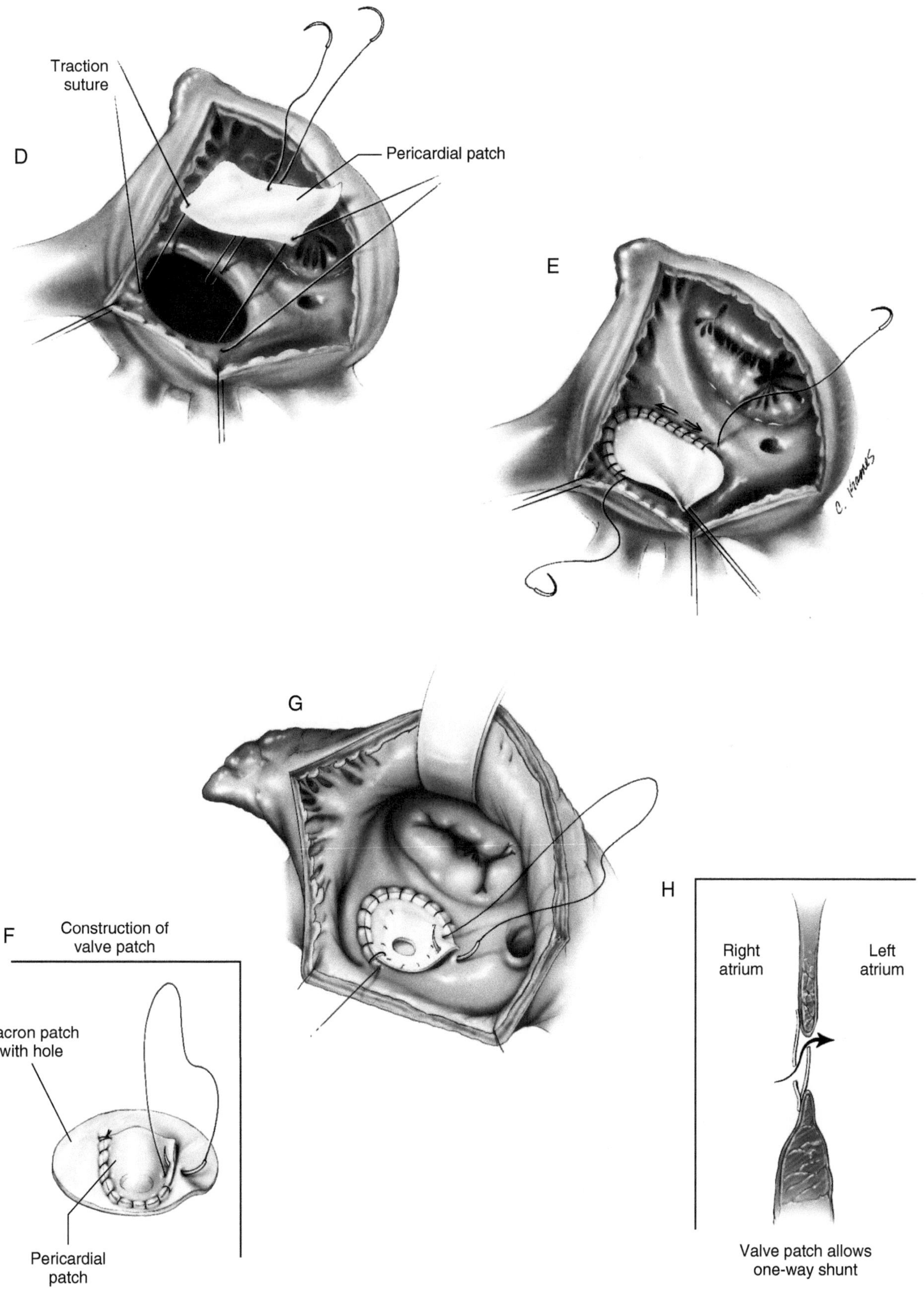
D
Traction suture
Pericardial patch
E
G
F
Construction of valve patch
Dacron patch with hole
Pericardial patch
H
Right atrium
Left atrium
Valve patch allows one-way shunt

Partial Atrioventricular Septal Defect

The partial atrioventricular septal defect involves the ostium primum defect in association with the six-leaflet common atrioventricular valve tethered to the crest of the ventricular septum.

Figure 4-3

A Partial atrioventricular septal defect, surgeon's view. This anatomic specimen, previously presented as Figure 4-1, *C*, has been rotated to appear as it would to the surgeon operating through a right atriotomy. It demonstrates an intact fossa ovalis with a small rim of septum that extends to the coronary sinus. This septal rim borders a low-lying atrial septal defect extending to the common atrioventricular valve. Right and left components of the atrioventricular valve are demonstrated. The left atrioventricular valve shows a prominent "cleft" in its septal portion, and the valve is fused to the ventricular septum; there is no septal defect on the ventricular side of the valve.

B The atrioventricular node is located within the triangle formed by the atrial defect, the attachment of the posterior bridging leaflet, and the ostium of the coronary sinus. The atrioventricular bundle (bundle of His) penetrates onto the crest of the ventricular septum at the apex of the triangle. In a partial atrioventricular septal defect, the bridging leaflets of the atrioventricular valve are joined and are adherent to the ventricular septum. A defect of the atrial portion of the atrioventricular septum is present (ostium primum atrial septal defect). In some instances interventricular communications may exist. The defect is exposed through a right atriotomy parallel to the atrioventricular groove. The atrial septal defect is identified, and its relation to the coronary sinus is determined. The atrioventricular node is located in the triangle of Koch. The characteristics of the right and left atrioventricular valves are examined and tested for competence by injecting saline through a catheter passed across the atrioventricular valve into the left ventricle. The point of contact of the anterior, posterior, and lateral components of the left atrioventricular valve is identified. The commissures of the valve extend radially from this point. Thus the "cleft" should actually be thought of as the septal commissure of the left atrioventricular valve, even though the edges of the leaflets are usually not very well supported by chordae tendineae. If the atrioventricular valve is competent, securing the septal commissure with a single stitch at the junction of the commissure and the septum may be sufficient.

C If the atrioventricular valve is incompetent, the "cleft" of the valve should be closed using interrupted stitches of 4/0 Cardionyl suture to approximate the apposing edges of the leaflet tissue, taking care not to create atrioventricular valve stenosis. It should be recognized that this repair cannot reproduce the appearance of the anterior leaflet of a normal mitral valve.

D Annuloplasty can be used to achieve better approximation of leaflet tissue by mattress stitches placed at the commissures. In older children or adults, an annuloplasty band may be employed.

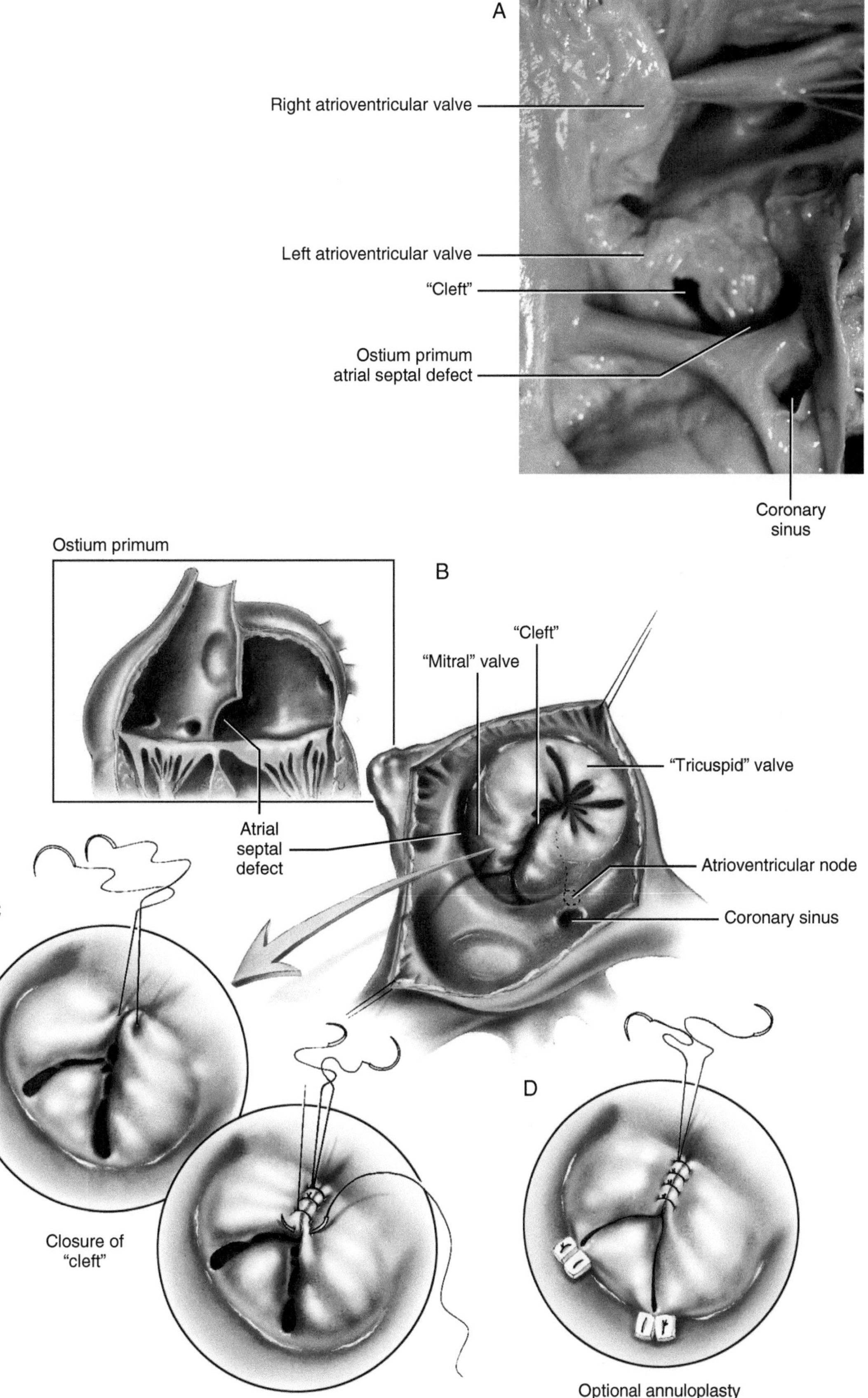
A
Right atrioventricular valve
Left atrioventricular valve
"Cleft"
Ostium primum atrial septal defect
Coronary sinus
Ostium primum
B
"Cleft"
"Mitral" valve
"Tricuspid" valve
Atrial septal defect
Atrioventricular node
Coronary sinus
C
Closure of "cleft"
D
Optional annuloplasty

Figure 4-3 (continued)

E The atrial septal defect is closed by a patch taken from the left side of the anterior pericardium. Retraction stitches of 4/0 polypropylene are placed at the lateral corners of the patch and through the lateral rim of the atrial septal defect. The patch should be large enough to include the coronary sinus and the nodal triangle within the suture line. A stitch of 4/0 polypropylene is used to join the central edge of the pericardial patch to the crest of the ventricular septum at the septal commissure of the atrioventricular valve. Conveniently, the stitch originally used to close the commissure can be used to begin the attachment of the pericardial patch. The stitch is placed through the patch before detaching it from the anterior pericardium so that the patch remains flat and properly oriented.

F The pericardial patch is secured to the crest of the ventricular septum between the right and left atrioventricular valves by continuous suture. The suture line is taken superiorly in a counterclockwise fashion onto the rim of the atrial septal defect. The stitches are placed securely into the strong tissue that bridges the two valves and is firmly adherent to the crest of the ventricular septum. Then the suture line is taken inferiorly in a clockwise fashion, placing the stitches superficially in the fibrous tissue that bridges the atrioventricular valves so as to protect the bundle of His. These stitches are best placed parallel to the crest of the ventricular septum to reduce the possibility of crossing the conduction tissue. Rather than risk injury to the atrioventricular node by placing stitches in the nodal triangle and crossing to the rim of the atrial septal defect, the suture line is taken inferior to the coronary sinus. The coronary sinus is left to drain into the left atrium as the suture line is brought around it and completed along the rim of the atrial septal defect.

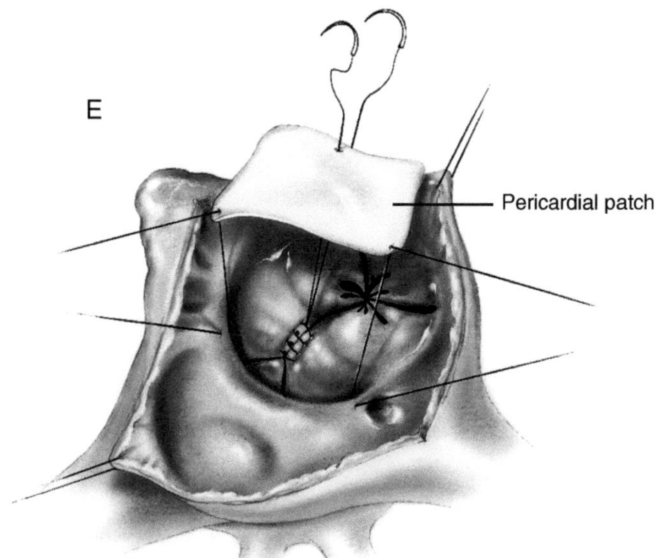
E
Pericardial patch

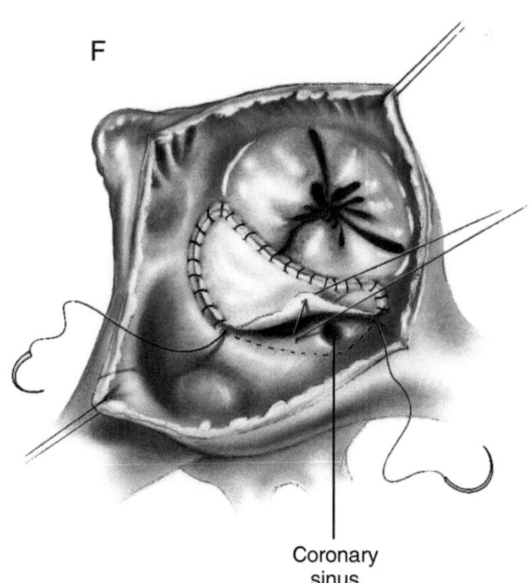
F
Coronary sinus

Complete Atrioventricular Septal Defect

In the complete form of the anomaly, the six-leaflet common atrioventricular valve guards a common atrioventricular orifice. There is an associated defect of the inlet ventricular septum, producing a characteristic scooped-out ventricular septal defect below the valve. The atrial septal defect is of the ostium primum type.

Figure 4-4

A An incision is made in the right atrium parallel to the atrioventricular groove. The characteristic six-leaflet common atrioventricular valve and the typical ostium primum atrial septal defect are identified. The inset demonstrates the vertical relationships of the septal defects and the atrioventricular valve.

B Retraction of the common atrioventricular valve exposes the scooped-out defect in the upper portion of the ventricular septum. The broken line defines the position of the bundle of His.

C Complete atrioventricular septal defect, anatomic specimen positioned to demonstrate the surgeon's view. The crest of the posterior portion of the ventricular septum is shown. The anterior leaflet of the common atrioventricular valve bridges the scooped-out ventricular septal defect. The location of the coronary sinus relative to the atrial portion of the atrioventricular septal defect is clearly seen, along with a small, fenestrated, secundum-type atrial septal defect.

D Complete atrioventricular septal defect, anatomic specimen positioned to demonstrate the surgeon's view. The bridging leaflet is retracted to expose the extent of the ventricular septal crest and a few chordae that attach the valve leaflet to the ventricular septum. The aortic valve is related to the atrioventricular valve at the hinge point at the septum. The bundle of His is located on the posterior portion of the ventricular septal crest. Anteriorly, there is no conduction system tissue, so the ventricular septal closure patch may be attached to the crest of the ventricular septum.

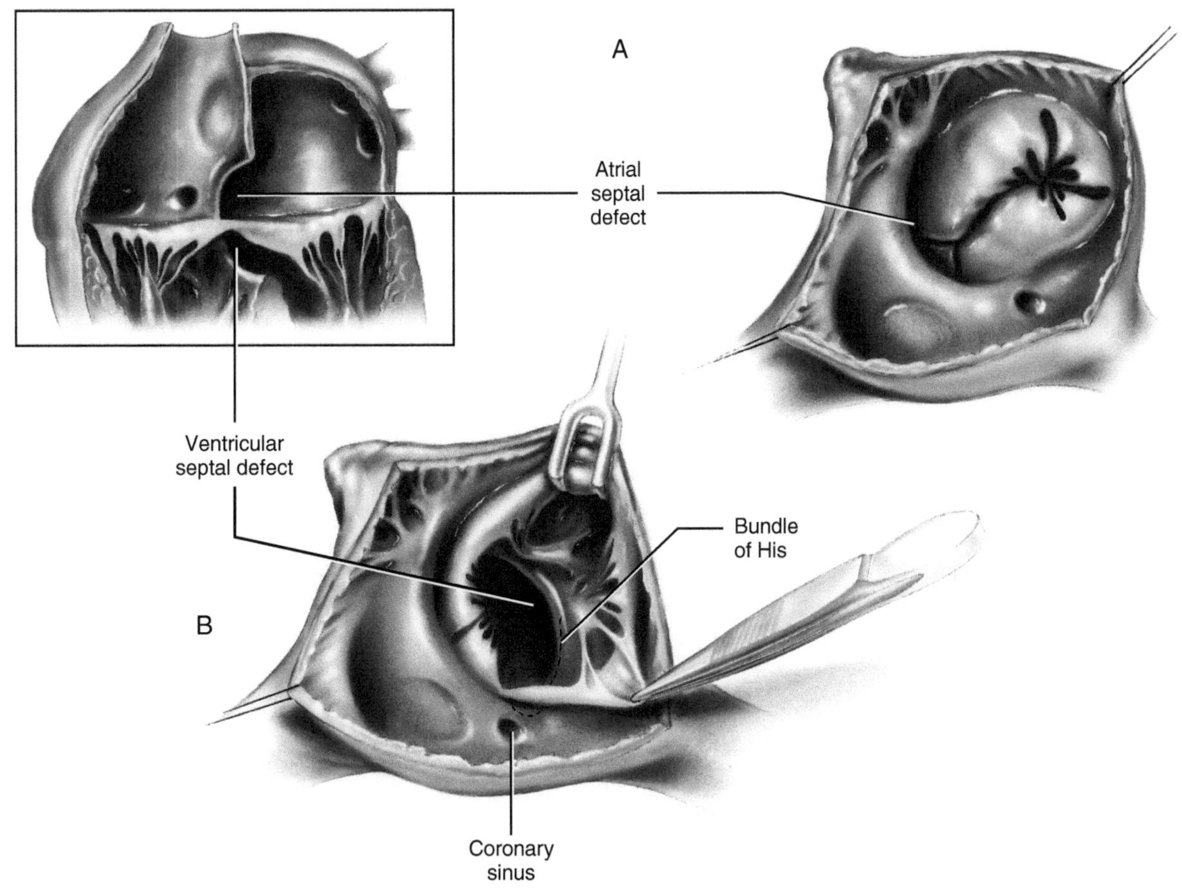
A
Atrial
septal
defect
Ventricular
septal defect
Bundle
of His
B
Coronary
sinus

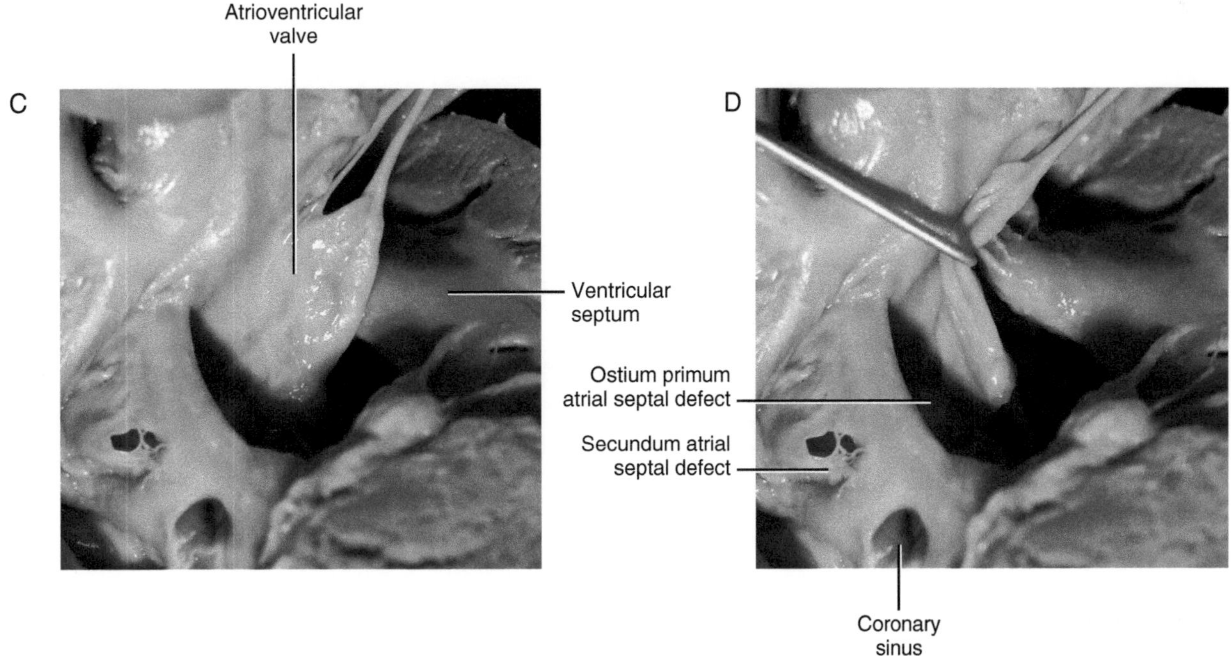
Atrioventricular
valve
C
D
Ventricular
septum
Ostium primum
atrial septal defect
Secundum atrial
septal defect
Coronary
sinus

Figure 4-4 (continued)

E The ventricular septal defect is closed with a half-circle patch constructed from flat, double-velour knit Dacron. Polypropylene suture (4/0) is used to join the Dacron patch to the ventricular septum, beginning at the lowest center point of the scooped-out defect in the septum. A small retractor or forceps is used to retract the septal portions of the atrioventricular valve to expose the crest of the septum.

F The suture line is initially taken superiorly along the ventricular septum, being careful to visualize the aortic valve during suture placement. The stitches are placed deeply into the septal myocardium for maximal security of the suture line. The final stitch is brought through the annulus of the atrioventricular valve into the right atrium, near the continuity with the annulus of the aortic valve.

G The suture line is then taken inferiorly on the right side of the ventricular septum to preserve the conduction system, which lies in the rim of the defect. The stitches are placed parallel to the rim of the defect to lie parallel to the bundle of His.

H The final stitch is brought into the right atrium at the annulus of the atrioventricular valve, to the right of the ventricular septum.

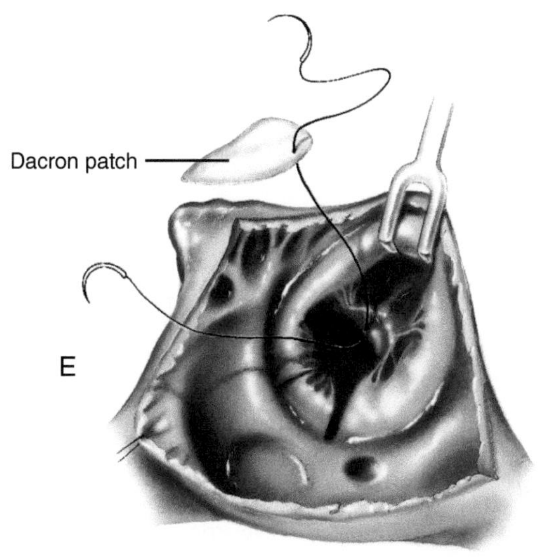
Dacron patch
E

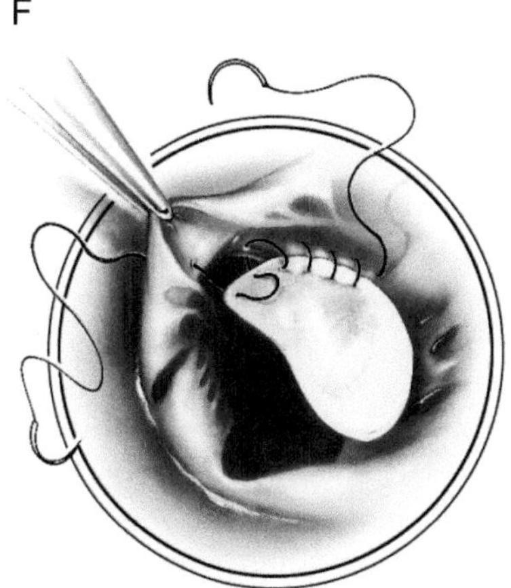
F

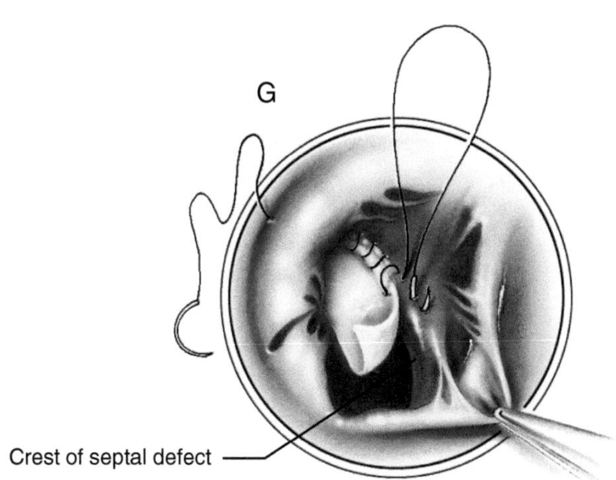
G
Crest of septal defect

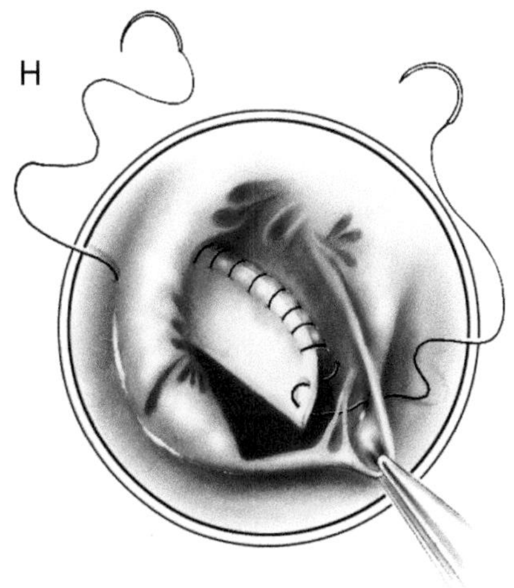
H

Figure 4-4 (continued)

I The bridging leaflets of the common atrioventricular valve are then attached to the crest of the Dacron "neoseptum." Saline solution is injected into the left ventricle to float the valve leaflets into apposition. The point of contact of the posterior and anterior leaflets is identified, along with this point's precise relation to the crest of the neoseptum. A stitch of 5/0 polypropylene is placed to join the two leaflets to the neoseptum at this exact point. The crest of the neoseptum should be at the level of the atrioventricular orifice to allow approximation to the valve without positional distortion.

J A series of mattress stitches of 5/0 polypropylene is then placed through the crest of the neoseptum and passed through the atrioventricular valve at the point of contact of the valve and the neoseptum. The stitches may be placed through the left edge of the anterior pericardium at this time to save the step of suture sorting. A pericardial patch is measured and cut from the anterior pericardium for closure of the atrial component of the defect. Traction sutures of 4/0 polypropylene placed in the lateral corners of the patch and in the lateral rim of the atrial septal defect help keep the patch flat and maintain its orientation.

K Tying of the sutures joins the three septal components: (1) the atrial pericardial patch, (2) the septal portions of the bridging leaflets of the atrioventricular valve, and (3) the superior edge of the Dacron patch used to close the ventricular septum. Thus the pericardial patch is used to reinforce the atrioventricular valve from above, and the Dacron patch reinforces the valve from below. The "cleft" or septal commissure of the component of the atrioventricular valve is then approximated using interrupted stitches of 4/0 Cardionyl. The apposing edges of the valve leaflets are brought together, taking care not to close too much of the valve orifice.

L The pericardial patch is folded back to close the atrial component of the defect. The stitches originally used to close the ventricular component and passed into the atrium at the annulus of the atrioventricular valve are used to close the atrial component of the defect. The superior stitch is taken in a counterclockwise fashion about halfway around the defect. The inferior stitch is used to approximate the pericardial patch to the atrial wall inferior to the coronary sinus and then to the rim of the atrial septal defect to complete the repair. The inferior portion of the repair is made in this manner to avoid placing stitches in the nodal triangle, which could injure the atrioventricular node.

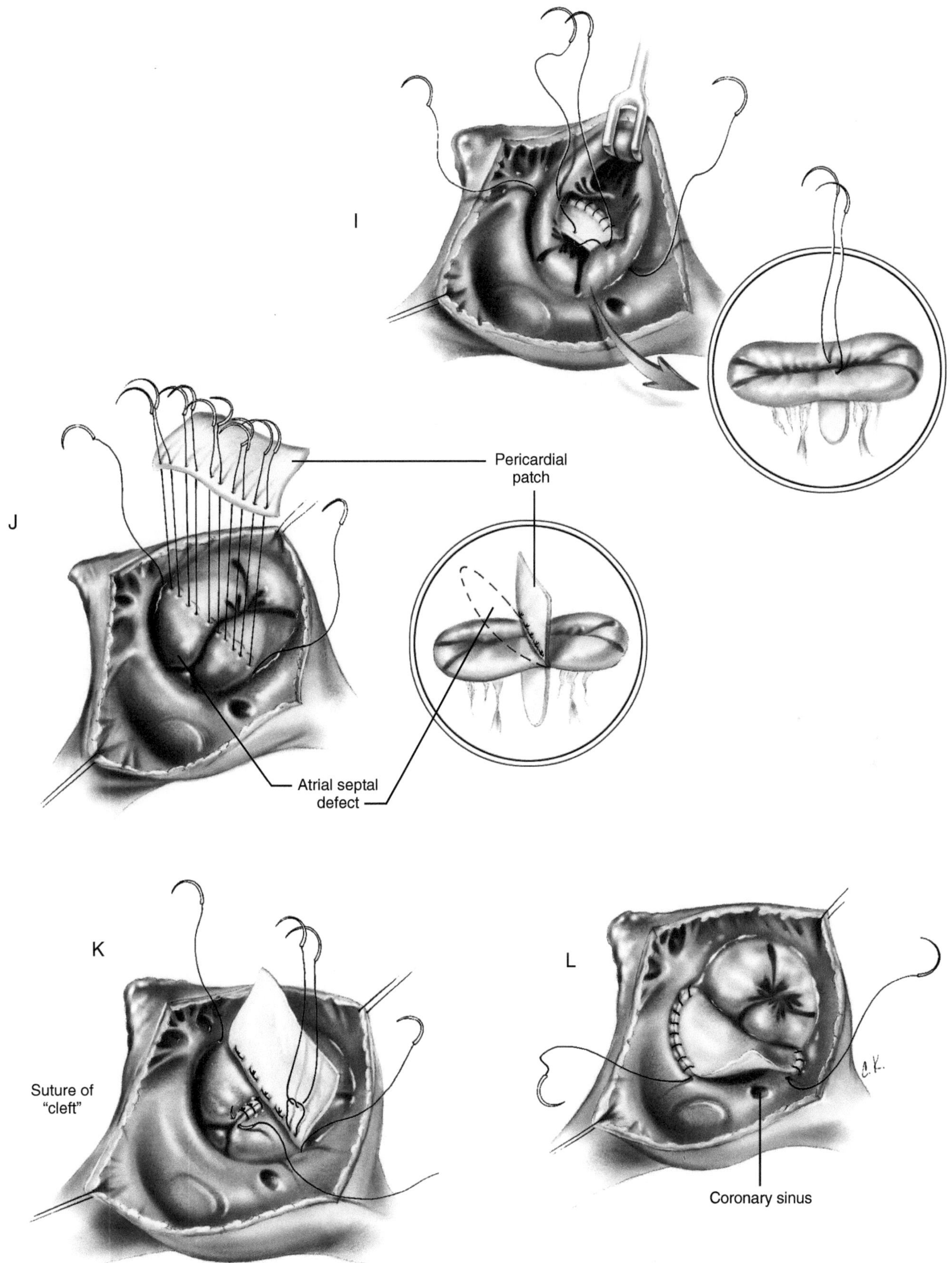
I
J
Pericardial patch
Atrial septal defect
K
Suture of "cleft"
L
Coronary sinus

Re-repair of Partial Atrioventricular Septal Defect

Severe left atrioventricular valve regurgitation requiring reoperation occurs in about 10% of patients 10-15 years after the repair of a partial atrioventricular septal defect. This is generally thought to be due to leaflet deficiency of the atrioventricular valve.

Figure 4-5

A The cause of left atrioventricular valve regurgitation following repair of a partial atrioventricular septal defect is a central deficiency of leaflet tissue, as illustrated here. An incision is made in the pericardial patch that was used to close the atrial septum at the previous operation, and the anterior aspects are retracted to provide good exposure of the left atrioventricular valve. The "cleft" has usually been repaired and may be involved in a cicatricial process, with retraction of leaflet tissue. There may be insufficient leaflet tissue opposite the "cleft," so the leaflets do not make contact centrally. Repair is commenced by incision of the atrioventricular valve leaflets along the septal attachment (*broken line*).

B As the leaflet tissue is mobilized and the subvalvar apparatus comes into view, the abnormal chordal attachments of the valve to the ventricular septum are usually found to be short and thick. Abnormal chordae restrict leaflet motion, contributing to valve regurgitation and, in severe cases, left ventricular outflow tract obstruction. The abnormal chordae are divided.

C A pericardial patch is obtained from whatever normal pericardium remains after the initial operation. This may require mobilization of pericardium from the diaphragm. The patch is treated with glutaraldehyde solution. The patch is used to augment the atrioventricular valve leaflets by attaching it to the leaflet tissue along the ventricular septum using continuous stitches of 5/0 Cardionyl.

D The pericardial patch is used to fill the defect in the anterior aspects of the left atrioventricular valve created by incision and mobilization of the valve. This allows increased flexibility and mobility of the valve and posterior displacement of the free edge to approximate its posterior aspects.

E The repair is supported with an annuloplasty ring attached to the valve annulus with interrupted stitches of 2/0 braided polyester.

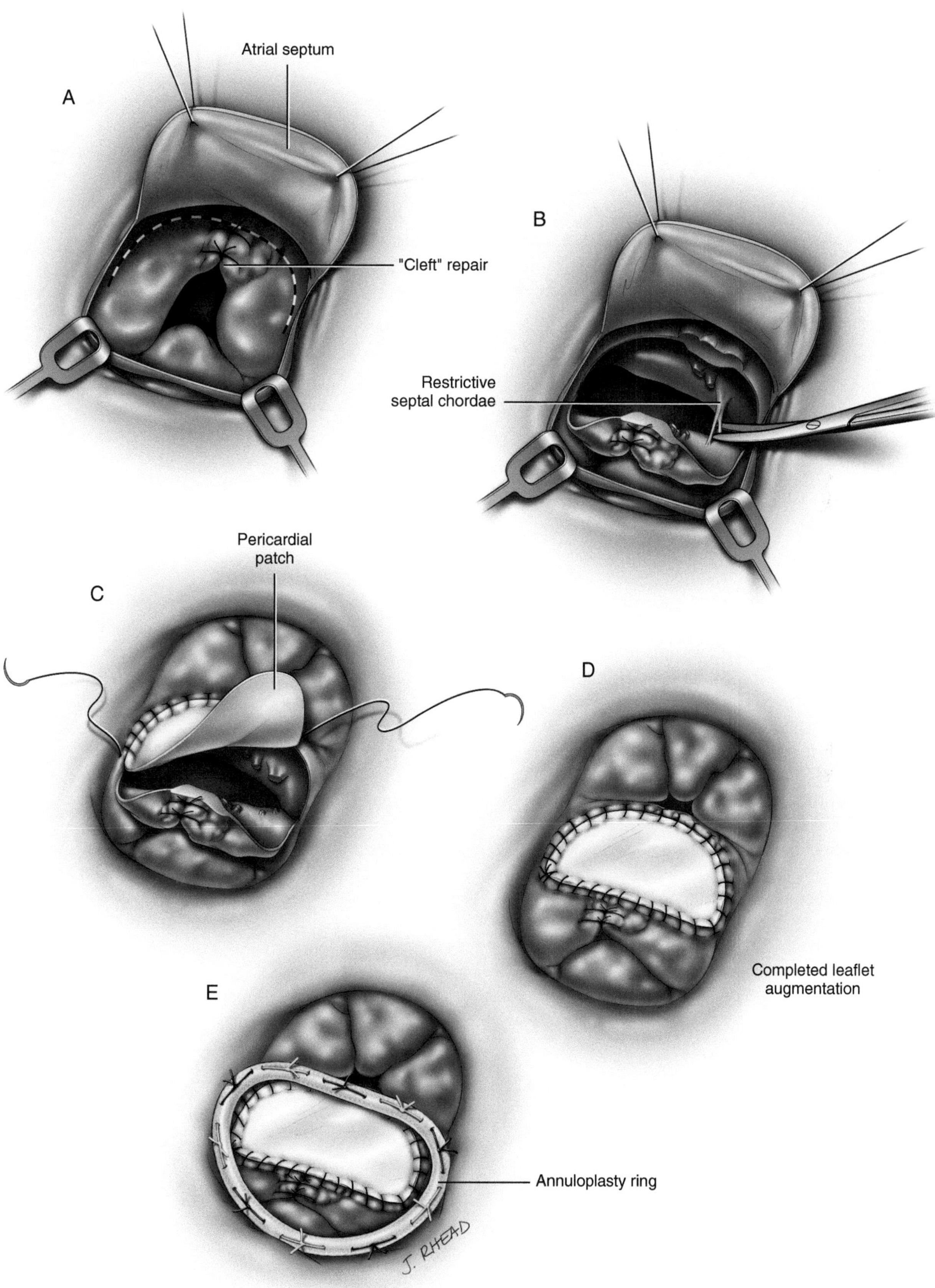
A
Atrial septum
"Cleft" repair
B
Restrictive septal chordae
C
Pericardial patch
D
Completed leaflet augmentation
E
Annuloplasty ring
J. RHEAD

chapter 5 VENTRICULAR SEPTAL DEFECT

Defects of the ventricular septum are among the most common congenital cardiac anomalies. Small ventricular septal defects are not associated with significant hemodynamic consequences and may close spontaneously. Large ventricular septal defects are associated with shunting of blood from the left-sided circulation to the right through the defect, resulting in heart failure and ultimately pulmonary hypertension.

Morphology

Ventricular septal defects are classified according to their location in the ventricular septum: (1) inlet, (2) perimembranous, (3) muscular, (4) outlet, or doubly committed subarterial.

Figure 5-1

A Inlet ventricular septal defect. This type of defect is located directly below the tricuspid valve in the inlet portion of the ventricular septum. It is associated with a complete atrioventricular septal defect, as described in chapter 4, Fig. 4-4D. The defect is high in the ventricular septum, scooped out, and associated with a common atrioventricular valve.

B This specimen (right ventricular view) shows three types of septal defects: a secundum-type atrial septal defect; a perimembranous ventricular septal defect, intimately associated with the tricuspid valve; and a large muscular ventricular septal defect in the body of the ventricle, meaning that all borders of the defect consist of ventricular septal myocardium.

C Perimembranous ventricular septal defect, left ventricular view. The defect is closely related to the aortic valve superiorly and the tricuspid valve, as seen through the defect. Its posterior inferior margin is ventricular septal myocardium, which contains the specialized tissues of the conduction system.

D Doubly committed subarterial ventricular septal defect. This defect is also known as an outlet or supracristal ventricular septal defect. It is directly below the aortic valve, which forms its superior margin. The pulmonary valve (not seen here) is also part of the superior margin. The close association of the semilunar valves to the margin of the defect affects the repair.

A

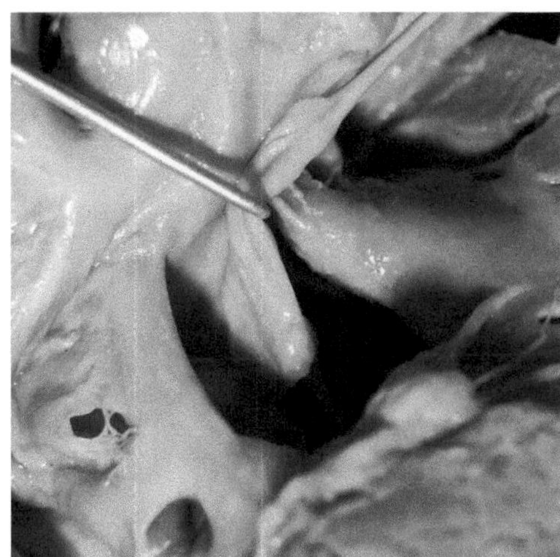

Inlet (atrioventricular septal) ventricular septal defect

B

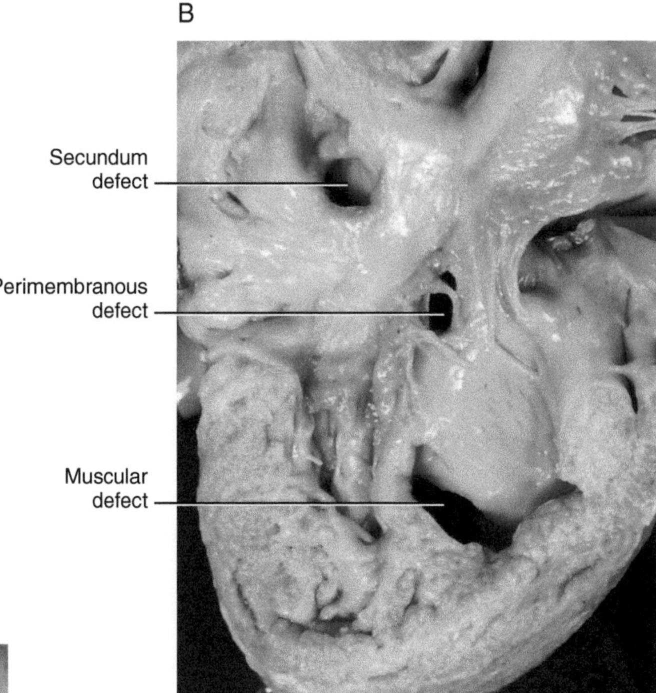

C

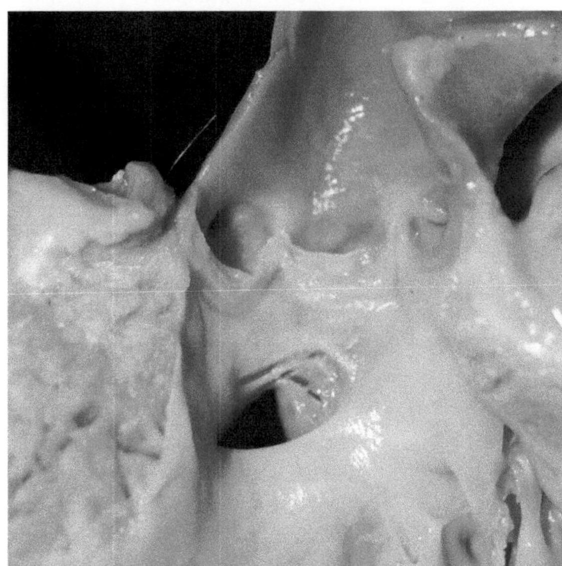

Perimembranous ventricular septal defect

D

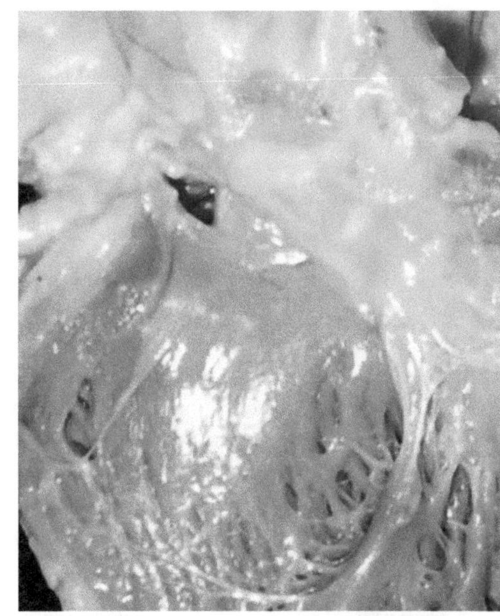

Doubly committed subarterial ventricular septal defect

Transatrial Approach

A ventricular septal defect located in the perimembranous portion of the ventricular septum and related to the tricuspid and aortic valves may be repaired through a right atrial or right ventricular approach. Preservation of right ventricular function is the main advantage of the right atrial approach; thus it is favored by most surgeons.

Figure 5-2

A Two retraction stitches are placed anteriorly near the annulus of the tricuspid valve, opposite the midportion of the anterior and posterior leaflets. A vent catheter is inserted through the fossa ovalis into the left atrium. The ventricular septal defect is exposed by placing a thyroid retractor through the tricuspid valve anteriorly and retracting the septal and anterior leaflets of the tricuspid valve with forceps. The bundle of His arises from the atrioventricular node in the most distal aspect of the triangle of Koch and penetrates the central fibrous body near the posterior inferior rim of the ventricular septal defect. The branches of the bundle of His are usually spread onto the ventricular septum posterior to the papillary muscle of the conus.

B A patch that is somewhat larger than the defect is fashioned from a tubular, crimped, weave-knit Dacron vascular prosthesis. A rectangular patch with the corner tips removed and rounded is quite satisfactory. The crimp ridges are oriented so that the patch can expand in a cephalocaudad direction, as this is the most difficult dimension to estimate. The continuous suture line is started with a deep stitch through the anterior rim of the ventricular septal defect at the 12 o'clock position, as viewed by the surgeon through the tricuspid valve. Double-needle 4/0 polypropylene suture material is used. The stitch is passed through the patch, back through the septum, and through the patch again. The suture is pulled tight as the patch is lowered into place.

C Retraction on the patch with forceps exposes the rim of the ventricular septal defect and provides good visibility of the next area to be stitched. The initial stitches are placed, working in a counterclockwise direction around the superior portion of the defect. The sutures must be woven around any tricuspid chordae tendineae overhanging the defect. The annulus of the aortic valve is carefully exposed and protected from injury. The junction of the aortic annulus, ventricular septal muscle, and tricuspid valve annulus is clearly identified.

D The final stitch on the superior rim is taken as a mattress stitch by reversing direction on the patch and then passing the needle through the aortic-tricuspid junction point at the base of the tricuspid annulus into the right atrium. With the other limb of the suture, the suture line is continued in a clockwise fashion, with stitches between the septum and the patch along the inferior rim of the defect.

E The stitches are placed around the papillary muscle of the conus, emerging progressively farther away from the rim of the defect so that the suture line is on the right side of the ventricular septum, 3 to 5 mm inferior to the rim of the defect. This suture line should preserve the conduction system by avoiding the area most likely occupied by the bundle of His. The stitches should be worked into the septum in a "wagon-wheel" fashion, with the stitches forming the "spokes" extending out from the defect (illustrated by the *broken line*), which is the "hub." Again, care is taken to weave the stitches beneath any overhanging tricuspid chordae tendineae.

F When the suturing between the septum and the patch has reached the junction point of the septum and the septal leaflet of the tricuspid valve, the suture is passed from ventricle to atrium through the base of the septal leaflet of the tricuspid valve, back from the atrial to the ventricular side, through the patch, and beneath any chordae. This stitch should obliterate the potential crevice between the ventricular septum and the hinge point of the septal leaflet of the tricuspid valve.

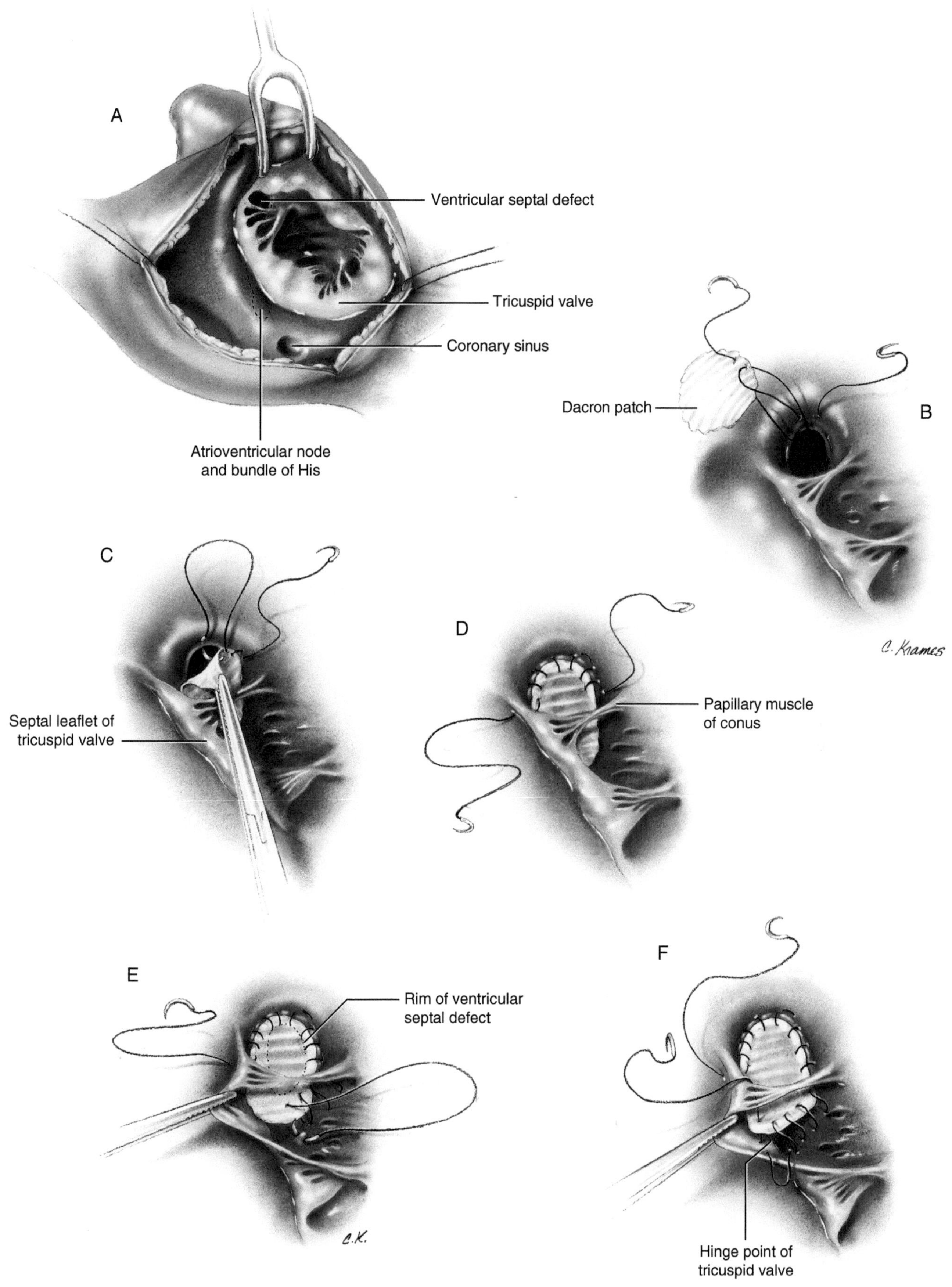
A
Ventricular septal defect
Tricuspid valve
Coronary sinus
Atrioventricular node
and bundle of His
Dacron patch
B
C
Septal leaflet of
tricuspid valve
D
Papillary muscle
of conus
C. Krames
E
Rim of ventricular
septal defect
C.K.
F
Hinge point of
tricuspid valve

Figure 5-2 (continued)

G The patch is then approximated to the base of the septal leaflet of the tricuspid valve with a running horizontal mattress stitch. Sutures are placed at the base of the leaflet rather than in the annulus to protect the conduction system from injury at the point where the bundle of His penetrates the central fibrous body. The final stitch along the base of the tricuspid valve septal leaflet is brought into the right atrium through the tricuspid annulus near the junction point of the tricuspid-aortic valves and the ventricular septal muscle, close to the other end of the suture left there during the initial part of the repair.

H The two ends of the suture are tied to complete the repair. Joining the two sutures has the effect of buttressing the patch onto the tissue at a potential weak point at the crevice where the valve tissue joins the ventricular septal muscle. The knot is placed well back in the floor of the atrium and thus cannot interfere with the tricuspid valve.

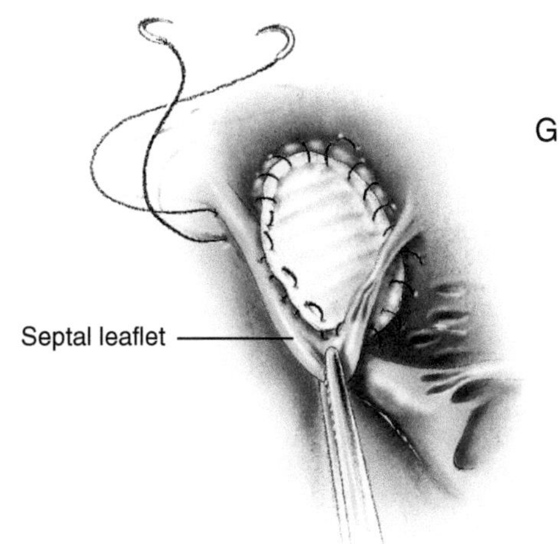
G
Septal leaflet

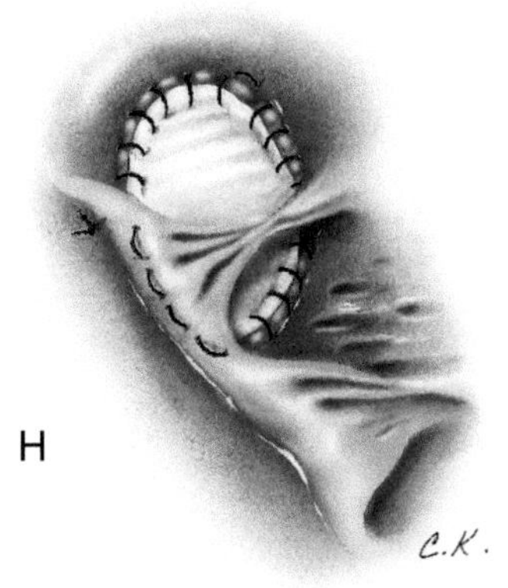
H
C.K.

Transventricular Approach

A transventricular approach is used when exposure of the ventricular septal defect through a right atriotomy and the tricuspid valve is inadequate. Defects of the ventricular septum that are not in a perimembranous location, hypertrophy of the parietal extension of the crista supraventricularis, associated right ventricular–pulmonary outflow tract pathology, and double-outlet right ventricle in which the ventricular septal defect is not committed to the aorta are indications for the transventricular approach when a transatrial approach is not advisable. A small right atriotomy can be made to determine the feasibility of a transatrial approach, and a vent catheter is inserted across the fossa ovalis into the left atrium even if the transventricular approach is chosen.

Figure 5-3

A A transverse right ventriculotomy is made parallel to the right ventricular branches of the right coronary artery. The incision should be placed on the surface of the ventricle to relate to the location of the ventricular septal defect. Four retraction stitches are placed—two at each apex of the incision—to open the ventriculotomy for exposure of the ventricular septal defect.

B The septal leaflet of the tricuspid valve overlies the defect and requires forceps retraction for optimal exposure of the posterior inferior rim of the defect. The specialized conduction system originates from the atrioventricular node in the most distal aspect of the triangle of Koch. The bundle of His penetrates the central fibrous body near the inferior rim of the ventricular septal defect. The bundle of His lies on the left ventricular aspect of the posterior inferior rim of the defect, and bundle branches are spread onto the ventricular septum posterior to the base of the papillary muscle of the conus.

C A patch that is somewhat larger than the defect is fashioned from a tubular, crimped, weave-knit Dacron prosthesis, orienting the crimp ridges so that the patch can expand in a cephalocaudad direction. The initial stitch is placed into the ventricular septum inferior to the rim of the ventricular septal defect, near the base of the septal leaflet of the tricuspid valve. One needle of a double-needle 4/0 polypropylene suture enters the septum 5 to 7 mm below the inferior rim of the defect and exits 3 to 5 mm below that rim. For the second stitch, the other needle is used to pass through the septal leaflet of the tricuspid valve close to the exit point of the first stitch. The stitch is passed from ventricle to atrium and then back through the base of the septal leaflet to the ventricular side. This seals off the potential crevice at the junction of the septal leaflet of the tricuspid valve and the ventricular septum, while avoiding the area most likely occupied by the bundle of His. Both needles are passed beneath any overhanging tricuspid chordae tendineae and then through the Dacron patch.

D The needle of the initial stitch is passed below the tricuspid chordae, and the suture is pulled tight to approximate the patch to the ventricular septum. Beneath the chordae tendineae of the tricuspid valve, three or four stitches are placed in a "wagon-wheel" fashion to a depth of about half the thickness of the ventricular septum, with the needle penetrating well below the defect and exiting 3 to 5 mm inferior to its rim. All the stitches are on the right side of the septum to preserve the conduction system.

E Once the base of the papillary muscle of the conus is passed, the stitches are brought progressively closer to the rim of the ventricular septal defect. The initial part of the suture line is completed at the septal extension of the crista supraventricularis.

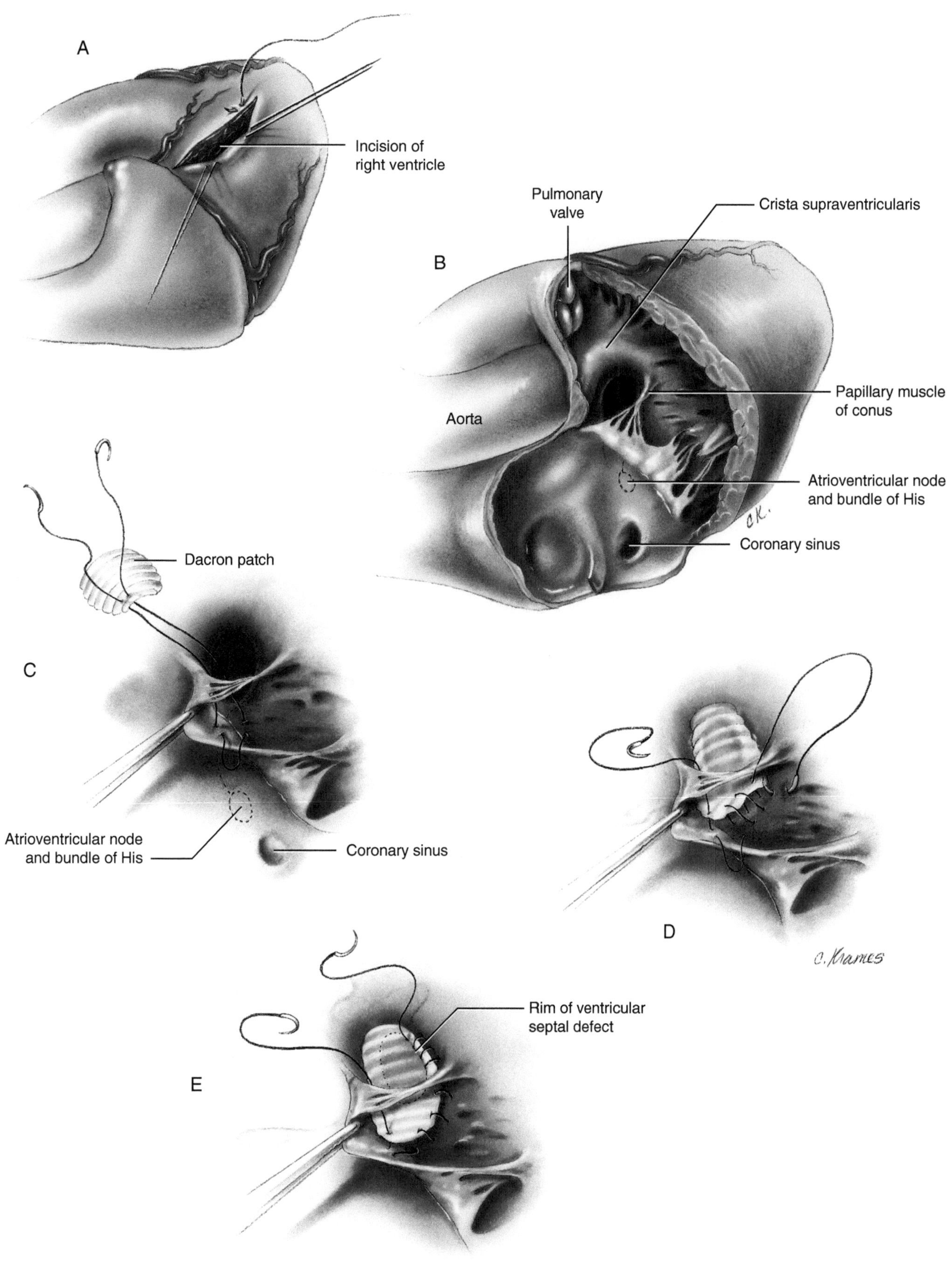
A
Incision of right ventricle
B
Pulmonary valve
Crista supraventricularis
Papillary muscle of conus
Aorta
Atrioventricular node and bundle of His
Coronary sinus
C
Dacron patch
Atrioventricular node and bundle of His
Coronary sinus
D
E
Rim of ventricular septal defect

Figure 5-3 (continued)

F The ventricular surface of the septal leaflet of the tricuspid valve is then exposed by forceps traction and countertraction on the Dacron patch. The hinge point of the septal leaflet on the annulus is identified so that stitches are placed in the base of the septal leaflet of the tricuspid valve slightly away from the annulus, thus preserving the conduction system by avoiding the point where the bundle of His penetrates the central fibrous body. A continuous horizontal mattress stitch is placed through the patch and the base of the septal leaflet of the valve by passing the needle from the ventricular side of the leaflet to the atrium and returning from the atrium to the ventricle. At the junction of the tricuspid valve septal leaflet and the annulus of the aortic valve, a transition stitch, in which the needle direction is reversed, is made by entering the fibrous continuity of the tricuspid and aortic valves and exiting deep into the muscle of the ventricle. The mattress stitch on the patch thus forms a buttress, sealing off the potential crevice at that point. The suture line is continued along ventricular septal muscle with substantial bites into the crista supraventricularis.

G With any overhanging tricuspid chordae protected, the repair is completed by joining the two ends of the suture.

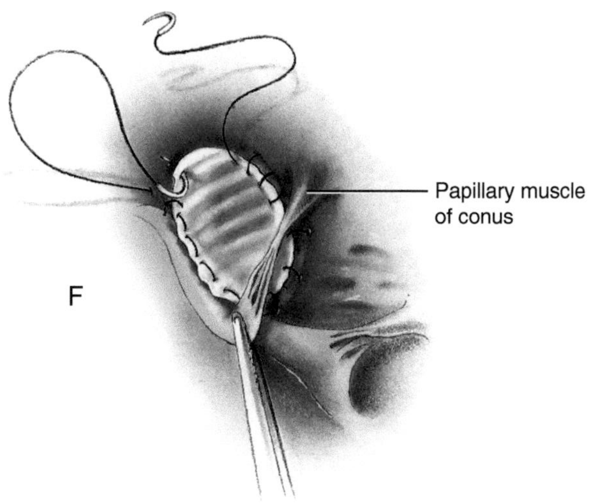
Papillary muscle
of conus
F

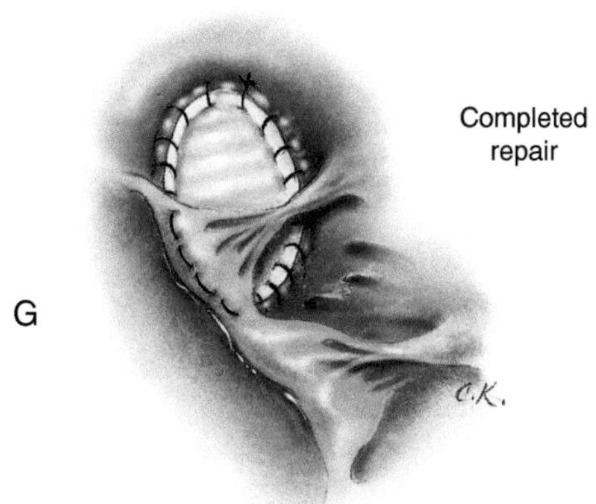
Completed
repair
G

Doubly Committed Subarterial Ventricular Septal Defect

Doubly committed subarterial (formerly called supracristal) ventricular septal defects are defects of the infundibular septum that are usually approached through an incision in the outflow tract of the right ventricle. Transpulmonary approaches are popular in Asia, where these defects are prevalent, but a transventricular approach provides somewhat better exposure of the defect.

Figure 5-4

A An incision is made in the outflow tract of the right ventricle below the pulmonary valve.

B These defects are located high in the ventricular septum, just below the pulmonary valve and above the crista supraventricularis. Because these defects are located a considerable distance from the tricuspid orifice, a transatrial approach is usually not possible. The defect is in close proximity to the fibrous support of both the pulmonary and aortic valves. The specialized conduction system of the heart is not related to the defect and is not at risk during repair.

C The defect is closed by prosthetic patch. A crimped Dacron patch is fashioned. Continuous suture technique is employed, using 4/0 polypropylene. Several suture loops are placed between the patch and the superior rim of the defect. These stitches may penetrate the fibrous hinge point of either the pulmonary valve or the aortic valve. If there is no myocardium at the superior rim, there may be fibrous continuity between the pulmonary and aortic valves, which must be partitioned by the patch. Thus, accurate visualization is required, as well as precise suture placement at the superior rim of the defect.

D The patch is lowered into the defect by pulling up the suture loops. Substantial needle bites into the infundibular septum are used to approximate the septal myocardium to the patch. The conduction system is well below the inferior rim of the defect, so it will not be injured during the repair.

E The completed repair should completely close the defect without distorting either the pulmonary valve or the aortic valve.

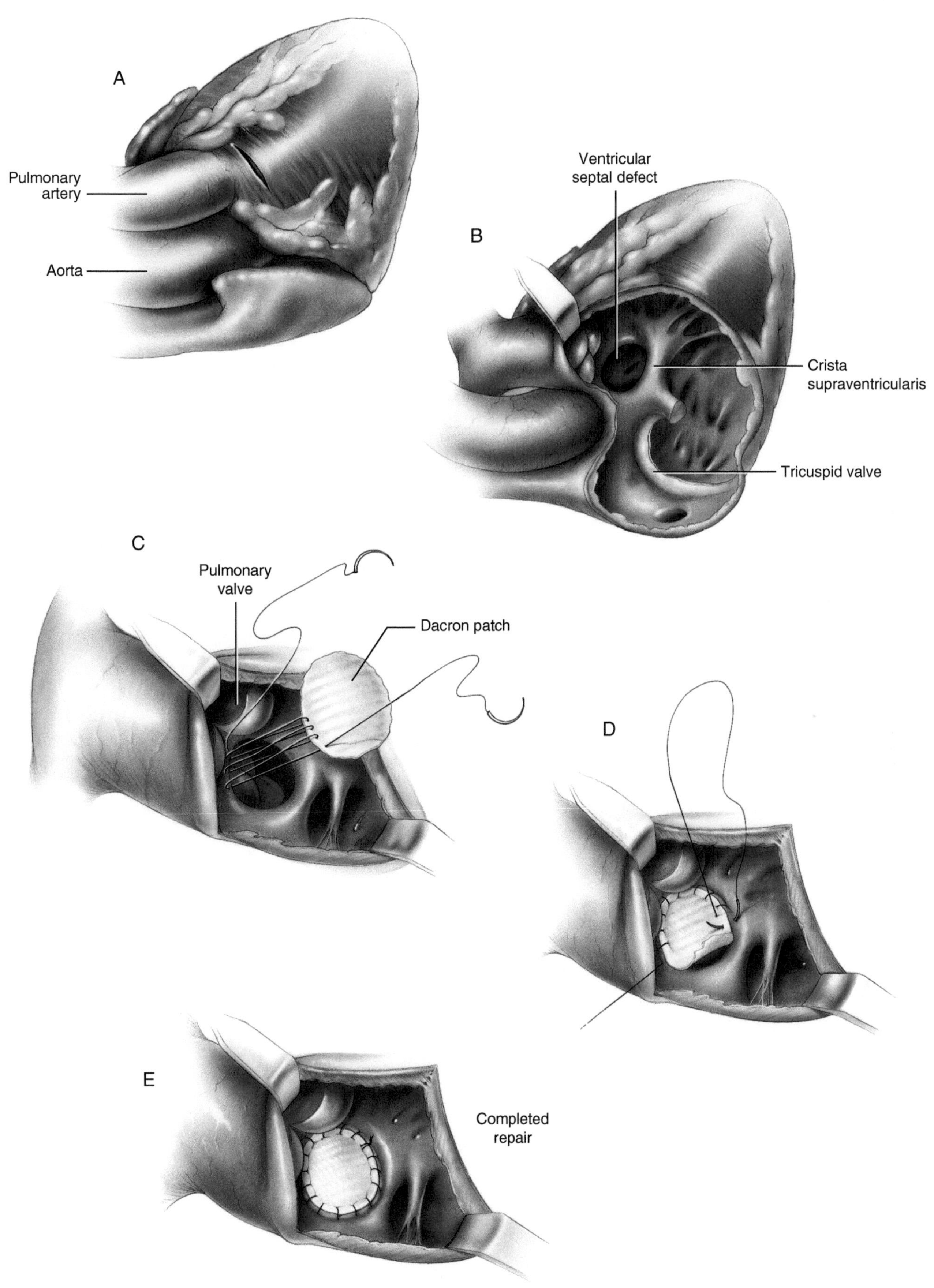
A
Pulmonary artery
Aorta
B
Ventricular septal defect
Crista supraventricularis
Tricuspid valve
C
Pulmonary valve
Dacron patch
D
E
Completed repair

chapter 6 AORTOPULMONARY SEPTAL DEFECT

Openings between the aorta and the pulmonary artery are described as aortopulmonary septal defects. There are three types of aortopulmonary septal defects, all of which share a common embryologic pathogenesis. Spiral septation of the truncus arteriosus occurs during the fifth to eighth weeks of fetal development. The aortic arch is formed from remnants of the third and fourth fetal arches, and the pulmonary artery is derived from the sixth arch. The aortopulmonary septum is formed from the conotruncal ridges, which fuse and separate the great vessels. Faulty formation of the aortopulmonary septum is the cause of these defects.

Morphology

Figure 6-1

A Aortopulmonary window. Incomplete septation results in the type I defect, or the typical aortopulmonary window. The type I defect is an opening between the aorta and the main portion of the pulmonary artery located just above the left sinus of Valsalva of the aortic valve. In this location, the defect is closely associated with the position of the left coronary artery.

B This specimen shows the aortopulmonary septum in profile, with a probe passing from aorta to pulmonary artery through the window above the aortic sinotubular junction.

C Aortopulmonary window visualized through the right ventricle and pulmonary artery.

D Should the right conotruncal ridge arise more posteriorly than normal, unequal partitioning of the aortopulmonary trunk may occur. The aorta may come in contact with the right sixth arch, destined to become the right pulmonary artery; as a result, the right pulmonary artery may connect with the main pulmonary artery as well as open into the aorta. This configuration results in the type II defect, which is located more distal on the ascending aorta and opens into the origin of the right pulmonary artery. An even more posterior position of the right conotruncal ridge and more dorsal development of the aorta may bring the right sixth arch in contact solely with the aorta, resulting in the type III defect, which is the anomalous origin of the right pulmonary artery from the ascending aorta (hemitruncus arteriosus).

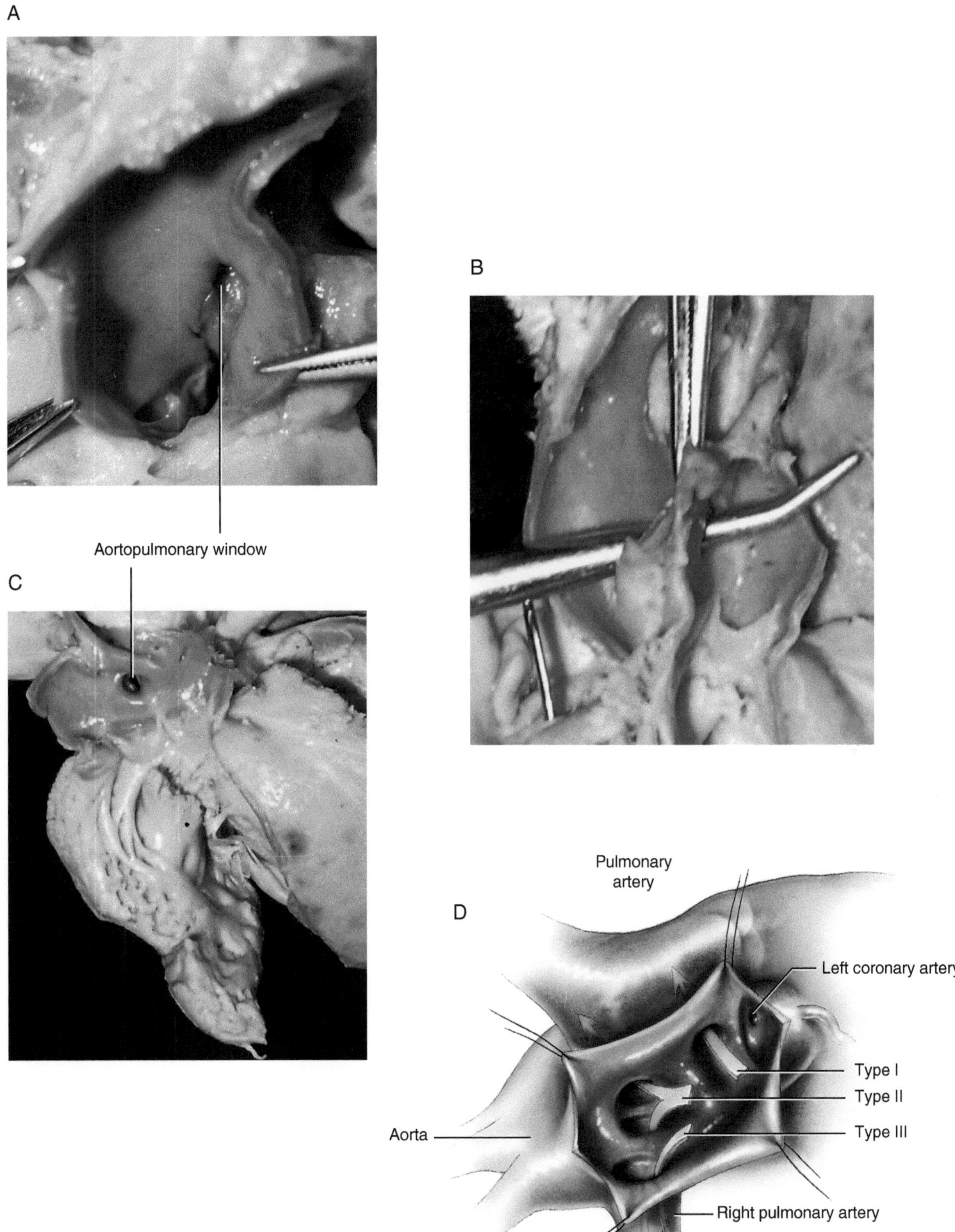
A
B
Aortopulmonary window
C
Pulmonary
artery
D
Left coronary artery
Type I
Type II
Type III
Aorta
Right pulmonary artery

Aortopulmonary Septal Defect—Type I
Figure 6-2

A The type I defect (aortopulmonary window) is repaired by placing an aortic perfusion cannula high on the ascending aorta. With the aorta occluded just below the perfusion cannula, a transverse incision is made that extends from the edge of the defect on the medial wall of the aorta and laterally across the ascending aorta. This incision provides good exposure of the defect, and all the structures of the aortic root can be clearly visualized. The condition of the aortic valve cusps should be noted, and the location of both coronary arteries must be identified prior to repair of the defect. Anomalous origin of the coronary arteries and ventricular septal defect may be associated with this defect.

B A patch is formed from crimped Dacron. A continuous stitch of 4/0 polypropylene is used to attach the Dacron patch to the edge of the defect. Care is taken while suturing around the rim, near the area associated with the ostium of the left coronary artery.

C Following closure of the defect, the aortotomy is closed by continuous suture.

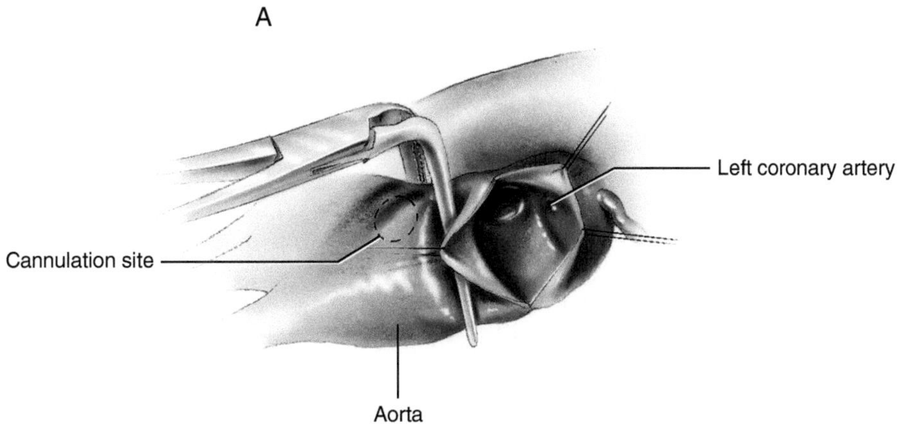
A
Left coronary artery
Cannulation site
Aorta

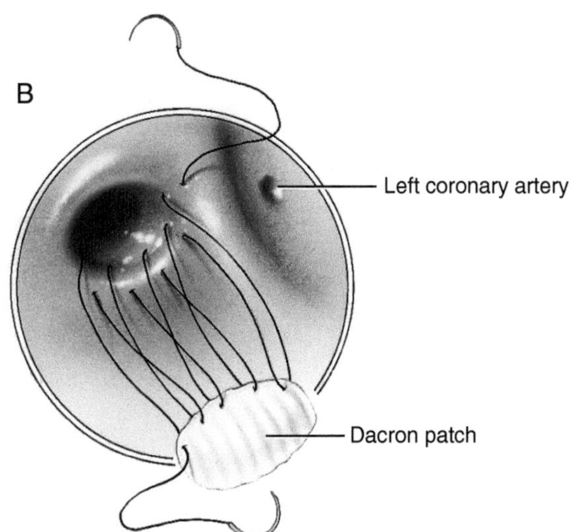
B
Left coronary artery
Dacron patch

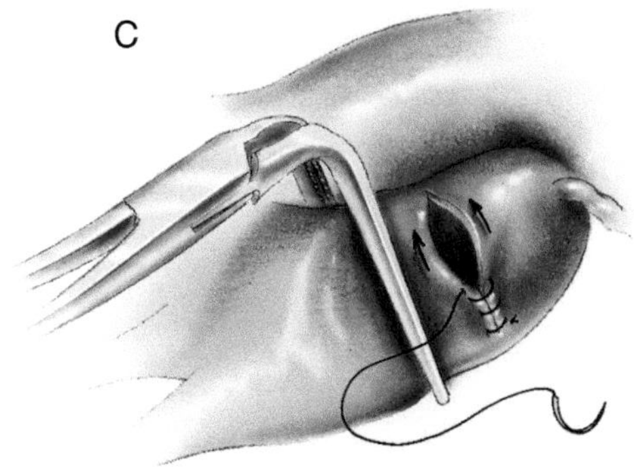
C
Close aortotomy

Aortopulmonary Septal Defect—Types II and III

For type II and III defects, complete exposure of more distal portions of the ascending aorta is required. For infants and small children, circulatory arrest under hypothermic conditions is generally the best approach. With circulatory arrest, it is not necessary to occlude the aorta, or it may be occluded across the arch branches. The perfusion cannula can be removed, providing maximal exposure of the entire ascending aorta. For older children, femoral artery or aortic arch perfusion may be considered, but this may not provide sufficient exposure of the distal portions of the ascending aorta with a cross-clamp in place.

Figure 6-3

A For repair of a type II aortopulmonary septal defect, a transverse incision is made in the ascending aorta, the defect is examined, and the location of the origin of the right pulmonary artery is clearly defined. The spur of the bifurcation of the pulmonary artery should be apparent.

B A patch is fashioned from a tubular graft of crimped Dacron for closure of the defect. The initial stitches are placed in the right lateral margin of the defect to attach the patch to the aorta without compromising the origin of the right pulmonary artery.

C The patch is secured to the rim of the defect by continuous stitches of 4/0 polypropylene.

D Following completion of the repair, the aortotomy is closed by continuous suture.

E Type III aortopulmonary septal defects (hemitruncus arteriosus) are generally repaired during circulatory arrest under hypothermic conditions. The aortic perfusion cannula can be removed to increase the exposure of the ascending aorta. The right pulmonary artery is detached from the posterolateral wall of the ascending aorta. The goal is to conserve as much of the length of the right pulmonary artery as possible; this is done by excising the pulmonary artery flush against the aorta or even by taking a bit of the aorta with the pulmonary artery.

F The defect in the aorta is closed with a patch of crimped Dacron, which is attached to the defect by continuous suture.

G The ascending aorta is retracted anteriorly to expose the main portion of the pulmonary artery. An incision is made in the pulmonary artery, and an end-to-side anastomosis of the right pulmonary artery to the main pulmonary artery is constructed by continuous suture. The suture line should be started at the superior end of the incision in the main pulmonary artery. A double-needle suture is used, passing each needle from the intimal surface to the outside on both the main pulmonary artery and the right pulmonary artery. The needle on the main pulmonary artery side is then brought from outside the right pulmonary artery to the intimal surface so that suturing can continue from the main pulmonary artery to the right pulmonary artery on the intimal surface. Careful planning of these initial stitches allows an accurate anastomosis in a very cramped location.

H A few interrupted stitches may be placed anteriorly to allow for growth of the anastomosis.

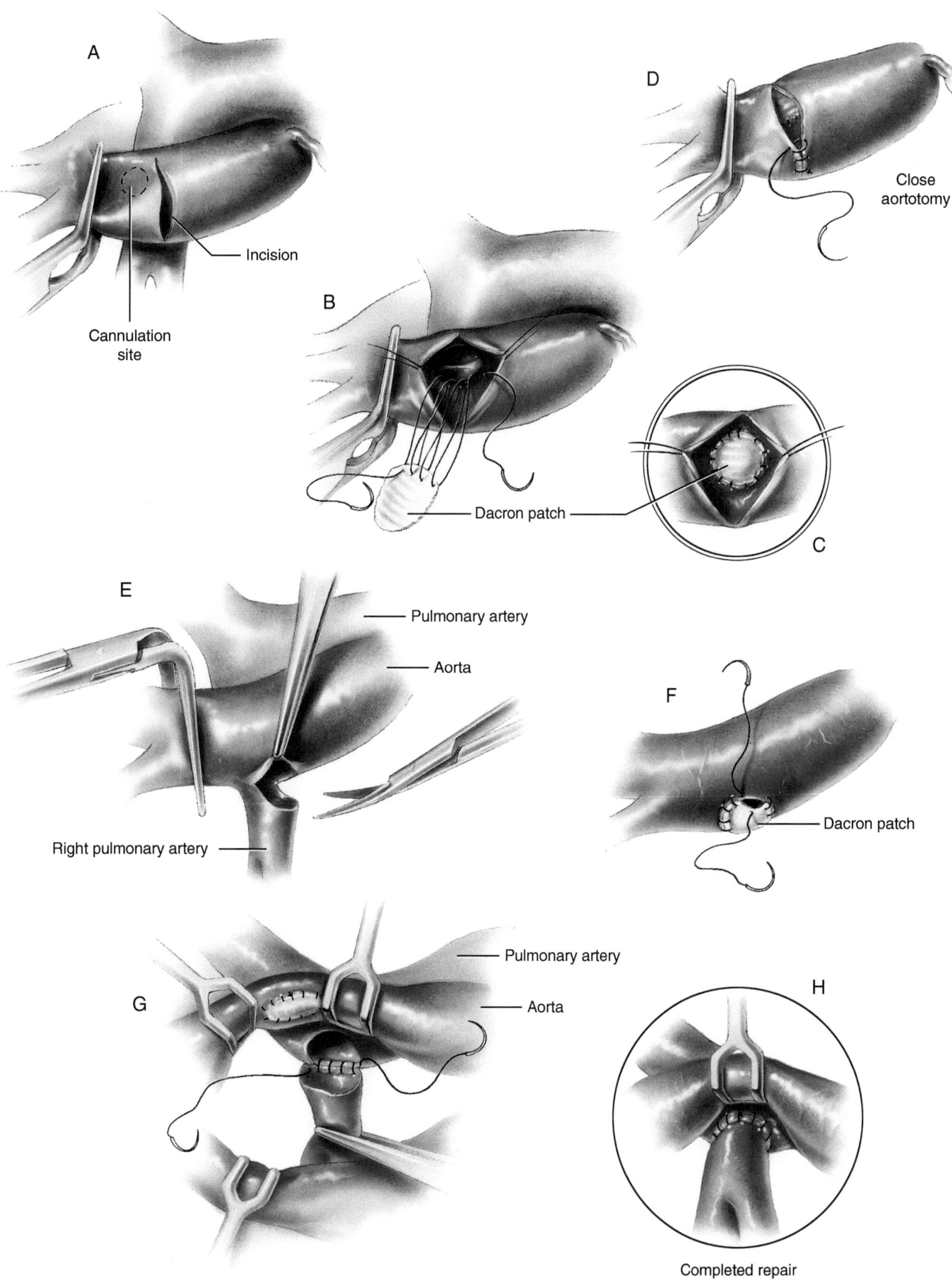
A
Incision
Cannulation site
D
Close aortotomy
B
Dacron patch
C
E
Pulmonary artery
Aorta
F
Dacron patch
Right pulmonary artery
Pulmonary artery
G
Aorta
H
Completed repair

part III

Anomalies of Pulmonary Venous Connection

chapter 7 PARTIAL ANOMALOUS PULMONARY VENOUS CONNECTION

Partial anomalous pulmonary venous connection is a group of anomalies in which the venous drainage from part or all of one lung is connected to the right atrium or to one of the major systemic veins leading to the right atrium.

Morphology

The three most common forms of partial anomalous pulmonary venous connection are discussed in this chapter, including a description of the morphology of each. Computed tomography (CT) scans and operative photographs are used to demonstrate the morphologic appearance.

Figure 7-1

A Contrast-enhanced CT scan of partial anomalous pulmonary venous connection—right superior pulmonary vein to superior vena cava. The right upper lobe branch of the right superior pulmonary vein is connected to the superior vena cava.

B Contrast-enhanced CT scan of partial anomalous pulmonary venous connection—right superior pulmonary vein to superior vena cava. The right middle lobe branch of the superior pulmonary vein is hypoplastic and connects normally to the left atrium. Hypoplasia of the right middle lobe vein is appreciated when compared with the normal-sized, unobstructed left superior pulmonary vein. This rare variant of partial anomalous pulmonary venous connection results in pulmonary venous obstruction from the right middle lobe. Collateral venous drainage is by way of the mediastinum, causing esophageal and tracheal varices associated with bleeding.

C Operative photograph of partial anomalous pulmonary venous connection—right superior pulmonary vein to superior vena cava. The right superior pulmonary vein is connected to the superior vena cava above the cavoatrial junction. The superior vena cava is enlarged due to the extra volume of blood flow entering the cava from the right superior pulmonary vein.

D Partial anomalous pulmonary venous connection—left pulmonary vein to innominate vein—viewed through a left thoracotomy. Branches of the left pulmonary vein are connected to a vein coursing vertically outside the pericardial sac. This vertical vein is the remnant of the left superior vena cava. It drains to the innominate (left brachiocephalic) vein. Pulmonary vein branches are controlled with vessel loops.

E Operative repair of partial anomalous pulmonary venous connection—left pulmonary vein to innominate vein. The vertical vein (left pulmonary vein) is rotated inferiorly and medially for anastomosis to the left atrial appendage, using a flap of the appendage to create a large anastomosis.

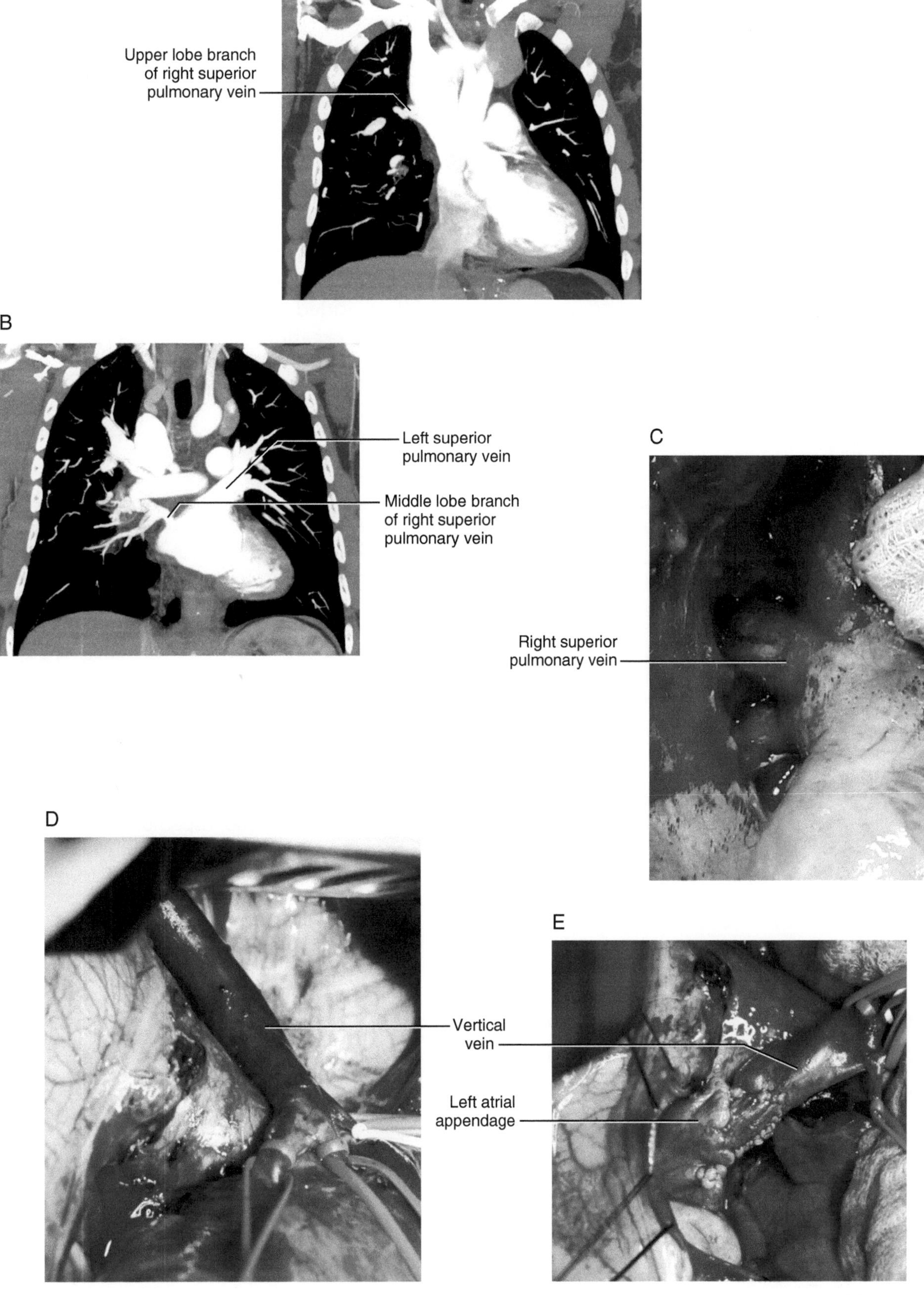
A
Upper lobe branch
of right superior
pulmonary vein
B
Left superior
pulmonary vein
Middle lobe branch
of right superior
pulmonary vein
C
Right superior
pulmonary vein
D
E
Vertical
vein
Left atrial
appendage

Right Superior Pulmonary Vein to Superior Vena Cava with Sinus Venosus Atrial Septal Defect

The sinus venosus type of atrial septal defect is located high in the atrial septum above the foramen ovale. It is often associated with an anomalous connection of the right superior pulmonary vein to the lateral aspect of the superior vena cava. The cava is enlarged to accommodate the increased flow added by the anomalous pulmonary vein. Correction of the defect involves the creation of a passageway within the vena cava to the high-lying atrial septal defect to divert pulmonary venous blood to the left atrium.

Figure 7-2

A Dissection of the superior vena cava at the pericardial reflection and above defines the limits of the anomalous connection between the pulmonary vein and the superior vena cava. The cannulation site for the superior vena cava is either through the atrial appendage, if the superior vena cava is large, or directly into the superior vena cava above the anomalous pulmonary venous connection. The inferior vena cava is cannulated through the right atrium. The primary incision into the right atrium is parallel to the atrioventricular groove. This incision is least likely to cause atrial arrhythmia. If the orifice of the right superior pulmonary vein at the point where it enters the superior vena cava is not easily visualized through the right atrial exposure, an optional counterincision can be made in the superior vena cava. When this incision is used, it must be entirely on the vena cava; it cannot be allowed to cross the cavoatrial junction or enter the area of the crista terminalis and possibly injure the sinoatrial node.

B With the right atrial wall removed for clarity, the sinus venosus atrial septal defect is shown high in the atrial septum above the foramen ovale. The right pulmonary vein enters the superior vena cava.

C A rectangular pericardial patch is fashioned from the anterior pericardium. With double, small-needle 4/0 polypropylene suture, four or five suture loops are placed from the pericardium to the superior rim of the orifice of the right superior pulmonary vein before the pericardial patch is pulled into the superior vena cava. This technique allows precise tissue approximation at the most difficult point of the repair. If exposure is compromised by the caval cannula, a short period of circulatory arrest with removal of the superior vena cava cannula may be used to enhance exposure.

D The suture line is continued in a clockwise fashion, with care taken not to compromise the orifice of the superior vena cava. The passageway created should occupy the posterior aspect of the vena cava. Placing the suture line in an anterior position should be avoided because it could obstruct the vena cava. In most cases the vena cava has been sufficiently enlarged by the increased blood flow to accommodate two blood flow passageways. Where there is a question about the adequacy of its diameter, the cava can be enlarged by a second pericardial patch in the caval counterincision. Repair is completed in a counterclockwise fashion, suturing around the inferior rim of the sinus venosus atrial septal defect. If the atrial septum is intact, the foramen ovale is excised to create an atrial septal defect that is closed in a similar fashion, bringing the right superior pulmonary vein in continuity with the left atrium through the atrial septal defect.

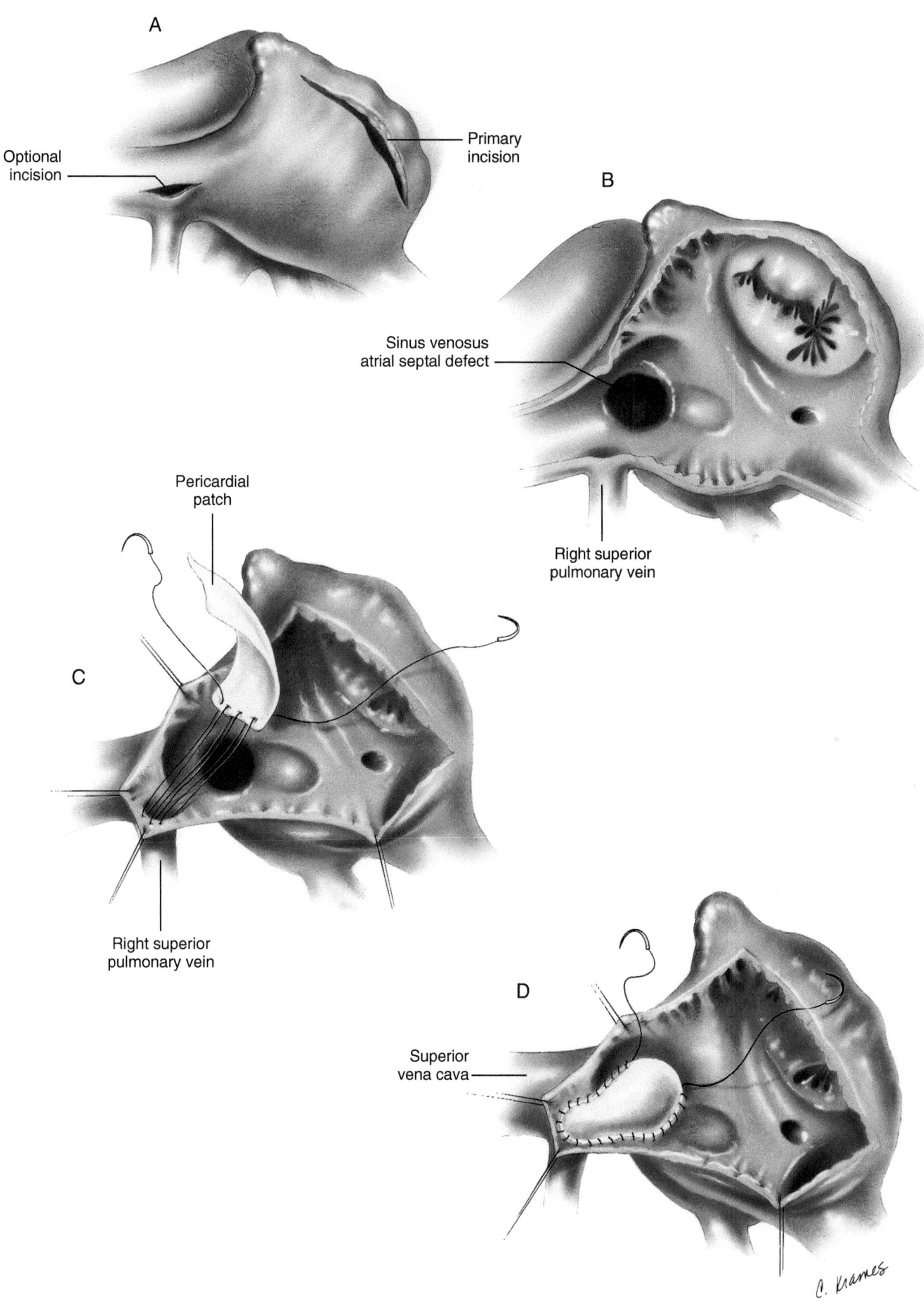
A
Optional
incision
Primary
incision
B
Sinus venosus
atrial septal defect
Right superior
pulmonary vein
Pericardial
patch
C
Right superior
pulmonary vein
D
Superior
vena cava

Right Pulmonary Vein to Inferior Vena Cava (Scimitar Syndrome)

In this defect, a single pulmonary vein drains the entire right lung and is connected to the inferior vena cava. It is often called the scimitar syndrome because of the appearance of the chest x-ray. There is typically a saber- or scimitar-like shape along the right cardiac border.

The anomalous vein enters the posterior aspect of the inferior vena cava at or somewhat below the diaphragm. This anomalous connection must be differentiated from the connection of the hepatic veins, which enter the vena cava anteriorly. The inferior vena cava is usually enlarged in proportion to the increased blood flow it must accommodate due to the anomalous pulmonary venous connection.

Figure 7-3

A The superior vena cava is cannulated through the right atrial appendage. The inferior vena cava (IVC) is cannulated through the right atrium sufficiently anterior to allow incision of the right atrium directly over the inferior vena cava posterior to the cannulation site. Tourniquets are placed on the venae cavae in the usual fashion, with the inferior vena cava tourniquet occluding it superior to the junction of the right pulmonary vein. Hypothermic perfusate lowers the body temperature to approximately 24°C.

B An atrial septal defect is created by excising the atrial septum in the area of the fossa ovale.

C Cardiopulmonary bypass is temporarily discontinued, and the inferior vena cava cannula is removed to allow access to the orifice of the right pulmonary vein. A rectangular pericardial patch is fashioned from the anterior pericardium. Several 4/0 polypropylene suture loops are placed between the pericardial patch and the inferior rim of the right pulmonary vein before the patch is pulled into the inferior vena cava.

D A tunnel is created by approximating the pericardium to the posterior wall of the inferior vena cava and the atrial septum medially and laterally, ensuring that the orifice of the inferior vena cava remains widely patent and allowing for unobstructed drainage of the right pulmonary vein. Because the inferior vena cava is already enlarged due to the increased blood flow, there is usually adequate exposure and working room, except in babies and small children. The lower rim of the anomalous venous connection must be accurately visualized, and the hepatic veins must be identified. The pericardial patch is placed between these structures while assuring adequate egress from the inferior vena cava. Once the suture line into the atrium is completed sufficiently to ensure that exposure will not be compromised by the venous uptake cannula, the inferior vena cava cannula is replaced, and the tourniquet is secured. Cardiopulmonary bypass is reestablished with warm perfusate to raise the body temperature to normal while the reconstruction proceeds.

E The repair is completed by approximating the pericardial patch to the superior rim of the atrial septal defect created previously, bringing the right pulmonary vein in continuity with the left atrium through the atrial septal defect. The suture line is positioned to the right of the coronary sinus so that the area of the atrioventricular node is not entered. The patch should be wide enough to allow it to bulge into the atrium and provide a totally unobstructed passageway for blood flow.

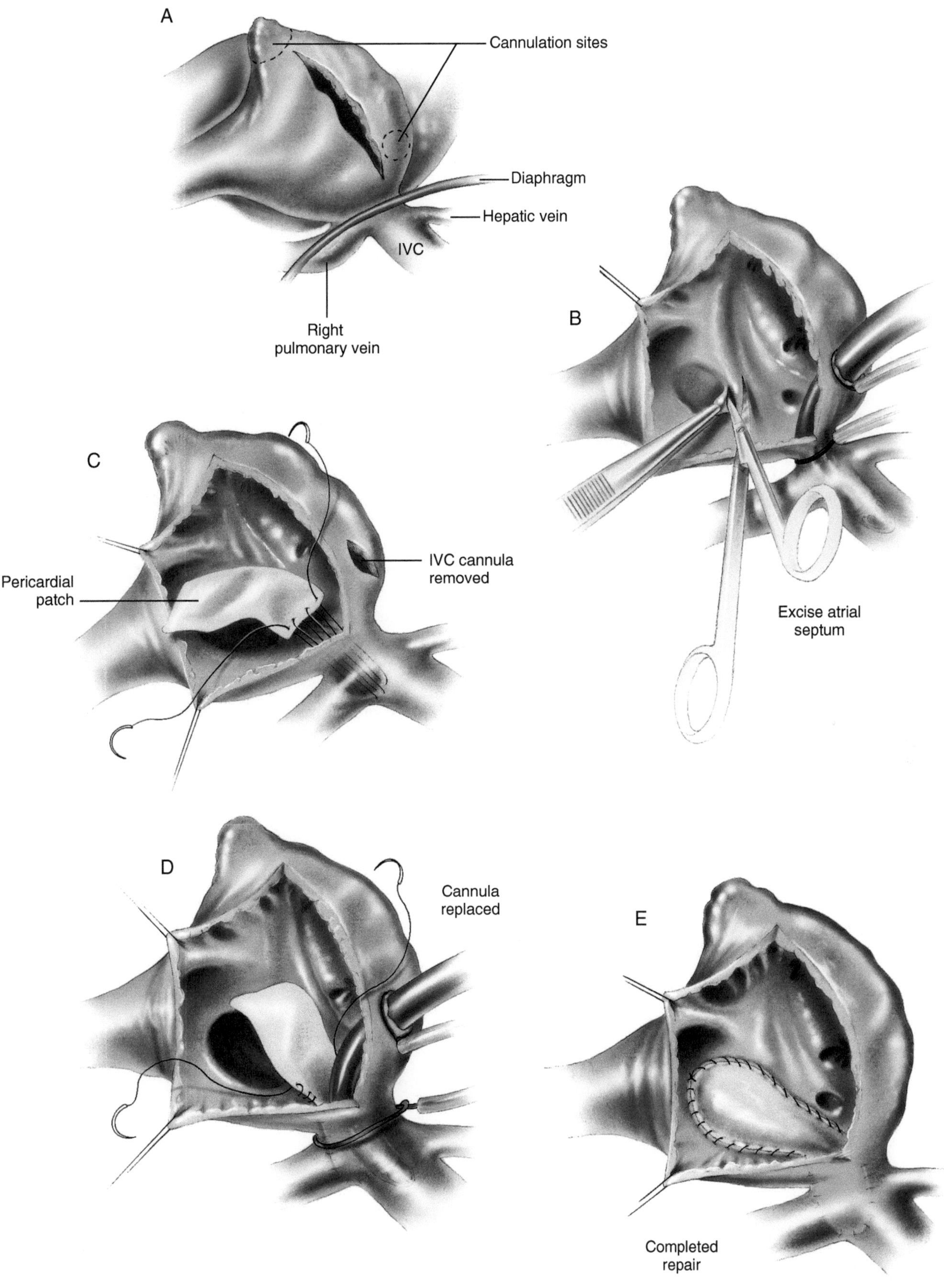
A
Cannulation sites
Diaphragm
Hepatic vein
IVC
Right pulmonary vein
B
Excise atrial septum
C
Pericardial patch
IVC cannula removed
D
Cannula replaced
E
Completed repair

Left Pulmonary Vein to Innominate Vein

In this defect, a single pulmonary vein drains the entire left lung and is connected to a vertical vein draining to the left innominate vein and then to the superior vena cava and the right atrium. That is, the left upper lobe pulmonary vein or the entire pulmonary venous drainage of the left lung is connected by a left vertical vein to the innominate (left brachiocephalic) vein. This vertical vein is the equivalent of a persistent left superior vena cava (see Figure 7-1, *D*).

Figure 7-4

A When this deformity is an isolated anomaly, the operation is performed through a left posterolateral thoracotomy. The chest is entered through the bed of the fourth or fifth rib. The vertical vein is completely mobilized. The pericardium is opened to expose the left atrial appendage. The vertical vein is ligated at its junction with the innominate vein. A vascular clamp is placed on the left pulmonary vein, and the vein is divided near the ligature to obtain maximal length.

B The vertical vein must be rotated inferiorly to approximate the left atrium. To lessen the substantial risk of kinking the vein during this maneuver, a venoplasty is performed. The vertical pulmonary vein is incised longitudinally. The venotomy is closed vertically.

C The left atrial appendage is occluded by a vascular clamp at the base. Parallel incisions are made on the lateral sides of the atrial appendage, beginning at the tip and extending toward the base. The incisions are joined at the base to create a flap of atrium. The interior of the appendage is carefully examined, and any trabeculae are excised. The pulmonary vertical vein is rotated inferiorly, and the anterior end is cut back (spatulated).

D A large anastomosis to the left atrium is created. The tip of the vein is anastomosed to the base of the left atrial appendage. Continuous stitches of 5/0 or 6/0 polypropylene are used.

E The flap of left atrium is worked into the spatulated pulmonary vein. This anastomosis is not circular, so there should be a reduced risk of late stenosis.

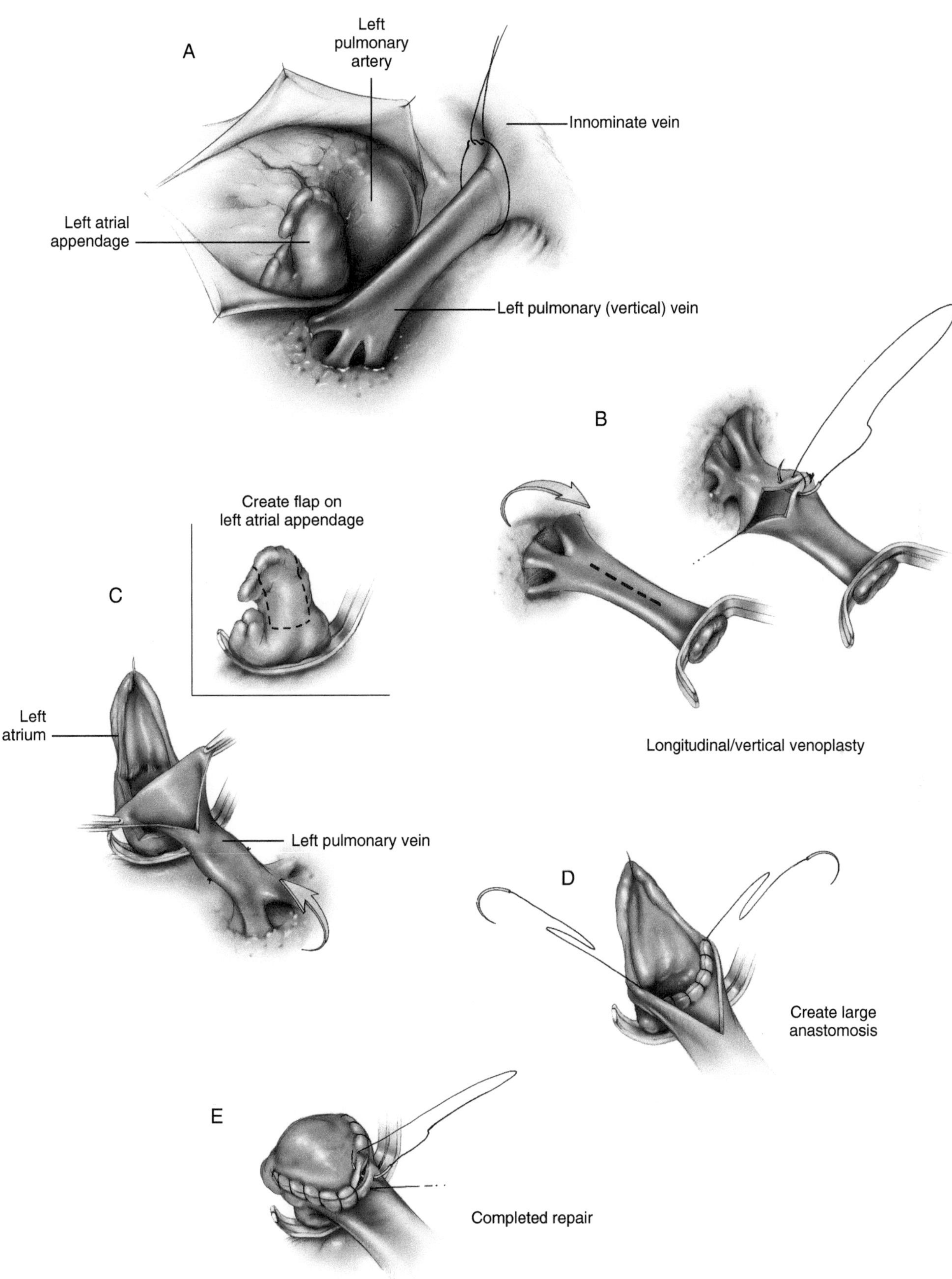
A
Left
pulmonary
artery
Innominate vein
Left atrial
appendage
Left pulmonary (vertical) vein
B
Longitudinal/vertical venoplasty
C
Create flap on
left atrial appendage
Left
atrium
Left pulmonary vein
D
Create large
anastomosis
E
Completed repair

Figure 7-4 (continued)

F If there is an atrial septal defect or another associated intracardiac lesion, the defect is repaired on cardiopulmonary bypass through a median sternotomy. A traction stitch is placed in the outflow tract of the right ventricle to allow the pulmonary artery to be retracted to the right, exposing the left atrial appendage. The pericardium is incised lateral and anterior to the pulmonary artery to expose the anomalous left pulmonary vertical vein. The anomalous pulmonary vein should be mobilized completely, to its junction with the innominate vein. The vertical vein is ligated close to the innominate vein and divided. Because the vertical vein is rotated inferiorly to approximate the left atrium, venoplasty is performed to reduce the chance of kinking. A longitudinal incision is made on the pulmonary vein as shown.

G The incision is closed vertically by continuous stitches of 6/0 polypropylene.

H The left atrial appendage is isolated by applying a vascular clamp at its base. The clamp is actually used to stabilize the appendage and deliver it upward for easier anastomosis. A flap of the lateral aspect of the appendage is created by parallel incisions from tip to base. The flap is released by joining the incisions near the base of the appendage. The pulmonary vein is cut back (spatulated) to provide a large perimeter for anastomosis.

I The tip of the pulmonary vein is anastomosed to the base of the left atrial appendage with continuous stitches of 5/0 or 6/0 polypropylene.

J A large anastomosis is created by working the flap of appendage into the spatulated pulmonary vein. After completion of the anastomosis, associated intracardiac defects are repaired in the usual manner.

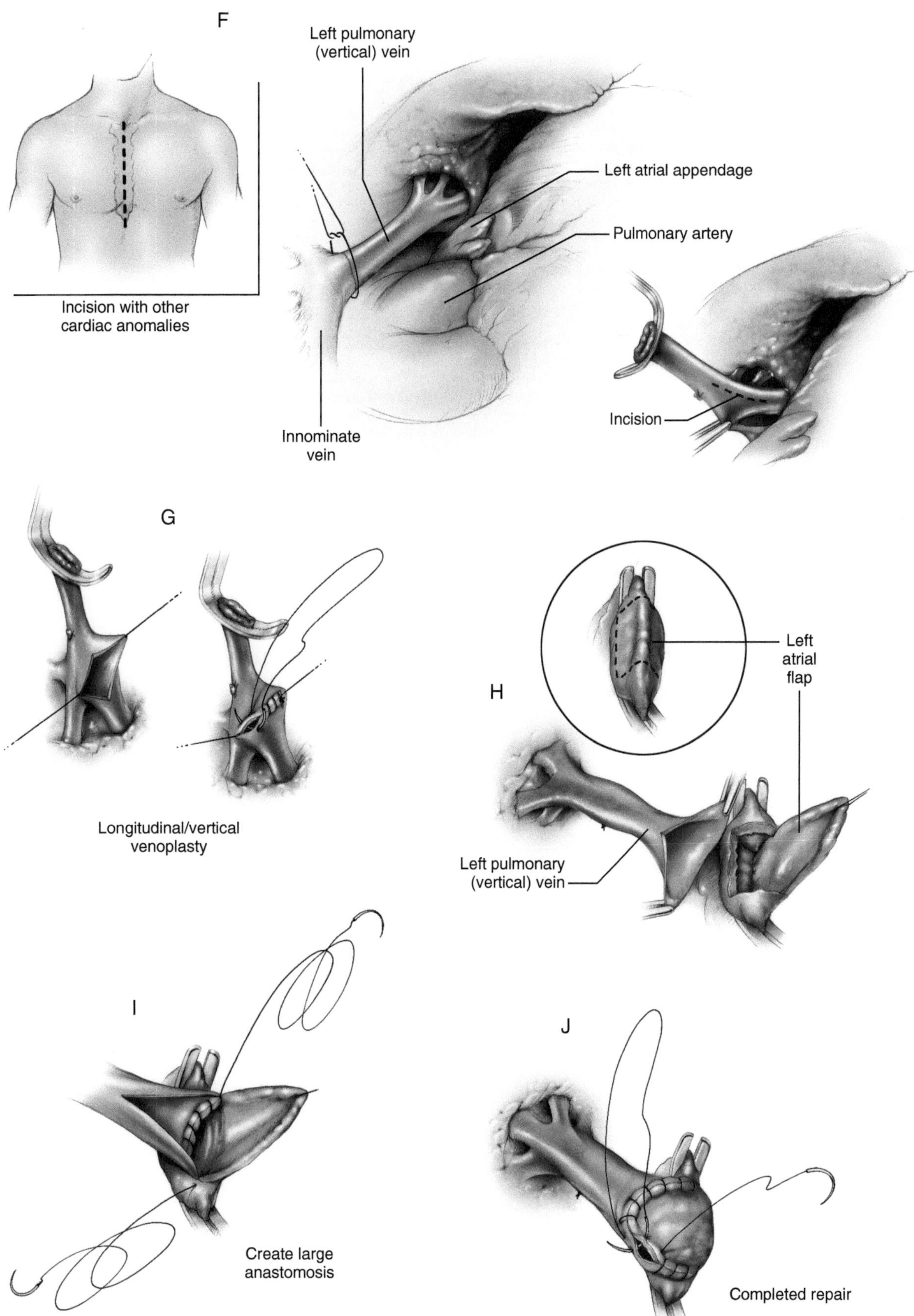
F
Incision with other cardiac anomalies
Left pulmonary (vertical) vein
Left atrial appendage
Pulmonary artery
Innominate vein
Incision
G
Longitudinal/vertical venoplasty
H
Left atrial flap
Left pulmonary (vertical) vein
I
Create large anastomosis
J
Completed repair

chapter 8 TOTAL ANOMALOUS PULMONARY VENOUS CONNECTION

Total anomalous pulmonary venous connection is defined as a malformation in which there is no direct connection between any pulmonary vein and the left atrium. The pulmonary veins connect either to the right atrium or to one of the major systemic veins that directs blood to the right atrium. For an infant with this defect to survive after birth, the foramen ovale or ductus arteriosus must remain patent.

Morphology

There are four types of total anomalous pulmonary venous connection. In the cardiac type, all pulmonary veins connect to the coronary sinus, and pulmonary venous drainage is directly to the right atrium. In the supracardiac type, all pulmonary veins connect to systemic veins superior to the heart. In the infracardiac type, all pulmonary veins enter systemic veins below the diaphragm. The mixed type is a combination of the others. Repair of the mixed type is most difficult and requires a combination of operative techniques employed in the other three types.

Figure 8-1

A Supracardiac type, anterior view. All pulmonary veins drain to a common vertical vein to the left of the midline. The ascending vein is the remnant of the left superior vena cava (SVC). The vertical vein is in continuity with the innominate (left brachiocephalic) vein, bringing pulmonary venous blood flow to the superior vena cava (right) and the right atrium (RA).

B Supracardiac type, posterior view. All four pulmonary veins are confluent posterior to the left atrium but are not connected to it.

C Infracardiac type, posterior veiw. Four pulmonary veins are confluent posterior to the left atrium. The forceps marks the vertical vein, which is directed inferiorly to connect with the portal vein or ductus venosus below the diaphragm.

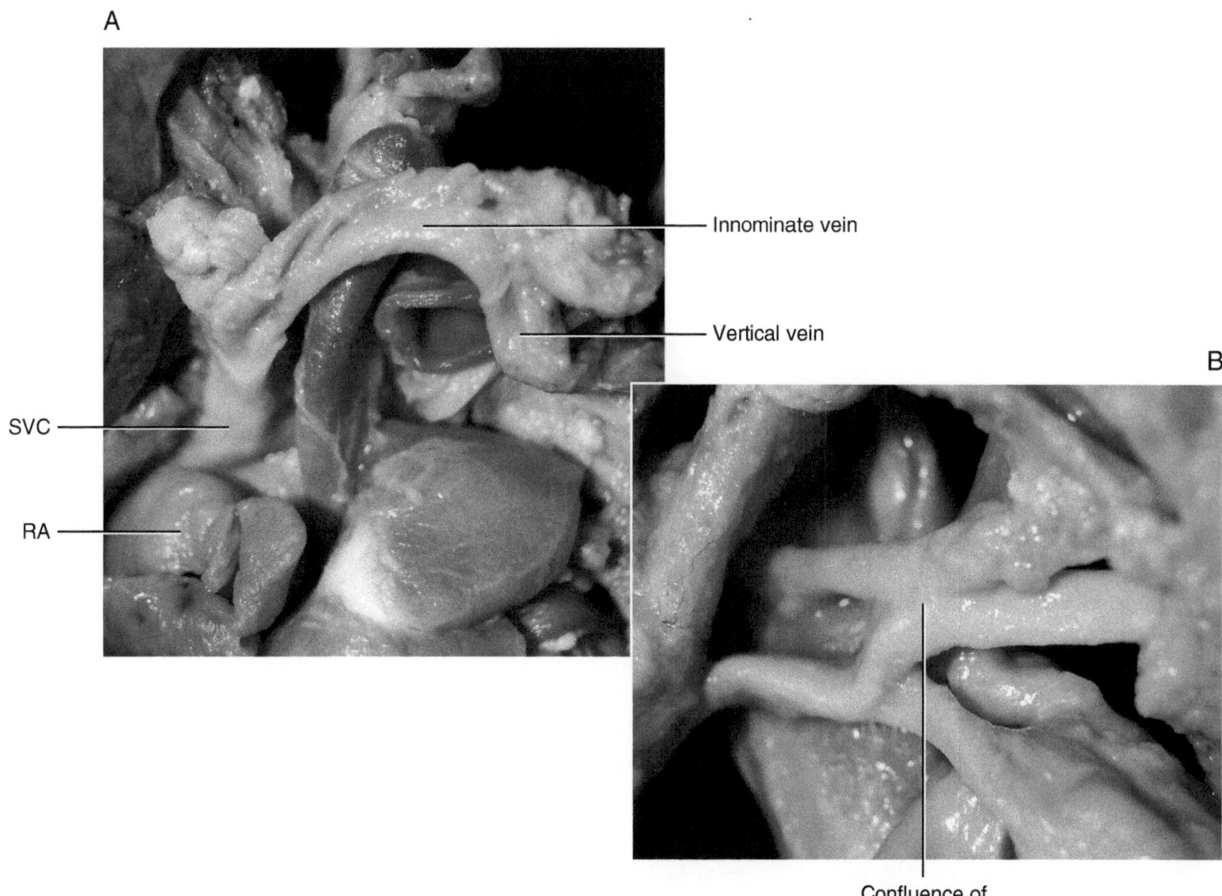
A
Innominate vein
Vertical vein
SVC
RA
B
Confluence of pulmonary veins

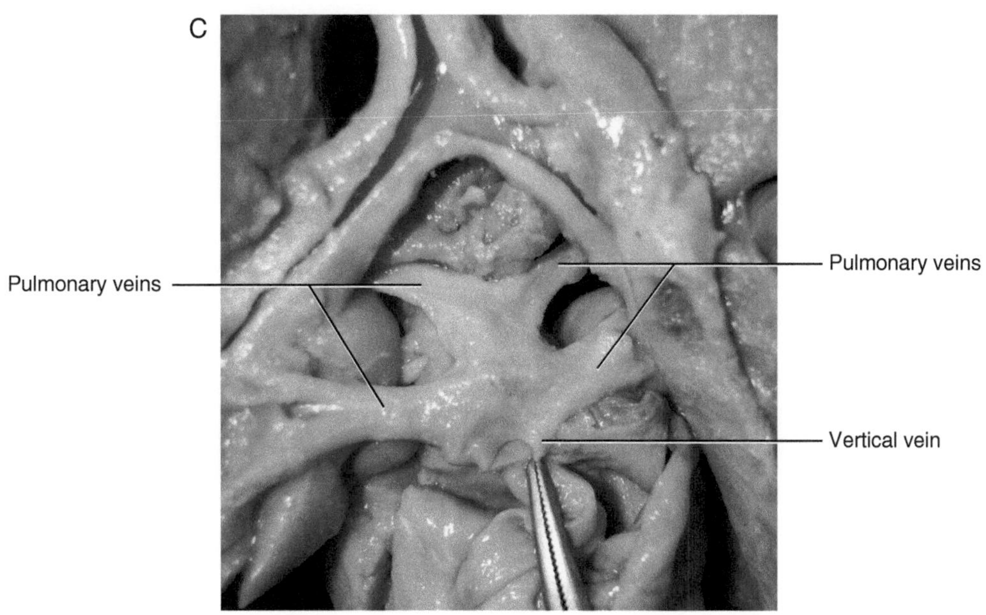
C
Pulmonary veins
Pulmonary veins
Vertical vein

Operations for total anomalous pulmonary venous connection can be performed with a single venous cannula in the right atrial appendage and the use of deep hypothermia and circulatory arrest so that the venous cannula can be removed to obtain optimal intracardiac exposure. Alternatively, two venous cannulae can be used, with the superior vena cava cannulated at the pericardial reflection.

Cardiac Type

In the cardiac type of defect, all pulmonary veins connect to the right atrium, usually via the coronary sinus. The object of operation is to redirect coronary sinus blood flow to the left atrium.

Figure 8-2

A An incision is made in the right atrium parallel to the atrioventricular groove. The large coronary sinus is identified, which is the point of the anomalous pulmonary venous connection. The membrane of the foramen ovale is excised to provide a large opening in the atrial septum. The common wall of the coronary sinus and left atrium is incised by placing scissors through the foramen ovale.

B The incision is made well back into the left atrium, to allow free drainage of the coronary sinus into the main portion of the left atrium. The atrioventricular node and bundle of His should be anterior to the incision and protected from injury.

C An appropriately sized pericardial patch is fashioned from the anterior pericardium to close the atrial septum. A continuous suture of double-ended 4/0 polypropylene is used to approximate the pericardium to the septum. In the area of the atrioventricular node, the suture line is placed a few millimeters deep, inside the cutback coronary sinus rather than on the coronary sinus rim in order to preserve the conduction system. The suture line is continued onto the lateral wall of the right atrium so as not to reduce the size of the left atrium.

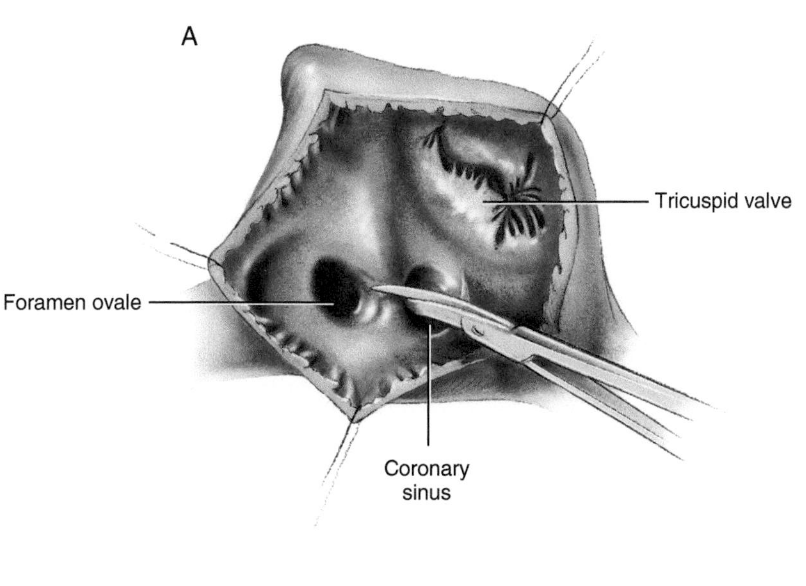
A
Tricuspid valve
Foramen ovale
Coronary sinus

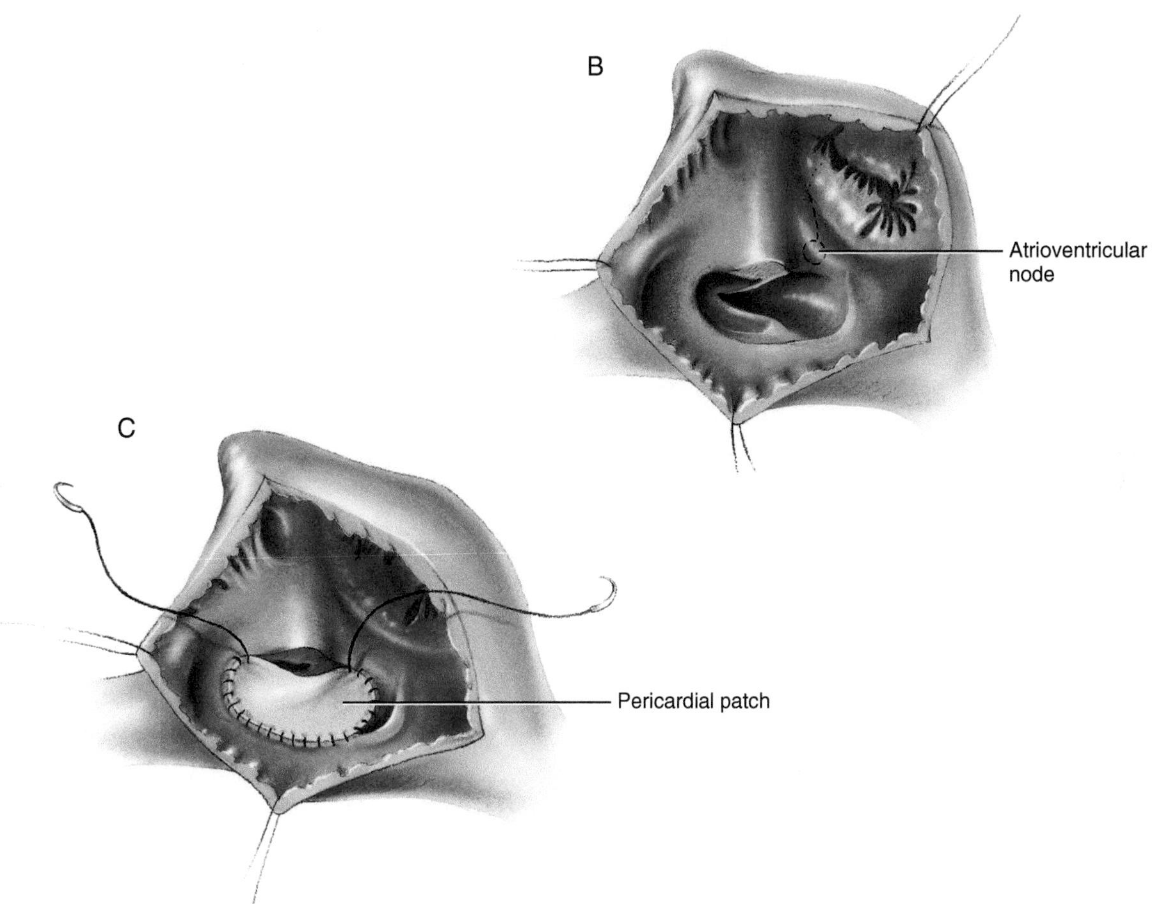
B
Atrioventricular node
C
Pericardial patch

Supracardiac Type

The pulmonary veins are confluent behind the left atrium in patients with the supracardiac type of total anomalous pulmonary venous connection. The confluent veins are connected to a vertical vein on the left side, which drains to the left innominate vein. The object of operation is to connect the confluent pulmonary veins to the left atrium.

Figure 8-3

A A right atriotomy parallel to the atrioventricular groove provides access to the atrial septum. The foramen ovale portion of the atrial septum is excised, exposing the posterior wall of the left atrium for the anastomosis. This approach provides maximal visualization of the area of anastomosis and reduces the possibility of distortion of the anastomosis because the repair is made in the natural anatomic position.

B A retractor placed on the atrial septum exposes the posterior wall of the left atrium. An incision is made through the posterior wall of the left atrium from the atrial septum on the right side to the base of the left atrial appendage. The incision can be extended into the left atrial appendage if more length is required. A retractor is placed on the superior margin of the left atriotomy to expose the common pulmonary vein, which lies directly behind the left atrium and is covered by the pericardium. An incision is made into the full length of the common pulmonary vein to approximate the size of the incision in the left atrium. The incision usually extends close to the bifurcation of the pulmonary vein on both the right and left sides. The continuity and position of the superior and inferior pulmonary veins on the right and left sides are confirmed, and the anomalous venous connection to the innominate vein (vertical vein) is ligated.

C The common pulmonary vein is anastomosed to the incision in the posterior wall of the left atrium, working through the right atrium and across the atrial septum. A continuous stitch of 6/0 or 7/0 polypropylene or polydioxanone is used. The anastomosis is started just superior to the left apex of the incision in the common pulmonary vein. The first two or three stitches are placed in a clockwise fashion around this apex. These stitches should be placed precisely and separately through the vein and the atrium to ensure accurate closure of the apex. Once these difficult stitches are established and pulled tight, the anastomosis lies directly in approximation, and an edge-to-edge anastomosis is readily accomplished. If desired, a few interrupted stitches can be placed at the superior rim of the incision in the common pulmonary vein before the anastomosis is completed.

D A generous pericardial patch is used to close the septum. This patch can be placed on the lateral wall of the right atrium anterior to the septum to avoid diminishing the size of the left atrium. A continuous stitch of 4/0 polypropylene is used for this anastomosis, which is begun anteriorly, with each end of the suture taken in opposite directions around the septal closure.

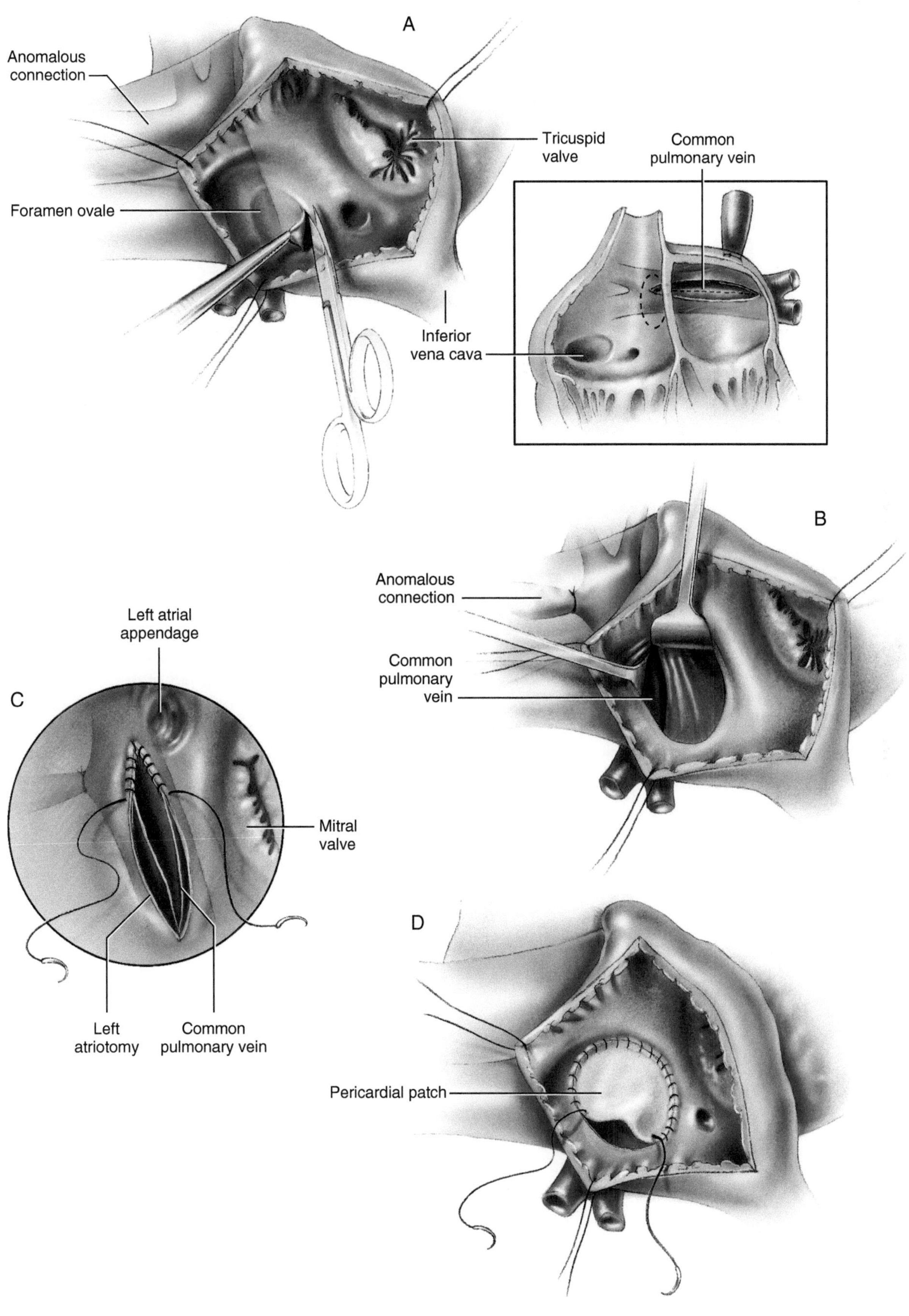
A
Anomalous connection
Tricuspid valve
Common pulmonary vein
Foramen ovale
Inferior vena cava
B
Anomalous connection
Common pulmonary vein
C
Left atrial appendage
Mitral valve
Left atriotomy
Common pulmonary vein
D
Pericardial patch

Infracardiac Type

In this anomaly, the pulmonary veins connect to a confluent vein, which courses posterior to the left atrium, behind the pericardium, and through the diaphragm to join the portal venous circulation. The object of operation is to connect the confluent pulmonary veins to the left atrium. The correction is made using deep hypothermia and circulatory arrest, with removal of the venous cannula to enhance exposure.

Figure 8-4

A A right atriotomy is made, and the atrial septum is excised in the area of the foramen ovale.

B The left atrium is approached through the resected atrial septum (*dashed circle*). An incision is made in the posterior wall of the left atrium over the confluent pulmonary veins. Incision of the pulmonary vein should be in a good position for the anatomically correct anastomosis of the pulmonary vein to the left atrium.

C Retractors are placed through the atrial septum to expose the posterior wall of the left atrium. An incision is made in the left atrium, extending from the atrial septum on the right side into the base of the appendage on the left side. Retractors are then placed into the left atrial incision to expose the confluent pulmonary vein posterior to the left atrium. A T-shaped incision is made in the common pulmonary vein, extending inferiorly along the confluent pulmonary vein and laterally toward the bifurcation of the pulmonary vein on the right and left sides. The precise junction of the superior and inferior pulmonary veins on the right and left sides must be located. The common pulmonary vein is ligated at the level of the diaphragm below the inferior pulmonary veins.

D The common pulmonary vein is anastomosed to the posterior wall of the left atrium with a running stitch of 6/0 or 7/0 polypropylene or polydioxanone. The anastomosis is started at the left apex of the incision in the left atrium, with stitches placed in a clockwise fashion to approximate the left atrium to the common pulmonary vein. The left atrium is sufficiently compliant to allow its accurate approximation to the T-shaped incision of the common pulmonary vein. A large anastomosis may be created.

E The atrial septum is repaired with a generous pericardial patch, which can be sutured to the lateral wall of the right atrium to avoid diminishing the size of the left atrium. A continuous stitch of 4/0 polypropylene is used.

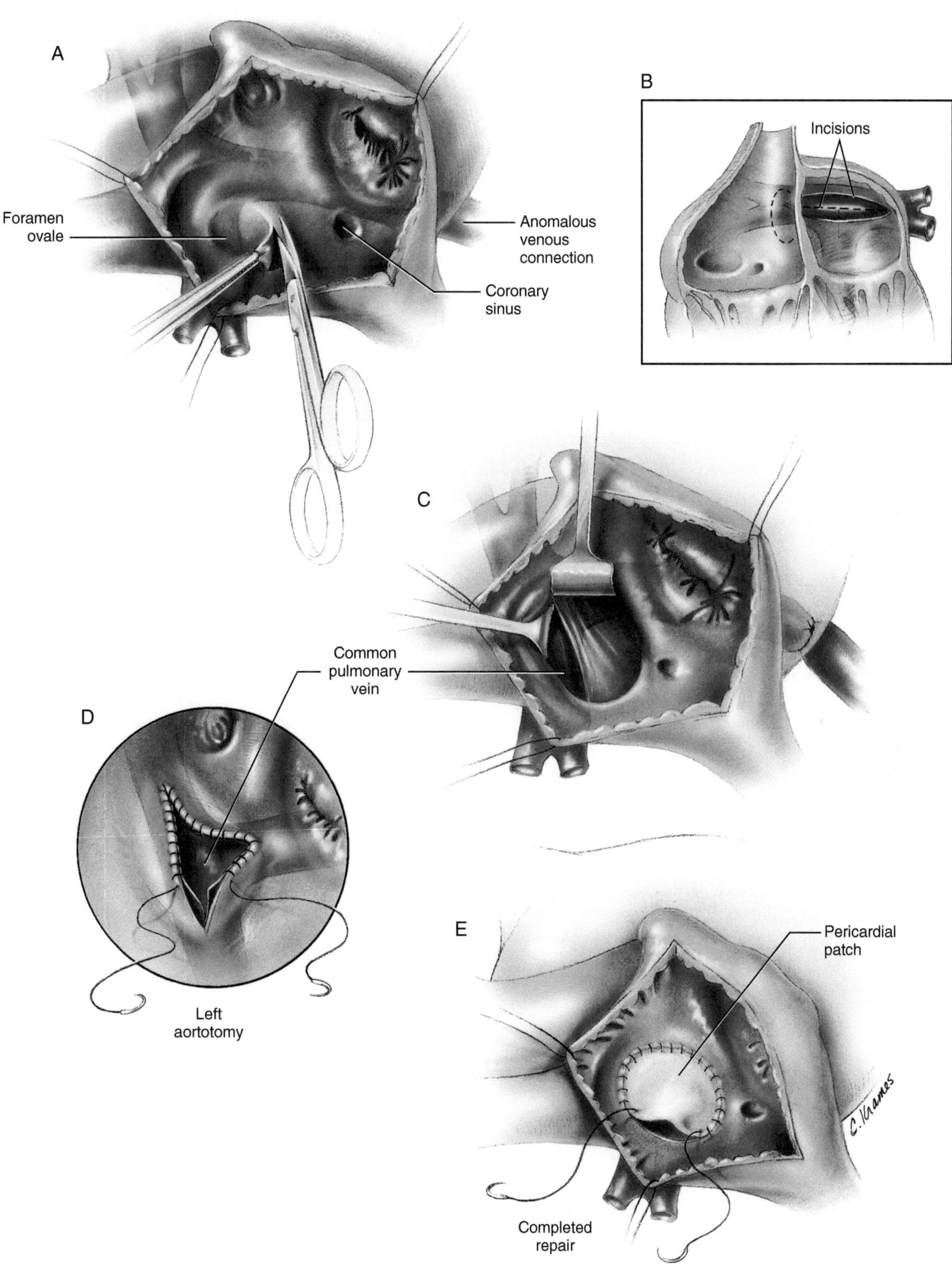
A
Foramen ovale
Anomalous venous connection
Coronary sinus
B
Incisions
C
Common pulmonary vein
D
Left aortotomy
E
Pericardial patch
Completed repair
C. Krames

chapter 9 COR TRIATRIATUM

Cor triatriatum is a rare congenital cardiac anomaly in which a membrane divides the left atrium into two chambers. The normal right atrium is the third chamber in the "triatrial" heart.

Morphology

The primary feature of cor triatriatum is a fibromuscular membrane that divides the left atrium into an upper or proximal chamber that receives the pulmonary veins and a lower or distal chamber that contains the atrial appendage and the mitral valve. The defect is the result of the embryonic failure of the common pulmonary vein to fuse properly to the left atrium. As the pulmonary vein fuses to the left atrium, the wall between the two is normally absorbed, leaving a common chamber. In cor triatriatum the absorption is incomplete, leaving a diaphragm dividing the left atrium.

Figure 9-1

A When the foramen ovale communicates with the upper chamber, the clinical features may simulate anomalous pulmonary venous connection.

B Occasionally, the foramen ovale provides communication between the distal chamber and the right atrium, so that the clinical features mimic mitral stenosis. The membrane or diaphragm that divides the left atrium is always intimately attached to the atrial septum on the medial side. On the lateral side, the diaphragm is attached to the left atrial wall just below the left pulmonary veins. The lateral area of attachment is somewhat difficult to identify from within the atrium and must be approached carefully, keeping in mind the relationships of the left pulmonary veins, mitral valve, atrial appendage, and coronary sinus.

C For older children and adults, an approach through the left atrium, similar to that for mitral valve operations, is quite satisfactory. Standard cardiopulmonary bypass with two venous cannulae is used. Caval tourniquets are necessary because there is always a patent foramen ovale. An incision is made in the left atrium on the right side, posterior to the interatrial groove.

D Anterior retraction of the atrial septum exposes the obstructing diaphragm with its central fenestration. The four pulmonary veins are easy to identify, but none of the other structures ordinarily visible in the left atrium can be seen at this point. The inability to visualize these structures is a significant drawback to this approach, but in larger hearts it should not hinder successful repair.

E Excision of the obstructing diaphragm is begun by creating an opening through the fenestration toward the left inferior pulmonary vein. The direction of this initial incision is convenient, but its length should be limited until the structures below the diaphragm are identified. Retraction and inspection through the incision in the diaphragm expose the mitral valve and allow the dissection to proceed safely. Care must be taken to protect the underlying mitral valve during excision of the obstructing diaphragm. As the dissection of the membrane approaches the left side, the close relationship of the left inferior pulmonary vein and the mitral valve can be identified, and the membrane should be removed from between them, taking care not to penetrate the free wall of the left atrium while achieving total excision of the diaphragm.

F Complete excision of the diaphragm places the pulmonary veins and the mitral valve in continuity and provides an unobstructed passageway for blood flow. The repair is completed by closure of the left atrial incision.

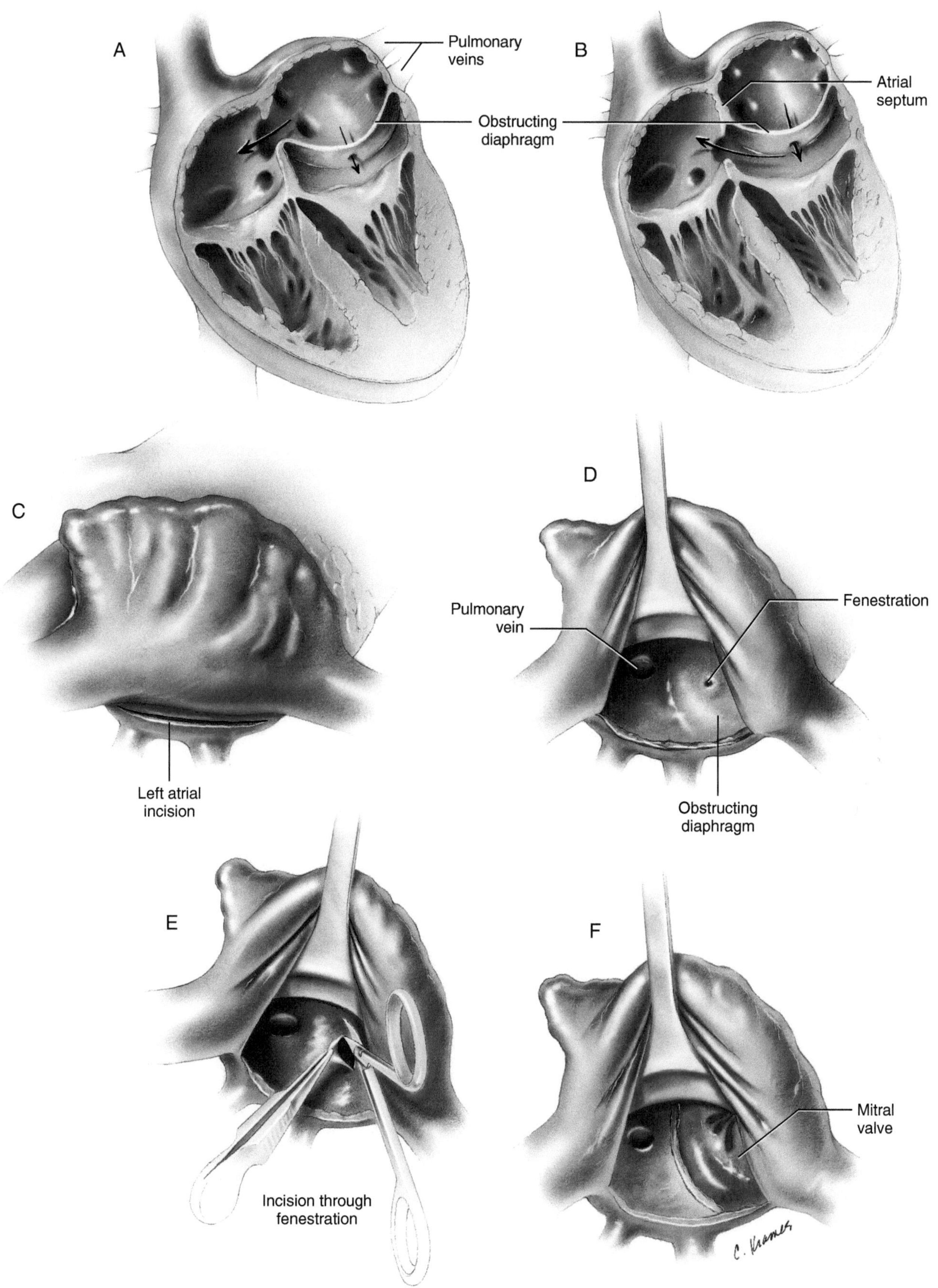
A
Pulmonary veins
B
Atrial septum
Obstructing diaphragm
C
Left atrial incision
D
Pulmonary vein
Fenestration
Obstructing diaphragm
E
Incision through fenestration
F
Mitral valve
C. Kramer

Figure 9-1 (continued)

G For infants and small children, the repair can be performed using deep hypothermia with circulatory arrest for maximal intraatrial exposure. A single venous cannula placed through the right atrial appendage can be removed to enhance exposure. A right atriotomy is made parallel and close to the atrioventricular groove. The atrial septum in the area of the foramen ovale is excised.

H As the atrial septum is excised, the point at which the obstructing membrane joins the atrial septum is exposed. Approaching the lesion through the atrial septum facilitates the identification of the intraatrial structures and greatly simplifies the repair of this defect in tiny hearts or even in older patients. A retractor placed anteriorly on the septum aids in exposing the obstructing diaphragm and its relations to the mitral valve and the left pulmonary veins.

I The four pulmonary veins should be clearly identified and probed to ascertain that they are all normally connected to the heart. The mitral valve may be difficult to visualize completely at first, but as the dissection of the diaphragm proceeds, it becomes more exposed. The mitral valve must be clearly visualized at its lateral aspect, where the diaphragm is attached close to the valve. The diaphragm is completely excised so that there is unobstructed blood flow from the pulmonary veins to the mitral valve. The dissection begins at the atrial septal attachment and proceeds posteriorly and anteriorly using scissors. The most difficult part of the operation is the excision laterally on the left atrial wall, where care must be taken to preserve the mitral valve and the left atrial attachment of the left inferior pulmonary vein. Depth of excision is difficult to gauge in this area, and the free wall of the posterior left atrium may be perforated. In addition, it is possible to enter the coronary sinus. The obstructing diaphragm must be completely removed to ensure the free flow of blood from the pulmonary veins to the mitral valve.

J The atrial septum is closed with a patch taken from the anterior pericardium. The patch is attached to the atrial septum using a continuous stitch of 4/0 polypropylene. The suture line is started anteriorly and initially proceeds in a counterclockwise direction around the superior rim of the defect below the superior vena cava. The repair is completed by taking the opposite end of the suture around the inferior aspect of the defect in a clockwise direction and joining the two ends of the suture.

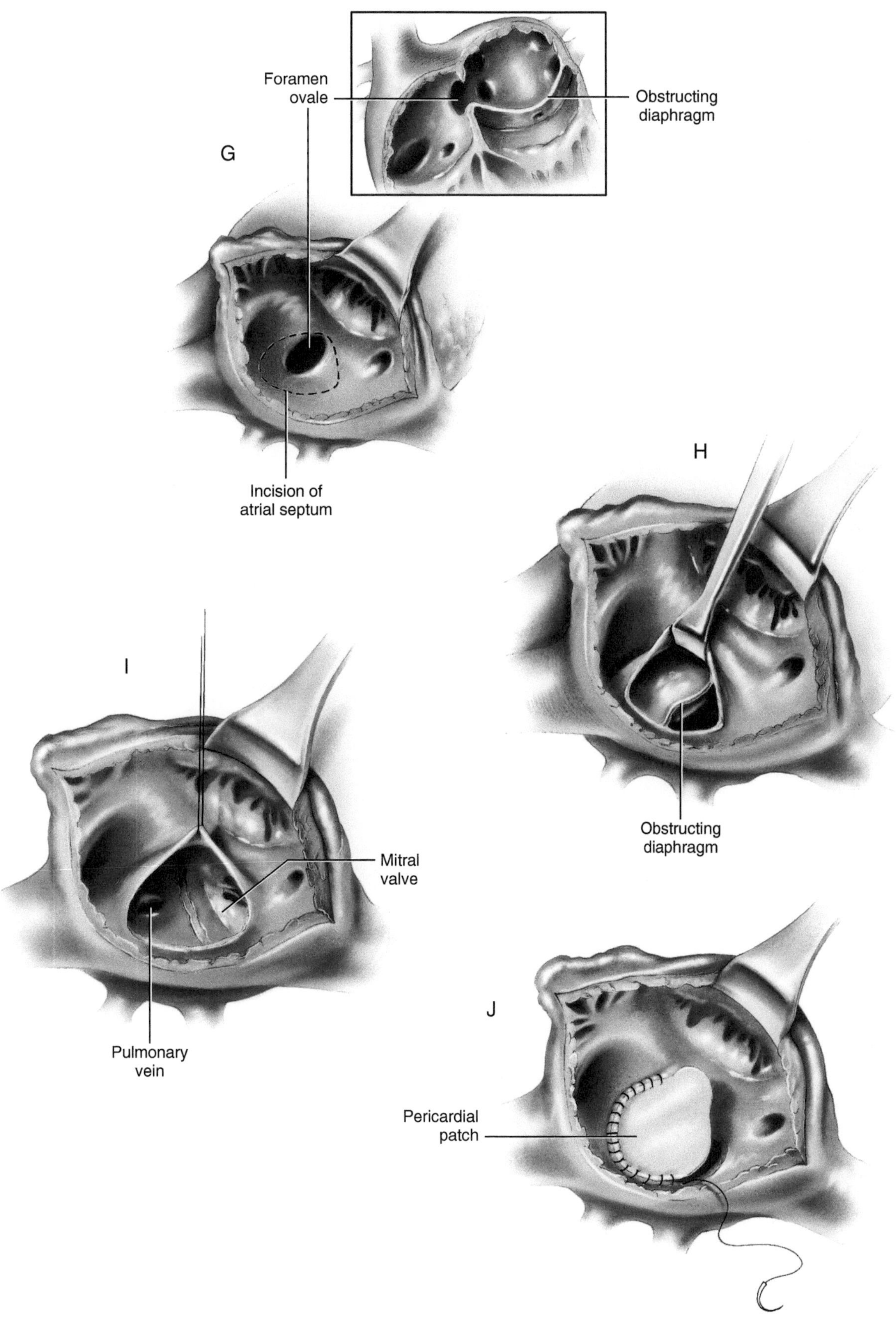
Foramen ovale
Obstructing diaphragm
G
Incision of atrial septum
H
Obstructing diaphragm
I
Mitral valve
Pulmonary vein
J
Pericardial patch

part IV

Right Heart Valve Lesions (Congenital)

chapter 10 PULMONARY VALVE STENOSIS

Pulmonary stenosis refers to congenital malformations of the pulmonary valve resulting in the obstruction of blood flowing from the right ventricle.

Morphology

The pulmonary valve is usually malformed, with fusion of the commissures resulting in stenosis of the valve orifice. The sinuses of Valsalva are usually formed, although they may be smaller than usual (hypoplastic). Valve leaflets are often thickened and malformed (dysplastic). There may be associated supravalvular stenosis at the sinuses' junction with the main pulmonary artery. The diameter of the right ventricular outflow tract at the level of the pulmonary valve may be small.

Figure 10-1

A Pulmonary valve stenosis, autopsy specimen. Valve leaflets are thick due to dysplasia. The supravalvular ridge is also thickened, resulting in an element of supravalvular stenosis and crowding of the valve leaflets.

B Neonatal pulmonary valve stenosis, operative image. The pulmonary valve leaflets are markedly dysplastic. Commissures are fused. Deformity of the valve is marked, and stenosis is severe.

C Pulmonary valve stenosis, operative image after pulmonary valvotomy. The anterior commissure has been opened by making an incision back to the wall of the pulmonary artery. Stenosis is reduced, but leaflet dysplasia remains.

A

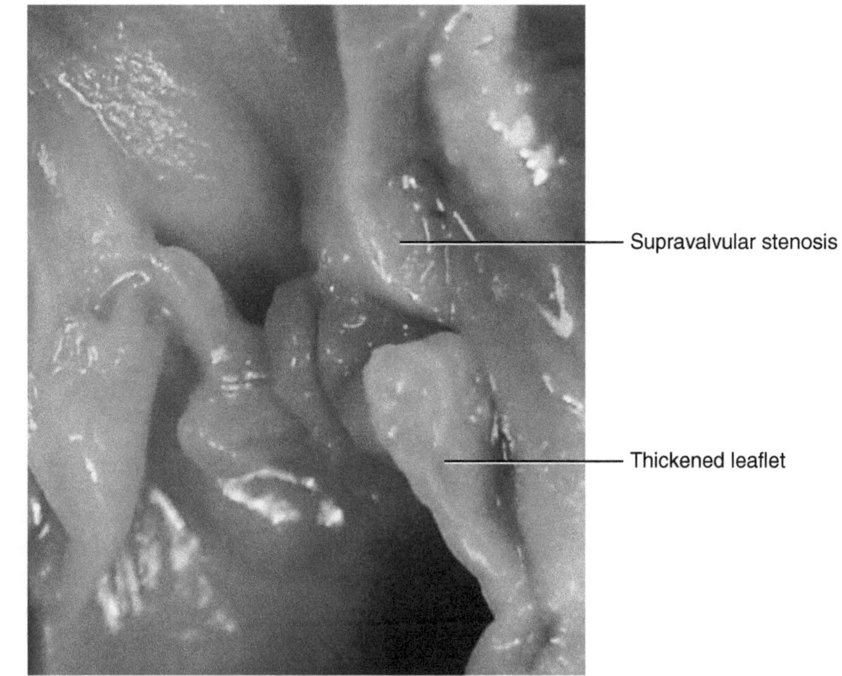
Supravalvular stenosis
Thickened leaflet

B

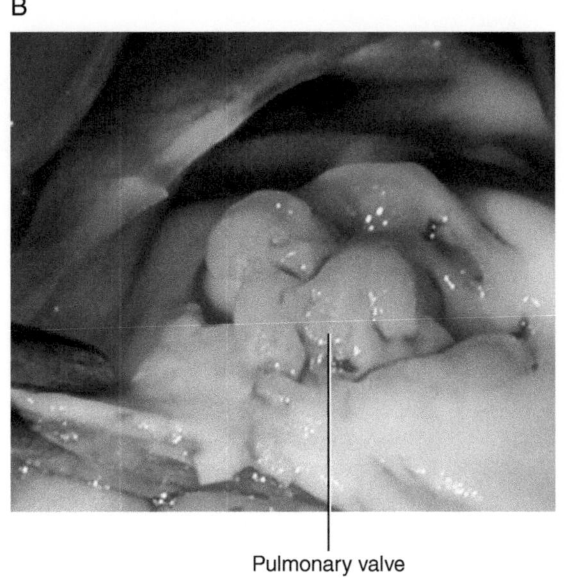
Pulmonary valve

C

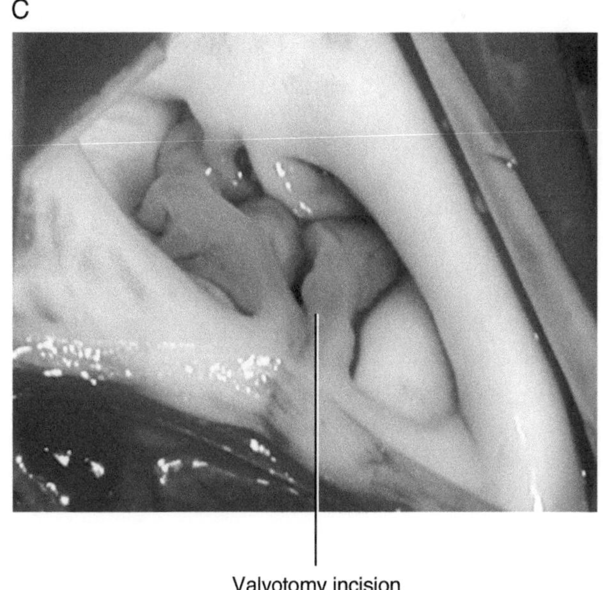
Valvotomy incision

Pulmonary Valvotomy

Pulmonary valvotomy to relieve stenosis may be performed for isolated pulmonary valve malformations or as part of another palliative operation for complex forms of right ventricular outflow tract obstruction. The operation has become less common since the advent and more widespread application of catheter balloon dilation.

Figure 10-2

A The open technique utilizes cardiopulmonary bypass, aortic occlusion, and cold cardioplegia for optimal exposure of the pulmonary valve. A traction suture is placed in the outflow tract of the right ventricle to expose the pulmonary artery. A vertical incision in the pulmonary artery may be extended into either of the anterior sinuses of Valsalva, alongside the anterior commissure of the pulmonary valve.

B A small retractor placed in the anterior sinus of Valsalva, aided by traction sutures, exposes the pulmonary valve. The pathology must be carefully assessed because there may be more than simply fusion of the commissures. The size of the supravalvular ring should be estimated, and small sinuses of Valsalva are a clue to more complex pathology. The actual diameter of the pulmonary annulus should be determined and compared with a chart of normal values based on patient size.

C Two forceps are used to align the cusps of the pulmonary valve. The commissures are sharply incised precisely along their line of fusion to the wall of the pulmonary artery using a No. 15 scalpel.

D Incision of all commissures completes the valvotomy. A nasal speculum can be used to inspect the subvalvular right ventricular outflow tract. The septal band of the crista supraventricularis can be incised, if necessary, to widen the subannular area.

E The pulmonary arteriotomy is closed by continuous suture.

F The closed technique utilizes a midline incision to expose the right ventricle and pulmonary outflow tract. A mattress stitch with a Teflon felt pledget is placed in the anterior wall of the right ventricle, preserving any right ventricular branches of the right coronary artery. A tourniquet is placed on the mattress stitch. A stab incision is made within the confines of the mattress stitch. Blood loss is controlled by digital pressure or, if necessary, closure of the tourniquet.

G A mosquito hemostat is preselected to perform the closed valvotomy. The hemostat should be long enough so that the tips can perforate the pulmonary valve while the hinge of the hemostat remains at approximately the level of the ventriculotomy. The hemostat is inserted through the ventriculotomy, across the outflow tract of the right ventricle, and pushed through the pulmonary valve.

H Forceful opening of the mosquito hemostat dilates the valve and its annulus. This should be performed in both the anteroposterior and lateral dimensions. During this maneuver, care must be taken to ensure that the hinge of the hemostat remains in the ventriculotomy so as not to dilate the incision in the right ventricle and cause unnecessary hemorrhage. Following the dilation valvotomy, the hemostat is removed, and the ventriculotomy is controlled with the tourniquet. Pressure gradient measurements are taken, and if they are satisfactory, the ventriculotomy is secured by tying off the pledgeted mattress stitch.

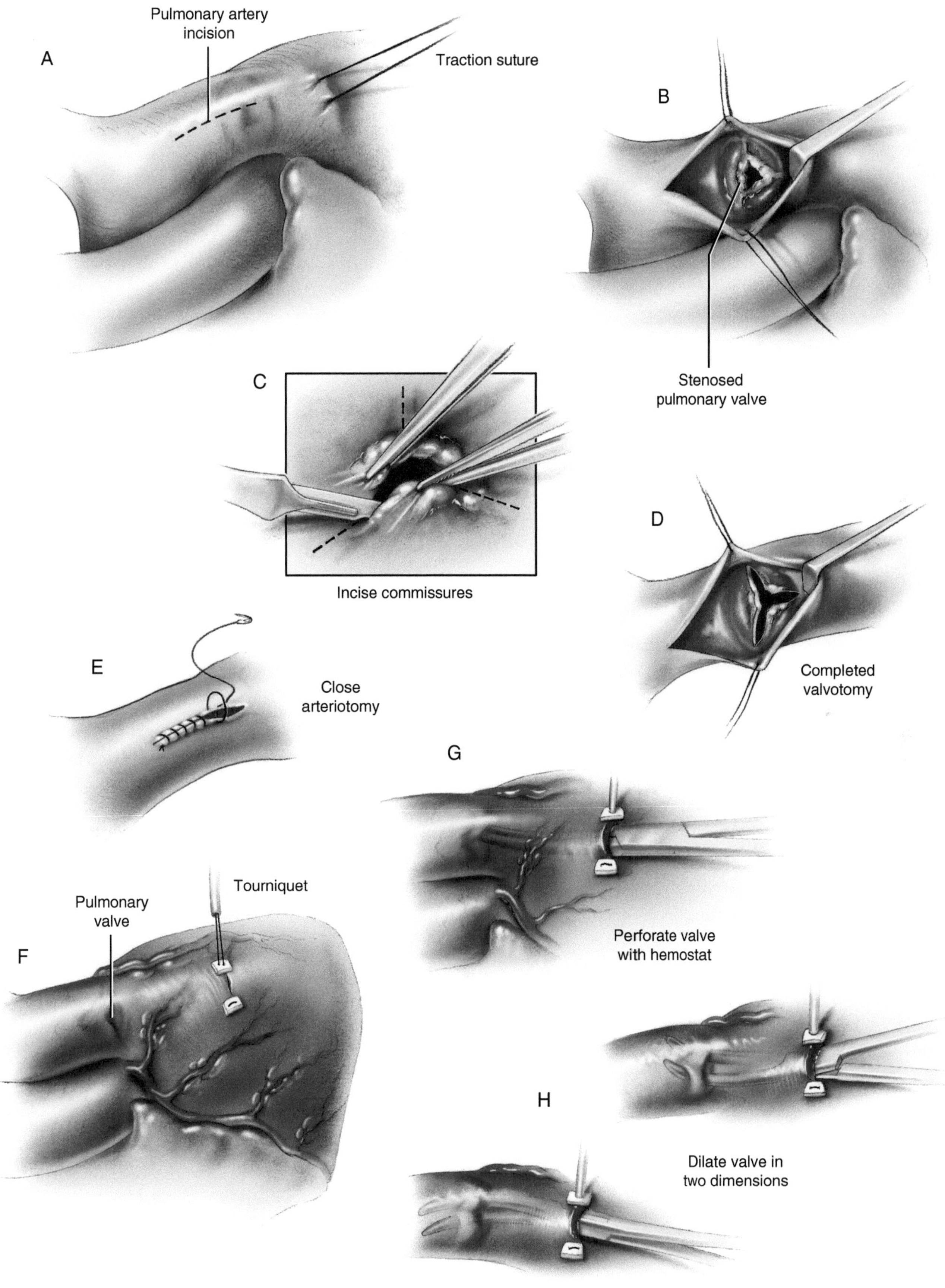
A
Pulmonary artery incision
Traction suture
B
Stenosed pulmonary valve
C
Incise commissures
D
Completed valvotomy
E
Close arteriotomy
F
Pulmonary valve
Tourniquet
G
Perforate valve with hemostat
H
Dilate valve in two dimensions

chapter 11 TETRALOGY OF FALLOT

Tetralogy of Fallot is a complex congenital anomaly that includes a malalignment-type ventricular septal defect, an aorta that overrides the septal defect, right ventricular outflow tract obstruction, and compensatory hypertrophy of the right ventricle. The defects are corrected at a single operation in most cases, although in small infants it may be better to perform a palliative operation and defer total correction until both the child and the heart are larger.

Morphology

Figure 11-1

A Tetralogy of Fallot results from embryologic underdevelopment of the infundibular portion of the right ventricle. The varying degree of hypoplasia of the right ventricular outflow tract results in a spectrum of severity. This figure shows an extreme form of infundibular hypoplasia resulting in a tiny opening from the body of the right ventricle (os infundibulum) to a small outflow portion of the right ventricle (infundibular chamber). Interestingly, the pulmonary valve leaflets appear normal, which is seen in about 25% of cases, even though the total area of the valve is usually smaller than normal.

B View of the os infundibulum through the opened right ventricle. Note the extreme hypertrophy of the right ventricular wall. The trabecula septomarginalis (septal extension) is displayed as hypertrophied myocardial bands coursing from the os infundibulum onto the ventricular septum. The hypertrophied bands of the ventriculoinfundibular fold (parietal extension) are seen opposite.

C Tetralogy of Fallot viewed from the left ventricular aspect. The ventricular septal defect with the aortic valve and aorta overriding the defect is clearly shown. Thus, the aorta receives blood flow directly from the right ventricle with each cardiac contraction.

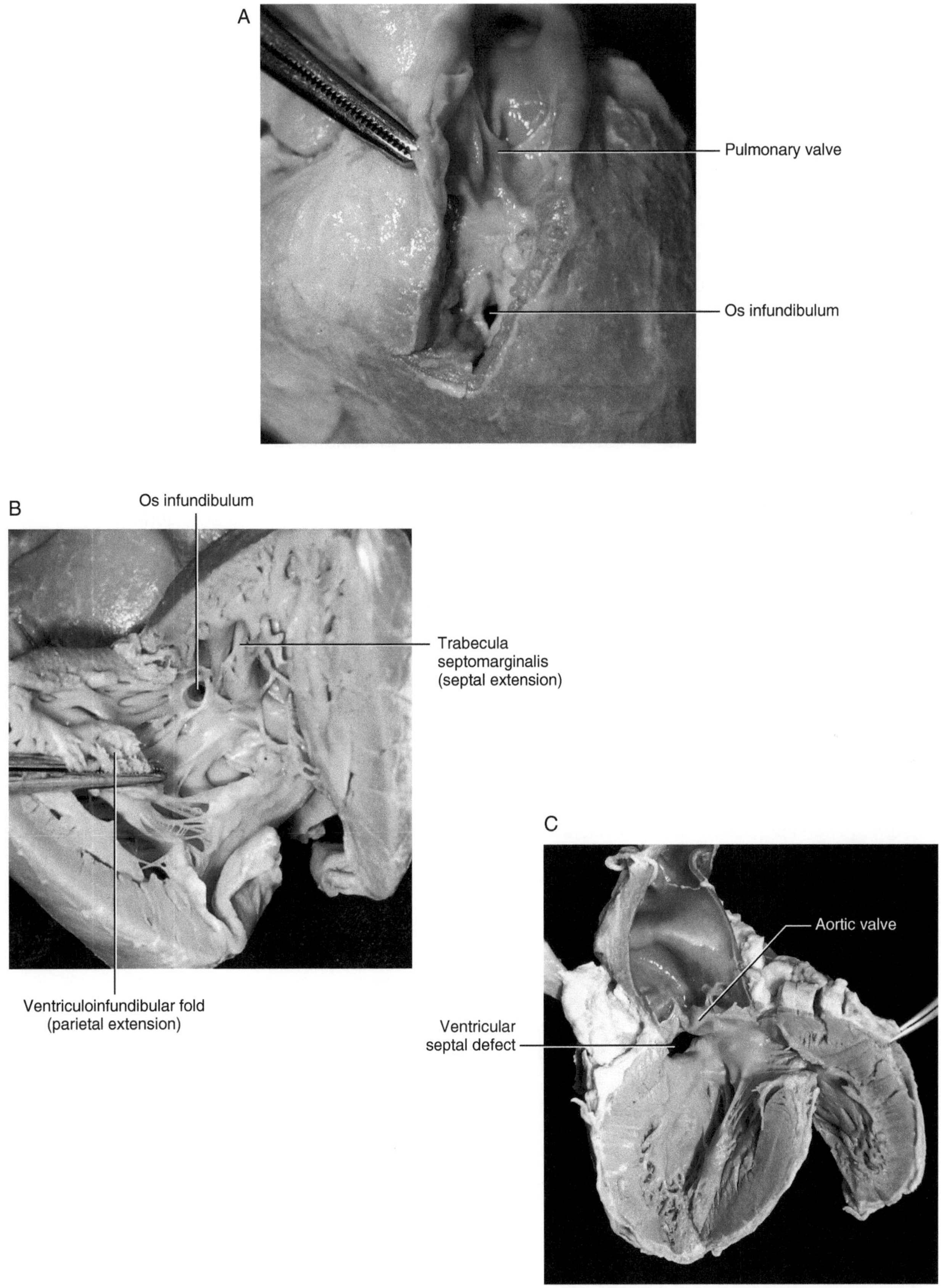

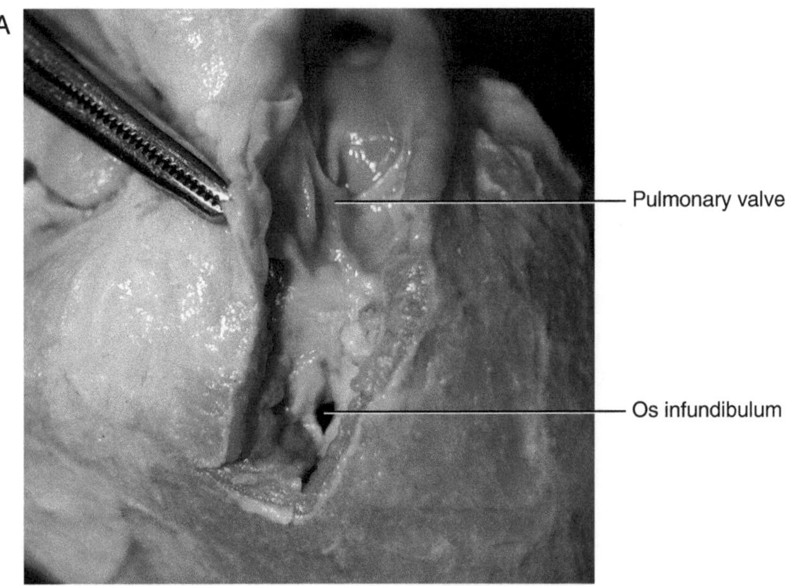

B
Os infundibulum
Trabecula septomarginalis (septal extension)
Ventriculoinfundibular fold (parietal extension)

C
Aortic valve
Ventricular septal defect

Right Atrial Approach

Operation to repair tetralogy of Fallot may be performed through a right atrial approach to avoid incision of the right ventricular myocardium. This approach is technically challenging because exposure of the muscle bundles obstructing the right ventricular outflow tract is difficult to manage.

Figure 11-2

A Anatomic relations of the components of tetralogy of Fallot. Blood flow (arrow) from the right atrium (RA) through the tricuspid valve (TV) to the right ventricle (RV) meets outflow resistance at the os infundibulum, which is narrowed due to hypertrophy of the septal and parietal myocardial extensions arising on the infundibular septum. Relief of this obstruction is required in all operations for tetralogy of Fallot. Not shown here are other commonly associated conditions, such as hypoplasia of the infundibular chamber, stenosis of the pulmonary valve, and hypoplasia of the pulmonary artery. Relationships of the ventricular septal defect (VSD) to the tricuspid valve are demonstrated.

B An incision is made in the right atrium parallel to the atrioventricular groove. The tricuspid valve is retracted to expose the elements of the defect below the valve. Serial repositioning of the retractors is required as the operation proceeds. The ventricular septal defect (VSD) is seen just below the tricuspid valve. The os infundibulum (opening from the body of the right ventricle to the infundibular chamber) is located anterior and medial to the ventricular septal defect. The os infundibulum is surrounded and obstructed by the parietal and septal extensions. The infundibular obstruction of the right ventricular outflow tract is relieved by dividing and resecting these extensions.

C Exposure and dissection of the parietal extension constitute the most difficult part of the right atrial approach because this extension is hidden by the tricuspid valve and the overlying anterior wall of the right ventricle. Superior retraction of the tricuspid valve exposes the parietal extension as it courses anteriorly from the infundibular septum above the ventricular septal defect. The parietal extension is divided close to the infundibular septum (shown by *broken lines*), sometimes called the crista supraventricularis. This myocardial band is dissected free of the anterior wall of the right ventricle as far anteriorly as possible; then it is divided to remove a segment of muscle. Once a segment of the parietal band is removed and out of the way, the septal extension lying on the ventricular septum and coursing anteriorly is exposed. A segment of the septal extension is then removed (shown by *broken lines*). The os infundibulum is enlarged by removal of these myocardial bands, ensuring an adequate passageway from the right ventricle to the infundibular chamber. Dissection of the septal and parietal extensions is less complete through a right atrial approach than through a right ventriculotomy, and it usually involves the removal of a segment of the muscle bundle rather than excision of the whole bundle. A fortuitous result of this less complete removal may be better right ventricular function, but this must be balanced against the possibility of leaving some infundibular obstruction.

D The ventricular septal defect (VSD) is closed with a prosthetic patch using the method described in Figure 5-2, with continuous stitches beginning anteriorly on the infundibular septum.

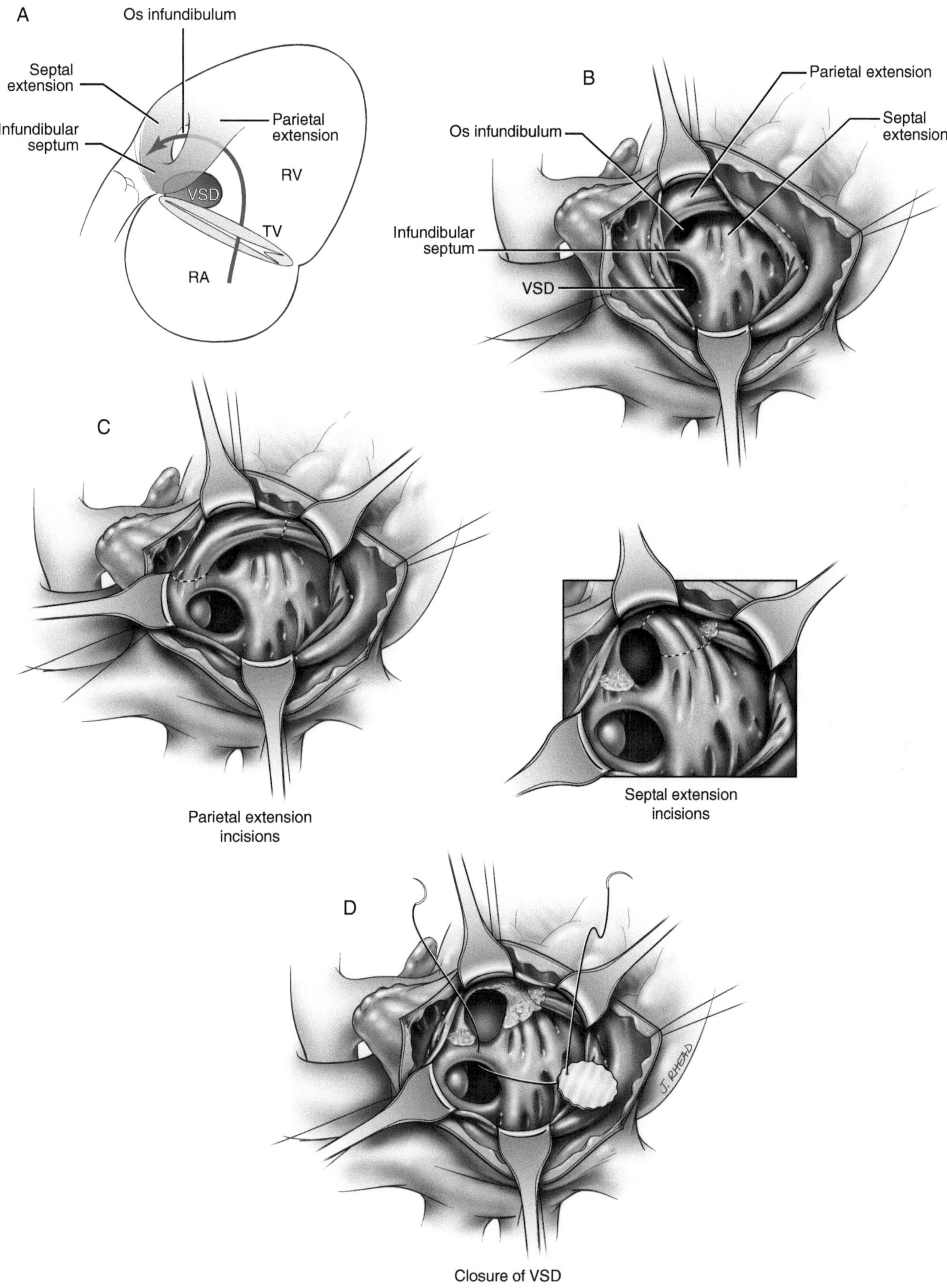

Parietal extension incisions

Septal extension incisions

Closure of VSD

Right Ventricular Approach

Repair of tetralogy of Fallot through an incision in the right ventricle offers the best exposure of the combination of defects. Resection of infundibular obstructing muscle bundles is complete. In cases of severe right ventricular outflow tract obstruction with combined infundibular obstruction and hypoplasia of the infundibular chamber, pulmonary valve, and pulmonary artery, incision and graft augmentation of all or various levels of the right ventricular outflow tract may be required. A single incision through all levels of obstruction or selective incisions including the right ventricle and pulmonary artery may be used.

Figure 11-3

A A vertical ventriculotomy incision is used in most cases of tetralogy of Fallot when the adequacy of the diameter of the pulmonary annulus or proximal pulmonary artery is questionable. The incision is made in the midportion of the outflow of the right ventricle. Coronary arteries are preserved, especially the anterior descending artery, which may have an anomalous origin. The incision is extended to the annulus of the pulmonary valve. The annulus is preserved if its diameter, determined using Hegar calibration dilators, compares favorably with normal values based on patient size. Pulmonary valvotomy is performed, achieving exposure from below by incising the valve commissures. In cases in which the pulmonary annulus remains narrow and obstructive after valvotomy, the ventriculotomy is extended across the annulus into the main portion of the pulmonary artery, widening the outflow tract. Subvalvular stenosis is relieved by excising hypertrophied infundibular myocardial bundles. The septal and parietal extensions of the crista supraventricularis are mobilized and excised. Trabecular clefts are lined with endocardium and can be used as guides to the depth of the excision to prevent septal perforation or septal coronary artery injury.

B The hypertrophied muscle bundles should be mobilized until the dissection plane reaches the limit of the trabecular clefts. At this point, the muscle bundle is excised flush with the ventricular septum. The crista supraventricularis can also be partly removed by wedge excision. Traction stitches placed at the annulus of the pulmonary valve, apex of the ventriculotomy, and base of the septal muscle band aid in exposing the ventricular septal defect.

C An optional transverse incision can be used when surface anatomy and preoperative imaging indicate that the pulmonary artery annulus and valve have an adequate diameter and can be preserved. An advantage of this incision is conservation of the coronary blood supply to the right ventricle. When inspection of the heart reveals a normal-sized pulmonary artery annulus, and the structure of the sinuses of Valsalva and pulmonary artery above the valve appears to be normal, it is possible to repair the intracardiac abnormalities through a transverse incision in the right ventricle. A transverse ventriculotomy is made parallel to the course of the ventricular branches of the right coronary artery. This type of incision may also have some hemodynamic advantages. After the usual infundibulectomy, the pulmonary valve is inspected from below. A vascular forceps is used to evert the pulmonary valve cusps to search for commissural fusion. The commissures can be accurately visualized using vascular forceps and precisely incised to the wall of the pulmonary artery. Additional widening of the pulmonary outflow tract is accomplished by dilating the pulmonary annulus in two planes using a hemostat.

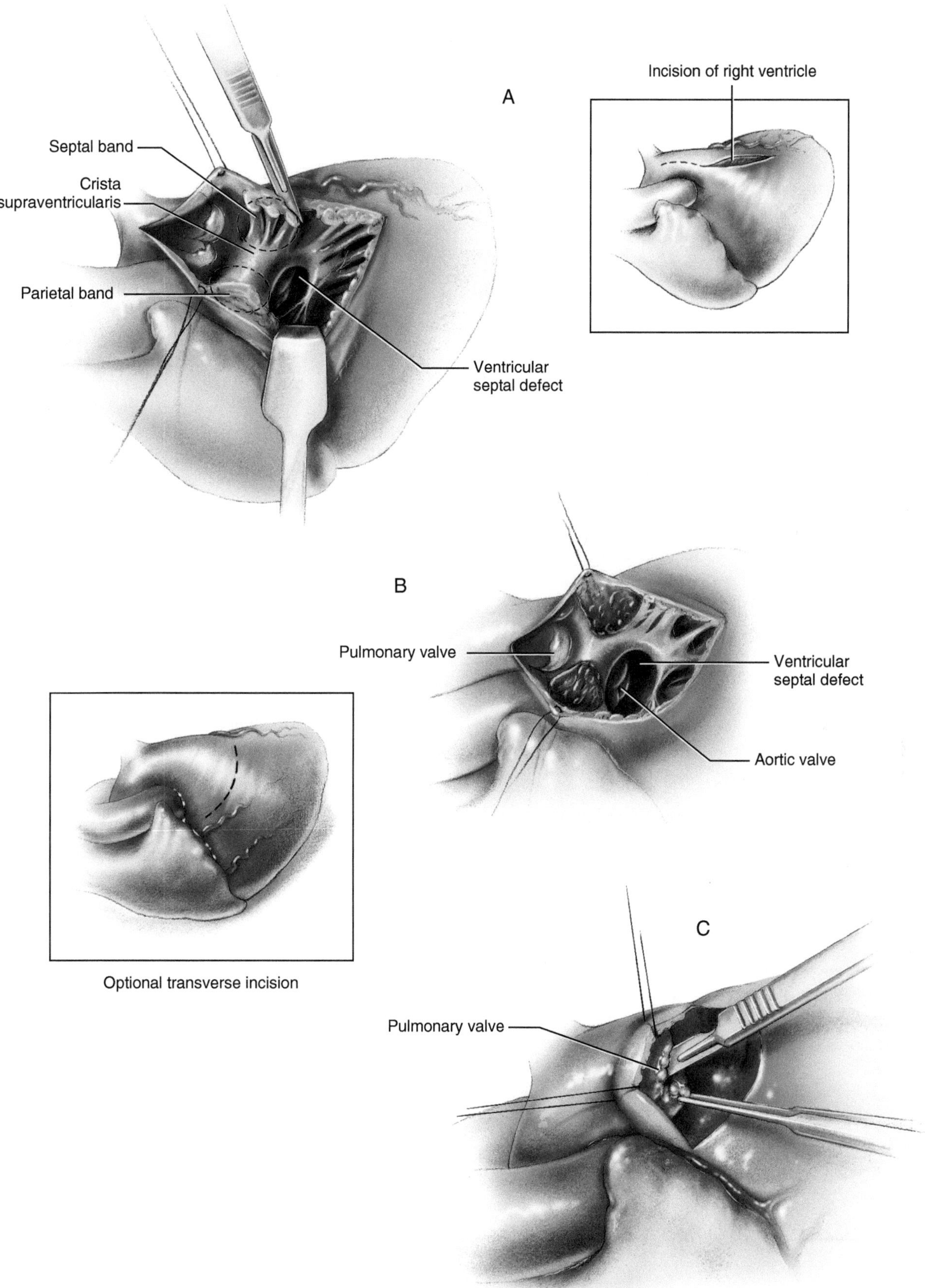
A
Incision of right ventricle
Septal band
Crista supraventricularis
Parietal band
Ventricular septal defect
B
Pulmonary valve
Ventricular septal defect
Aortic valve
Optional transverse incision
C
Pulmonary valve

Figure 11-3 (continued)

D The septal leaflet of the tricuspid valve overlies the defect and requires forceps retraction for optimal exposure of the posterior inferior rim of the defect. The specialized conduction system originates from the atrioventricular node in the most distal aspect of the triangle of Koch. The bundle of His penetrates the central fibrous body near the inferior rim of the ventricular septal defect and courses along the left ventricular aspect of the posteroinferior rim of the defect. The bundle branches spread onto the ventricular septum posterior to the base of the papillary muscle of the conus. A patch is fashioned from a tubular, crimped, weave-knit Dacron prosthesis, making the patch slightly larger than the defect and orienting the crimp ridges so that the patch can expand in a superior-inferior direction. The needle of double-ended 4/0 polypropylene suture enters the ventricular septum 5 to 7 mm below the inferior rim of the defect and exits 3 to 5 mm below the inferior rim, near the base of the septal leaflet of the tricuspid valve. The opposite needle is passed through the septal leaflet of the tricuspid valve close to the exit point of the first stitch, from ventricle to atrium and back through the base of the septal leaflet to the ventricular side. This seals off the potential crevice at the junction of the septal leaflet of the tricuspid valve and the ventricular septum, while avoiding the area most likely occupied by the bundle of His. Both needles are passed beneath any overhanging tricuspid chordae and through the Dacron patch.

E With the needle used for the initial stitch, three or four stitches are placed in a "wagon-wheel" fashion to a depth of about half the thickness of the ventricular septum. The needle must penetrate well below the ventricular septal defect so as to exit 3 to 5 mm inferior to its rim and preserve the conduction system.

F Once the base of the papillary muscle of the conus is passed, the stitches are brought progressively closer to the rim of the ventricular septal defect. The initial part of the suture line is completed at the septal extension of the crista supraventricularis.

G The ventricular surface of the septal leaflet of the tricuspid valve is exposed by forceps traction and countertraction on the Dacron patch. The hinge point of the septal leaflet on the annulus is identified so that stitches are placed in the base of the septal leaflet of the tricuspid valve, slightly away from the annulus, to avoid placing stitches at the point where the bundle of His penetrates the central fibrous body, thus preserving the conduction system. A continuous horizontal mattress stitch is created through the patch and the base of the septal leaflet of the valve by passing the needle from the ventricular side of the leaflet to the atrium and then returning from atrium to ventricle. At the junction of the septal leaflet of the tricuspid valve and the annulus of the aortic valve, a transition stitch is made that reverses the needle direction, entering the fibrous continuity of the tricuspid and aortic valves and exiting deep into the muscle of the ventricle. The mattress stitch on the patch then forms a buttress to seal off any potential crevice at that point.

H The suture line is continued along ventricular muscle, with substantial bites into the crista supraventricularis. Any overhanging tricuspid chordae are protected. The repair is completed by joining the two ends of the suture.

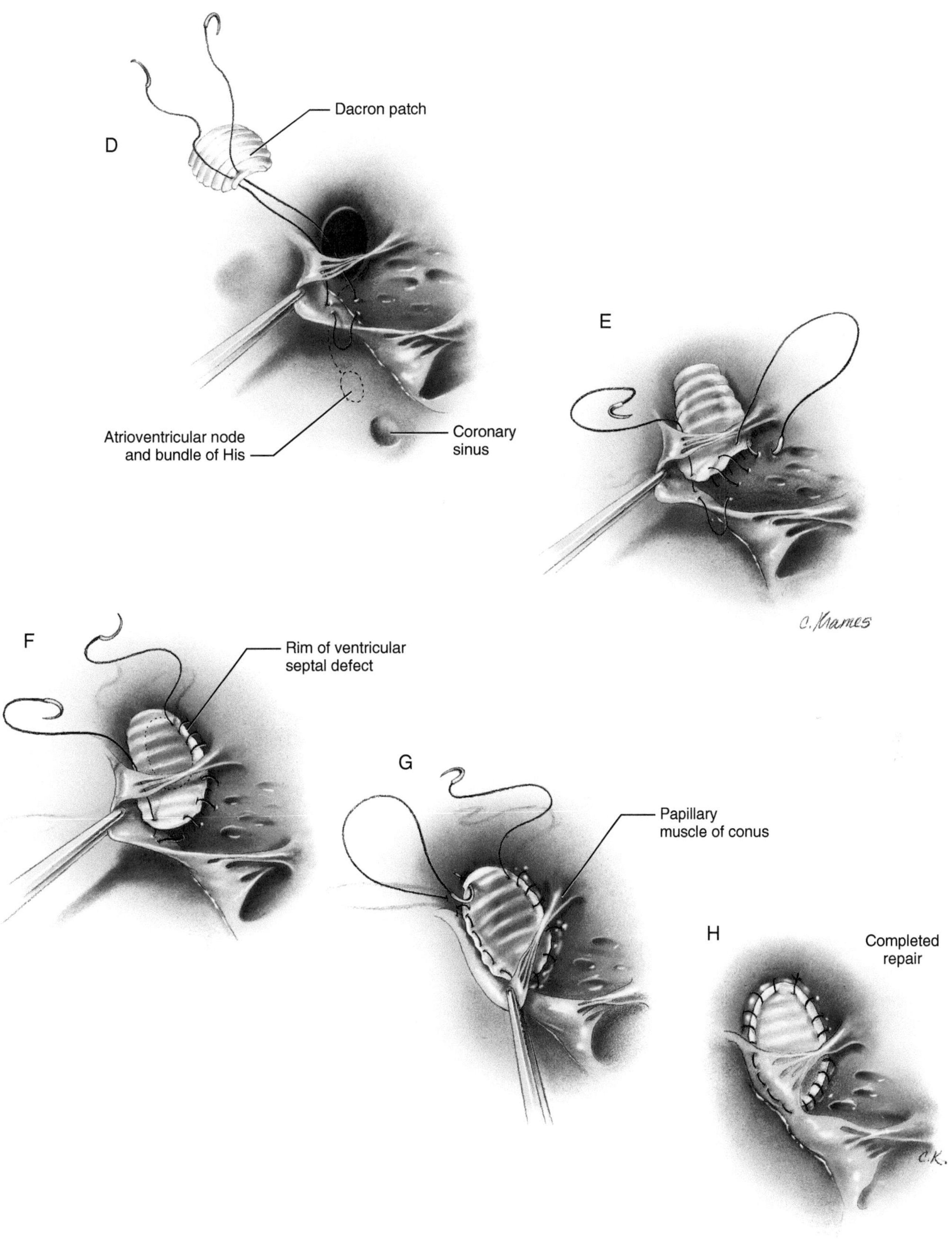
D
Dacron patch
Atrioventricular node
and bundle of His
Coronary
sinus
E
C. Kramer
F
Rim of ventricular
septal defect
G
Papillary
muscle of conus
H
Completed
repair
C.K.

Figure 11-3 (continued)

I When the incision has been extended across the pulmonary annulus, the pulmonary arteriotomy and ventriculotomy are closed using a prosthetic outflow patch. The patch is constructed from a tubular graft of crimped, collagen-sealed, knitted velour Dacron. Some surgeons prefer polytetrafluoroethylene (PTFE) grafts for this purpose, but needle hole bleeding may be a problem with this material. A continuous stitch of 4/0 polypropylene is used. Five stitch loops are placed around the apex of the pulmonary arteriotomy and through the graft before approximating the graft and the artery. This ensures accurate closure of the suture line.

J The suture loops are pulled up securely, and the suture line is continued to the annulus of the pulmonary valve on the right side and then on the left side. The stitches are placed slightly wider on the graft than on the pulmonary artery so that sufficient graft length is available in the outflow tract to allow anterior bulging for maximal cross-sectional area when the outflow tract is filled with blood. The suture line can be tied off at the pulmonary annulus and a larger suture used to approximate the graft to the myocardium, or the suture line can simply be continued to completion around the rest of the ventriculotomy.

K An alternative approach is preferable when elevated pressure in the right ventricle is anticipated following repair. Mattress stitches reinforced with Teflon pledgets are used to approximate the graft to the ventriculotomy to obtain maximal strength of suture closure in the myocardium. Individual primary mattress sutures tend to "bunch up" the suture link, resulting in closure to a cuff of myocardium. A smoother, more uniform closure results when mattress sutures are used to supplement primary closure by continuous suture.

L When hypoplasia affects the right and left branches of the pulmonary artery beyond the bifurcation, the incision is extended into the right and left pulmonary arteries until satisfactory widening of the outflow tract is achieved. The spur of the bifurcation of the pulmonary artery presents some problems in terms of accurate reconstruction of the outflow tract when extension of the incision is required.

M A tubular graft of crimped Dacron or PTFE is used for the reconstruction. Extensions of the graft to cover the branch incisions of the pulmonary artery are constructed, and a small wedge is taken from the distal end to accommodate the spur of the bifurcation of the pulmonary artery. This prevents buckling of the graft at the bifurcation, which could result in residual obstruction. Five stitches are taken around the extensions of the graft and the apex of the incision in each of the pulmonary arteries before pulling the graft into the pulmonary arteriotomy. Integrity of the distal ends of the suture line is assured, and the pulmonary arteries are accurately reconstructed and widened. It may be necessary to work posterior and to the right of the aorta when right pulmonary artery hypoplasia extends a considerable distance beyond the bifurcation. Sutures and graft must be passed behind the aorta to complete the central portion of the repair. Separate sutures used for each branch of the pulmonary artery are joined at the bifurcation.

N The suture line is continued along the right and left edges of the pulmonary arteriotomy to the annulus of the pulmonary valve and then completed around the ventriculotomy.

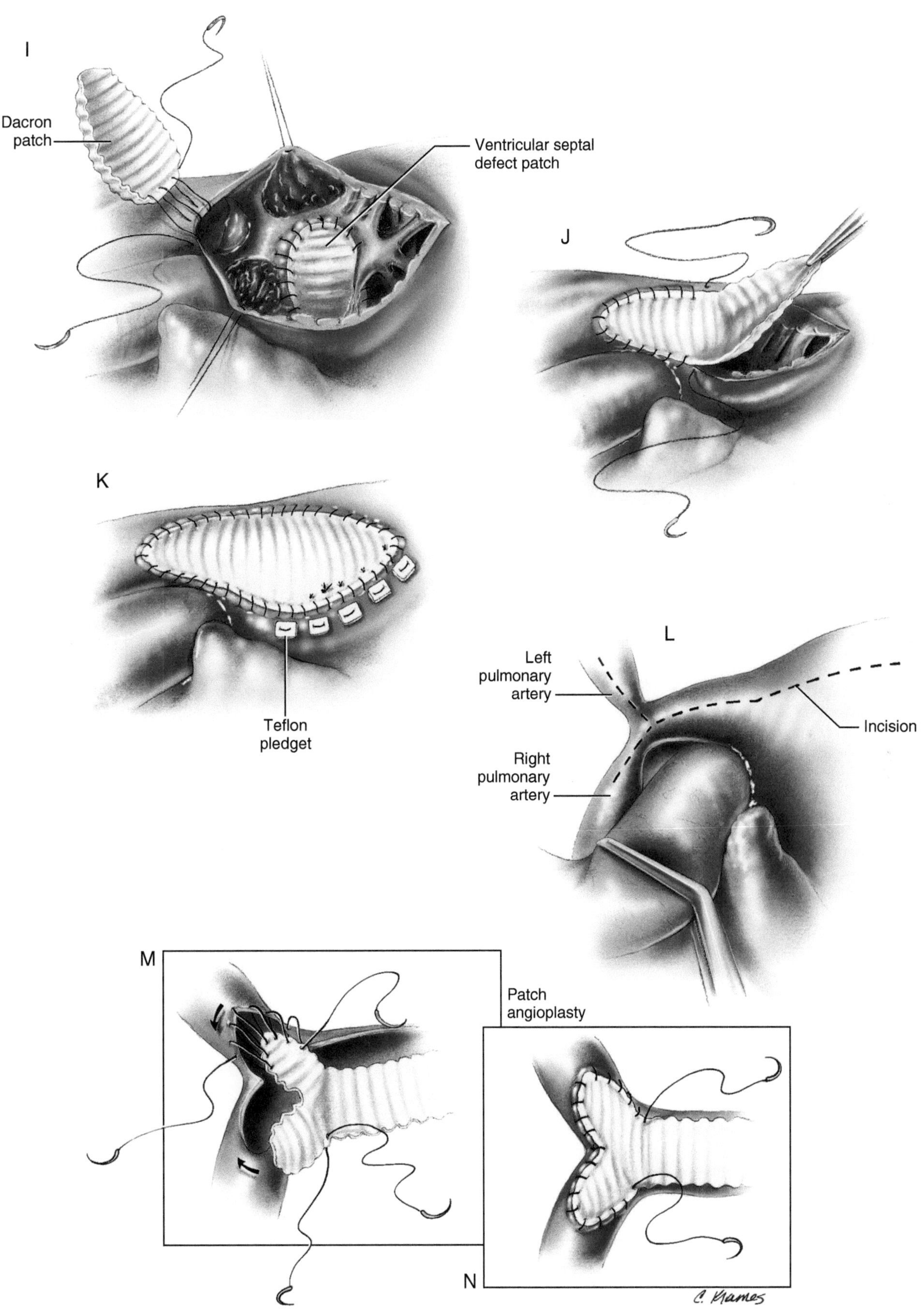
I
Dacron patch
Ventricular septal defect patch
J
K
Teflon pledget
L
Left pulmonary artery
Incision
Right pulmonary artery
M
Patch angioplasty
N
C. Hames

chapter 12 RIGHT VENTRICLE–PULMONARY ARTERY DISCONTINUITY

Congenital cardiac anomalies in which there is no usable connection of the pulmonary artery to the heart are treated by establishing a conduit between the right ventricle and the pulmonary artery.

Morphology

Included in this group of anomalies are conditions in which there is no connection (pulmonary atresia, truncus arteriosus) and those in which pulmonary outflow is so obstructed or stenosed that bypass is a more efficient means of restoring right ventricular–pulmonary continuity than reconstruction of the pulmonary outflow tract. This operation is also used in patients with transposition of the great arteries associated with ventricular septal defect and pulmonary stenosis. In this context the operation is referred to as the Rastelli procedure.

Figure 12-1

A Truncus arteriosus type I. This anomaly demonstrates the morphology of the group of defects that can be corrected by creating a conduit from the right ventricle to the pulmonary artery. There is a single great artery, the truncus arteriosus, which is connected to the left ventricular outflow tract. The pulmonary trunk takes its origin from the aorta just above the sinotubular junction. The valve guarding the truncal orifice in this specimen is a normal three-leaflet semilunar valve. There is a defect located high in the ventricular septum just below the truncal valve that communicates between the left and right ventricles.

B Truncus arteriosus type I. Magnified view of the truncus arteriosus showing the origin of the pulmonary artery from the aorta, the normal truncal valve, an outlet-type ventricular septal defect, and continuity of the mitral valve with the truncal valve.

C Truncus arteriosus type I. Magnified view of another specimen demonstrates the origin of the pulmonary artery from the truncus arteriosus above the sinotubular junction, the dysplastic truncal valve, and a high-lying ventricular septal defect.

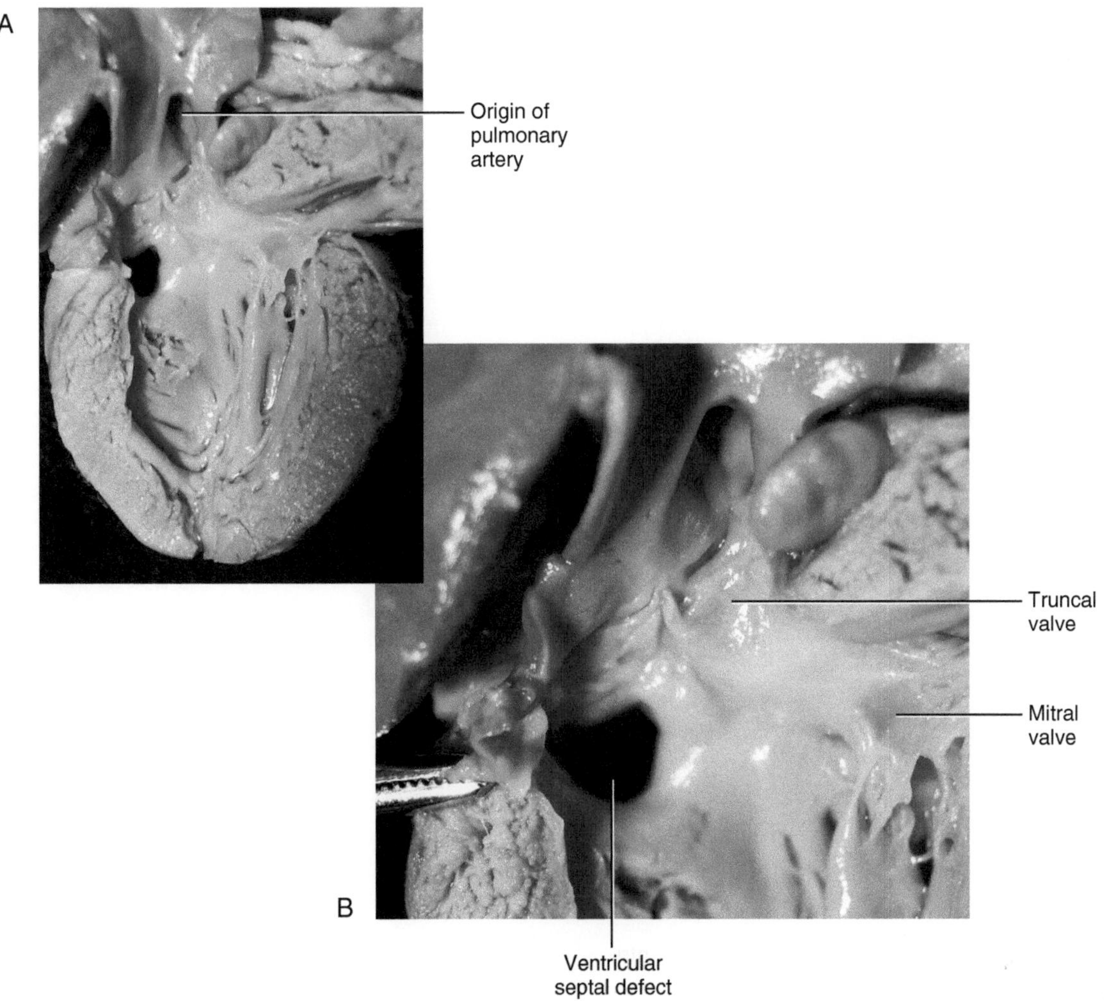
A
Origin of pulmonary artery
Truncal valve
Mitral valve
B
Ventricular septal defect

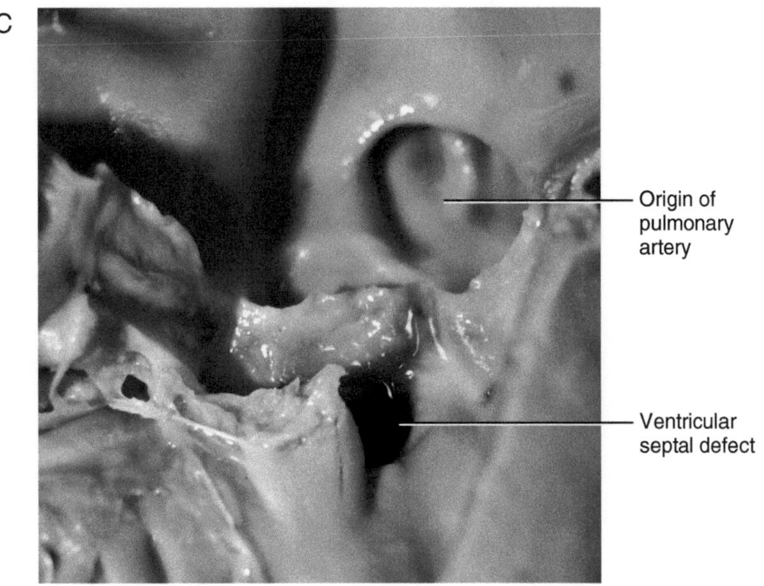
C
Origin of pulmonary artery
Ventricular septal defect

Figure 12-1 (continued)

D Truncus arteriosus type II. This type is defined by the side-by-side origin of the right and left pulmonary arteries from the aorta. The truncal valve has four dysplastic leaflets. The ventricular septal defect is just below the truncal valve.

E Truncus arteriosus type II. Magnified view shows greater detail of the dysplastic four-leaflet truncal valve.

F Truncus arteriosus type II, right ventricular view. The right and left pulmonary arteries are shown in their defined side-by-side relationship, originating from the aorta.

G Truncus arteriosus type II. Magnified view demonstrates greater detail of the origins of the right and left pulmonary arteries and the dysplastic truncal valve.

H Truncus arteriosus. The truncus arteriosus is continued as the ascending aorta and arch, with cut-off arch branch arteries on the left side of the image. On the right side are the pulmonary arteries joined with the lungs.

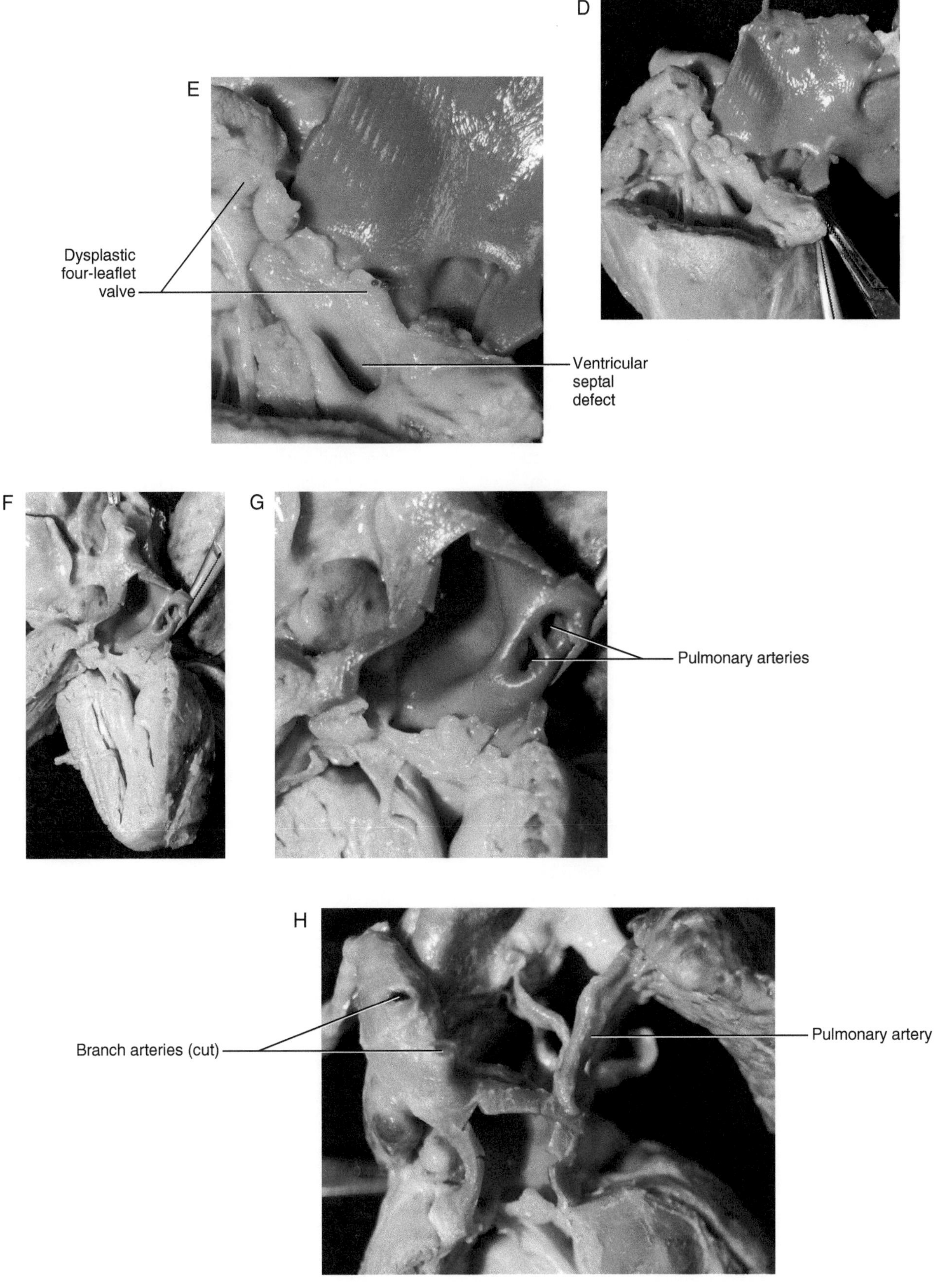
D
E
Dysplastic
four-leaflet
valve
Ventricular
septal
defect
F
G
Pulmonary arteries
H
Branch arteries (cut)
Pulmonary artery

Closure of Ventricular Septal Defect
Figure 12-2

A A right atriotomy is the initial step of the operation. Through the atriotomy a vent catheter is placed across the foramen ovale into the left atrium. To verify the diagnosis and determine whether complete repair is feasible, the intraventricular anatomy is inspected by retracting the tricuspid valve. A short transverse ventriculotomy is made parallel to the right ventricular branches of the right coronary artery to preserve the blood supply to the right ventricle. The ventriculotomy should be made as close as possible to the ventricular septal defect; its location is estimated based on the surface coronary artery anatomy. The edges of the ventriculotomy are undercut, thinning out the myocardium to the thickness of the normal right ventricle. Unobstructed egress from the body of the right ventricle must be achieved. Traction stitches are placed at the edges of the ventriculotomy to expose the ventricular septal defect.

B Closure of the ventricular septal defect varies according to the type of anomaly. For patients with pulmonary atresia–tetralogy of Fallot, the defect is closed by prosthetic patch, with the stitches placed to the right of the septum and inferior to the posterior rim of the ventricular septal defect to preserve the bundle of His, which courses along the rim of the defect. On the superior edge of the defect, the stitches are placed to the right of the aortic valve annulus in the crista supraventricularis to correct the dextroposition of the aorta.

C For patients with truncus arteriosus, the defect may be high in the ventricular septum, which means that the conduction system may not be in the rim of the defect. If the papillary muscle of the conus is located a significant distance from the rim of the defect, the sutures can be placed in the inferior rim of the defect. When the papillary muscle of the conus is located in the usual position relative to a perimembranous defect, suture placement is as usual for that type of defect. Superiorly, the stitches are placed to the right of the aortic valve annulus.

D For D-transposition of the great arteries with ventricular septal defect and pulmonary stenosis or atresia, the defect is a perimembranous type and is closed by prosthetic patch, with the stitches placed to the right of the septum and inferior to the posterior rim of the defect. Different rules apply to L-transposition anomalies. In these cases, the suture line is deviated from the edge of the ventricular septal defect superiorly onto the subaortic conus. The stitches are placed to the right of the aortic valve annulus, creating a passageway through the subaortic conus, which brings the ventricular septal defect in continuity with the aortic valve annulus.

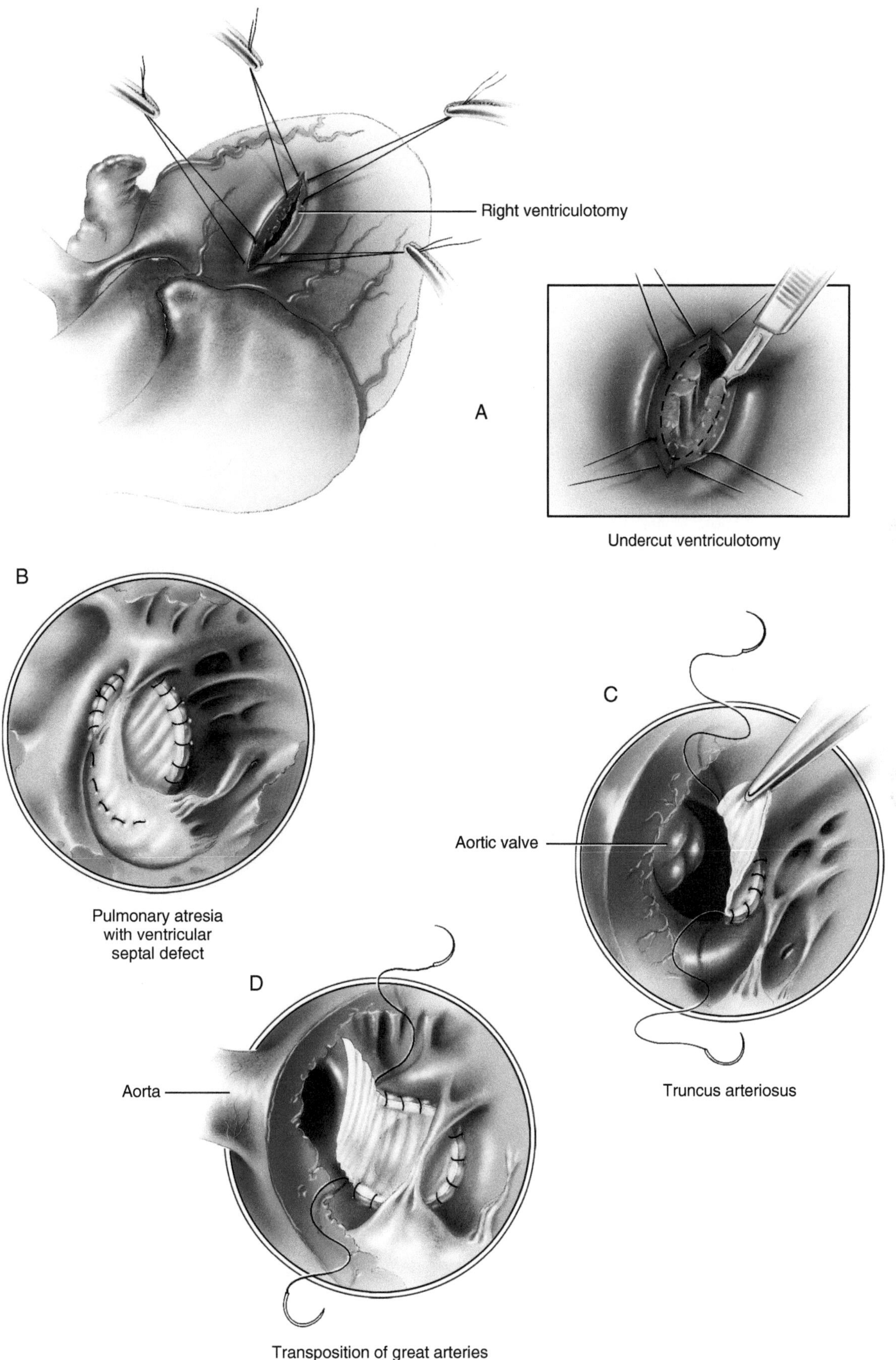
Right ventriculotomy
A
Undercut ventriculotomy
B
Pulmonary atresia
with ventricular
septal defect
C
Aortic valve
Truncus arteriosus
D
Aorta
Transposition of great arteries

Right Ventricle–to–Pulmonary Artery Conduit
Figure 12-3

A An incision is made into the confluent portion of the pulmonary artery. If necessary to achieve adequate length, the incision is extended onto the left pulmonary artery.

B The distal end of a prosthetic valved conduit is shortened to a point just above the heterograft valve. The conduit shown here is meant to be generic; valves from a variety of species have been employed. The composite valved conduit is approximated to the pulmonary artery by continuous suture. To ensure accurate closure, several suture loops are placed around the apex of the incision onto the left pulmonary artery before the prosthesis is pulled into the arteriotomy. Generous bites of tissue are taken in each stitch, including as much of the overlying pericardial tissue as possible to strengthen the anastomosis and ensure a tight tissue-to-graft approximation. The pulmonary artery is often thin and fragile, making it extremely important to use accurate suture technique and follow the arc of the needle precisely. Low-flow cardiopulmonary bypass or short periods of circulatory arrest, which reduce the amount of blood in the pulmonary artery due to aortopulmonary collateral flow, are useful to achieve optimal visualization of the anastomosis. The suture line is continued in a counterclockwise fashion about halfway around the anastomosis.

C The suture line is completed in a clockwise fashion anteriorly. Placing the valve portion of the conduit close to the pulmonary artery avoids compression of either the valve or the surface coronary arteries.

D The proximal end of the composite conduit is shortened and beveled for approximation to the right ventriculotomy. A continuous stitch of 4/0 polypropylene is used to anastomose the conduit to the surface of the right ventricle. Several suture loops are placed at the heel of the conduit to ensure accurate approximation.

E The suture line is taken in a counterclockwise fashion to the right lateral margin of the ventriculotomy. The anastomosis of the conduit to the surface of the right ventricle is completed in a clockwise fashion around the toe of the valved conduit. Several interrupted pledget-reinforced mattress stitches are placed to reinforce the anastomosis if the branch pulmonary arteries are small or if there is evidence of obstructive pulmonary vascular disease, which will likely result in high postoperative right ventricular pressure.

F Allograft tissue can be used for the conduit. Both aortic and pulmonary allografts have been used for this purpose, but the pulmonary allograft may be preferred because of its favorable anatomic structure. The graft usually consists of a portion of the outflow tract of the right ventricle, the pulmonary valve, and the pulmonary artery, including the right and left branches. The myocardium of the outflow tract is trimmed, leaving the scalloped pulmonary valve hinge point ("annulus"). A polytetrafluoroethylene (PTFE) graft of appropriate size is fashioned to match the scallop of the pulmonary valve and is attached by continuous suture to the pulmonary allograft. An externally reinforced graft can be used if there is concern that anterior chest call compression might occur after repair. The pulmonary artery bifurcation is opened by incision of the superior aspect between the right and left branches of the pulmonary artery.

G The reconstruction is performed as described previously, with incisions in the right ventricle and pulmonary artery confluence.

H The allograft is fashioned to fit into and widen the pulmonary artery confluence. Its anatomic shape conforms nicely for this purpose. Continuous suture is used for reconstruction of the pulmonary bifurcation. The proximal PTFE portion of the graft is shortened and beveled appropriately and anastomosed to the right ventriculotomy to complete the repair.

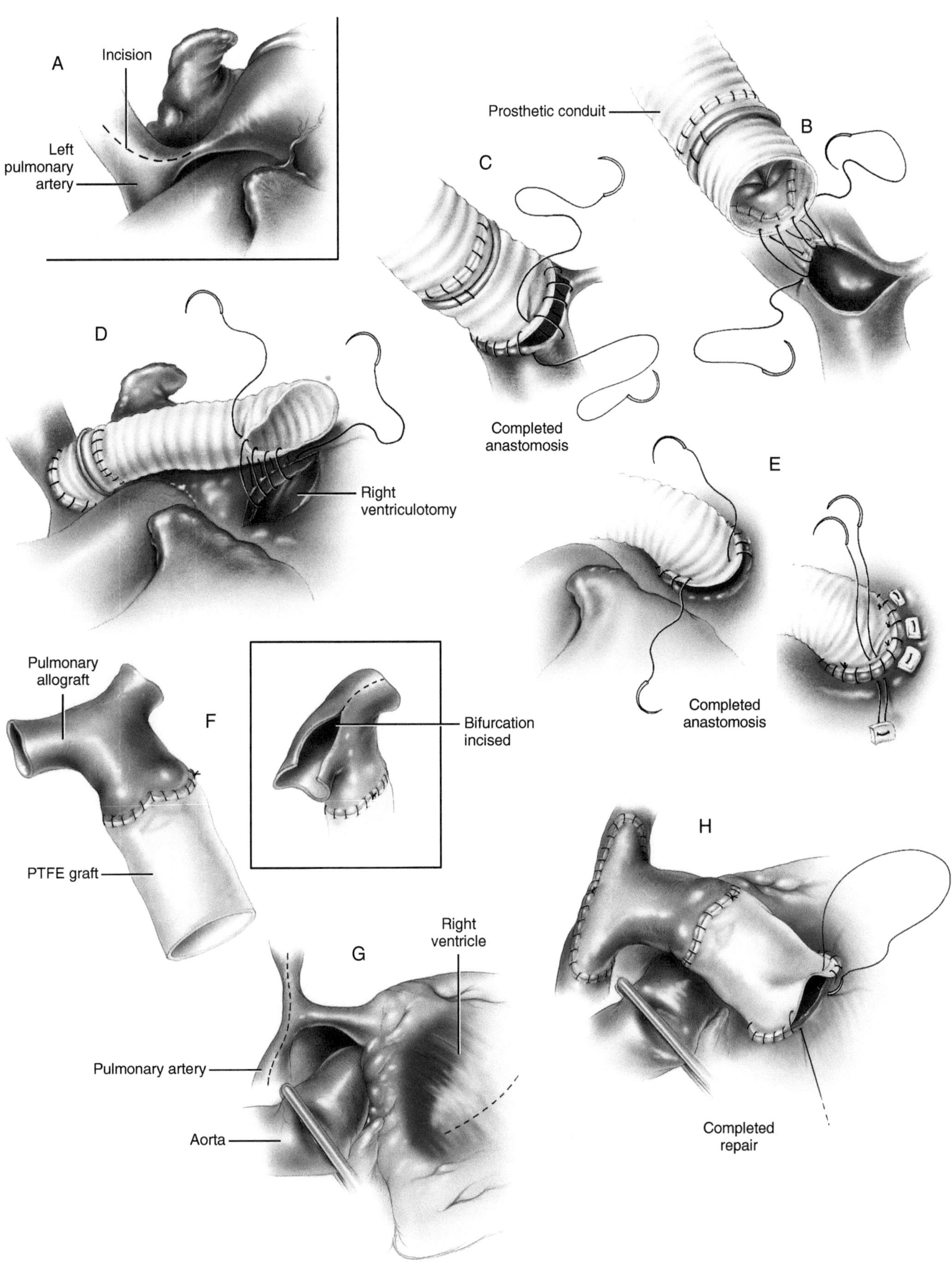
A
Incision
Left
pulmonary
artery
Prosthetic conduit
B
C
D
Completed
anastomosis
E
Right
ventriculotomy
Pulmonary
allograft
F
Bifurcation
incised
Completed
anastomosis
H
PTFE graft
Right
ventricle
G
Pulmonary artery
Aorta
Completed
repair

chapter 13 EBSTEIN'S ANOMALY

Ebstein's anomaly encompasses a spectrum of abnormalities that have in common the distal displacement and abnormal attachment of the tricuspid valve.

Morphology

In mild to moderate forms, the posterior leaflet and part of the septal leaflet are displaced and attached below the annulus. The portion of the ventricle between the annulus and the valve attachment is thinned and shows anatomic atrialization. In the most severe forms, the anterior leaflet is abnormally attached to a shelf-like structure in the right ventricle, so that the tricuspid valve acts as a barrier to the passage of blood from the right atrium to the right ventricle.

Figure 13-1

A Ebstein's anomaly, mild form. The septal leaflet of the tricuspid valve is attached to the right ventricle on the septum. There is minimal displacement of the tricuspid annulus. The anterior leaflet of the valve is enlarged compared with the other leaflets. There is an atrial septal defect.

B Ebstein's anomaly, mild form. Magnified view demonstrates the details of the septal attachment of the tricuspid valve.

C Ebstein's anomaly, moderate form. There is denser attachment of the tricuspid valve to the ventricular septum. Valve leaflet tissue is inadequate to occlude the valve orifice. Marked right ventricular hypertrophy and an atrial septal defect are present.

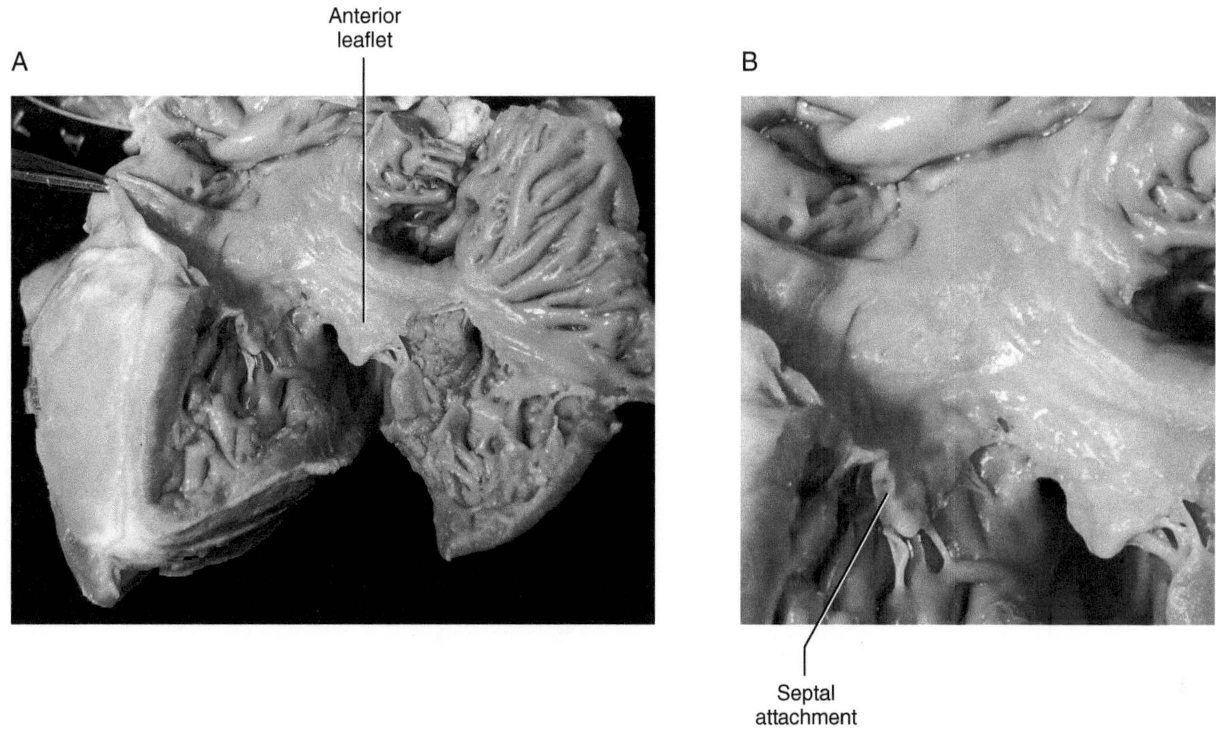
A
Anterior
leaflet
B
Septal
attachment

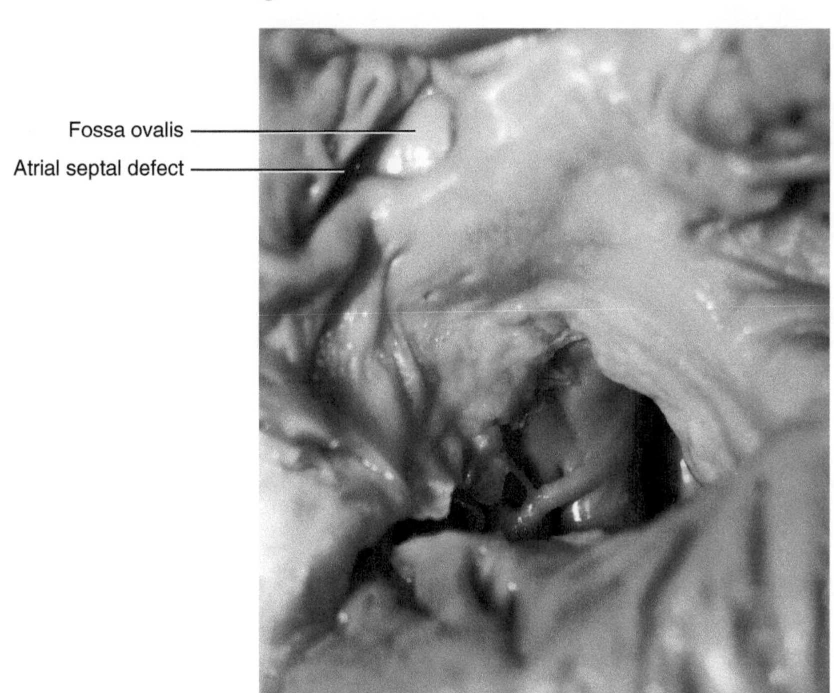
C
Fossa ovalis
Atrial septal defect

Tricuspid Repair or Replacement

Severe forms of Ebstein's anomaly must be treated by valve replacement or the Fontan procedure. Moderate forms are treated by valvuloplasty-annuloplasty techniques. The principles of repair are based on plication of the atrialized portion of the right ventricle and a posterior tricuspid annuloplasty to create a monocusp valve from the sail-like anterior leaflet or rearrangement of the anterior and free portions of the posterior leaflets to better occlude the right atrioventricular orifice.

Figure 13-2

A Pledget-reinforced mattress stitches are placed through the base of the anterior and posterior leaflets of the tricuspid valve.

B Several stitches are taken through the atrialized portion of the ventricle. Sutures are passed through the true annulus of the tricuspid valve and through a Carpentier tricuspid annuloplasty ring.

C When the sutures are tied down to the annuloplasty ring, the atrialized ventricle is plicated, and the aneurysmal portions of the right ventricle are eliminated. Reduction of the size of the tricuspid annulus brings the anterior leaflet in contact with the ventricular septum to function as a monocusp valve.

D Valve replacement is performed when the tricuspid valve leaflets are insufficient to occlude the tricuspid orifice. The tricuspid valve remnants are excised in the usual fashion.

E Pledget-reinforced mattress stitches of 2/0 braided suture are placed in the anterior leaflet annulus. The atrialized portion of the ventricle is plicated to the annulus with the valve attachment sutures. The repair is secured to a prosthetic valve. A large prosthesis is usually required because of the extensive dilation of the tricuspid orifice.

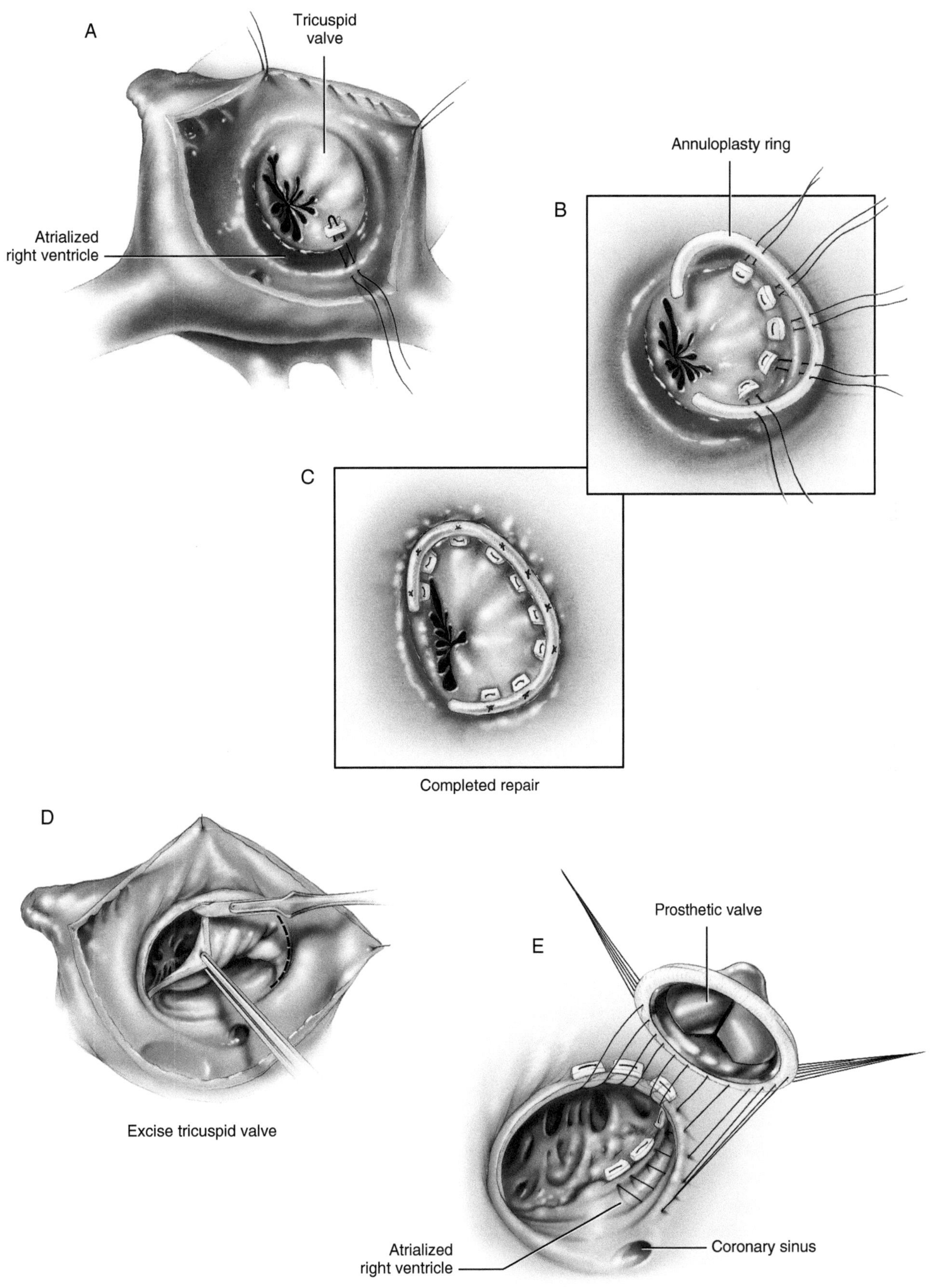
A
Tricuspid valve
Atrialized right ventricle
Annuloplasty ring
B
C
Completed repair
D
Excise tricuspid valve
Prosthetic valve
E
Atrialized right ventricle
Coronary sinus

Rotation Valvuloplasty-Annuloplasty (Carpentier Method)

Classic repairs of Ebstein's anomaly plicate the atrialized portion of the ventricle to the tricuspid annulus in a horizontal fashion. Carpentier introduced vertical plication of the atrialized ventricle and the accompanying narrowing of the annulus. The tricuspid valve may be rotated to more completely occlude the tricuspid orifice.

Figure 13-3

A Ebstein's anomaly of the tricuspid valve. The septal and posterior leaflets of the tricuspid valve are displaced into the ventricle and attached to the ventricular wall. The space occupied by the valve attachment below the annulus is called the atrialized portion of the ventricle. The anterior leaflet is usually enlarged and sail-like. The tricuspid orifice is often greatly dilated.

B The anterior leaflet of the tricuspid valve is detached from the annulus. The incision is continued to the point where the valve begins to be displaced onto the ventricular wall.

C The detached anterior leaflet is pulled toward the septum to expose the support mechanism. There is usually chordal fusion, which may be marked in some cases. Fenestrations are made in the support mechanism to lengthen the chordae tendineae and relieve obstruction below the leaflets.

D Pledget-reinforced mattress stitches of 2/0 braided suture are placed to create a vertical plication of the atrialized portion of the ventricle. The stitches are continued through the level of the annulus and above, into the right atrium. The stitches can be woven across the atrialized portion or placed from edge to edge as shown here.

E The plication stitches are tied down, forcing the atrialized portion to the outside in a vertical fashion. The annulus is significantly narrowed by the plication.

F The detached portion of the anterior leaflet is rotated clockwise to reach the usual location of the commissure between the septal and posterior leaflets or beyond, as far as the anterior leaflet reaches on the septum. The anterior leaflet is reattached to the annulus in the new orientation. Continuous stitch of 4/0 Cardionyl or polypropylene is used for leaflet reattachment.

G The repair is supported by an appropriately sized Carpentier tricuspid annuloplasty ring, attached to the annulus using mattress stitches of 2/0 braided suture.

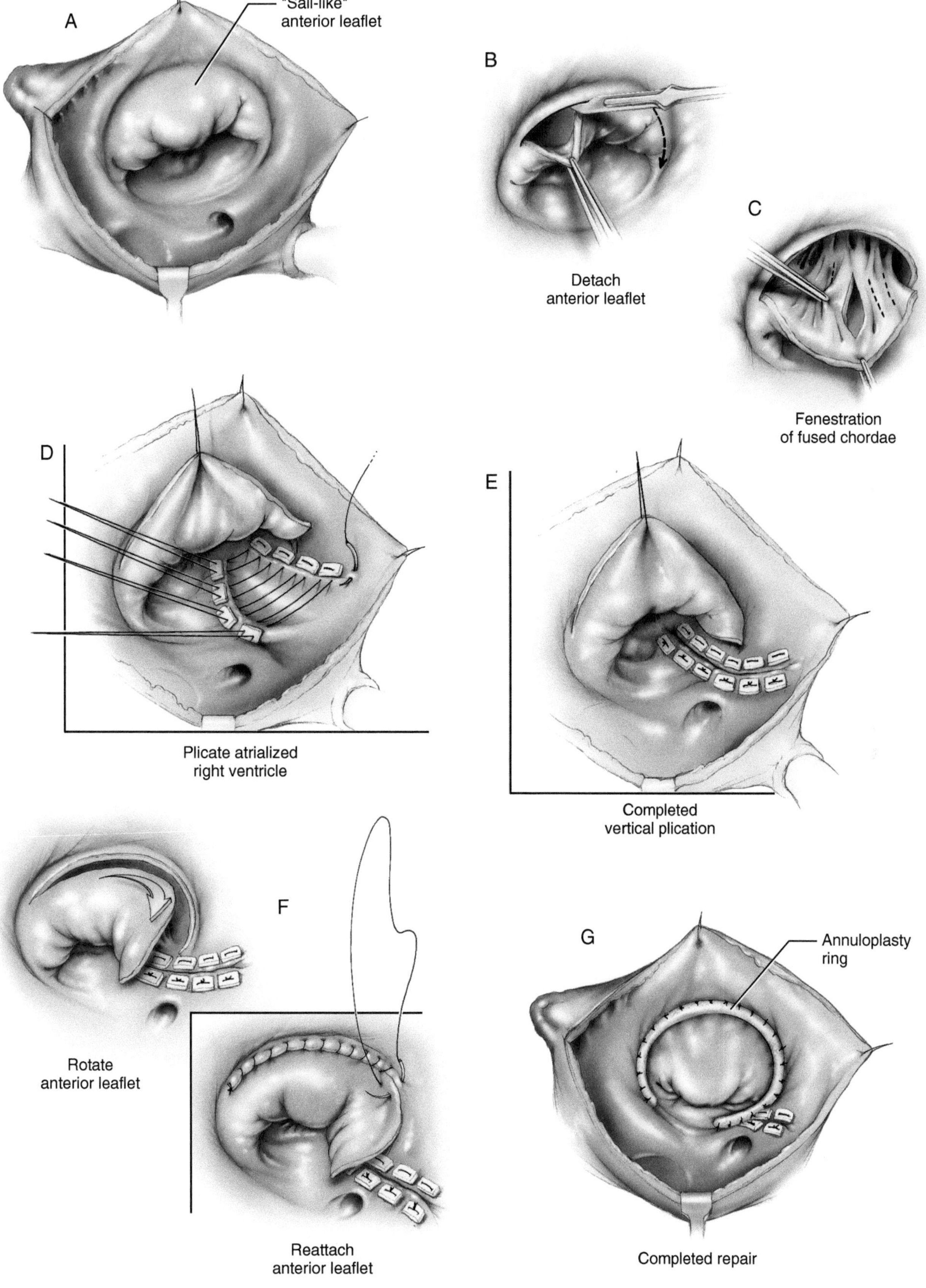
A
"Sail-like" anterior leaflet
B
Detach anterior leaflet
C
Fenestration of fused chordae
D
Plicate atrialized right ventricle
E
Completed vertical plication
F
Rotate anterior leaflet
Reattach anterior leaflet
G
Annuloplasty ring
Completed repair

part V

Left Heart Valve Lesions (Congenital)

chapter 14 AORTIC VALVE STENOSIS

Aortic valve stenosis is the most common form of congenital left ventricular outflow tract obstruction. Patients with congenital aortic valve stenosis may require operative intervention at any time. As a general rule, more severe lesions require earlier intervention.

Morphology
Figure 14-1

A Aortic valve stenosis, severe. The aortic valve is bicuspid, with fusion of the commissures, resulting in severe stenosis of the valve orifice. Generalized cardiomegaly accompanies this severe stenosis.

B Aortic valve stenosis, severe. This magnified image shows a bicuspid aortic valve, thickening of the leaflet tissue, and hypoplastic sinuses of Valsalva. The commissures of the valve are fused, and the orifice is severely stenotic.

C Severe aortic valve stenosis, left ventricular view. The left ventricular outflow tract is severely stenosed, and the left ventricle is markedly hypertrophied. The endocardium is normal, not showing any evidence of the endocardial fibroelastosis that commonly accompanies severe aortic valve stenosis in neonates.

D Severe aortic valve stenosis, left ventricular outflow tract, magnified image. The left ventricular outflow tract is severely obstructed by a small aortic valve annulus and dysplastic valve leaflet tissue.

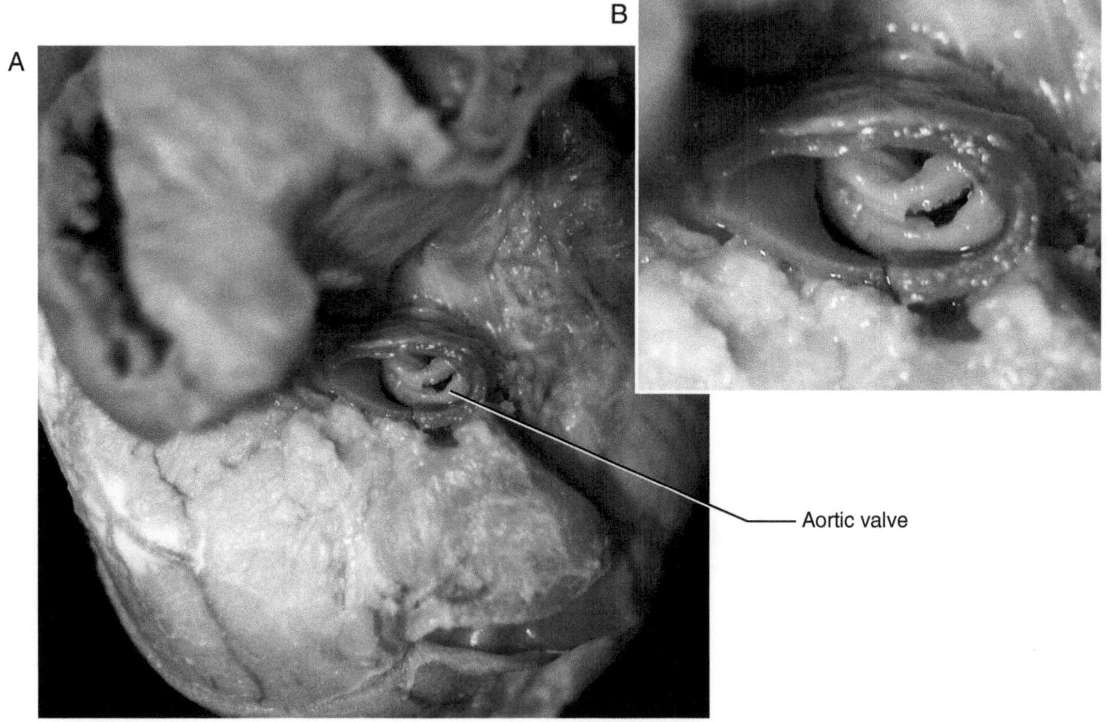
A
B
Aortic valve

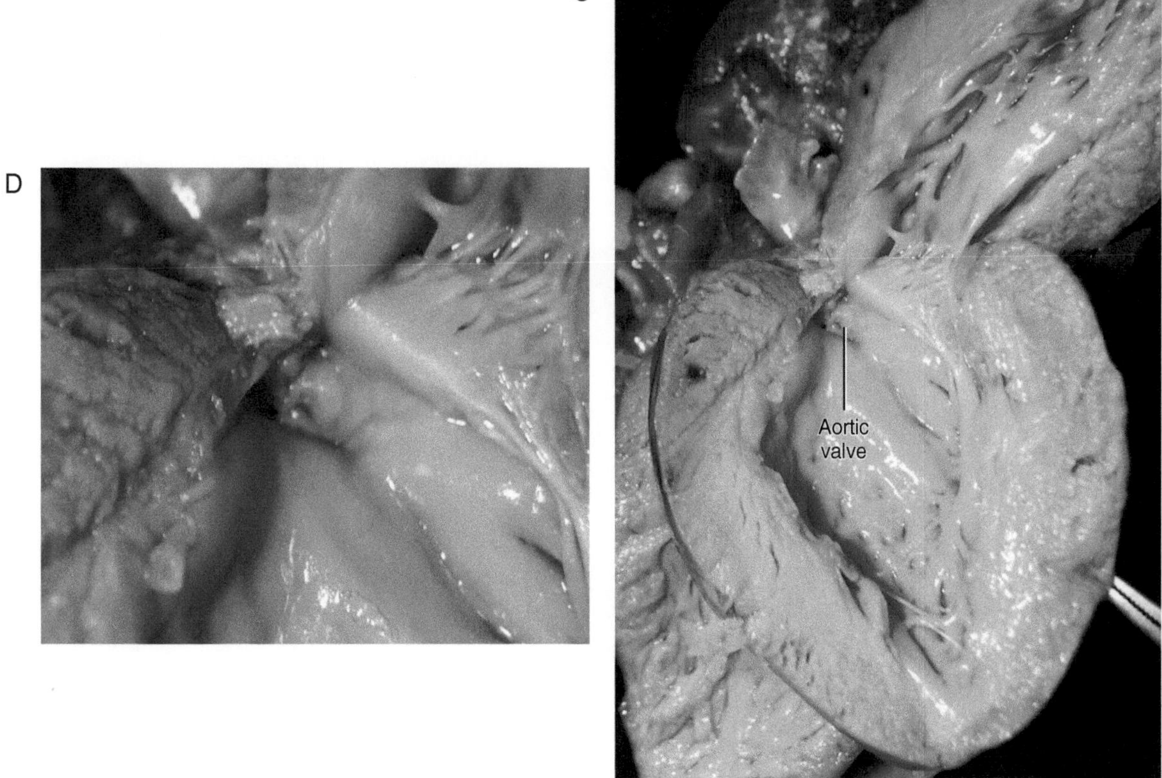
C
D
Aortic valve

Aortic Valvotomy

The operation is palliative, with the goal being to relieve left ventricular outflow tract obstruction without creating aortic valve incompetence. It is thought that the more complete the relief of obstruction, the longer the interval until a second operative intervention is required.

Figure 14-2

A The patient is placed on cardiopulmonary bypass, the aorta is cross-clamped, the left side of the heart is vented through the left atrium, and hypothermic cardioplegia is administered. A transverse incision is made in the ascending aorta above the sinuses of Valsalva. The incision is extended close to but not into the noncoronary sinus.

B A retractor is placed into the right coronary sinus of Valsalva to expose the congenitally stenosed valve. The valve almost always has a bicuspid configuration. After careful inspection of the valve, a decision is made as to which of the commissures to incise. A general principle is to avoid incising too much so that an incompetent aortic valve is created.

C While two forceps are used to align the cusps of the aortic valve, the chosen commissure is carefully incised to the wall of the aorta using a No. 15 scalpel. Optical magnification is helpful to ensure that the incision is placed accurately in the commissure to avoid detaching either of the cusps from the aortic wall. The valvuloplasty is completed, and the aortic valve is tested for approximation and competence by flooding the aortic root with saline. The valve orifice can be calibrated with Hegar dilators. The subvalvular area is examined for any associated lesions before the aortotomy is closed by continuous suture.

D Some patients present with a type of aortic stenosis in which the valve is bicuspid and commissural fusion is minimal. The left coronary sinus of Valsalva is small and may actually be hypoplastic. There is a prominent supravalvular ridge that shortens the distance between the commissures bordering the left sinus, producing deformity of the free edge of the aortic valve cusp. This morphology may be suspected from preoperative aortography, which reveals the typical supravalvular ridge over the left sinus and a slit-like deformity of the hypoplastic left sinus.

E As usual for valvular aortic stenosis, the initial oblique incision extends to the superior margin of but not into the sinus of Valsalva. When this morphology is confirmed, the aortotomy is extended onto the posterior wall of the aorta in a spiral fashion. The supravalvular ring is divided to the left of the posterior commissure. The incision is continued into the left coronary sinus, slightly to the left of and parallel to the commissure. The left coronary artery ostium is located to the left of the incision, and the leftward course of the artery prevents injury to it.

F A tubular, crimped Dacron prosthesis is used for the reconstruction and to enlarge the left sinus. A spiral-shaped graft is taken from the wall of the tubular graft. This graft will be used to close and widen the spiral incision in the left coronary sinus of Valsalva. Before the graft is pulled into position, four or five suture loops are placed in the graft and in the apex of the incision into the left coronary sinus of Valsalva.

G The suture line is continued along both edges of the aortotomy incision and is completed on the anterior wall of the aorta.

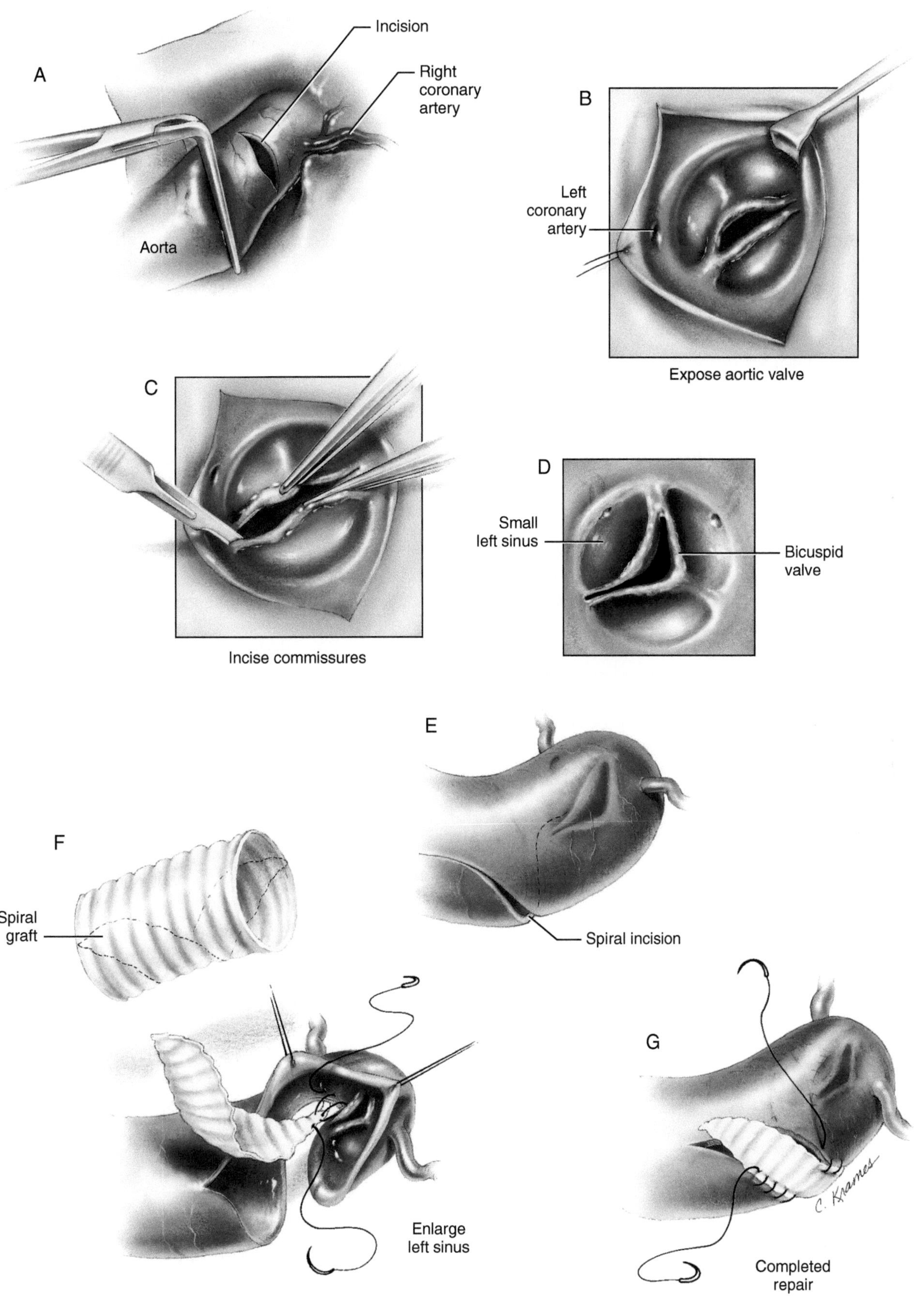
A
Incision
Right coronary artery
Aorta
B
Left coronary artery
Expose aortic valve
C
Incise commissures
D
Small left sinus
Bicuspid valve
E
Spiral incision
F
Spiral graft
Enlarge left sinus
G
C. Krames
Completed repair

Figure 14-2 (continued)

H In cases in which the left sinus is markedly hypoplastic and there is a prominent supravalvular ridge that brings the bordering commissures close together, there may be buckling of the free edge of the left cusp of the aortic valve. The valve is likely to be thickened, which, in combination with the buckling and folding effect, creates a major obstruction of the left ventricular outflow tract, even though there may be only minor commissural fusion. In these cases it is desirable to relocate the posterior commissure to straighten the free edge of the left cusp and achieve the best possible anatomic reconstruction.

I The spiral incision is made on the posterior aspect of the aorta and into the left sinus, alongside and to the left of the posterior commissure. A second incision is made into the noncoronary sinus just to the right of the posterior commissure.

J When these two incisions are extended deep into the sinuses to the level of the aortic annulus, they provide complete mobilization of the posterior commissure, allowing it to be repositioned to a more lateral and anterior location. This permits the left coronary cusp to achieve its full length at the free edge.

K A spiral graft is constructed from a tubular, crimped Dacron graft. The base of the graft is cut wide enough to span between the apices of the incision in the left and noncoronary sinuses. The aorta, with the attached posterior commissure, is retracted anteriorly to expose the external surface of the aorta. The spiral graft is attached to the aortic annulus on the exterior surface by continuous suture technique, placing deep stitches into the annulus from the outside.

L The suture line is continued along the lateral margins of the sinus incisions until the superior margin of the sinuses of Valsalva is reached. The posterior commissure is repositioned onto the spiral graft in a location that achieves the best possible anatomic appearance and thus the best function of the aortic valve. Any commissural fusion is incised. The aorta with attached posterior commissure is sutured to the graft in its new, more desirable position using continuous suture technique. A Teflon pledget can be placed at the top of the commissure for additional strength and security of its position.

M The repair is completed by approximating the graft to the edges of the aortotomy on the anterior aspect of the aorta.

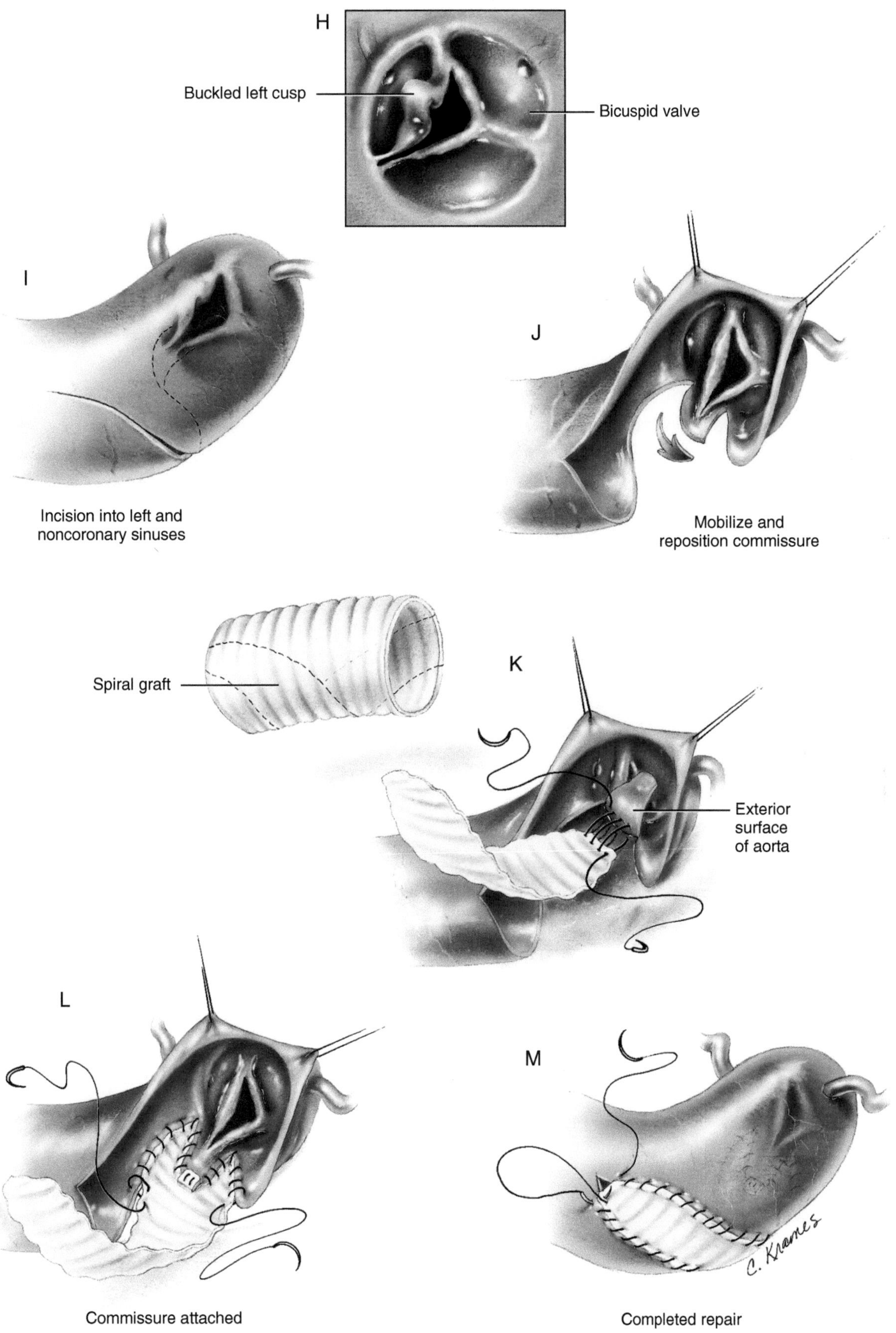

Incision into left and noncoronary sinuses

Mobilize and reposition commissure

Commissure attached

Completed repair

chapter 15 SUPRAVALVULAR AORTIC STENOSIS

Supravalvular aortic stenosis is the least common form of left ventricular outflow obstruction.

Morphology

There are two forms of the defect: localized and diffuse. The localized form encompasses the so-called hourglass and membranous forms. The diffuse form involves not only the sinus rim but also the ascending aorta, arch, and arch arterial branches. Supravalvular aortic stenosis should be thought of as a complex anomaly of the aortic root. The narrowing and thickening of the sinus rim are fundamental to the defect's morphology. The aortic valves are involved because the relationships of the commissures are distorted as they are drawn close together by the shortened and thickened sinus rim. This distortion produces a characteristic buckling of the free edge of the aortic valve because the normal length adjusts for the shortened space at the sinus rim. The buckled aortic cusps become part of the obstruction in a space too small to accommodate them. The free edge of the aortic cusps is usually a normal length in young patients.

Figure 15-1

A Left ventricular outflow tract obstruction caused by the localized form of supravalvular aortic stenosis can often be relieved simply by placing a diamond-shaped patch across the sinus rim in the noncoronary sinus of Valsalva. This is the classic operation, and it usually reduces or eliminates pressure gradients between the left ventricle and the ascending aorta. Unfortunately, this operation accomplishes little in terms of rebuilding or remodeling the other aortic root abnormalities that usually accompany thickening and narrowing of the sinus rim.

B Operations that achieve the best reconstruction of the entire aortic root have the best chance of giving the patient a good early result and a longer interval until a secondary operation on the aortic valve or aortic root becomes necessary. The authors proposed an extended patch aortoplasty to achieve a more symmetric reconstruction of the aortic root. The sinus rim is divided at two points opposite each other, and the incisions are extended into both the noncoronary sinus and the right coronary sinus between the right coronary ostium and the commissure between the left and right cusps of the aortic valve. Dividing the sinus rim at two points allows the noncoronary cusp and the right coronary cusp of the aortic valve to stretch out to a normal length. Buckling of the valve is relieved as the halves of the aorta are separated anteriorly and posteriorly. The aortic root is reconstructed by extended patch angioplasty. The patch is fashioned so that it extends into each of the incised sinuses.

C Brom described an operation in which incisions are made into all three aortic sinuses after transection of the aorta. Pericardial patches are inserted to widen the sinus and sinus rim and achieve symmetric reconstruction of the aortic root.

D Myers reported a method called the V-Y flap technique. The thickened and stenosed sinus rim is resected by aortic transection. The three sinuses are incised (V). The ascending aorta is completely mobilized and then cut back to create flaps (Y), which are then advanced into the incisions in the aortic sinuses. This method does not employ prosthetic material and may be better at retaining the elastic properties of the aortic root.

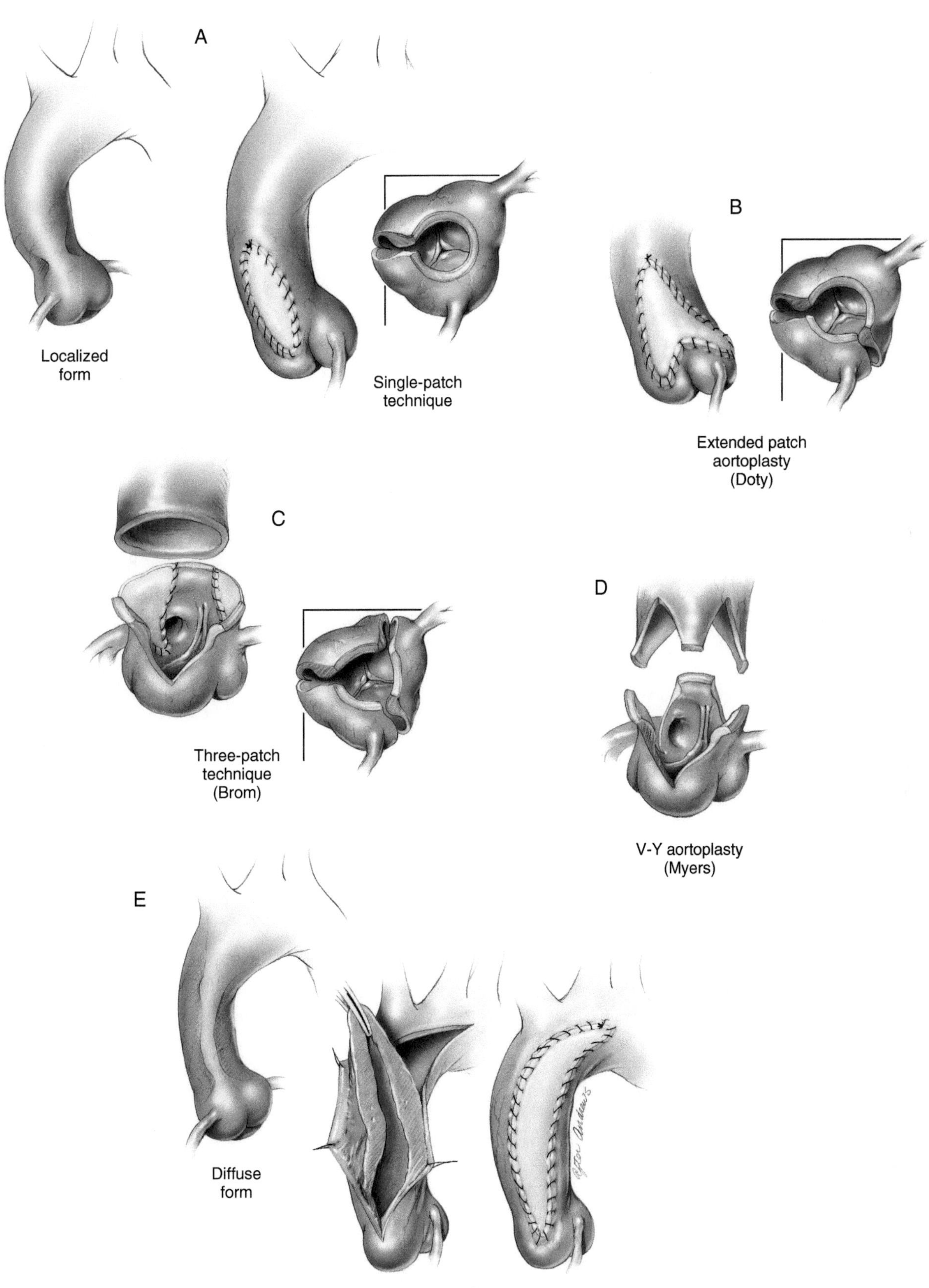
A
Localized form
Single-patch technique
B
Extended patch aortoplasty (Doty)
C
Three-patch technique (Brom)
D
V-Y aortoplasty (Myers)
E
Diffuse form
Endarterectomy-aortoplasty

Figure 15-1 (continued)

E Operations to correct the diffuse form of supravalvular aortic stenosis are less well defined. The diffuse form has been treated by a variety of operations, including patch aortoplasty, left ventricular apex–to–aorta conduits, aortic resection with graft replacement, and extensive endarterectomy of the ascending aorta and arch with patch aortoplasty. The last method seems to be promising because it is directed at the diffuse pathology of the anomaly. It is known that the morphologic defect involves the media and intima, so it is logical to remove that portion of the aortic wall by endarterectomy. Patch aortoplasty that does not widen the entire ascending aorta and aortic arch, however, may not correct the aortic valve obstruction.

Extended Aortoplasty

Extended aortoplasty is performed in patients with the localized or hourglass form of supravalvular aortic stenosis. This operation opens the stenotic ring at two points and achieves symmetric reconstruction of the aortic root.

Figure 15-2

A The patient is placed on cardiopulmonary bypass, the aorta is occluded, the left heart is vented through the left atrium, and the heart is arrested by cold cardioplegia. An oblique incision is made in the ascending aorta toward the noncoronary sinus of Valsalva. The extent of the supravalvular deformity can be assessed through this incision. The fibrosing supravalvular ring is located at the superior margin of the sinuses of Valsalva (sinotubular junction). The leaflets of the valve are secondarily involved because the commissures are drawn close together by the stenosing ring. This causes buckling of the free edge of the valve cusps. There is usually some fibrosis and thickening of the leaflets secondary to turbulent blood flow, but the edges of the cusps generally retain a normal length unless the fibrotic process is advanced. Once the presence of the usual hourglass type of supravalvular stenosis is confirmed, the stenosing ring must be incised at least twice. Incision of the aorta at two opposite points on the ring allows the anterior portion of the ring to move farther anteriorly, for symmetric widening of the aorta. The first incision is made across the stenosing ring into the center of the noncoronary sinus of Valsalva to the level of the aortic annulus. The second incision is made into the right coronary sinus just anterior to the commissure between the left and right coronary cusps.

B If these two incisions do not produce adequate widening of the aortic outflow tract, a third incision can be made in the left coronary sinus, close and parallel to the commissure between the left and right coronary sinuses. These incisions should allow the normal length of the aortic leaflets to be achieved.

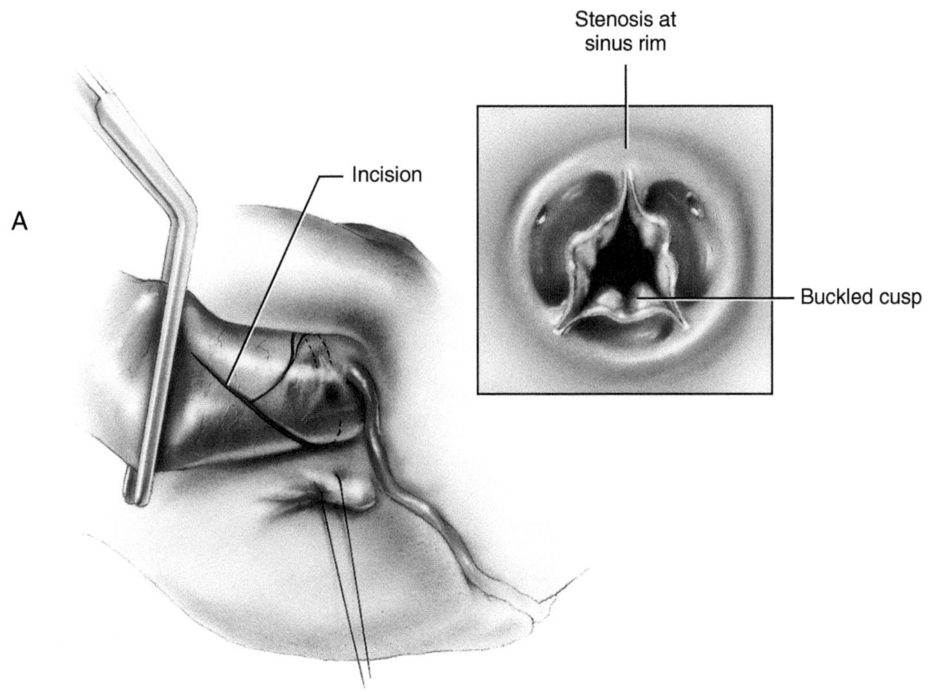
A
Incision
Stenosis at
sinus rim
Buckled cusp

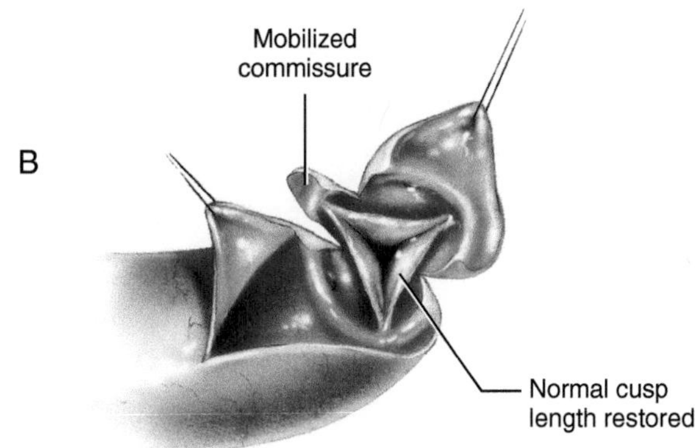
B
Mobilized
commissure
Normal cusp
length restored

Figure 15-2 (continued)

C A tubular graft of crimped Dacron is used to create the patch for the aortoplasty. Two extensions of the graft are fashioned to reconstruct the right and noncoronary sinuses of Valsalva, and a wedge of the graft is excised to accommodate the anterior wall of the aorta, which contains the right coronary artery. Sufficient graft length is retained to allow adequate anterior bulging of the reconstructed aorta.

D The graft is sutured to the aortic annulus behind the commissure of the left and right coronary cusps using a continuous stitch of 4/0 polypropylene. These stitches are placed from the adventitial surface of the aorta, taking care to attach the patch firmly.

E The suture line is continued along the aortic incision, in the right coronary sinus, and in the left coronary sinus of Valsalva above the level of the supravalvular ring.

F A second suture is used to approximate the graft to the aortic wall to which the commissure between the right and left cusps is attached, in an appropriate orientation for correct coaptation of the valve leaflets. The final stitch can be placed through a Teflon felt pledget to bolster the attachment of the top of the commissure. The stitch is passed to the outside of the Dacron graft.

G The opposite limb of the graft is then placed into the noncoronary sinus of Valsalva and sutured into position with a running stitch of 4/0 polypropylene. Several suture loops are placed into the apex of the incision to ensure that the graft is correctly approximated to the aorta before the suture loops are pulled up.

H The suture line is continued across the aorta above the right coronary artery and completed anteriorly. The suture line is then continued along the aortotomy incision and completed at the superior end. Care is taken to place sufficient graft material into the aortotomy to allow anterior bulging of the graft once the aorta is filled with blood.

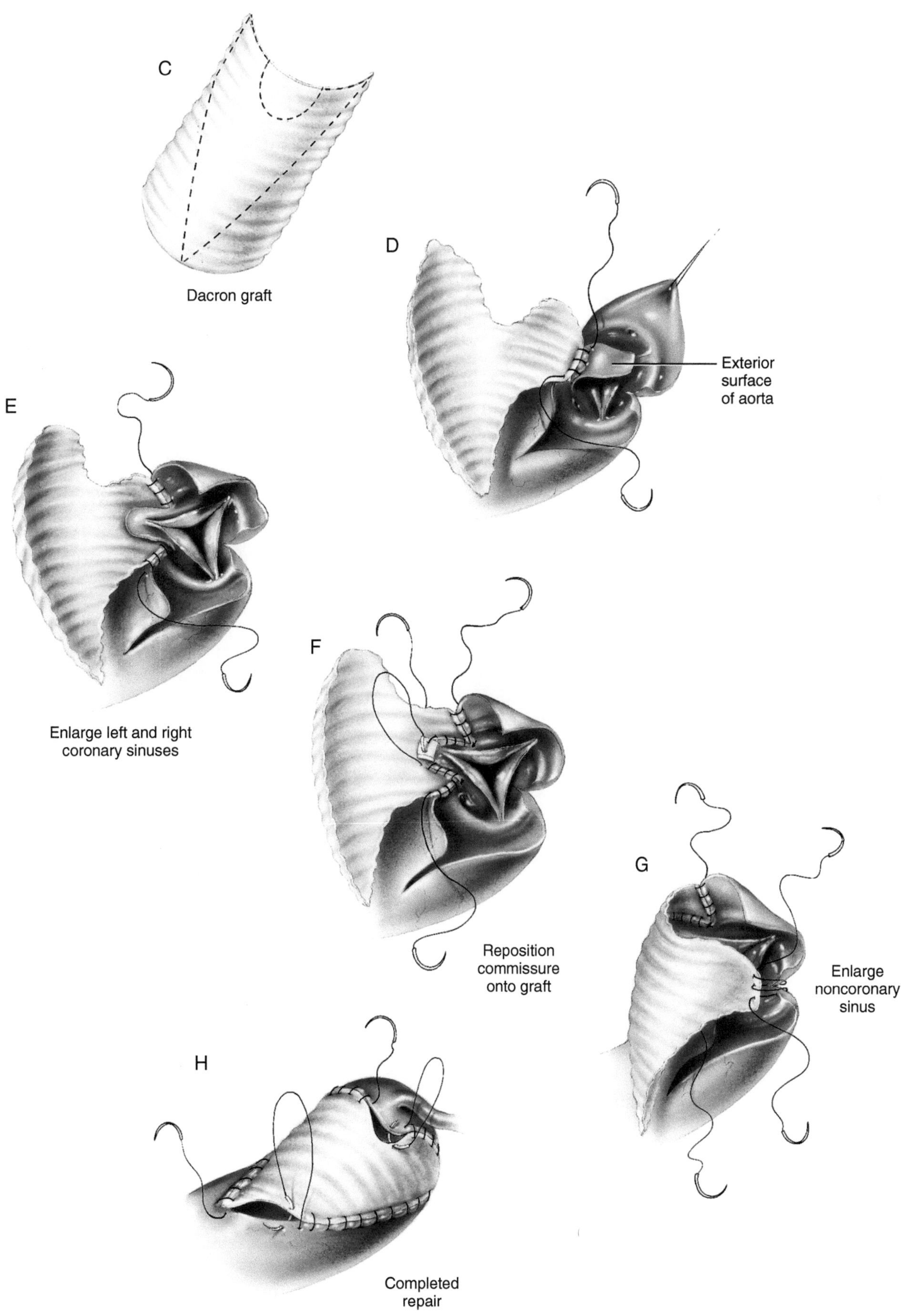
C
Dacron graft
D
Exterior
surface
of aorta
E
Enlarge left and right
coronary sinuses
F
Reposition
commissure
onto graft
G
Enlarge
noncoronary
sinus
H
Completed
repair

chapter 16 SUBVALVULAR AORTIC STENOSIS

Subvalvular aortic stenosis includes anomalies causing left ventricular outflow obstruction that are located primarily below the aortic valve. It is customary to divide subvalvular aortic stenosis into two types: the localized membranous or fibromuscular (fixed) type and the diffuse or tunnel type. The membranous or fibromuscular type is represented by the formation of a discrete fibrous circumferential diaphragm that extends from the septum onto the anterior leaflet of the mitral valve.

Localized Fibromuscular Type
Figure 16-1

A The aorta is occluded, and the heart is arrested by the infusion of cold cardioplegia. A transverse incision is made in the ascending aorta, extending toward the noncoronary sinus of Valsalva.

B The aortic valve is inspected for any associated abnormality. The cusp structure is examined, and the sinuses of Valsalva are inspected for associated supravalvular abnormalities. The right coronary cusp of the aortic valve is retracted anteriorly, exposing the subvalvular fibromuscular ring. While working through the aortic valve, the surgeon must take care not to injure the cusps of the valve. A retractor placed against the right coronary cusp provides exposure and protection of the right coronary cusp. The proposed area of septal excision should be located anterior to the membranous portion of the ventricular septum and away from the course of the bundle of His. In general, the portion of the fibromuscular ring from the commissure of the left and right coronary cusps of the aortic valve to the midportion of the right cusp can be safely excised.

C With a No. 11 scalpel, a wedge excision of the fibromuscular ring is performed anterior to and to the left of the conduction system. The center of the right coronary cusp is used as a reference point for the initial incision into the fibromuscular ring. The second point of penetration is below the commissure between the right and left coronary cusps. Deep incisions into the septum at these points provide a significant wedge of septum for excision. The scalpel is thrust into the fibromuscular obstruction and drawn posteriorly into the outflow tract to cut parallel grooves in the septum. The tissue in between can be removed as a wedge. A septal myotomy can be continued to the base of the anterior papillary muscle of the mitral valve if there is associated septal hypertrophy.

D Débridement of the obstructing fibrous portion of the subvalvular ring must be performed with great care because the fibrous ring is attached to the annulus of the mitral valve. Deep excision of the fibrous ring may detach the anterior leaflet of the mitral valve, producing mitral valve insufficiency. Débridement of the subvalvular ring in the area of the anterior leaflet of the mitral valve must be superficial to avoid including the full thickness of the mitral leaflet or annulus.

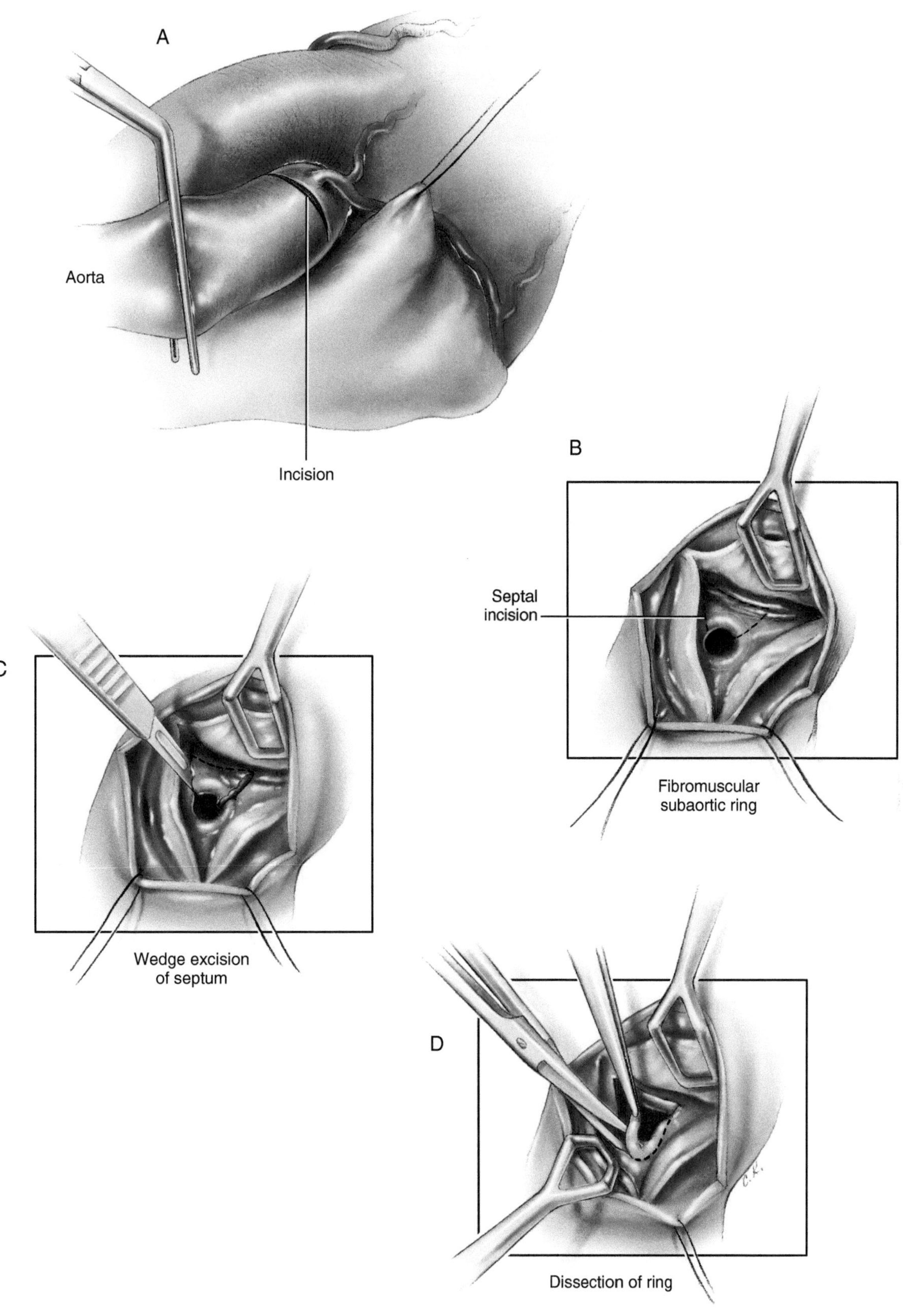
A
Aorta
Incision
B
Septal incision
Fibromuscular subaortic ring
C
Wedge excision of septum
D
Dissection of ring

Diffuse or Tunnel Type

This group of cardiac defects represents a spectrum of anomalies, including fibrous tunnel subaortic stenosis with a normal-sized aortic valve or hypoplastic aortic root and myocardial (muscular) abnormalities of localized or diffuse hypertrophic obstructive cardiomyopathy (HOCM). These various types of diffuse subaortic stenosis often blend imperceptibly, expressing some characteristics of the fibrous or muscular forms. There is even some evidence that the fibrous forms of diffuse or tunnel subaortic stenosis and HOCM represent different degrees of expression of the same genetically transmitted disease.

Illustrated here is asymmetric septal hypertrophy (also known as idiopathic hypertrophic subaortic stenosis), one form of the diffuse or tunnel type of subaortic stenosis.

Figure 16-2

A Aortic occlusion and arrest of the heart by the infusion of cold cardioplegia not only protect the ischemic heart but also greatly enhance subaortic exposure. A transverse incision is made in the ascending aorta, extending toward the noncoronary sinus of Valsalva.

B The aortic valve is inspected for any associated abnormality. The right coronary cusp of the aortic valve is retracted anteriorly, exposing the subvalvular shelf of hypertrophied septum. While working through the aortic valve, the surgeon must take care not to injure the cusps of the aortic valve. The tips of instruments, especially the scalpel, must be strictly controlled to prevent inadvertent perforation of the cusps. A retractor placed against the right coronary cusp provides both exposure and protection. A narrow, malleable ribbon retractor can be placed in the outflow tract to apply counterpressure to displace the left coronary cusp of the aortic valve posteriorly, protecting the valve cusp and providing additional exposure. The proposed area of septal excision should be located well anterior to the membranous portion of the ventricular septum to avoid interrupting the course of the bundle of His. In general, the portion of the hypertrophied septum from the commissure of the left and right coronary cusps of the aortic valve to the midportion of the right cusp can be safely excised.

C A No. 11 scalpel is used to perform a rectangular excision of the hypertrophied septum anterior to and to the left of the conduction system. The center of the right coronary cusp is used as a reference point for the initial incision into the septum. The second point of penetration is below the commissure between the right and left coronary cusps. Deep incisions into the septum at these points provide a significant groove for excision. The scalpel is thrust into the septum and drawn posteriorly into the outflow tract to cut parallel grooves in the septum. The tissue in between the incisions is joined by a transverse incision and the muscle bar is removed, creating a deep passageway in the septum and enlarging the outflow tract.

D The septal myotomy is continued to the base of the anterior papillary muscle of the mitral valve. The depth of the septal myotomy can be gauged by placing the index finger of the left hand into the outflow tract and palpating the exterior anterior wall of the heart with the thumb. Débridement of the obstructing muscle of the subvalvular ring should be as deep and complete as feasible, without perforating the septum. Deep excision of the septum should provide a rectangular channel that is not obliterated when the anterior leaflet of the mitral valve approximates the septum during systole.

E In some situations the mitral valve and its supporting structure compound the left ventricular outflow tract obstruction in patients with asymmetric septal hypertrophy. The anterior leaflet of the mitral valve may be markedly displaced into the left ventricular outflow tract so that it approximates the septum during ventricular systole. The mitral valve may also be incompetent. In this case, mitral valve replacement with septal myectomy is performed.

F Septal myectomy is performed by working through the aortic valve. The septal excision is taken to the base of the anterior papillary muscle of the mitral valve. Mitral valve replacement is then performed in the usual fashion, approaching the valve via the left atrium. The chordae tendineae of the mitral valve are preserved, except for any that may be located in the left ventricular outflow tract.

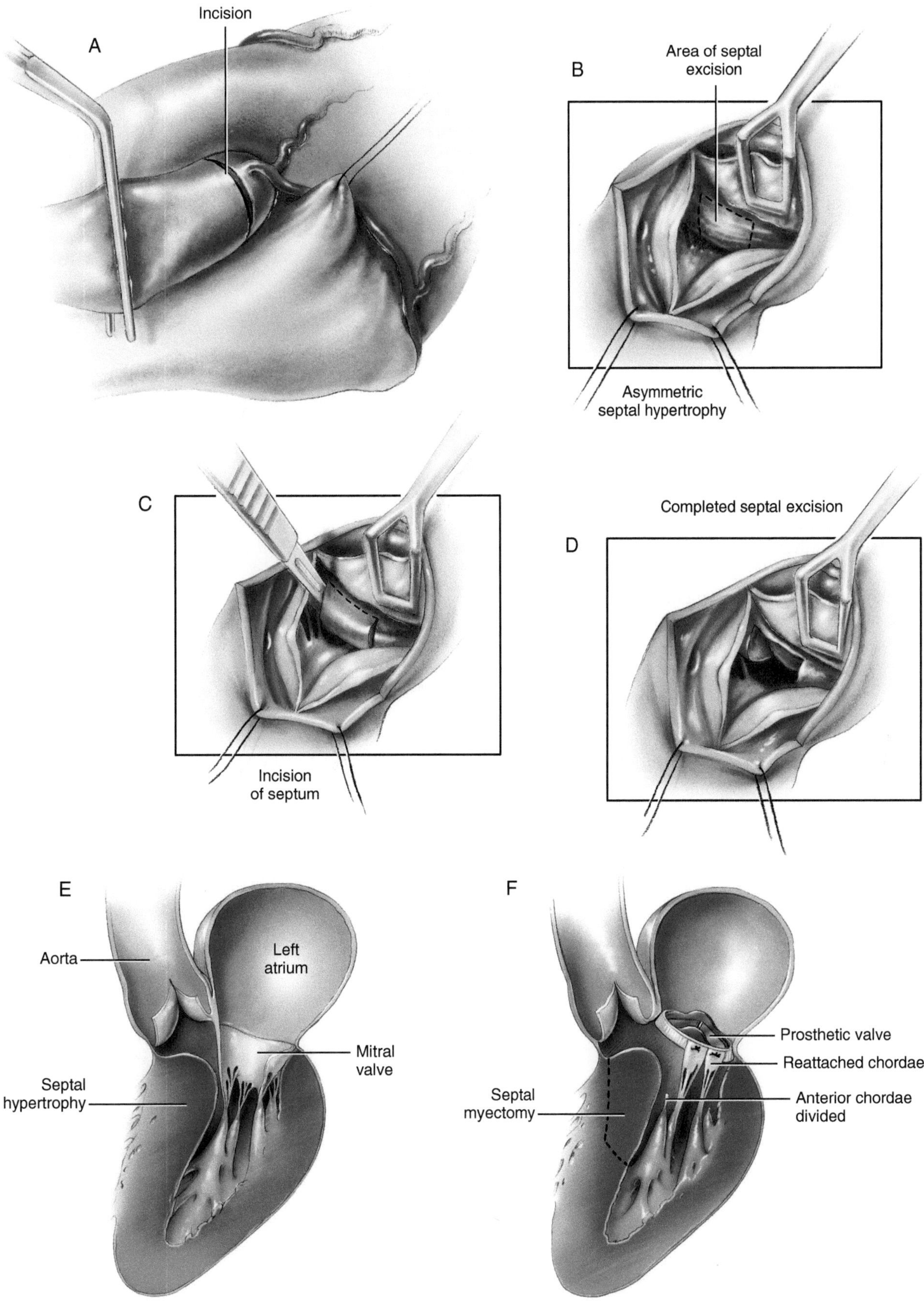
A
Incision
B
Area of septal excision
Asymmetric septal hypertrophy
C
Incision of septum
Completed septal excision
D
E
Aorta
Left atrium
Mitral valve
Septal hypertrophy
F
Prosthetic valve
Reattached chordae
Septal myectomy
Anterior chordae divided

chapter 17 LEFT VENTRICULAR OUTFLOW TRACT OBSTRUCTION

Types of Operations

There are a number of options available to enlarge an obstructed left ventricular outflow tract.

Figure 17-1

A This illustration shows the aortic root and the various points at which the aortic annulus can be divided to open the left ventricular outflow tract. The options include an anterior incision medial to the orifice of the right coronary artery (Konno-Rastan operation), an anterior incision through the medial commissure of the aortic valve (Vouhe operation), and posterior enlargement incisions. An incision into the posterior commissure and the interleaflet triangle below it has been described by Manougian and Nunez; an incision at the low midpoint in the noncoronary sinus is attributed to Nicks.

B The Konno-Rastan operation is commonly referred to as an aortoventriculoplasty because the incision extends from the aorta medially across the aortic annulus into the right ventricular outflow tract and the ventricular septum.

C The Vouhe operation is also an aortoventriculoplasty. The aortic incision is through the commissure between the left and right coronary cusps of the aortic valve. Thus, the incision into the right ventricle is made in the outlet portion and into the infundibular septum. This offers the option of preserving the aortic valve if it is normal or repairable.

D In the Manougian operation, an incision is extended from the aorta through the posterior commissure between the left and noncoronary cusps of the aortic valve, into the interleaflet triangle, and across the mitral annulus about 1 cm into the middle of the anterior leaflet of the mitral valve. The left atrium is also opened.

E In the Nunez operation, described 4 years after the Manougian operation, an incision is also made through the posterior commissure into the interleaflet triangle, but it stops short of entering the mitral valve and the left atrium.

F The Nicks operation extends an aortic incision across the aortic valve annulus at the midpoint of the noncoronary sinus into the anterior aspect of the anterior leaflet of the mitral valve. The left atrium is also opened.

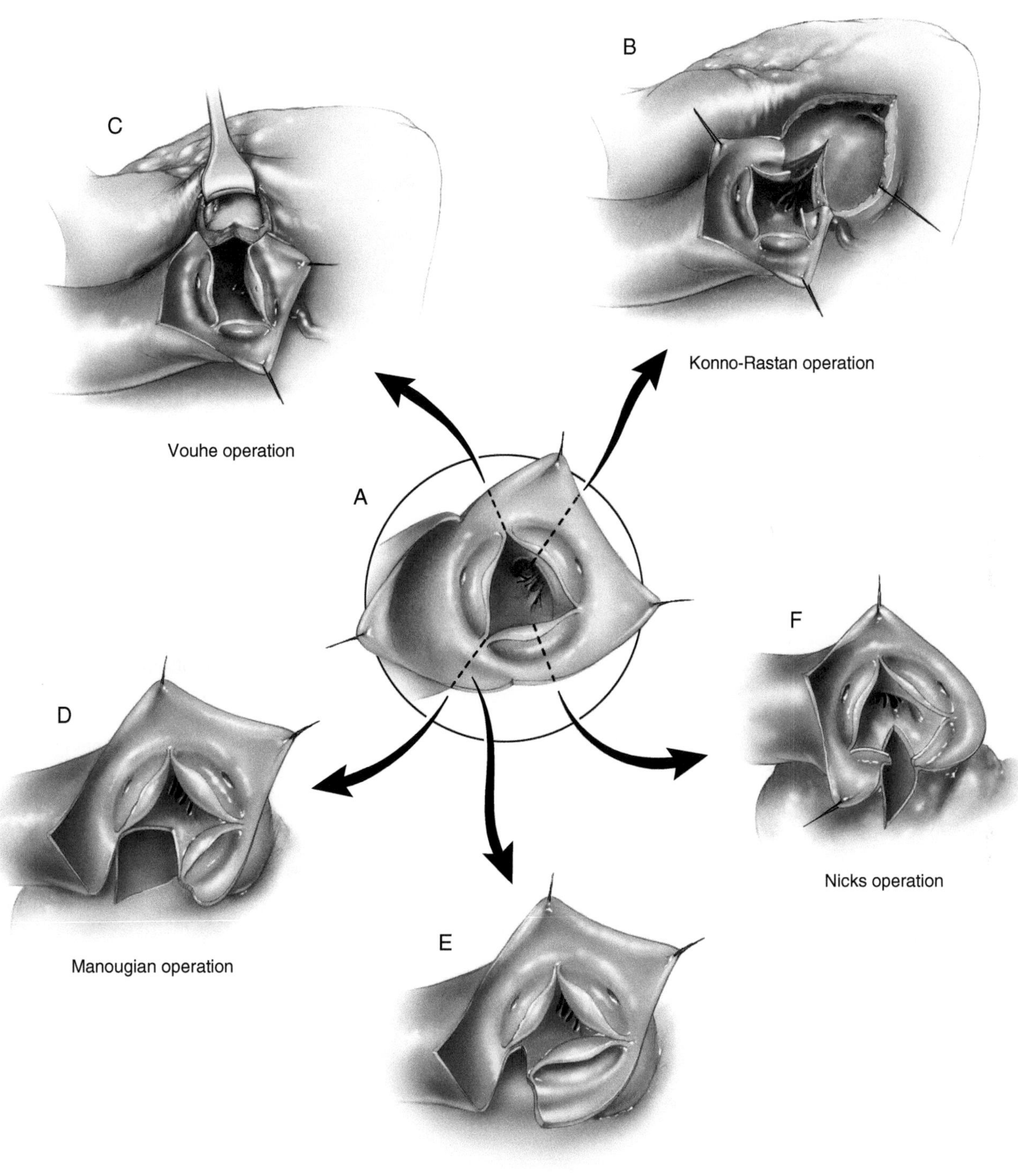
B
C
Konno-Rastan operation
Vouhe operation
A
F
D
Nicks operation
E
Manougian operation
Nunez operation

Posterior Enlargement of Left Ventricular Outflow Tract: Manougian and Nunez Operations

These operations are the most anatomic methods to enlarge the left ventricular outflow tract because the incisions follow natural paths and do not interrupt basic anatomic structures. The aortic incision is made through the posterior commissure into the interleaflet triangle (Nunez). The incision may be extended into the middle of the anterior leaflet of the mitral valve and posteriorly on the roof of the left atrium (Manougian) if a greater enlargement is desired.

Figure 17-2

A The Nunez operation involves an aortotomy extended through the commissure, which separates the left and noncoronary cusps of the aortic valve. The incision is made into the interleaflet triangle. Because the tissues in the interleaflet triangle are not supported by dense, fibrous tissues, they are flexible, compliant, and easily separated. With this incision, the diameter of the left ventricular outflow tract is enlarged as much as 2 to 3 mm. The aorta of the noncoronary sinus and the supporting dense, fibrous tissues of the noncoronary cusp of the aortic valve may be partially or completely excised to gain additional space.

B A prosthetic patch is attached to the aortic-mitral valve continuity by interrupted mattress stitches of 2/0 braided suture supported by Teflon pledgets. The patch may be collagen-sealed, knitted, double-velour Dacron, or a composite patch of autogenous pericardium backed with Teflon felt. The mattress stitches used to attach the patch are also passed through the sewing ring of a prosthetic valve of the appropriate diameter.

C The rest of the circumference of the prosthetic valve is attached to the annulus of the aortic valve in the usual fashion, using continuous or interrupted mattress stitches. The valve is seated in the left ventricular outflow tract in the interannular position.

D The prosthetic patch is used to close all or part of the aortotomy, using continuous stitches of 4/0 polypropylene.

E In the Manougian operation, the aortic incision extends through the interleaflet triangle, across the annulus of the mitral valve into the midportion of the valve's anterior leaflet, and posteriorly on the roof of the left atrium. This operation is used when greater enlargement of the left ventricular outflow tract diameter is required. The degree of enlargement is related to the depth of incision into the anterior leaflet. A 4- to 5-mm increase in diameter is possible with an aggressive incision to the free edge of the mitral valve.

F The defect in the anterior leaflet of the mitral valve is repaired with a prosthetic patch, which is extended across the mitral and aortic annulus into the aorta. Interrupted stitches of 4/0 Cardionyl suture are used to attach the patch to the mitral leaflet tissues. It may be tempting to use continuous stitches, but they are less desirable than simple interrupted stitches in terms of strength and accuracy of the repair.

G Interrupted mattress stitches of 2/0 braided suture with Teflon felt pledgets are used to approximate an appropriately sized prosthetic valve to the prosthetic patch. These stitches may be started in the rim of the left atrial defect if the atrial tissues are sufficiently flexible to allow approximation to the prosthetic patch without tension. Otherwise, the atrial defect is filled in with a separate patch of autogenous pericardium treated with glutaraldehyde solution.

H The prosthetic patch is tailored to close all or part of the aortotomy.

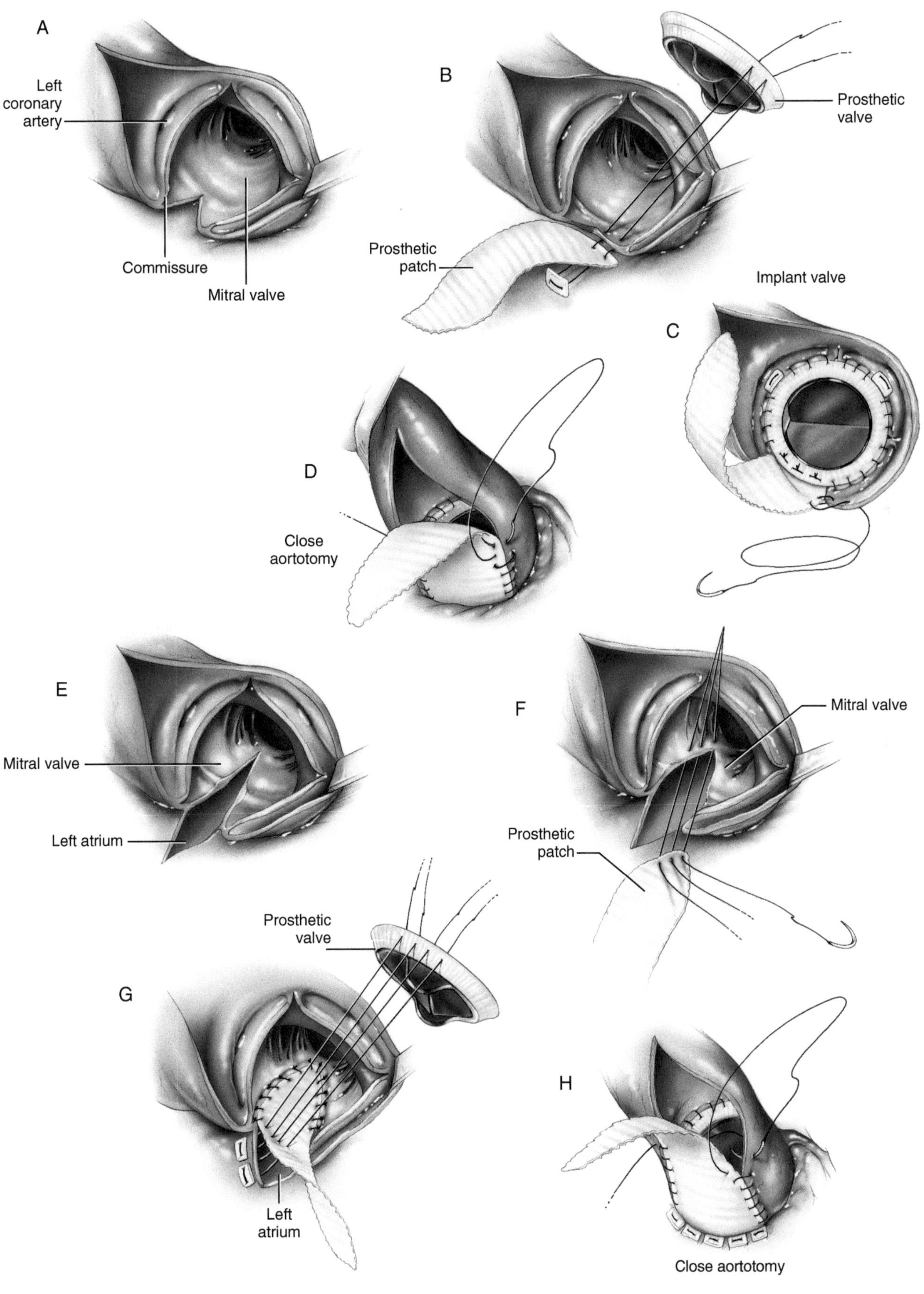
A
Left coronary artery
Commissure
Mitral valve
B
Prosthetic valve
Prosthetic patch
Implant valve
C
D
Close aortotomy
E
Mitral valve
Left atrium
F
Mitral valve
Prosthetic patch
Prosthetic valve
G
Left atrium
H
Close aortotomy

Posterior Enlargement of Left Ventricular Outflow Tract: Nicks Operation

Among the operations covered in this chapter, this was the first to be described. It has been widely employed for enlarging the left ventricular outflow tract. The only problem with this method is that the incision of the anterior leaflet of the mitral valve is off center. The diameter of the left ventricular outflow tract can be enlarged by 2 to 4 mm using the Nicks operation.

Figure 17-3

A A transverse incision is made in the ascending aorta and extended into the noncoronary sinus of Valsalva to the aortic annulus.

B The left atrium is opened laterally, opposite the aortic incision. With the left atrium and the aorta open, the anterior leaflet of the mitral valve is clearly visualized. The aortic annulus is divided, extending the incision into the anterior leaflet of the mitral valve. The mitral valve can be incised extensively; the off-center entry at the annulus is shifted to the exact midposition of the anterior leaflet as the incision is taken almost to the free edge of the anterior leaflet. This incision achieves maximal separation and widening of the aortic annulus.

C A patch is constructed from a tubular graft of collagen-sealed, knitted, double-velour Dacron. The graft is cut to an appropriate shape that approximates the incision in the mitral valve. As shown here, a continuous stitch of 4/0 polypropylene can be used to approximate the Dacron graft to the anterior leaflet of the mitral valve. Although this is acceptable, it is probably better to use interrupted stitches of 4/0 Cardionyl suture to reduce the risk of dehiscence. The suture line is taken to the aortic annulus.

D The aortic annulus is calibrated, and an appropriately sized prosthetic valve is selected for replacement of the aortic valve. Mattress stitches with pledgets are passed first through the left atrial wall, then through the prosthetic patch, and finally through the sewing ring of the prosthetic valve. This closes the left atrium in the area of the noncoronary sinus and approximates the prosthetic valve to the reconstructed left ventricular outflow tract.

E The prosthetic valve can be attached to the remainder of the natural aortic annulus using interrupted mattress stitches with pledgets or continuous suture technique.

F The remainder of the left ventricular outflow tract patch is approximated to the aortotomy with a running stitch of 4/0 polypropylene, completing the repair.

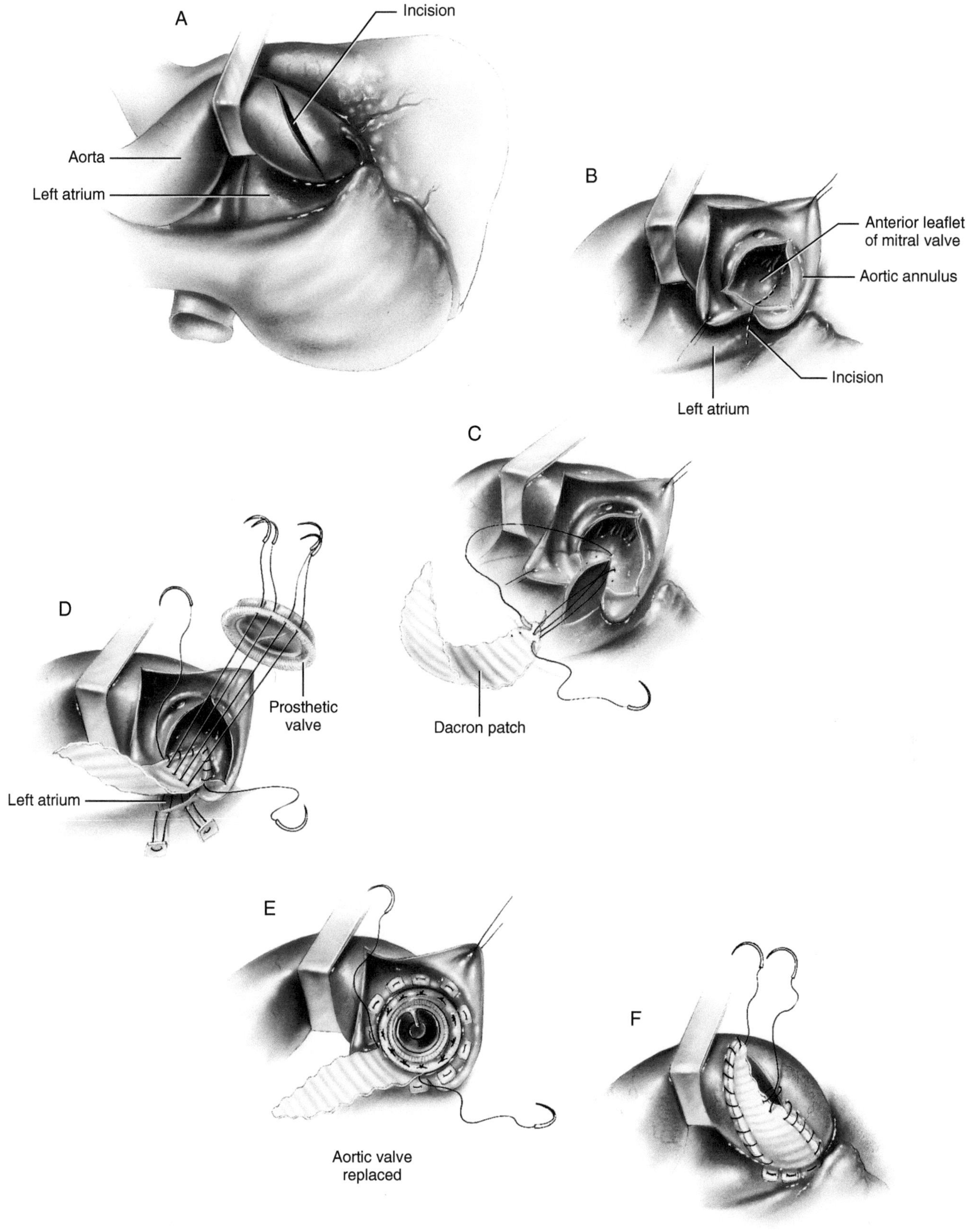
A
Incision
Aorta
Left atrium
B
Anterior leaflet of mitral valve
Aortic annulus
Incision
Left atrium
C
Dacron patch
D
Prosthetic valve
Left atrium
E
Aortic valve replaced
F
Completed repair

Anterior Enlargement of Left Ventricular Outflow Tract: Konno-Rastan Aortoventriculoplasty

The left ventricular outflow tract is enlarged anteriorly when widening of more than 2 to 4 mm in diameter is required. Because much greater diameters can be accomplished with aortoventriculoplasty, this operation is usually chosen for small children to allow placement of a prosthetic valve that is sufficient to accommodate the child's growth and thus delay the need for subsequent valve replacement. This operation is substantially more complex than posterior enlargement procedures and has a much greater potential for problems related to hemorrhage, septal patch dehiscence, conduction system injury, and reduced left ventricular performance. Nevertheless, when significant enlargement of the left ventricular outflow tract is required, this operation is useful.

Figure 17-4

A The aorta is dissected in the groove between the aorta, right ventricle, and pulmonary artery, to the left side of the right coronary artery. The dissection extends to the aortic annulus. A vertical incision is made in the aorta, extending to the annulus in the right coronary sinus of Valsalva, just anterior to the commissure between the left and right coronary cusps. The right ventricular outflow tract is opened by extending the aortotomy incision into the right ventricle anteriorly. The ventricular septum is incised from the aortic annulus into the ventricular septum, anterior and to the left of the bundle of His of the conduction system.

B As the incisions in the right ventricular outflow tract and the ventricular septum are extended, the outflow tract below the aorta is greatly widened, allowing the annulus of the aortic valve to separate widely. The cusps of the aortic valve are excised.

C The left ventricular outflow tract is reconstructed using a patch fashioned from a graft of collagen-sealed, knitted, double-velour Dacron. The patch is cut in roughly a diamond shape. The ventricular septum is closed to the patch with a running stitch of 3/0 or 4/0 polypropylene suture, with deep bites taken into the septum for maximal security of the closure. The suture line is continued to the level of the aortic annulus.

D The diameter of the aortic annulus is measured, and an appropriately sized prosthetic valve is selected for replacement of the aortic valve. A second prosthetic patch shaped like a triangle is fashioned to widen the right ventricular outflow tract. Interrupted mattress stitches with Teflon felt pledgets are used to join this patch to the prosthetic left ventricular outflow tract patch, and the stitches are continued through the prosthetic aortic valve.

E The aortic valve prosthesis is approximated to the aortic annulus using interrupted mattress stitches with pledgets. An alternative technique is to use a running stitch if the aortic annulus is of adequate strength. As the prosthetic valve is tied into the aortic annulus, it is joined securely to the prosthetic outflow tract patches.

F The right ventricular outflow tract patch is approximated to the right ventriculotomy with a running stitch of 4/0 polypropylene suture. Sufficient patch length is required to create the proper contour of the right ventricular outflow tract. This portion of the cardiac anatomy may become distorted as the left ventricular outflow tract is widened by the patch in the septum, and it should be accurately reconstructed by the right ventricular outflow patch. Special attention should be paid to the initial suture placement in the area of the aortic annulus where the transition to the right ventricle is made, because this is the weakest point of the entire repair. Hemorrhage from this area is especially troublesome. The left ventricular outflow tract patch is approximated to the aortotomy with a running stitch of 4/0 polypropylene, completing the repair. Use of BioGlue reduces hemorrhage from multiple needle holes, adding safety to any aortic root reconstructive procedure.

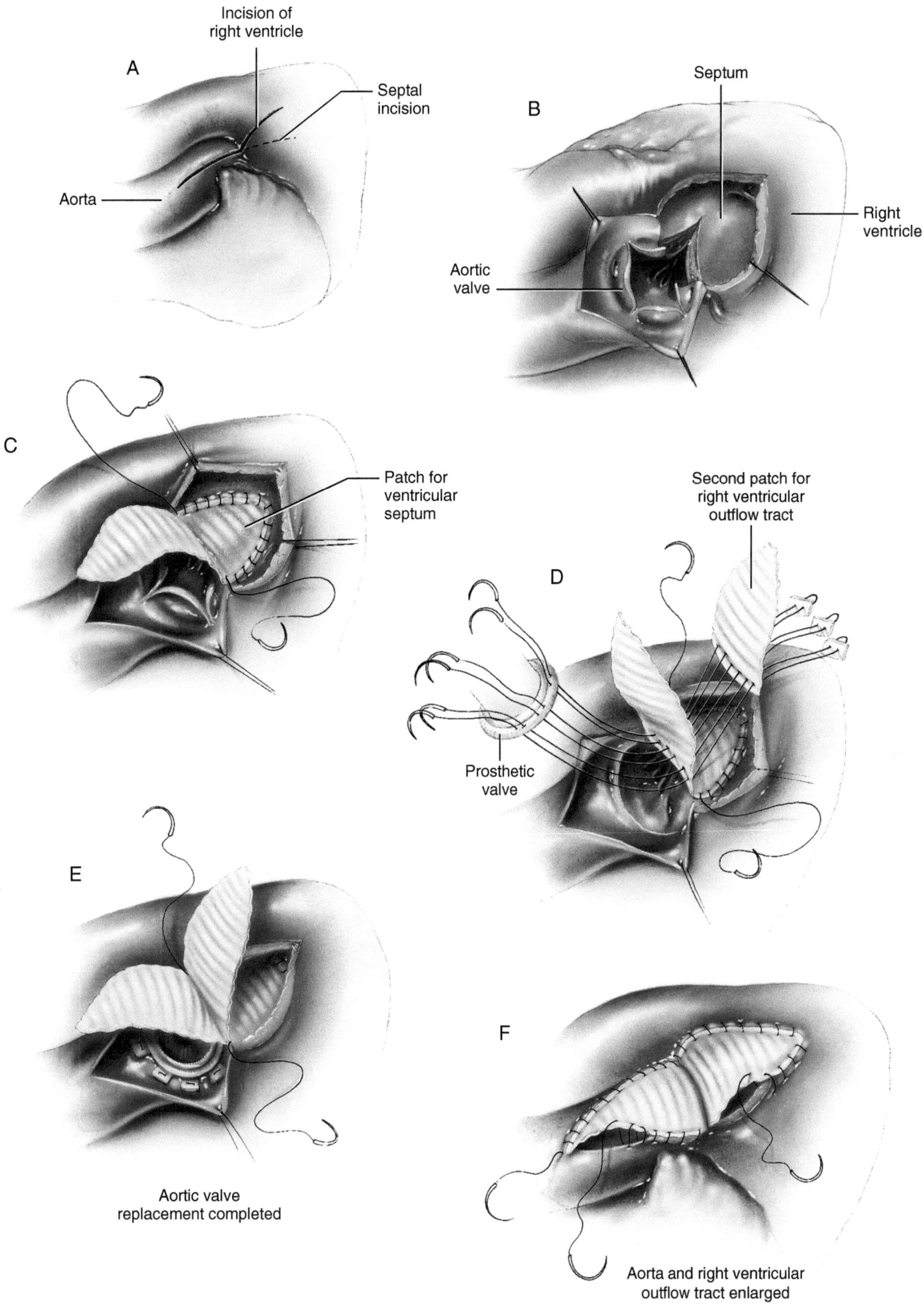
A
Incision of right ventricle
Septal incision
Aorta
B
Septum
Right ventricle
Aortic valve
C
Patch for ventricular septum
D
Second patch for right ventricular outflow tract
Prosthetic valve
E
Aortic valve replacement completed
F
Aorta and right ventricular outflow tract enlarged

Anterior Enlargement of Left Ventricular Outflow Tract: Vouhe Aortoventriculoplasty

As noted earlier, the left ventricular outflow tract is enlarged anteriorly when widening greater than 2 to 4 mm is required, such as in small children. In some cases the left ventricular outflow tract obstruction may be entirely subvalvular, and the aortic valve may be normal or repairable. The Vouhe operation offers the option of preserving the aortic valve. Also, because the incision is into the infundibular septum, it protects against injury to the conduction system.

Figure 17-5

A The aorta is dissected in the groove between the aorta, right ventricle, and pulmonary artery, to identify fibers of the infundibular septum. An oblique incision is made in the aorta. The aortic valve morphology is studied. The aortic incision is extended into the commissure between the left and right coronary cusps of the aortic valve into the interleaflet triangle. The outflow chamber of the right ventricle is opened transversely. The hypertrophied infundibular septum is opened by extending the aortotomy across and into the opened right ventricle and the underlying left ventricle.

B The thickness of the hypertrophied ventricular septum is reduced by cutting away the left ventricular side of the septum to relieve the left ventricular outflow tract obstruction. If the obstruction is removed by ventricular septectomy and the aortic valve is normal, the ventricular septum is repaired by direct suture, using continuous or interrupted stitches up through the incision in the aortic commissure.

C The incision in the right ventricle is closed with a separate suture. The aorta is closed as a continuation of the suture line in the aortic valve commissure.

D If the aortic valve is part of the left ventricular outflow tract obstruction or it has been irreversibly damaged by turbulent blood flow over time, or if the left ventricular outflow tract is not sufficiently enlarged by ventricular septectomy, the left ventricular outflow tract is reconstructed using a patch fashioned from a graft of collagen-sealed, knitted, double-velour Dacron. The patch is cut in roughly a diamond shape. The ventricular septum is closed to the patch with a running stitch of 3/0 or 4/0 polypropylene suture, with deep bites taken into the septum for maximal security of the closure. The suture line is continued to the level of the aortic annulus. The diameter of the aortic annulus is measured, and an appropriately sized prosthetic valve is selected for replacement of the aortic valve. A second prosthetic patch shaped like a triangle is fashioned to widen the right ventricular outflow tract. Interrupted mattress stitches with Teflon felt pledgets are used to join this patch to the prosthetic left ventricular outflow tract patch, and the stitches are continued through the prosthetic aortic valve. The aortic valve prosthesis is approximated to the aortic annulus using interrupted mattress stitches with pledgets. An alternative technique is to use a running stitch if the aortic annulus is of adequate strength. As the prosthetic valve is tied into the aortic annulus, it is joined securely to the prosthetic outflow tract patches.

E The right ventricular outflow tract patch is approximated to the right ventriculotomy with a running stitch of 4/0 polypropylene. The left ventricular outflow tract patch is approximated to the aortotomy with a running stitch of 4/0 polypropylene, completing the repair. Use of BioGlue reduces hemorrhage from multiple needle holes, adding safety to any aortic root reconstructive procedure.

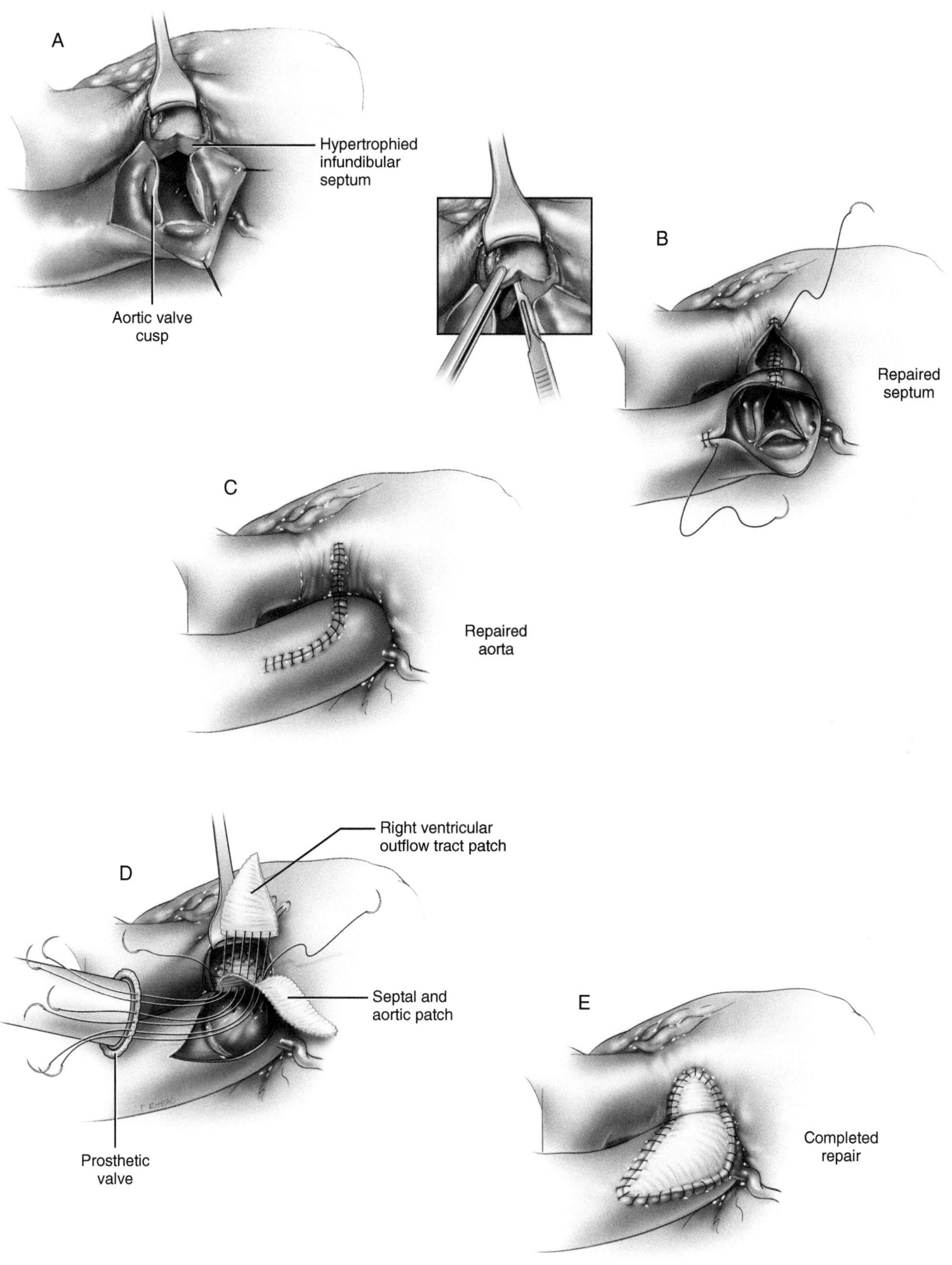
A
Hypertrophied infundibular septum
Aortic valve cusp
B
Repaired septum
C
Repaired aorta
D
Right ventricular outflow tract patch
Septal and aortic patch
Prosthetic valve
E
Completed repair

Apex Left Ventricle–to–Aorta Conduit

In some cases a direct approach to the left ventricular outflow tract obstruction is not advisable. An example is recurrence of an obstruction after complex repair. These patients can be treated easily and safely by placing a conduit between the left ventricle and the aorta, thus bypassing the obstruction.

Figure 17-6

A A midline incision that extends from the suprasternal notch to the umbilicus is made. The peritoneal cavity is opened in continuity with the pericardium. The colon and small intestine are packed away in the lower abdomen. The triangular ligament of the left lobe of the liver is incised and mobilized to the midline.

B The left lobe of the liver is retracted to the right, exposing the supraceliac abdominal aorta. The aortic crus of the diaphragm is retracted, and the segment of the aorta between the diaphragm and the celiac artery is mobilized.

C A partial-occlusion clamp is placed on the aorta above the celiac artery. A longitudinal incision is made in the aorta. The distal end of a composite valved conduit is shortened appropriately so that the valve will be relatively near the aorta. A continuous stitch of 4/0 polypropylene suture is used to anastomose the composite valved conduit to the aorta in an end-to-side fashion. Two double-needle sutures are used. All the stitches are placed around each apex, working in a clockwise and counterclockwise fashion from the center point of the incision on the left side to the center point of the incision on the right. The valved conduit is held away from the aortotomy until all the suture loops are placed, to achieve maximal exposure. The conduit is approximated to the aorta by pulling up the suture loops. A nerve hook is useful for achieving proper tension on the suture loops. The ends of the continuous suture are joined to complete the anastomosis.

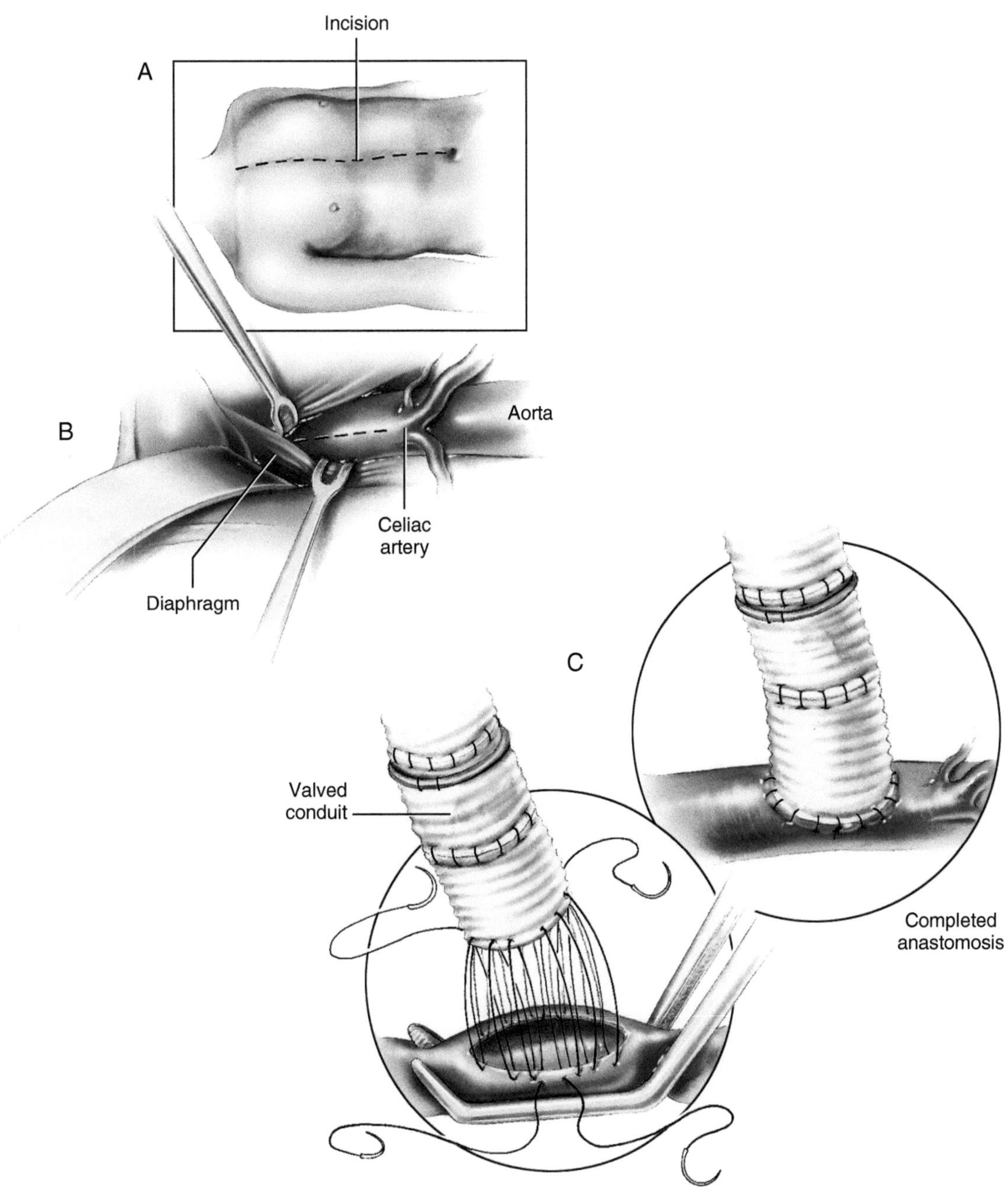
Incision
A
B
Aorta
Celiac
artery
Diaphragm
C
Valved
conduit
Completed
anastomosis

Figure 17-6 (continued)

D With the patient on cardiopulmonary bypass, the left side of the heart is vented, the ascending aorta is occluded, and hypothermic cardioplegic arrest of the heart is induced. The left ventricular apex is exposed by retracting the heart superiorly and to the right. An incision is made in the apex of the left ventricle. The orientation of the ventriculotomy is determined by the distribution of the surface coronary arteries, ensuring that the blood supply to the apex of the left ventricle will be preserved.

E The edges of the ventriculotomy are undermined to enlarge the opening into the left ventricle. The apex connector device is then inserted into the left ventricle through the ventriculotomy. A continuous stitch of 3/0 polypropylene is used to approximate the sewing ring of the apex connector to the edges of the ventriculotomy. The anastomosis is reinforced with pledget mattress sutures.

F The left ventricle is returned to its natural position in the pericardium, and the diaphragm is incised using the electrocautery at a point directly opposite the apex connector. The apex connector is drawn through the hole in the diaphragm. The apex connector, or the composite valved conduit or both are shortened appropriately to allow a uniform conduit loop across the upper portion of the peritoneal cavity below the diaphragm. An end-to-end anastomosis of the apex connector to the composite valved conduit is constructed with a running stitch of 3/0 or 4/0 polypropylene to complete the repair.

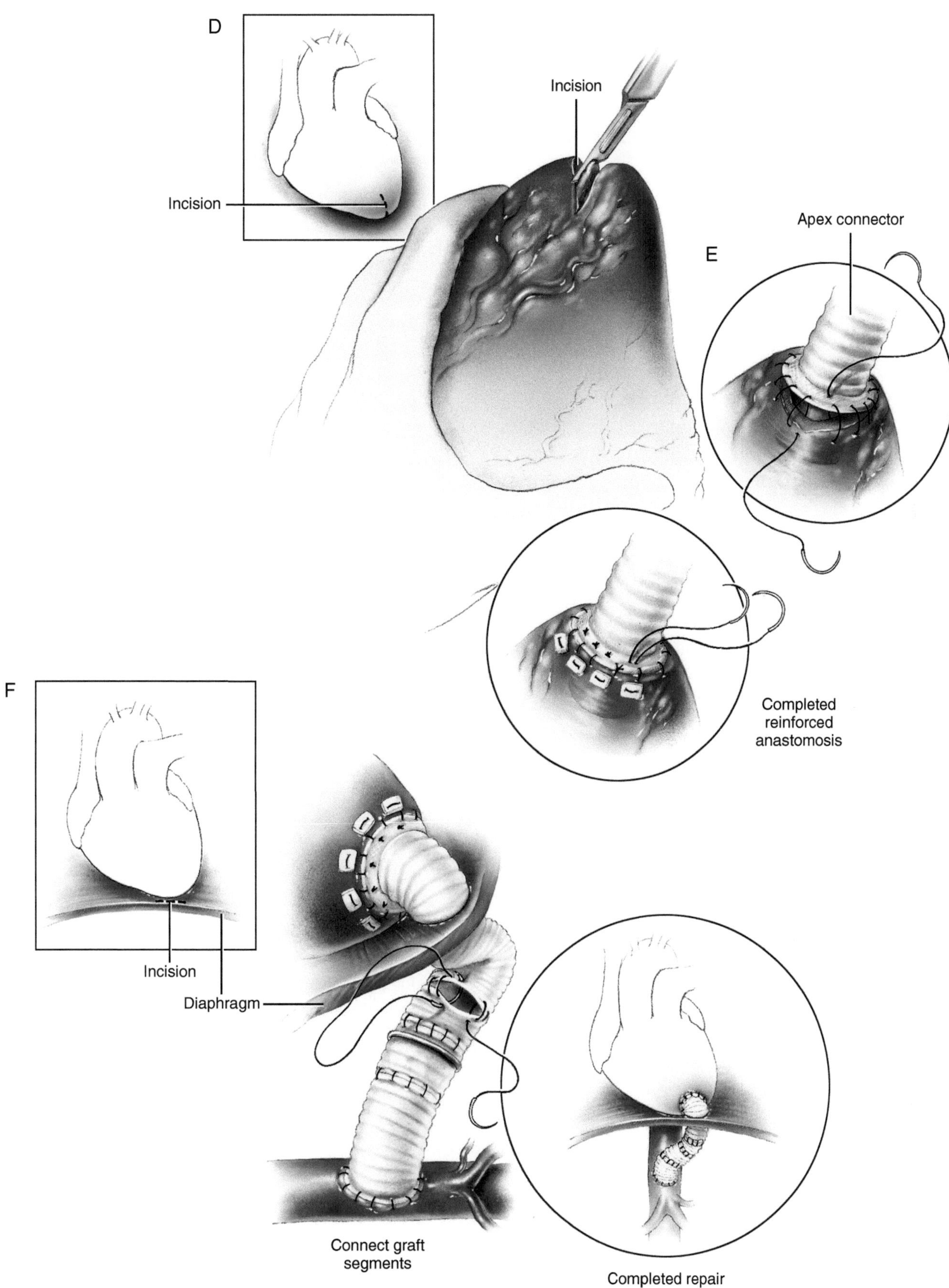
D
Incision
Incision
Apex connector
E
Completed
reinforced
anastomosis
F
Incision
Diaphragm
Connect graft
segments
Completed repair

chapter 18 SINUS OF VALSALVA ANEURYSM AND FISTULA

Sinus of Valsalva aneurysm or fistula is the result of the inherent weakness of fibromuscular tissues at the fibrous hinge point of the aortic valve.

Morphology

Sinus of Valsalva aneurysm presents as a depression at the base of the sinus of Valsalva. The fistula has a characteristic windsock appearance and is usually located in the right ventricular outflow tract, but it may present in any other cardiac chamber, depending on which sinus is involved. There may be an associated ventricular septal defect, in which case the annulus of the aortic valve separates the sinus aneurysm from the ventricular septal defect.

Figure 18-1

A In cases in which there is no associated ventricular septal defect and the sinus of Valsalva defect is not ruptured or obstructive, the anomaly can be approached directly through an incision in the ascending aorta made just above the sinuses.

B The sinus defect is examined by retracting the aortic valve cusps. The defect consists of a separation of the fibrous tissue of the aortic annulus from the fibrous tissue of the sinus of Valsalva. Correction of the defect involves closing the sinus opening without distorting the aortic cusps, while at the same time strengthening and supporting the aortic annulus. In most cases correction is best accomplished by inserting a prosthetic patch that maintains the cup-like structure of the sinus of Valsalva and avoids shortening the aortic annulus.

C An appropriately sized patch is fashioned from a Dacron graft. The patch is sutured to the aortic annulus and to the edge of the sinus defect with a continuous suture of 4/0 polypropylene.

D Incisions for the repair of a sinus of Valsalva fistula depend on which sinus is involved and the chamber to which the aneurysm ruptures. In general, the right ventricle and the right coronary sinus of Valsalva are involved. There may be a fistula to the right atrium when the noncoronary sinus is involved. A transverse incision is made in the ascending aorta above the sinuses of Valsalva. Depending on the cardiac chamber involved, a transverse incision is made in the outflow tract of the right ventricle, preserving the surface coronary arteries, or in the right atrium parallel to the atrioventricular groove.

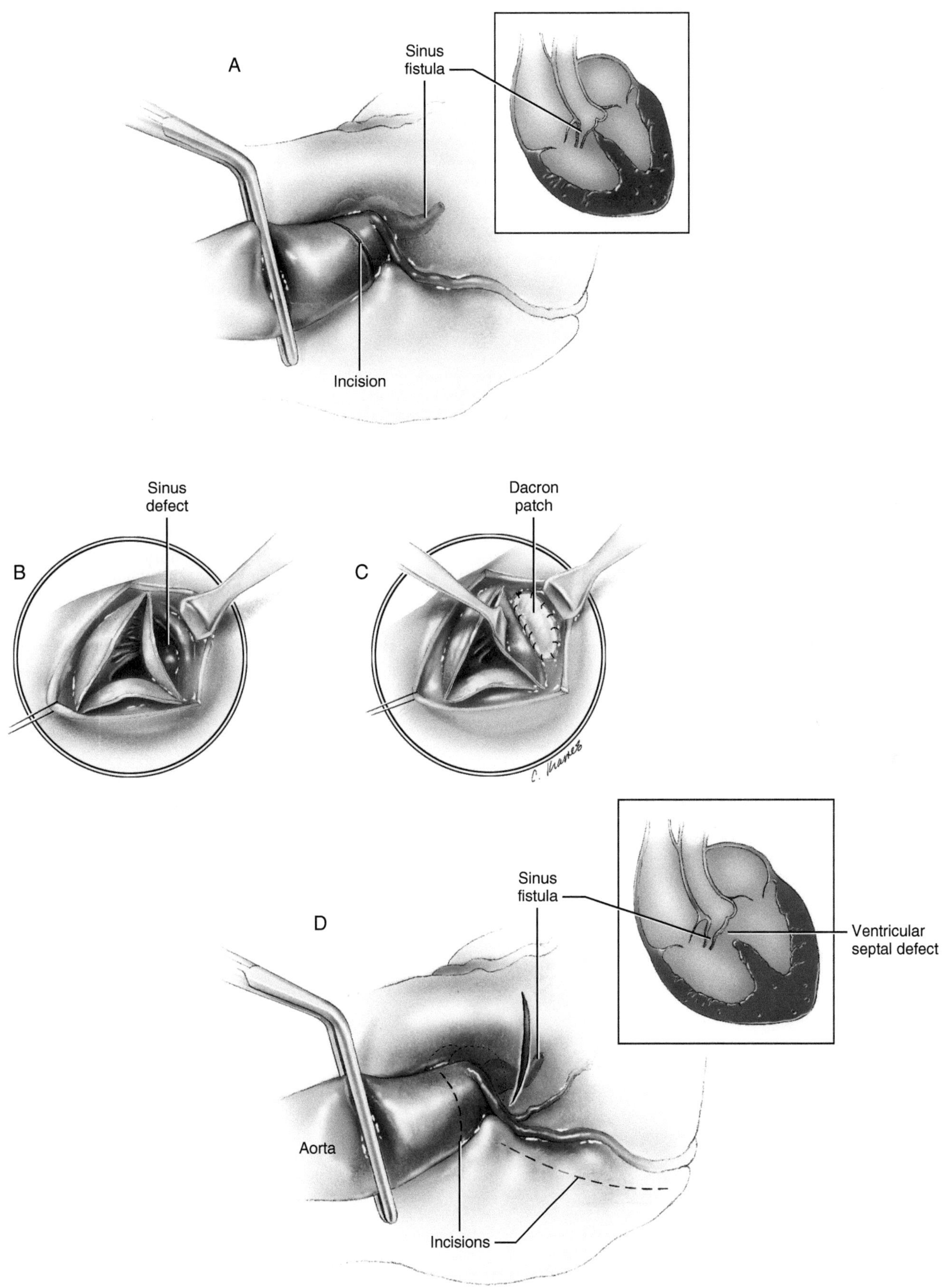
A
Sinus fistula
Incision
Sinus defect
B
Dacron patch
C
C. Kramer
Sinus fistula
D
Ventricular septal defect
Aorta
Incisions

Figure 18-1 (continued)

E The fibrous tissue of the windsock is excised flush with the ventricular septum.

F When there is an associated ventricular septal defect, the repair must not only close the sinus fistula and the ventricular septal defect but also provide proper support of the aortic annulus.

G An appropriately sized patch is fashioned from a tubular graft of crimped, collagen-sealed, double-velour Dacron. Careful inspection of the ventricular septal defect provides clues to the location of the conduction system. Usually the ventricular septal defect is of the perimembranous type; therefore the initial stitches for closure of the defect should be placed to the right side of the ventricular septum beneath the septal leaflet of the tricuspid valve and inferior to the rim of the defect. Stitches placed in this fashion will not penetrate the area of the conduction system. Continuous suture technique with 4/0 polypropylene is used.

H The ventricular septal defect is closed along the posteroinferior rim of the defect in a counterclockwise fashion to the level of the annulus of the aortic valve, using the usual technique for ventricular septal defect repair. A running mattress suture is placed through the septal leaflet of the tricuspid valve in the usual method of septal defect closure, until the junction with the aortic annulus is reached.

I To support the aortic valve, several interrupted mattress stitches are placed in a precise manner where the aortic annulus and the Dacron patch are approximated. These stitches must be accurately placed to avoid distorting the aortic valve and shortening the annulus.

J The repair is completed by continuing the suture line around the edges of the defect in the sinus of Valsalva. The completed repair should be checked through both the aortic exposure and the cardiac chamber that was opened to assist in the repair. The two incisions provide maximal exposure for correct orientation and reconstruction of the defect.

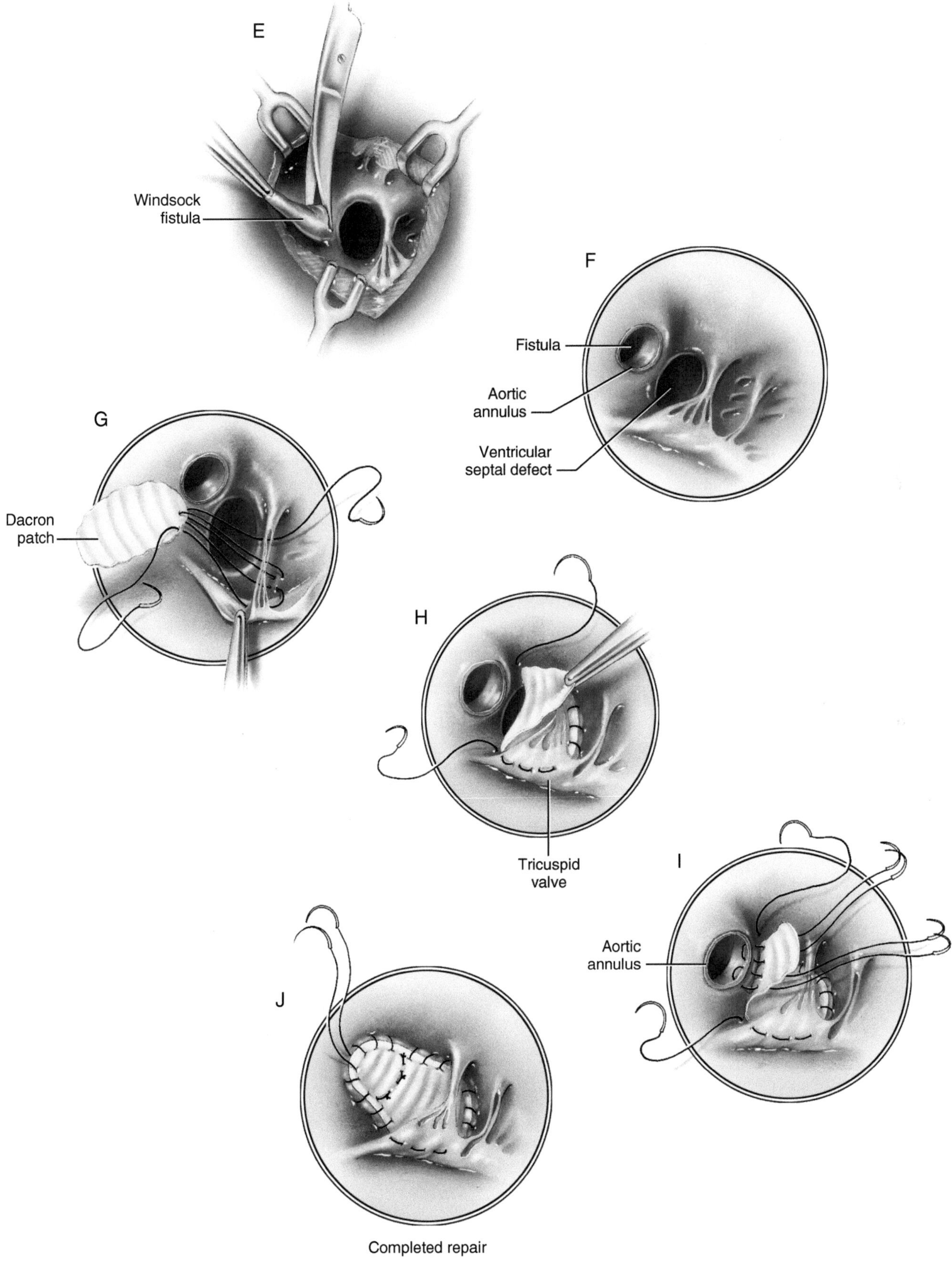
E
Windsock fistula
F
Fistula
Aortic annulus
Ventricular septal defect
G
Dacron patch
H
Tricuspid valve
I
Aortic annulus
J
Completed repair

Yacoub Aortoplasty

An aortoplasty technique devised by Yacoub addresses the primary defect of separation of the fibrous aortic valve support tissue from the fibrous tissue of the sinus of Valsalva and the lack of support of the aortic valve by the void of the closely associated ventricular septal defect.

Figure 18-2

A The exposure is through an anterior transverse aortotomy. The ventricular septal defect is seen directly below the retracted right coronary leaflet of the aortic valve. The close proximity of the ventricular septal defect results in loss of support for the aortic valve, which is already compromised by the sinus of Valsalva aneurysm or fistula.

B The repair is done using 4/0 polypropylene suture with needles at each end and a small, centrally mounted pledget. Three or four sutures are used. Pledgets are the only prosthetic material employed. The suture is placed as a mattress stitch to the right side of the rim of the ventricular septal defect. The stitch is placed accurately through the fibrous tissue of the hinge point of the aortic valve leaflet. The stitch is continued, reefing the weakened tissues of the sinus of Valsalva aneurysm to the normal fibrous tissues of the aortic sinus above the defect. This point is below the sinus rim (aortotubular junction). The second needle is used to duplicate the pathway of the first needle but is separated from it by 2 mm. The inset diagram shows the completed initial stitch.

C Three or four mattress stitches are used for the repair. All are placed in an identical fashion with uniform separation. The repair is completed by tightening and securing the suture to achieve approximation of the ventricular septal defect to the aortic hinge point and the reefed up tissues of the aortic sinus. The inset diagram shows that three mattress sutures were used, for a total of six reefing stitches, equally spaced in the aortic sinus.

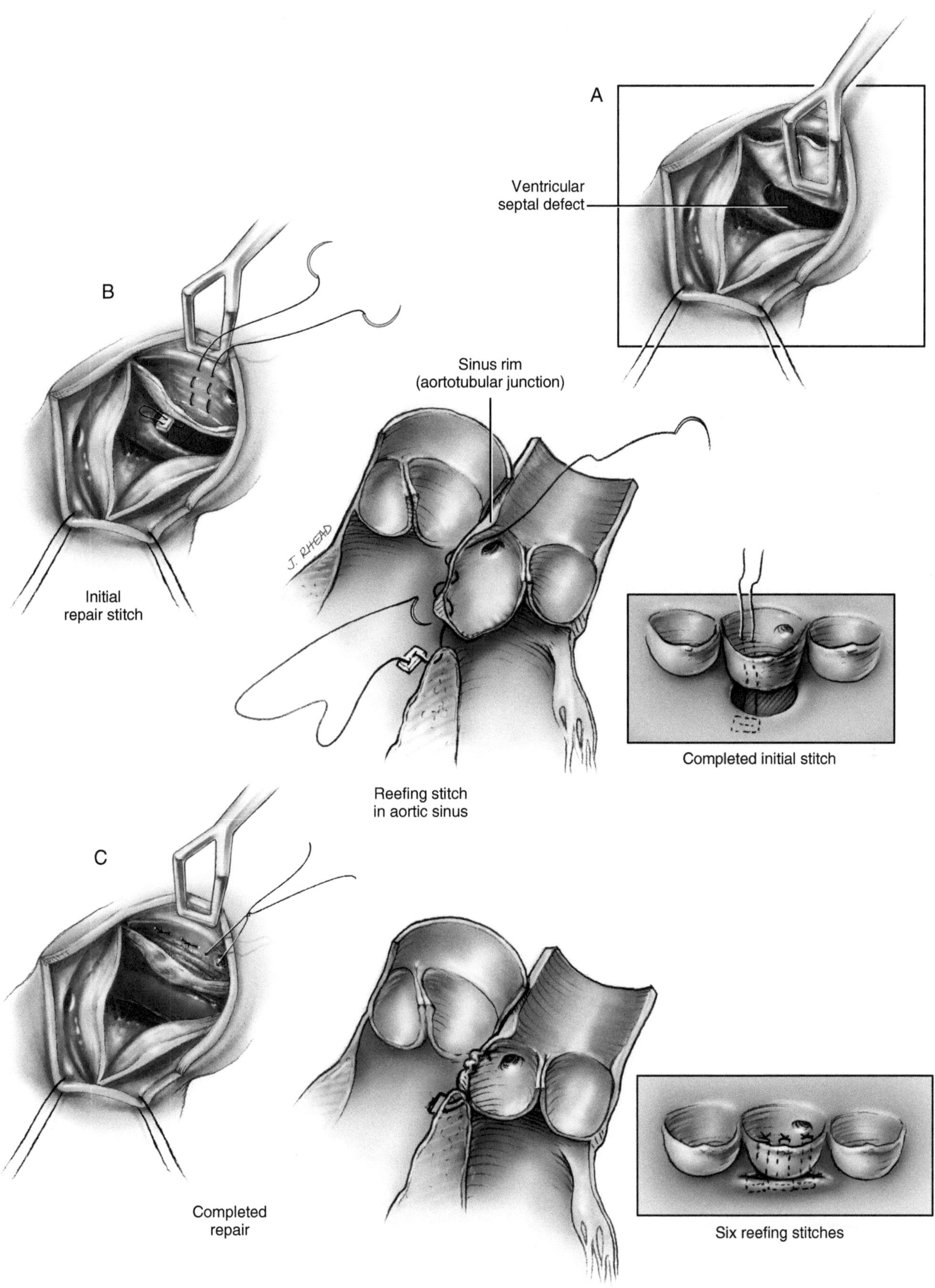
A
Ventricular septal defect
B
Initial repair stitch
Sinus rim (aortotubular junction)
J. RHEAD
Completed initial stitch
Reefing stitch in aortic sinus
C
Completed repair
Six reefing stitches

part VI

Single Ventricle

chapter 19 SEPTATION OF THE UNIVENTRICULAR HEART

A univentricular heart is defined as a single ventricular chamber that receives the input of the two atria through two atrioventricular valves. The great arteries may be normally related or transposed, and one of the great vessels originates from a small outlet chamber that communicates with the single ventricle via the bulboventricular foramen.

Morphology

Figure 19-1

A Univentricular heart defects with L-transposition of the great arteries are most amenable to correction by septation procedures. The aorta in L-transposition originates from the small outlet chamber and is anterior and to the left of the pulmonary artery. The pulmonary annulus is posterior and to the right of the aorta and is wedged deeply between the two atrioventricular valves, with a variable amount of subannular or infundibular myocardium separating it from the annulus of the right atrioventricular valve. The posterior papillary muscle of the right atrioventricular valve and the anterior papillary muscle of the left atrioventricular valve are closely related and may share a common base. The atrioventricular bundle originates from an anterior atrioventricular node in the floor of the right atrium near the atrioventricular valve and courses anterior to the pulmonary annulus in the subendocardium. The atrioventricular bundle courses along the right side of the anterior rim of the bulboventricular foramen. Operative exposure for septation procedures is through an incision in the right atrium parallel to the atrioventricular groove.

B The right atrioventricular valve is retracted, and all the intracardiac structures are identified. Hypothermic cardioplegic technique provides excellent pliability of the myocardium, making extended exposures through the right atrioventricular valve possible. The entire defect cannot be seen through a single exposure. With several sequential changes in the position of the retractors and some patience, complete definition of the anatomy is possible, and the septal partition can be performed entirely via the right atrioventricular valve.

C The two atrioventricular valves are visualized quite readily at the base of the heart. The only intraventricular area not adequately exposed is anterior and to the right of the pulmonary annulus. Because the suture line in this procedure passes posterior to the pulmonary annulus, lack of exposure of this region is not important.

D A patch of collagen-sealed, knitted, double-velour Dacron is fashioned for the septum. Working through the right atrioventricular valve, the surgeon sutures the patch into the ventricle to divide it into right and left chambers of roughly equal size. A continuous suture line of 3/0 polypropylene is used to attach the patch to the ventricular wall. The suture line is started anterior and to the right of the bulboventricular foramen and continued anteriorly to the apex, where the papillary muscles of the two atrioventricular valves are inserted into heavy trabeculated muscle. The patch is worked between the sets of papillary muscles to preserve function of the atrioventricular valves. The suture line is then continued along the posterior wall of the ventricle superiorly to the fibrous junction of the two atrioventricular valves. The anterior suture line is carried superiorly to the right of the rim of the bulboventricular foramen and then across the area of the bundle of His to the posterior aspect of the pulmonary annulus. Superficial sutures should preserve the conduction system. The suture line is continued posteriorly along the pulmonary annulus to the fibrous junction of the two atrioventricular valves. The septation is completed by attaching the patch to the fibrous continuity between the atrioventricular valves. Permanent ventricular pacing electrodes are attached in most cases because of the conduction system's tendency to spontaneously deteriorate.

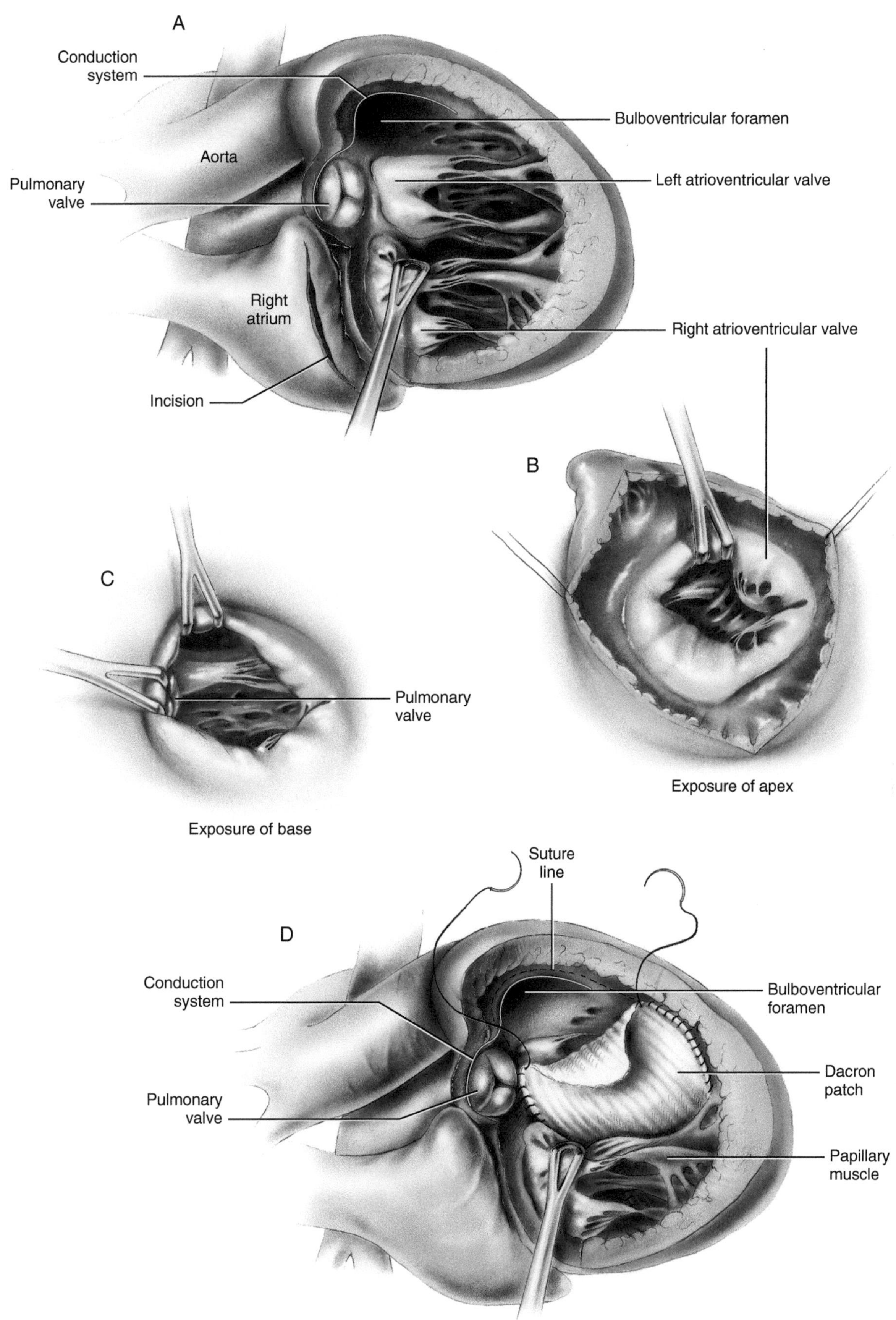
A
Conduction system
Bulboventricular foramen
Aorta
Pulmonary valve
Left atrioventricular valve
Right atrium
Right atrioventricular valve
Incision
B
C
Pulmonary valve
Exposure of apex
Exposure of base
Suture line
D
Conduction system
Bulboventricular foramen
Dacron patch
Pulmonary valve
Papillary muscle

chapter 20 MODIFIED FONTAN PROCEDURE

Fontan and Baudet described an operation to bypass the right ventricle for physiological correction of tricuspid atresia. Subsequent modifications devised to connect the right atrium to the pulmonary artery or the right ventricular outflow tract are called modified Fontan procedures. The trend in these operations has been to use only autogenous materials and to eliminate valves because the patients are young and may outgrow prosthetic devices, and the durability of biological valve prostheses is unknown.

Morphology

Various modified Fontan procedures that shunt systemic venous return directly to the pulmonary arteries have been applied to nearly all single-ventricle anomalies involving hypoplastic right or left hearts. The best functional results have been achieved with Fontan procedures for tricuspid atresia, probably because the single ventricle has a left ventricular morphology.

Figure 20-1

A Tricuspid atresia. The right atrium is cut away to expose the atrial septum and the floor of the right atrium. There is no atrioventricular (tricuspid) valve visible.

B Tricuspid atresia. Magnified view with a probe in the patent foramen ovale. The atrioventricular valve is absent.

C Tricuspid atresia (severe hypoplasia). The right atrial free wall has been removed to demonstrate the atrial septum and floor of right atrium. There is a patent foramen ovale. The tricuspid valve is extremely hypoplastic, with only a small circular annulus covered by a thin membrane in which there is a tiny perforation.

D Tricuspid atresia (severe hypoplasia), ventricular view. This is the same specimen as in C, with the single ventricle opened. The ventricle surrounding the hypoplastic right atrioventricular valve demonstrates the coarse trabeculation of a morphologic right ventricle; the rest of the ventricle has a finely trabeculated left ventricular morphology. The bulboventricular foramen leads to a small outlet chamber beneath the aorta.

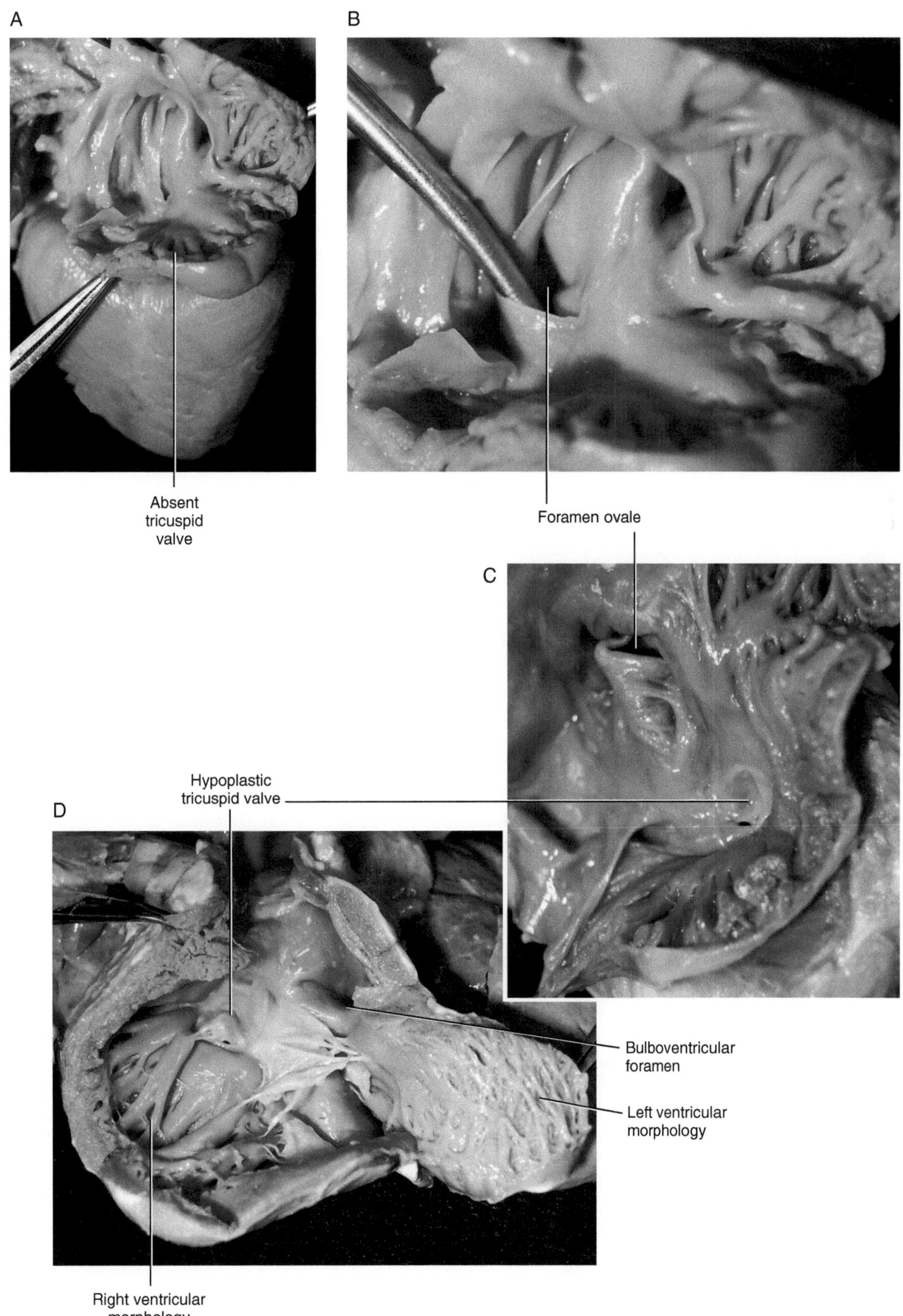
A
B
C
D
Absent tricuspid valve
Foramen ovale
Hypoplastic tricuspid valve
Bulboventricular foramen
Left ventricular morphology
Right ventricular morphology

Total Cavopulmonary Connection/ Fenestrated Atrial Septum

After many modifications of the Fontan procedure were introduced, total cavopulmonary connection was developed to streamline venous blood flow to the pulmonary artery and to obviate problems associated with complex intraatrial septation. Providing a small, controlled atrial septal defect (fenestrated Fontan procedure) has also been beneficial in controlling elevated systemic venous pressure postoperatively. The fenestrated Fontan procedure has several modifications, but the principle is standard.

Figure 20-2

A The remnant of the atrial septum is excised (*dashed line*) to create a wide opening to the left atrium. This passageway conducts coronary sinus blood flow to the left side in cases of tricuspid atresia or brings the pulmonary venous return to the right atrioventricular valve in cases of aortic or mitral atresia and other forms of hypoplastic left heart syndrome. The superior vena cava is divided at the level of the right pulmonary artery, preparatory to the construction of an anastomosis to provide bidirectional flow to the pulmonary artery. The *dotted line* demonstrates the suture line for the septal partition. The passageway created between the inferior vena cava and the superior vena cava should be smooth, straight, cylindrical, and as short as possible. The septal partition can be created from the right atrial free wall or by a prosthetic patch or conduit connecting the venae cavae inside the atrium or externally.

B A right atrial flap can be created to partition the atrium and create an intraatrial conduit that connects the inferior vena cava to the superior vena cava. Continuous stitches of 4/0 polypropylene are used to connect the atrial flap to the floor of the right atrium at the right margin of the atrial septal defect.

C A short segment of polytetrafluoroethylene (PTFE) is commonly used to partition the atrium and create the conduit. A patch of the appropriate size is fashioned from a tubular graft, using as short a segment of prosthetic material as possible to join the venae cavae. The patch is attached to the atrium by a continuous stitch of 4/0 polypropylene.

D The suture line proceeds using a double-needle suture until a small space remains at the midpoint laterally. The sutures are tied, leaving a small defect in the suture line. A mattress stitch of 4/0 polypropylene reinforced by Teflon felt pledgets is placed around this residual defect and is brought outside the right atrium. Silastic tourniquet tubing is placed over the suture to allow later closure of the defect in the atrial septum. The tourniquet must be long enough so that its end reaches the upper abdominal midline. The tourniquet and the suture are left in this position for easy access at a later time. Alternatively, the residual defect can be closed later by a percutaneous catheter closure device.

E Incisions are made in the superior and inferior aspects of the right pulmonary artery. The upper end of the superior vena cava is anastomosed to the superior incision in the pulmonary artery using 6/0 polypropylene or polydioxanone suture. A similar anastomosis of the lower end of the superior vena cava to the inferior aspect of the right pulmonary artery is constructed. This portion of the operation is commonly referred to as a bidirectional Glenn anastomosis, and it may be performed as a preliminary staged procedure.

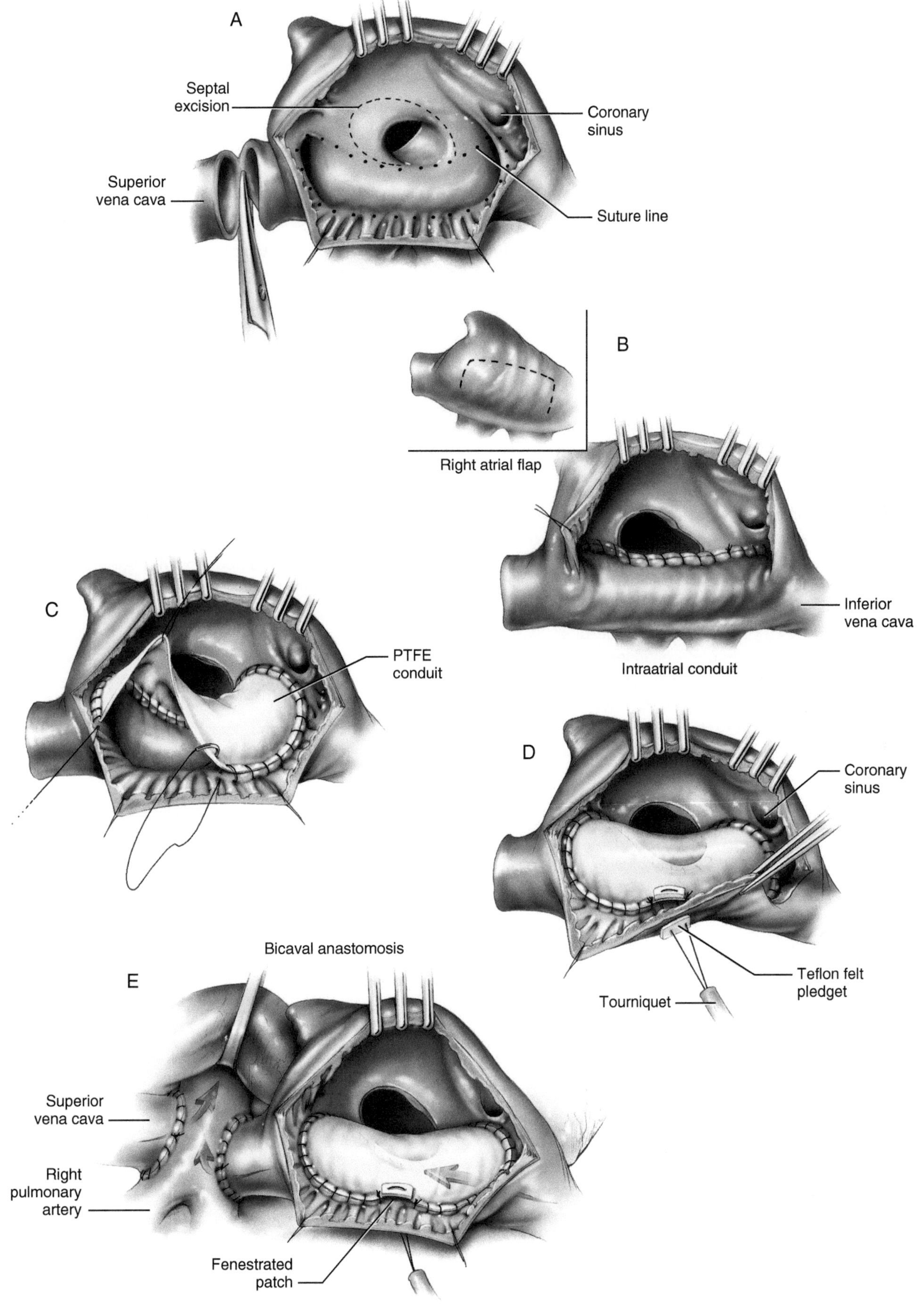
A
Septal excision
Coronary sinus
Superior vena cava
Suture line
B
Right atrial flap
Inferior vena cava
Intraatrial conduit
C
PTFE conduit
D
Coronary sinus
Teflon felt pledget
Tourniquet
Bicaval anastomosis
E
Superior vena cava
Right pulmonary artery
Fenestrated patch

chapter 21 HYPOPLASTIC LEFT HEART SYNDROME

Hypoplastic left heart syndrome includes a spectrum of conditions involving the underdevelopment of the left-sided heart structures and the aortic outflow tract, including (1) aortic valve atresia and hypoplasia of the ascending aorta, (2) mitral valve atresia or hypoplasia, and (3) diminutive left ventricle. Patent ductus arteriosus is essential for survival, and there is usually a patent foramen ovale. Coarctation of the aorta is frequently associated with the lesion and may seriously impair retrograde blood flow to the ascending aorta, which functions as a common coronary artery.

Morphology

Figure 21-1

A The enlarged right ventricle (RV) occupies all of the anterior and lateral heart. The left ventricle is not defined externally. The right ventricle gives origin to an enlarged pulmonary artery (PA). The right and left pulmonary arteries are normal. The patent ductus arteriosus (PDA) originates at the bifurcation of the pulmonary artery and continues as the descending aorta. The ascending aorta (Ao) is markedly hypoplastic, wrapping around the right pulmonary artery. The arch portion is larger than the ascending aorta and gives origin to normal arch branches.

B A closer view of the specimen demonstrates a hypoplastic ascending aorta (Ao) and its relation to and size in comparison with the right pulmonary artery. Continuation of the patent ductus arteriosus (PDA) as the descending aorta is demonstrated.

C The aortic arch (Ao) is opened and reflected inferiorly and to the left.

D The interior of the aortic arch and the junction with the descending aorta show typical evidence of coarctation of the aorta.

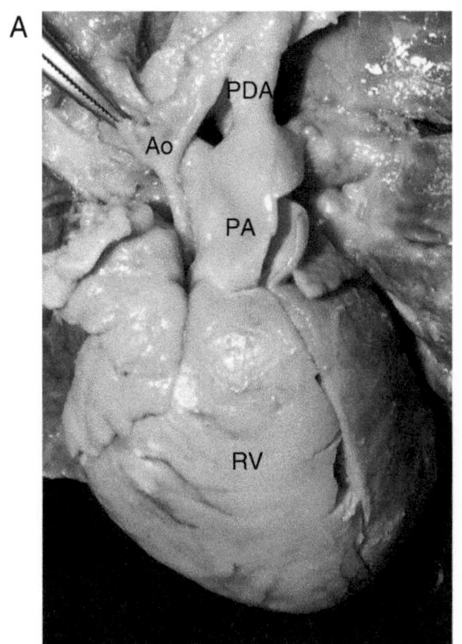
A
PDA
Ao
PA
RV

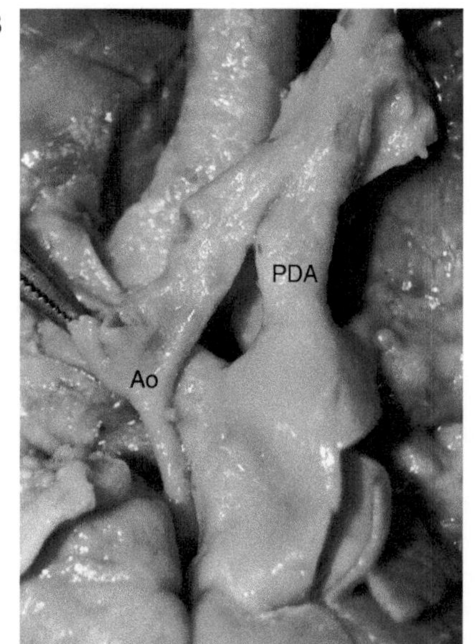
B
PDA
Ao

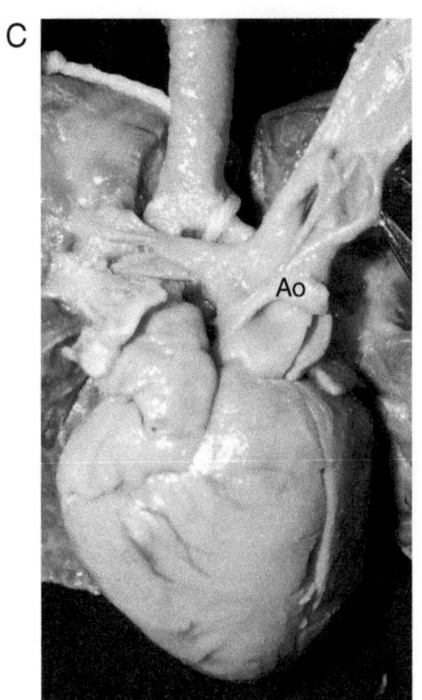
C
Ao

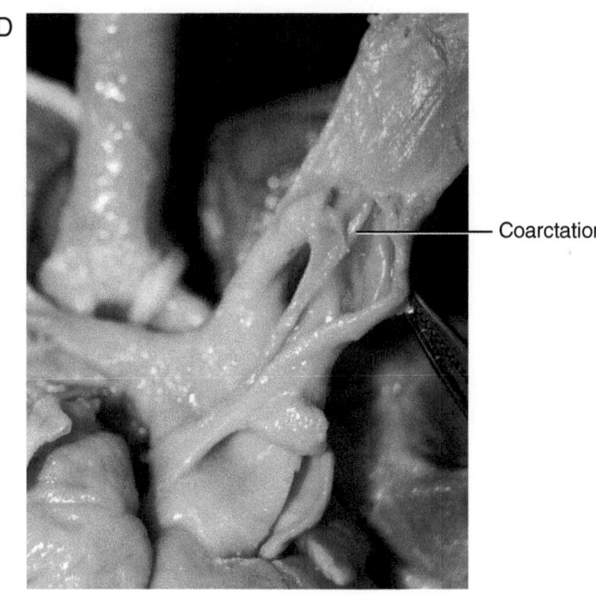
D
Coarctation

Figure 21-1 (continued)

E Normal left atrium and mitral valve open to a hypoplastic left ventricle.

F Mitral valve leaflet tissue is nearly normal, but the subvalvular supporting structure is abnormal due to hypoplasia of the left ventricle.

G Right ventricle in hypoplastic left heart syndrome. The ventricle is enlarged and hypertrophied. Similarly, the tricuspid valve is enlarged. The right ventricular outflow tract is unobstructed and leads to the enlarged pulmonary artery. The pulmonary valve is normal. The ductus arteriosus is off the top of the pulmonary artery at the bifurcation. The aortic arch is to the right of the ductus arteriosus.

H Palliative operation for hypoplastic left heart syndrome—the modified Norwood operation. This view at operation demonstrates severe hypoplastic left heart syndrome with a severely hypoplastic ascending aorta to the right of a greatly dilated pulmonary trunk. A "collar" (pulmonary artery allograft) has been used to connect the pulmonary artery to the aortic arch. The ascending aorta is not included in the aortoplasty; rather, it has been left as a common coronary artery from the aortic arch. A polytetrafluoroethylene (PTFE) graft in the upper left is used for a modified Blalock-Taussig shunt to control pulmonary blood flow.

I Palliative operation for hypoplastic left heart syndrome—the Sano procedure. Aortic reconstruction is achieved by attaching a patch (*light color*) to the ascending aorta (*darker color*) and the arch. Two leaflets of normal pulmonary valve are seen through which the right ventricle ejects to the aorta. A PTFE conduit connects the right ventricle to the pulmonary artery.

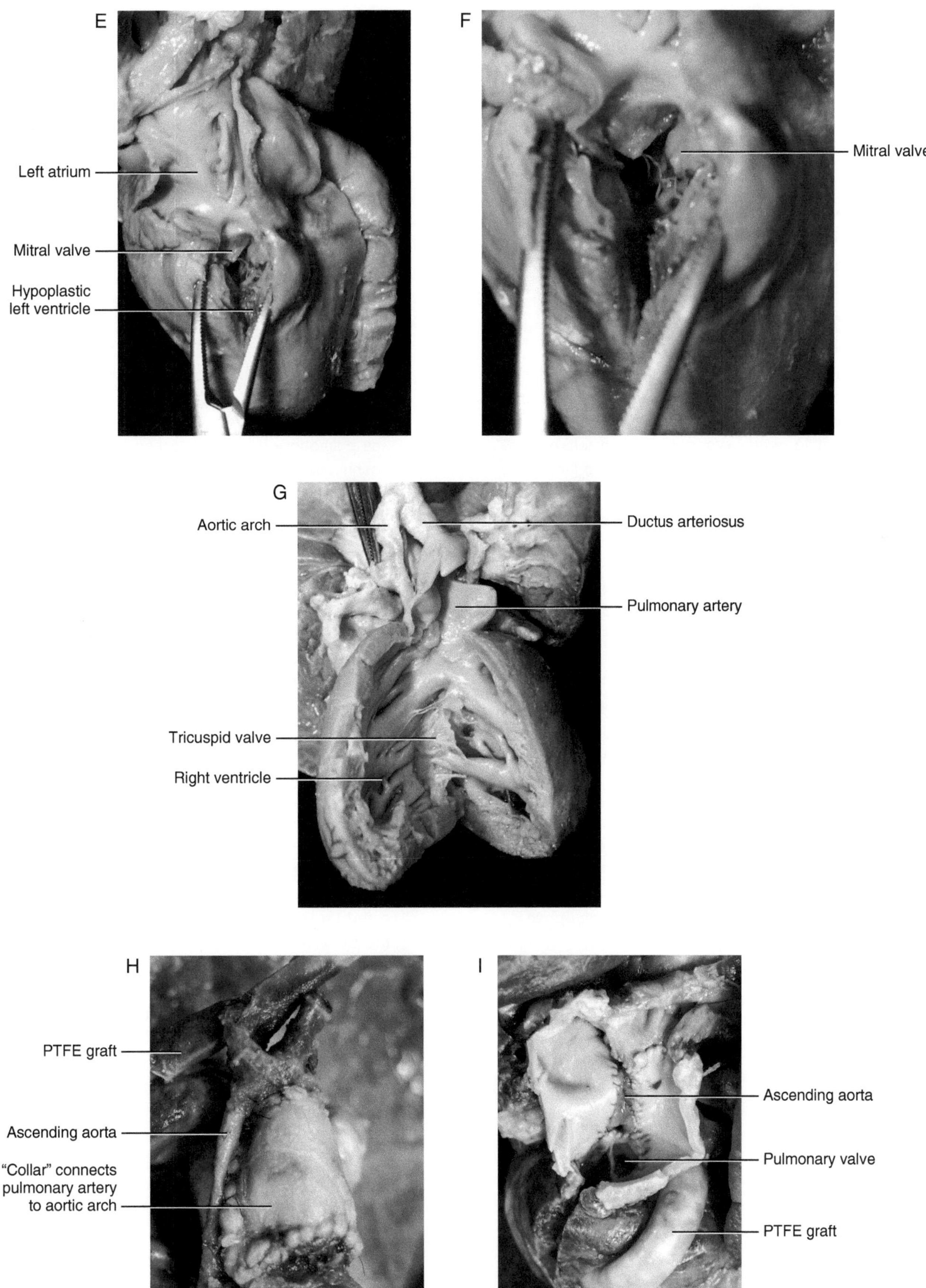
E
Left atrium
Mitral valve
Hypoplastic
left ventricle
F
Mitral valve
G
Aortic arch
Ductus arteriosus
Pulmonary artery
Tricuspid valve
Right ventricle
H
PTFE graft
Ascending aorta
"Collar" connects
pulmonary artery
to aortic arch
I
Ascending aorta
Pulmonary valve
PTFE graft
Right ventricle

Norwood Operation

A number of palliative operations have been proposed. The Norwood operation is the one used most frequently.

Figure 21-2

A The operation is performed with the patient under deep hypothermia and circulatory arrest. Perfusion for cooling and rewarming is provided via a single venous cannula, with oxygenated blood returned to a cannula in the pulmonary artery passed through the ductus arteriosus to the aorta. The pulmonary artery is divided just above the sinuses of Valsalva. A long incision is made in the aorta from just above the sinus rim, through the ascending aorta and transverse arch, and into the upper portion of the descending aorta, past the region of coarctation (if present).

B The ductus arteriosus is ligated. The distal end of the pulmonary artery is closed by continuous suture, with attention paid to preserving the confluence between the right and left pulmonary arteries.

C A collar is fashioned from allograft pulmonary artery or polytetrafluoroethylene (PTFE) to enlarge the ascending aorta and aortic arch. A mattress stitch of 6/0 or 7/0 polypropylene is placed at the critical, delicate apex of the incision in the upper portion of the descending aorta.

D The collar is attached to the edges of the aortotomy by continuous suture. The suture line is placed from within the aorta and continued into the ascending aorta to a point opposite the right pulmonary artery.

E The pulmonary artery is attached to the collar using a continuous suture. The posterior wall of the pulmonary artery is attached to the portion of the collar connected to the posterior aortotomy.

F The anterior wall of the pulmonary artery is sutured to the collar attached to the anterior aortotomy. The tissue at the apex of the incision in the aortic sinuses is carefully attached to the collar and the pulmonary artery to create a wide opening between the pulmonary artery and the aorta while avoiding any narrowing of the sinuses.

G The anastomosis of the aorta to the pulmonary artery is completed by suturing the remainder of the collar to the lateral rim of the incision in the ascending aorta. The completed repair creates a common trunk of the aorta and proximal pulmonary artery. Blood flow to the distal pulmonary artery is restored in a controlled fashion by the creation of a right subclavian artery-to-right pulmonary artery anastomosis (Blalock-Taussig shunt). This is readily accomplished by dissecting the subclavian artery distal to the brachiocephalic artery and connecting the subclavian artery to the right pulmonary artery medial to the superior vena cava.

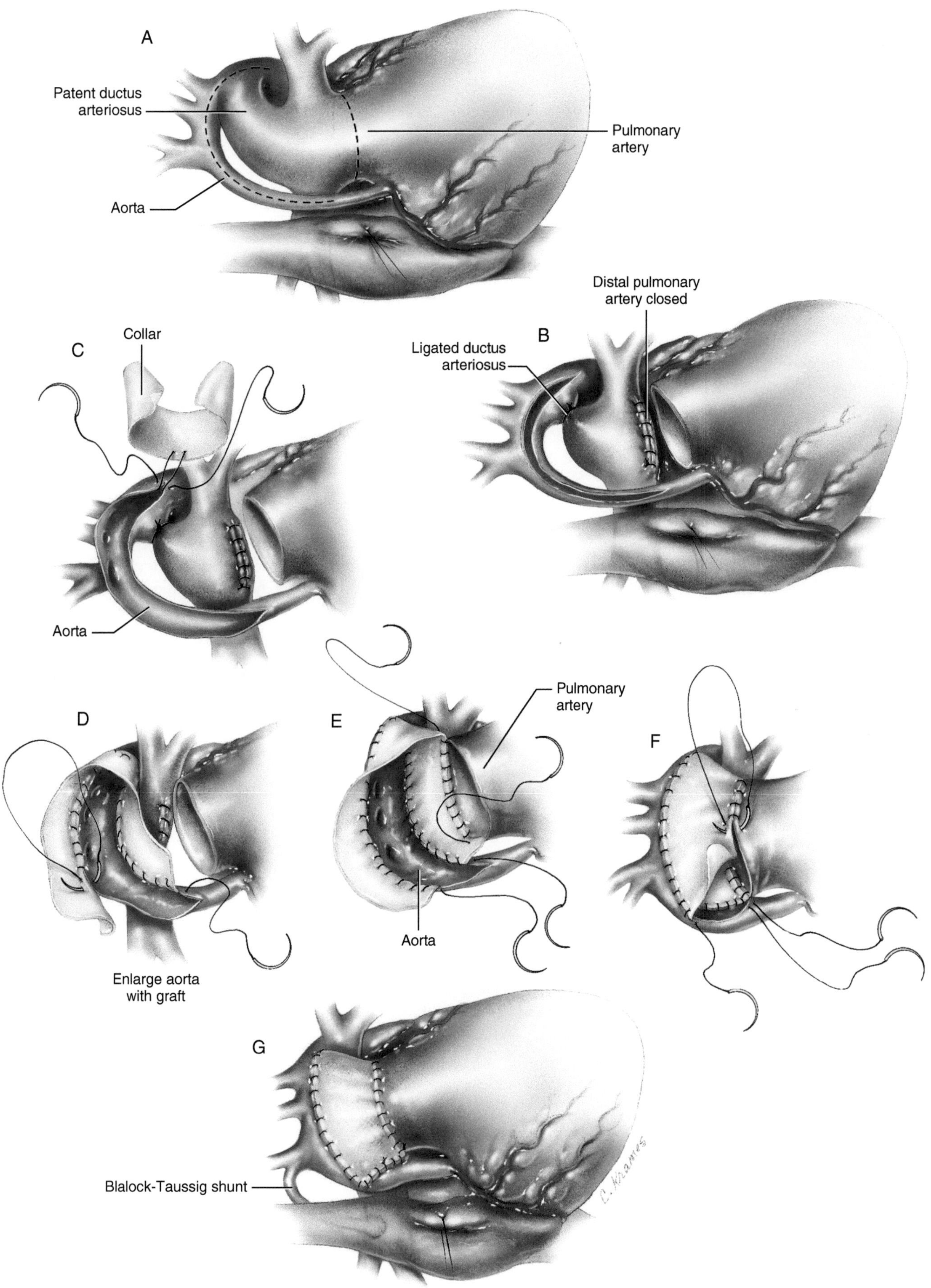
A
Patent ductus arteriosus
Pulmonary artery
Aorta
Distal pulmonary artery closed
C
Collar
B
Ligated ductus arteriosus
Aorta
D
E
Pulmonary artery
F
Aorta
Enlarge aorta with graft
G
Blalock-Taussig shunt
C. Kramer

Figure 21-2 (continued)

H A tapered patch can also be used. The patch is attached to the upper portion of the descending thoracic aorta beyond any coarctation segment.

I The patch is anastomosed to the sides of the aortotomy. The patch becomes wider proximally so that the opening diameter is sufficient to approximate the diameter of the pulmonary artery. The apex of the aortotomy is attached to the end of the pulmonary artery. The patch is attached to the pulmonary artery to create a common pulmonary artery and aorta.

J An alternative means of controlling pulmonary blood flow is to use the left subclavian artery as a central shunt. The initial aortic incision is made posterior to the origin of the left subclavian artery as the aortic arch is opened. This pathway was suggested by Hawkins, based on anatomic studies of cadaveric hearts with hypoplastic left heart syndrome.

K The posterior deviation of the aortic arch incision around the origin of the left subclavian artery leaves the left subclavian artery with the inferior rim of the aortotomy. Distal ligation and division of the left subclavian artery allow the artery to be rotated inferiorly so that the end faces the distal pulmonary artery. The pulmonary artery is partially closed by direct suture.

L An end-to-side anastomosis of the subclavian artery to the pulmonary artery is constructed using a combination of continuous and interrupted stitches of 7/0 polypropylene. A few stitches must be taken near the origin of the subclavian artery to create a more uniform edge for the anastomosis to the prosthetic collar and reconstruction of the common aortic trunk.

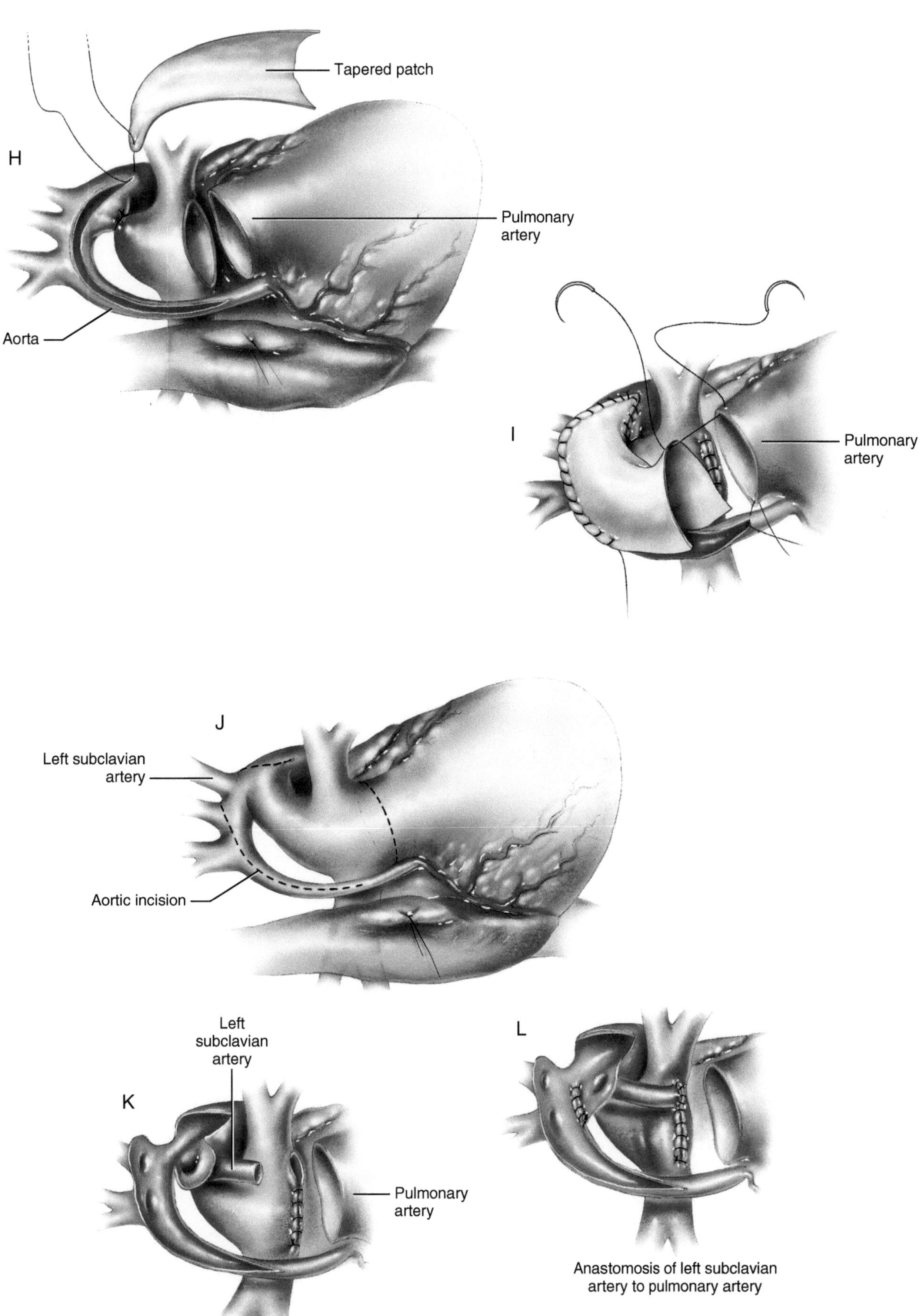
H
Tapered patch
Pulmonary artery
Aorta
I
Pulmonary artery
J
Left subclavian artery
Aortic incision
K
Left subclavian artery
Pulmonary artery
L
Anastomosis of left subclavian artery to pulmonary artery

Figure 21-2 (continued)

M Controlled pulmonary blood flow can also be accomplished using a polytetrafluoroethylene (PTFE) graft (modified Blalock-Taussig shunt). A 4-mm tubular PTFE graft is anastomosed to the side of the right brachiocephalic artery using continuous stitches of 6/0 or 7/0 polypropylene. The opposite end of the graft is anastomosed to the superior aspect of the right pulmonary artery in end-to-side fashion.

N Many surgeons currently prefer to achieve balanced pulmonary and aortic blood flow using a valveless conduit between the right ventricle and the pulmonary artery. This is called the Sano procedure. The distal pulmonary artery is not closed following division of the pulmonary artery in the initial stages of the operation. After the creation of the common aorta and pulmonary artery, a PTFE patch is used to close the distal pulmonary artery. A small ventriculotomy is made in the right ventricular outflow tract below the pulmonary valve.

O A 4 mm opening is made in the patch used to close the distal pulmonary artery. A 4-mm tubular PTFE graft is anastomosed to the patch in the pulmonary artery in an end-to-side fashion, using continuous stitches of 6/0 polypropylene. The tubular graft is anastomosed to the right ventriculotomy with continuous stitches of 4/0 polypropylene.

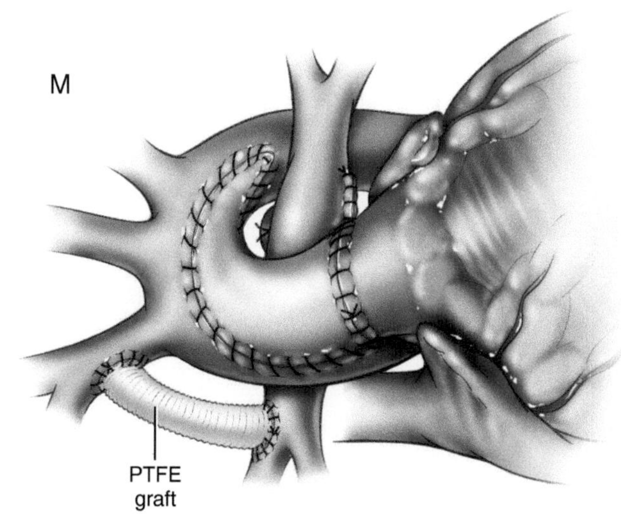

Modified Blalock-Taussig shunt

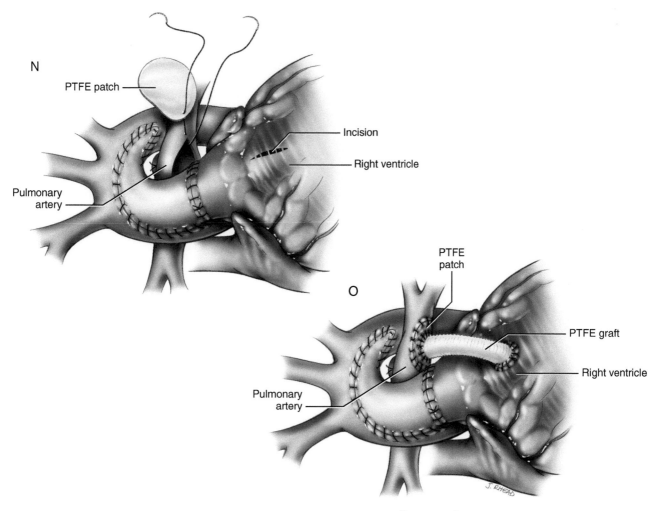

N
PTFE patch
Incision
Right ventricle
Pulmonary
artery

PTFE
patch
O
PTFE graft
Right ventricle
Pulmonary
artery

J. RHEAD

Sano procedure

part VII

Malposition of the Great Arteries

chapter 22

TRANSPOSITION OF THE GREAT ARTERIES

Transposition of the great arteries is a congenital cardiac anomaly defined by origin of the aorta from the right ventricle and origin of the pulmonary trunk from the left ventricle. The ventricular septum may be intact (simple transposition of the great arteries), or there may be a defect in the ventricular septum (transposition with ventricular septal defect).

Morphology

Figure 22-1

A Transposition of the great arteries, external view. The aorta originates from the right ventricle (ventriculoarterial discordant connection). It is anterior and to the right of the pulmonary artery, which arises from the left ventricle.

B Transposition of the great arteries, right ventricular view. The heavily trabeculated anatomic right ventricle is enlarged and hypertrophied. The right ventricular outflow tract, with its well-defined crista supraventricularis and ventricular infundibular fold, is in continuity with the aorta. The ostia of the coronary arteries confirm that this is the aorta. The aortic valve is normal.

C Transposition of the great arteries, left ventricular view. The finely trabeculated left ventricle is in continuity with the pulmonary trunk. The pulmonary valve is continuous with the mitral valve. The left ventricle has a thin wall because it pumps blood to the low-pressure pulmonary circulation.

D Transposition of the great arteries with ventricular septal defect. The aorta originates anteriorly from the right ventricle. The pulmonary trunk arises from the left ventricle and is located posterior to and to the left of the aorta. There is a ventricular septal defect in the membranous portion of the septum. The left ventricle is hypertrophied.

E Transposition of the great arteries with ventricular septal defect, magnified view. This view shows details of the close relationship between the ventricular septal defect and the pulmonary valve. The pulmonary valve is normal.

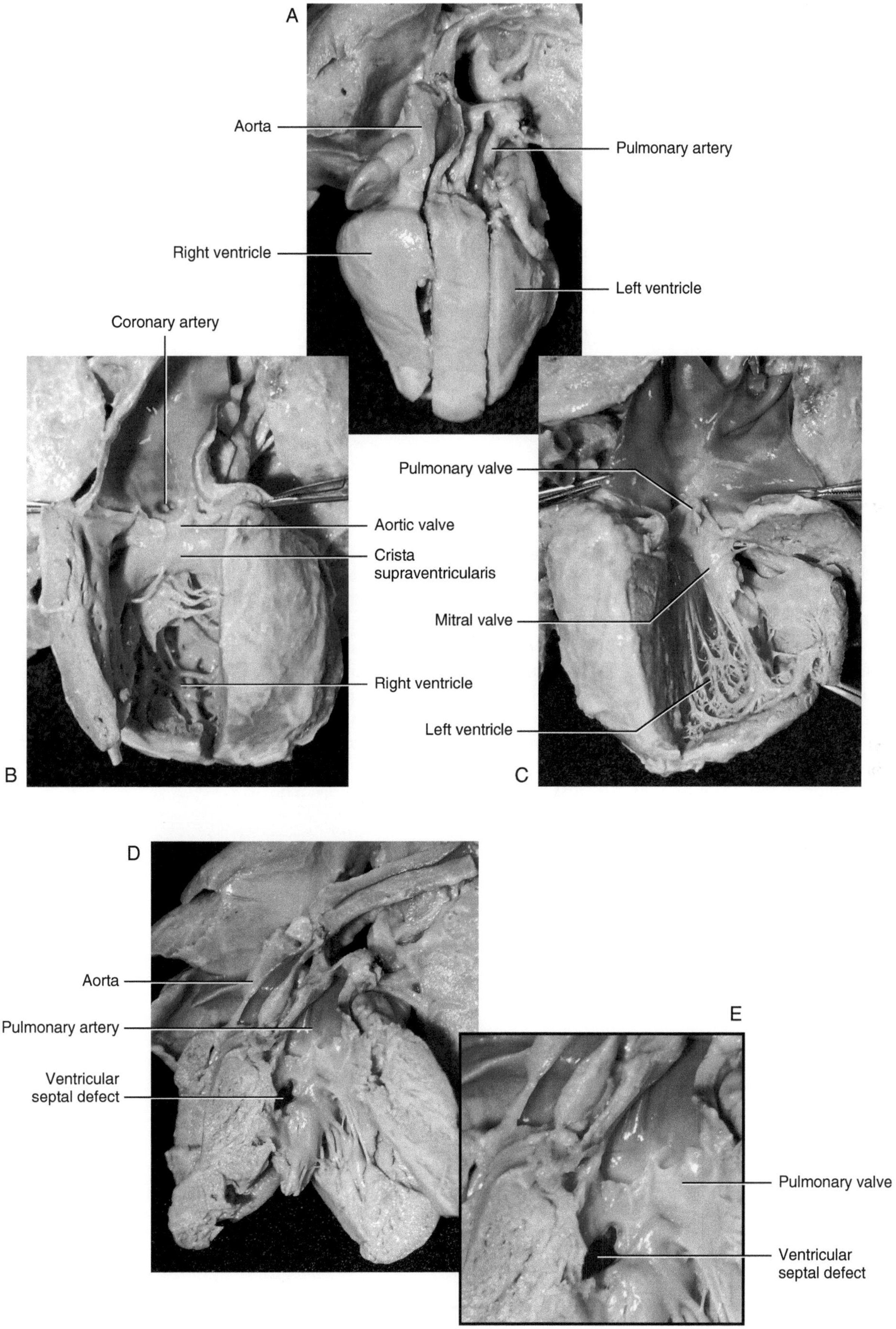

A
Aorta
Pulmonary artery
Right ventricle
Left ventricle

Coronary artery
Aortic valve
Crista supraventricularis
Right ventricle
B

Pulmonary valve
Mitral valve
Left ventricle
C

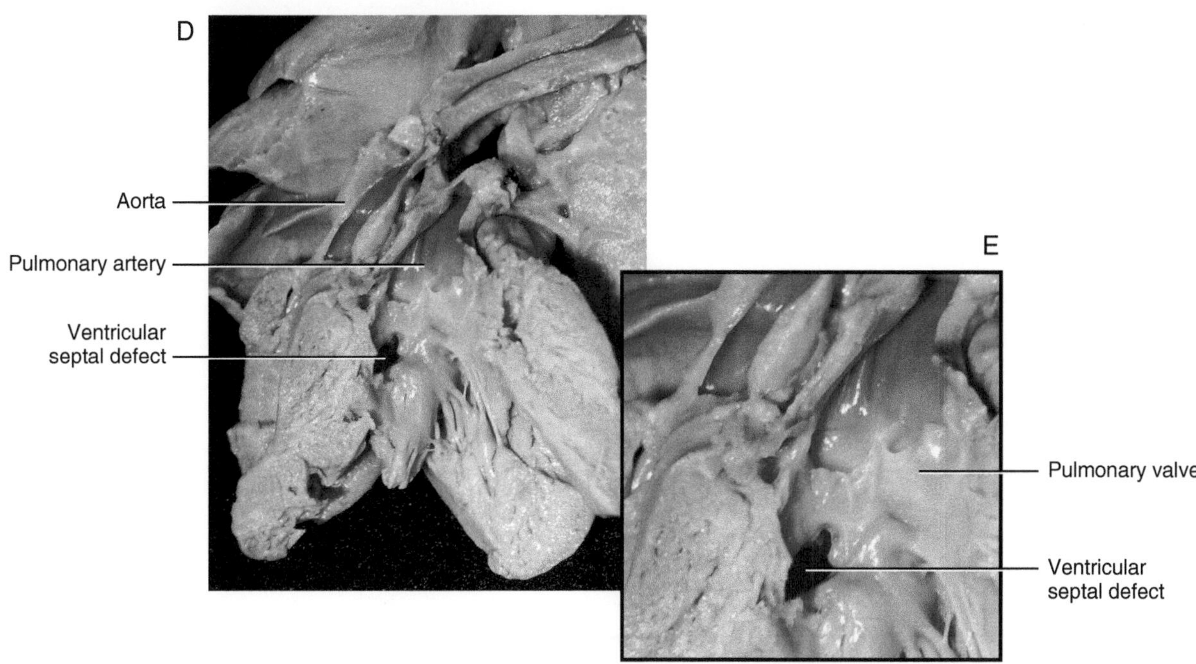

Arterial Repair

Arterial repair of transposition of the great arteries has its greatest application in patients presenting with an associated ventricular septal defect or those with an intact ventricular septum in the first month of life. In the former group, the left ventricle is enlarged and hypertrophied due to the ventricular septal defect, so it is well prepared to function as the systemic ventricle. Likewise, in the latter group there is normal fetal development of the left ventricle, which has not had time to involute as it naturally would because it functions as the pulmonary ventricle in transposition of the great arteries.

Figure 22-2

A The unique arrangement of the coronary arteries in transposition of the great arteries makes it possible to exchange the positions of the great vessels and transfer the coronary arteries to effect an anatomic correction. The aortic root is usually located directly anterior to the pulmonary trunk, and the coronary arteries originate from the posterior sinuses of Valsalva. The coronary ostia are in close approximation to the anterior wall of the pulmonary artery in most cases. Even though there are variations in the anatomic arrangement of the coronary arteries, in nearly all cases of transposition of the great arteries it is possible to transfer the coronary arteries to the pulmonary artery.

B The aorta and pulmonary arteries are divided. The aorta is divided above the sinuses of Valsalva, leaving it slightly longer anteriorly. The pulmonary artery is divided above the valve at a level approximating that of the aorta, taking into account the origin of the right pulmonary artery. The aorta is mobilized completely away from the pulmonary artery. The pulmonary artery is then divided under full exposure. The ligamentum arteriosum is mobilized and divided.

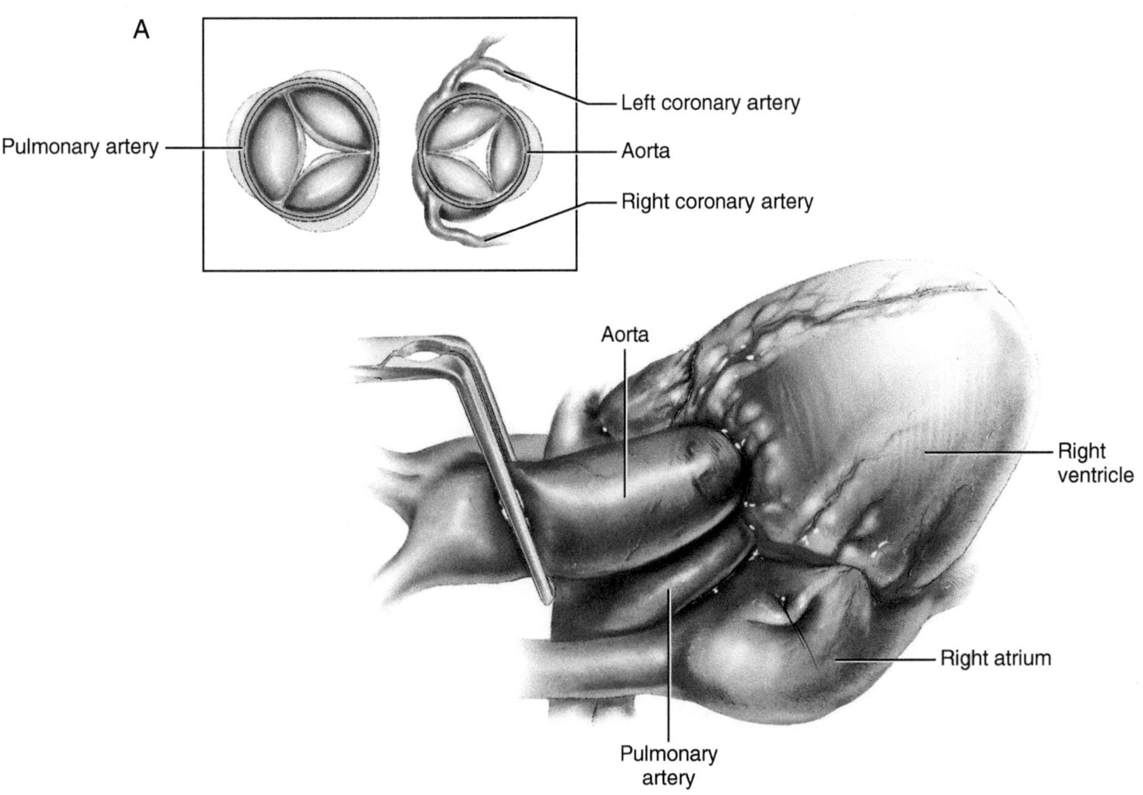
A
Left coronary artery
Pulmonary artery
Aorta
Right coronary artery
Aorta
Right ventricle
Right atrium
Pulmonary artery

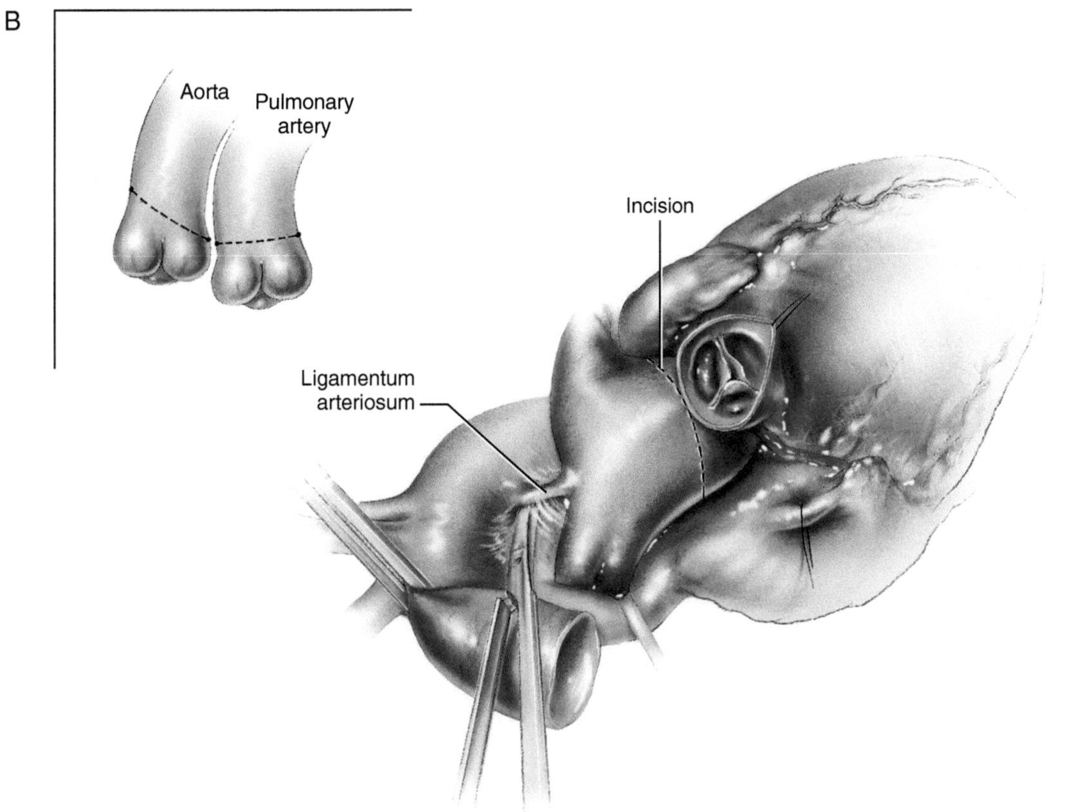
B
Aorta
Pulmonary artery
Incision
Ligamentum arteriosum

Figure 22-2 (continued)

C The right and left pulmonary arteries are completely mobilized. The right and left coronary arteries are removed from the aorta, along with a generous amount of sinus aorta, cutting into the sinus from the free edge of the divided aorta. The proximal coronary arteries are mobilized minimally, if at all.

D Similar excisions of the pulmonary artery in the sinuses adjacent to the coronary arteries are made. The coronary arteries are rotated slightly to approximate the openings in the pulmonary artery. The coronary arteries are anastomosed to the pulmonary artery using continuous stitches of 6/0 to 7/0 polypropylene, depending on the thickness of the tissue. Polydioxanone suture material can also be considered for this anastomosis because growth of this part of the repair remains an unknown factor in late results. Suturing is started at the lowest point in the sinus opening and continues in both directions to a knot at the top edge of the pulmonary artery.

E The distal aorta is drawn behind the bifurcation of the pulmonary artery (LeCompte maneuver). An anastomosis is created between the proximal pulmonary artery and the distal aorta. A double-needle 5/0 to 6/0 polypropylene or polydioxanone suture is started posteriorly, placing several suture loops before drawing the arteries together. The suture line is continued to completion anteriorly. At this point the aortic occlusion clamp can be removed temporarily to check these critical posterior suture lines.

F The defects in the aortic sinuses created by excision of the coronary arteries are filled in with pericardium or polytetrafluoroethylene (PTFE) graft.

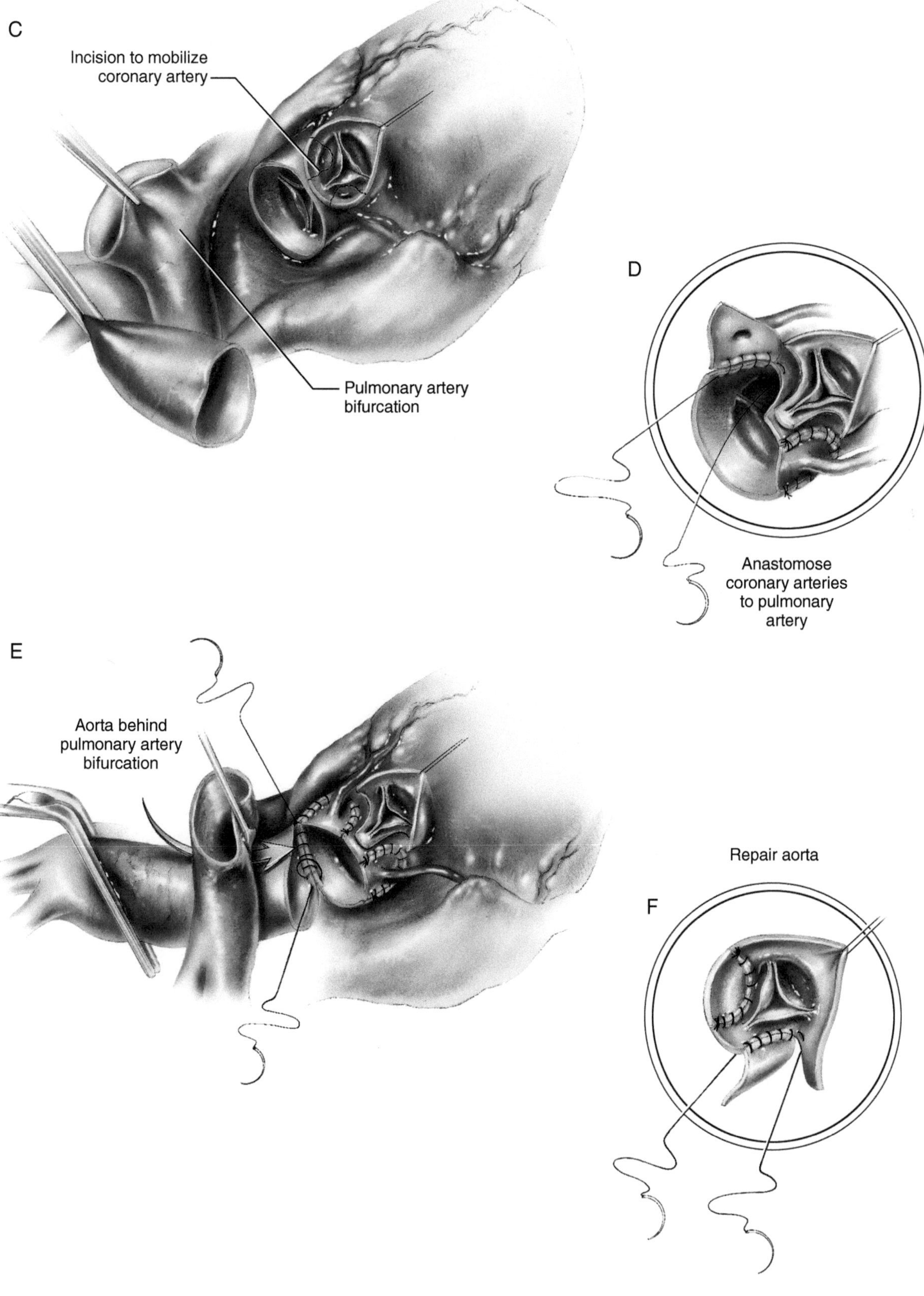
C
Incision to mobilize coronary artery
Pulmonary artery bifurcation
D
Anastomose coronary arteries to pulmonary artery
E
Aorta behind pulmonary artery bifurcation
Repair aorta
F

Figure 22-2 (continued)

G An anastomosis is created between the proximal aorta and the distal pulmonary artery. The pulmonary artery bifurcation lying anterior to the distal aorta is usually long enough to reach to the aorta, especially if the aorta was left with a slightly longer anterior portion when divided. The anastomosis is performed using 5/0 to 6/0 polypropylene or polydioxanone suture material in continuous stitches. The suture line is started posteriorly, and several suture loops are placed prior to drawing the ends of the arteries together.

H The completed repair is an anatomic correction of the defect, in that the left ventricle becomes the systemic ventricle and the right ventricle becomes the pulmonary ventricle.

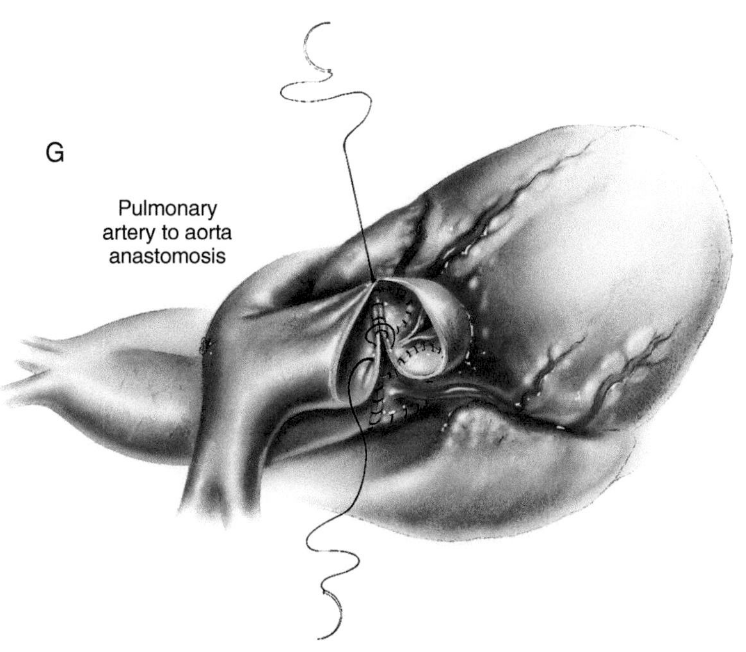

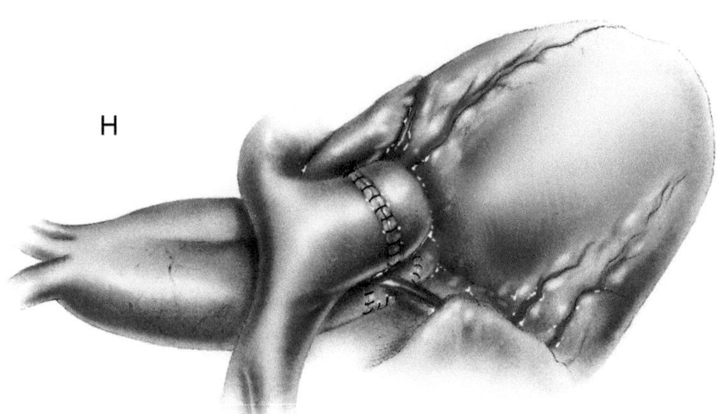

Completed repair

Atrial Repair: Senning Operation

Atrial repair of transposition of the great arteries has become less frequent as arterial repair has become more popular. Nevertheless, there are circumstances when atrial repair is desirable. Atrial repair by the Senning operation may be preferred in patients who present with transposition of the great arteries after the first month of life or in those referred for operation after successful palliation by atrial septectomy or balloon septostomy.

Figure 22-3

A The superior vena cava is cannulated directly using a right-angled cannula through a purse-string stitch of 3/0 polypropylene at the pericardial reflection. The inferior vena cava is cannulated through the right atrium just above the diaphragm. An incision is made in the right atrium anterior and parallel to the crista terminalis. The incision should be sufficiently anterior to the interatrial groove to provide a strip of right atrium at least as wide as the venae cavae. The incision is extended around the base of the right atrial appendage and into the tip of the appendage on its medial wall. The incision should be anterior to the sinoatrial node. The right atrium is mobilized off the anterior wall of the left atrium by dissection in the interatrial groove. An incision is made in the anterior wall of the left atrium in a location as medial as possible. The incision may be extended to the right superior pulmonary vein to achieve maximal opening.

B With a retractor placed in the tricuspid valve, the atrial septum can be visualized. The foramen ovale atrial septal defect is identified. The atrial septum is mobilized by incising the septum anterior and superior to the septal defect, creating a flap of the atrial septum. A small patch is fashioned from double-velour knitted Dacron to fill in the atrial septal defect. A PTFE patch could also be used.

This patch should be just large enough to fill in the defect; it should not enlarge the atrial septum. The patch is sutured to the lateral wall of the right atrium and to the septal flap with a continuous stitch of 4/0 polypropylene. When an atrial septectomy (Blalock-Hanlon operation) has been performed previously, a larger, trapezoid-shaped patch is used.

C The retractor is moved into the mitral valve orifice, posterior to the remnant of the atrial septum. This exposes the posterior wall of the left atrium, the left atrial appendage, and the left pulmonary veins. The mobilized portion of the atrial septum is displaced posteriorly and attached to the left atrial wall, anterior to the left pulmonary veins and posterior to the left atrial appendage and the mitral valve. A continuous stitch of 4/0 polydioxanone is used to attach the atrial septum to the left atrial wall. This slowly absorbable suture should allow better growth potential. The suture line is started anterior to the left pulmonary veins and continued to the right side of the atrium, posterior to the superior and inferior caval orifices. As the suture line proceeds laterally, the stitches are kept close to the venae cavae so that a wide channel is maintained posteriorly between the suture lines. The opening into the left atrium will be widened as the right atrial wall is pulled medially, along with the atrial septum as it is displaced to be attached to the left atrial wall. The size of the prosthetic patch added to the septum must therefore be kept small to ensure this effect.

D With the retractor returned to the tricuspid valve, the size of the passageway from the venae cavae to the mitral valve beneath the atrial septal remnant is determined. If it is judged adequate, a suture line can be placed along the atrial septal remnant and to the right of the coronary sinus, which reduces the possibility of injury to the atrioventricular node and proximal conduction bundle. If the passageway seems too narrow, it can be enlarged by dividing the common wall between the coronary sinus and the inferior wall of the left atrium. The caval passageway is thereby enlarged equivalent to the circumference of the coronary sinus.

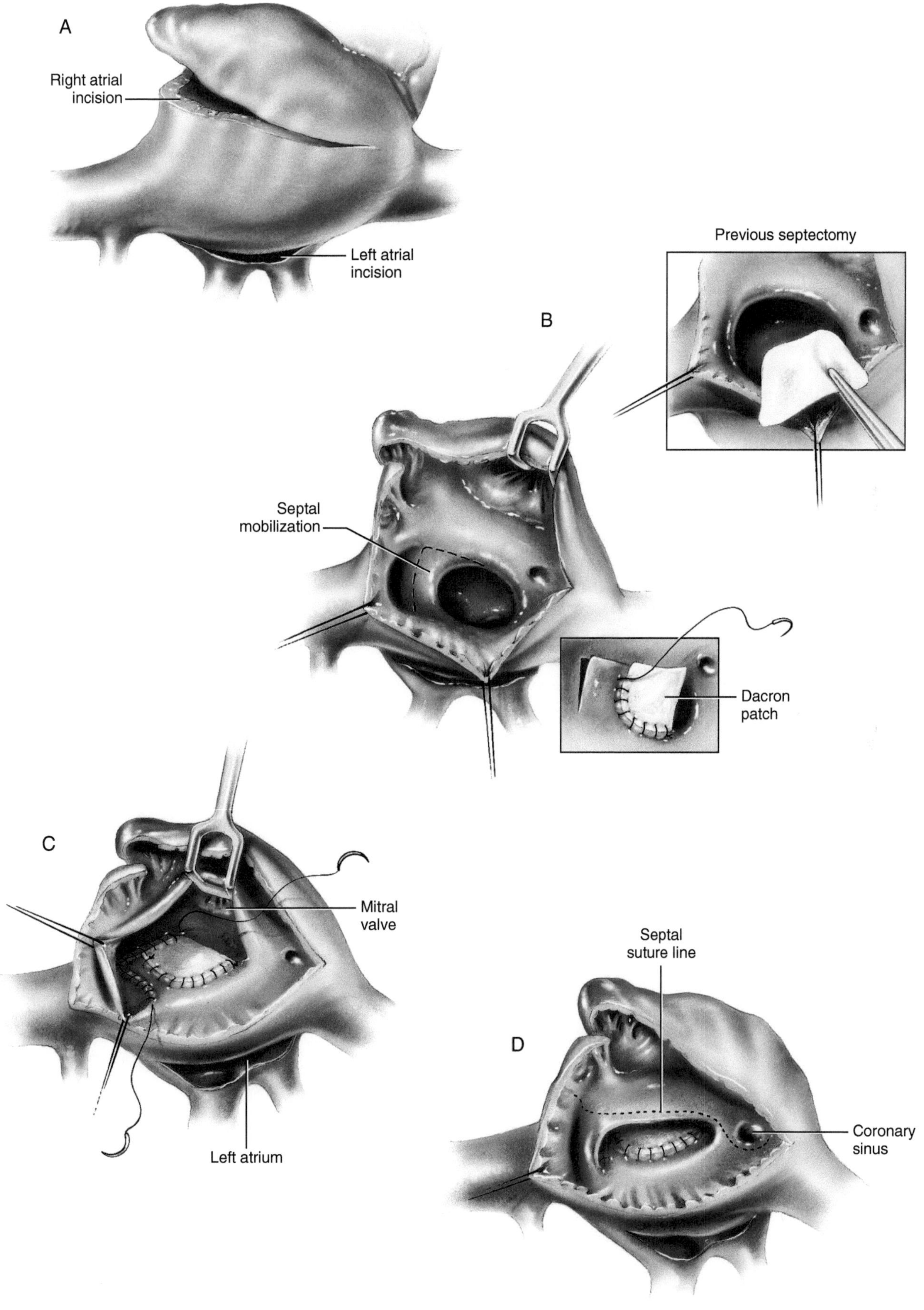
A
Right atrial incision
Left atrial incision
Previous septectomy
B
Septal mobilization
Dacron patch
C
Mitral valve
Left atrium
Septal suture line
D
Coronary sinus

Figure 22-3 (continued)

E The posterior rim of the right atriotomy is attached to the atrial septal remnant with a continuous stitch beginning at the superior end of the atriotomy. A Hegar dilator is passed into the superior vena cava to ensure an adequate caval orifice. The sinoatrial node is located posterior to the suture line. Another suture line is started inferiorly, attaching the posterior rim of the atriotomy to the eustachian valve or the floor of the right atrium and the lateral rim of the coronary sinus. This creates a passageway for blood to flow from the venae cavae to the left atrioventricular valve between the atrial septal remnant and the posteriorly displaced atrial septum.

F The anterior rim of the right atriotomy is attached to the lateral rim of the left atriotomy by continuous suture. Several loops of 4/0 polydioxanone suture are placed between the atrial flap and the right pulmonary veins prior to approximating these structures. The suture line should be placed only on the lateral half of the left atrial orifice to avoid creating a circumferential closure, which might constrict the left atrial opening. A transition must be made across pericardial-mediastinal tissues to reach the vena cava or right atrium at the halfway point. At the superior end, the suture line crosses a tenuous point along the roof of the left atrium, right pulmonary artery, and posterior aspect of the superior vena cava. Adequate tissue to hold the suture and to conform the atrial flap closure to the irregular contour must be ensured. Extra length of the atrial flap should be worked into the area over the superior vena cava to avoid tension. The suture line is cephalad to the sinoatrial node. A similar transition across the interatrial groove to the right atrial wall must be accomplished inferiorly. The completed repair directs blood flow from the left atrium to the right atrioventricular valve.

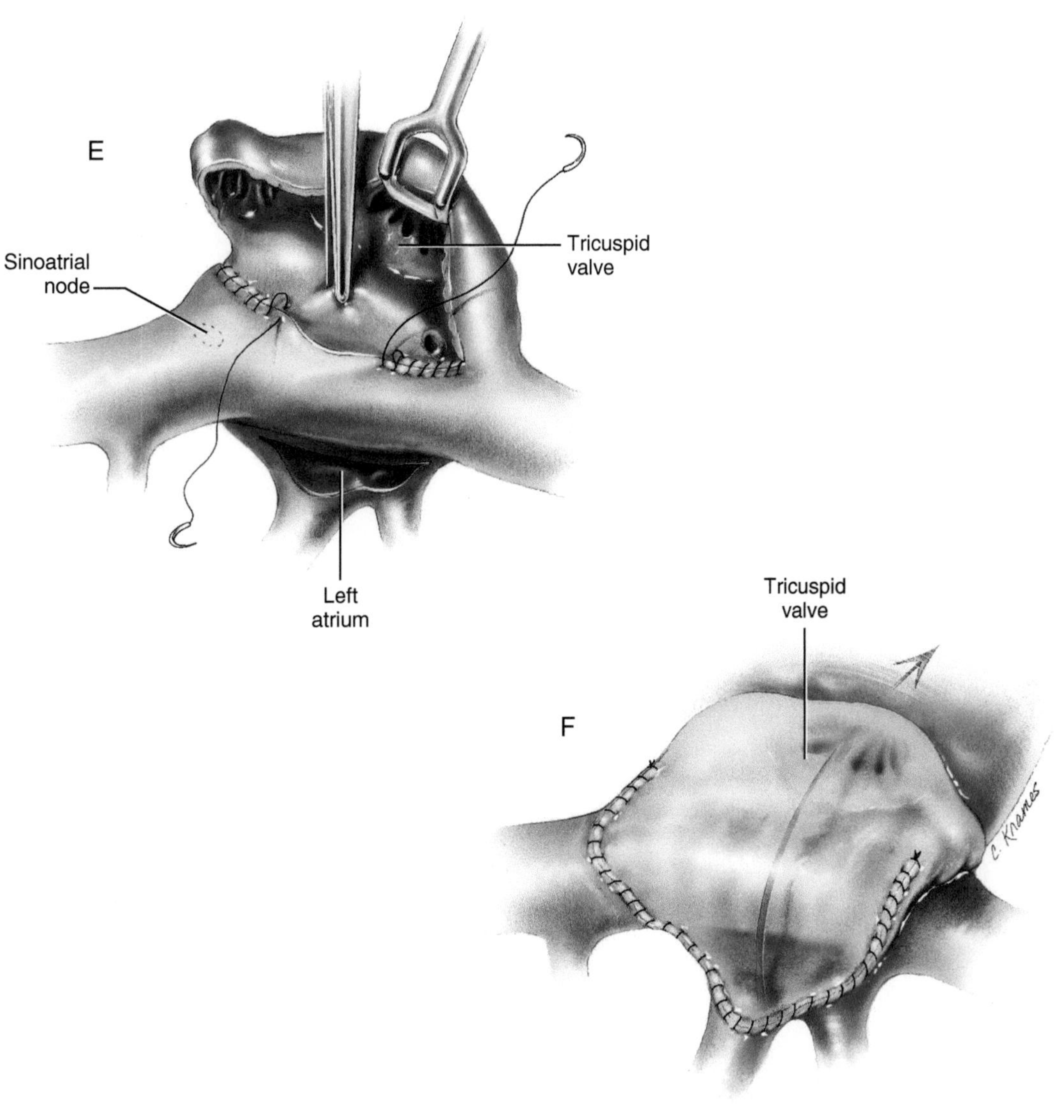
E
Sinoatrial node
Tricuspid valve
Left atrium
Tricuspid valve
F
Completed repair

Atrial Repair: Mustard Procedure

This operation had widespread application at one time, and although it is performed less often today, it still has utility. It is also important to know the details of this operation because the systemic ventricle is the right ventricle, which is subject to failure after some years. Cardiac transplantation may be required after the Mustard procedure, and knowledge of how the operation was performed helps the surgeon take it apart efficiently and safely.

Figure 22-4

A A rectangular patch is fashioned from the anterior pericardium. The pericardium for the intraatrial baffle is excised over the great vessels superiorly, to the level of the diaphragm inferiorly. This pattern of excision provides the heart's appropriate premeasured length as contained within the pericardium. The width of the rectangular pericardial patch is about two-thirds the length. The superior vena cava is cannulated directly through a purse-string stitch at the pericardial reflection. The inferior vena cava is cannulated through the right atrium above the diaphragm. An incision is made in the right atrium parallel to the atrioventricular groove.

B A retractor is placed in the tricuspid valve, exposing the atrial septum. The atrial septum is excised superiorly and laterally to the right atrial wall. The medial portions of the atrial septum are preserved.

C The pericardial patch is attached to the left atrium using double-armed 4/0 polypropylene suture. The suture line is begun anterior to the left pulmonary veins and posterior to the left atrial appendage.

D The suture line is taken along the superior wall of the left atrium, posterior to the superior vena cava orifice, to the junction of the atrial septal remnant and the right lateral wall of the right atrium. The suture line is taken inferiorly along the wall of the left atrium, posterior to the mitral valve, and posterior to the inferior vena cava orifice, to the septal remnant at the right side of the atrium. An incision is made in the pericardial patch approximately halfway across it to form two limbs and to shorten the waist of the pericardial patch so that it will not bulge into the pulmonary venous outflow. With the suture line beginning at the apex of the incision in the patch, the pericardium is attached to the midportion of the septal remnant.

E The suture line is taken superiorly along the edge of the septal remnant near the commissure of the septal and anterior leaflets of the tricuspid valve. At this point the suture line is taken across the right atrial wall and around the orifice of the superior vena cava anteriorly.

F The suture line is taken inferiorly along the septal remnant and to the right side of the coronary sinus. It is continued across the floor of the right atrium and anterior to the orifice of the inferior vena cava to complete the repair.

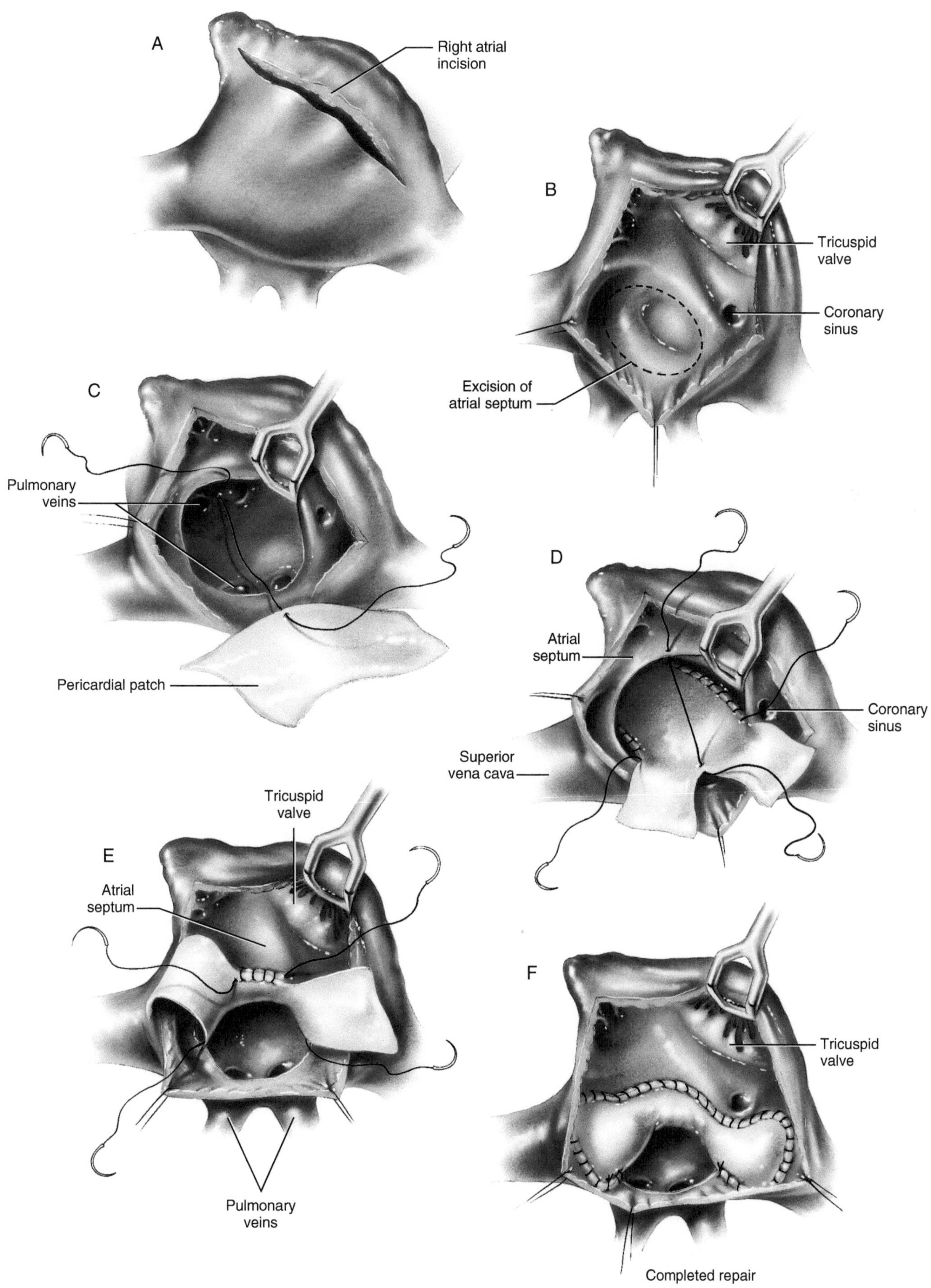
A
Right atrial incision
B
Tricuspid valve
Coronary sinus
Excision of atrial septum
C
Pulmonary veins
Pericardial patch
D
Atrial septum
Coronary sinus
Superior vena cava
E
Tricuspid valve
Atrial septum
Pulmonary veins
F
Tricuspid valve
Completed repair

chapter 23 TRANSPOSITION WITH VENTRICULAR INVERSION (CORRECTED TRANSPOSITION)

The aorta originates from the morphologic right ventricle and is located in levoposition anterior and to the left of the pulmonary artery, which originates from the morphologic left ventricle (discordant ventriculoarterial connection). There is a discordant connection of the atria and ventricles (ventricular inversion), meaning that the morphologic right atrium connects to the morphologic left ventricle, and in like manner, the left atrium connects with the right ventricle. Thus, the transposition of the great arteries is "corrected" in terms of blood flow through the heart. Ventricular septal defect and pulmonic stenosis are the intracardiac defects most commonly associated with corrected transposition of the great arteries.

Morphology
Figure 23-1

A Transposition with ventricular inversion (corrected transposition), right heart. This specimen demonstrates the trabeculated right atrium connected to the finely trabeculated morphologic left ventricle. The ventricular wall has the typical thickness of a left ventricle. The right atrioventricular valve separating the right atrium from the left ventricle is a typical mitral valve. This valve is supported by chordae tendineae and papillary muscles of a mitral valve. There is a ventricular septal defect high in the septum.

B Transposition with ventricular inversion (corrected transposition), magnified view. This view shows the details of the high-lying ventricular septal defect. The bundle of His is located in the subendocardial tissue of the anterior rim of the ventricular septal defect. Details of the mitral-type leaflets of the right atrioventricular valve, with its chordae tendineae and papillary muscles, are demonstrated.

C Transposition with ventricular inversion (corrected transposition), left heart. The left atrium is not seen in this view. The inlet to the ventricle is through the left atrioventricular valve, which has the anatomic characteristics of a tricuspid valve. The ventricle is heavily trabeculated, typical for a morphologic right ventricle. The aorta is connected to this morphologic right ventricle (transposition of great arteries, discordant ventriculoarterial connection).

D Transposition with ventricular inversion (corrected transposition), left atrioventricular valve. The morphologic details of the left atrioventricular valve are shown in this magnified view. The three leaflets of a tricuspid-type atrioventricular valve are clearly demonstrated.

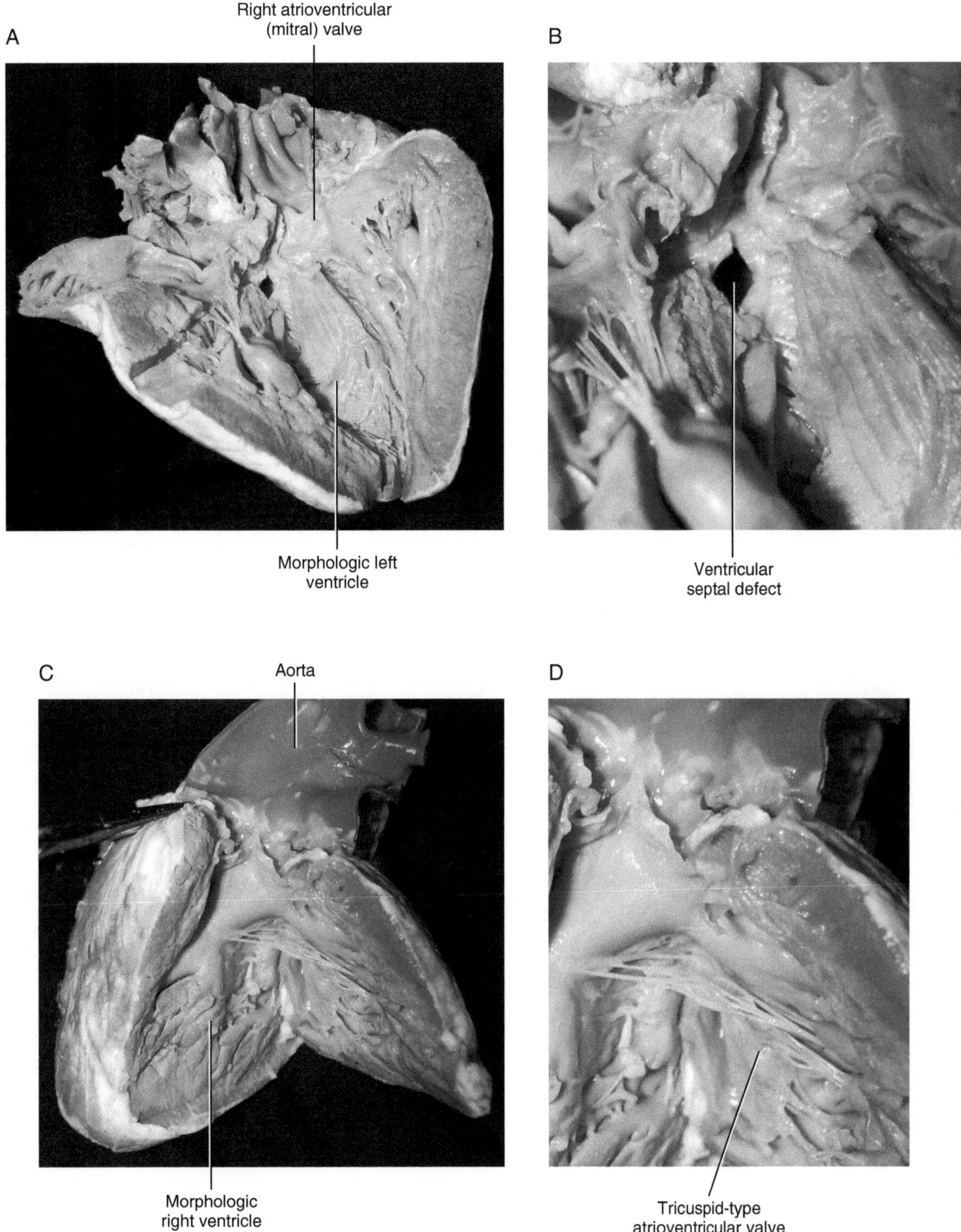
A
Right atrioventricular
(mitral) valve
Morphologic left
ventricle
B
Ventricular
septal defect
C
Aorta
Morphologic
right ventricle
D
Tricuspid-type
atrioventricular valve

Correction of Ventricular Septal Defect

The operative situations encountered when correcting the intracardiac defects associated with transposition with ventricular inversion are related primarily to the unique location of the specialized electrical conduction system of the heart in this anomaly.

Figure 23-2

A Intracardiac defects can usually be repaired through an incision in the right atrium parallel to the atrioventricular groove, with no need to incise the ventricles.

B Inside the morphologic right atrium, the right atrioventricular valve has the structure of an inverted mitral valve, since it leads to the morphologic left ventricle. Retraction of this valve to adequately expose the intraventricular structures can generally be accomplished safely under cardioplegic conditions without splitting the commissure or detaching the valve leaflet. The atrioventricular node is usually located anteriorly in the floor of the atrium, close to the commissure between the septal and anterior leaflets of the right atrioventricular valve. There may be a second atrioventricular node in the usual location near the coronary sinus.

C The bundle of His courses through the subendocardial tissue anterior to the annulus of the pulmonary artery and in the anterior rim of the ventricular septal defect on the right side of the septum. Sutures placed in the usual manner to close a perimembranous-type ventricular septal defect would interrupt the bundle of His.

D The ventricular septal defect is closed using a prosthetic patch fashioned from crimped, knitted, double-velour polyester (Dacron). Working through the ventricular septal defect, the surgeon places a continuous stitch of 4/0 polypropylene between the left side of the ventricular septum and the prosthetic patch. A small Teflon pledget in the center of the suture prevents it from cutting the septum and allows two or three suture loops to be placed on both sides of the center. Tension on the suture loops provides exposure for succeeding stitches. Three groups of suture loops are placed, with the patch held away from the ventricular septum. Placing the sutures in this manner provides good exposure and allows all the stitches to be placed deeply in the left side of the septum around the anterior margin of the ventricular septal defect before the patch is approximated to the ventricular septum. Sutures should also be placed on the left side along the posteroinferior margin of the ventricular septal defect; this area is less important, however, and stitches may be placed in the rim of the defect. Between the two atrioventricular valves, the stitches should be placed securely into the fibrous connective tissue separating the valves.

When all the stitches are in place, the suture loops are pulled up through the tissue, positioning the patch to the left side of the ventricular septum. The ends of the suture groups are joined to finish the repair.

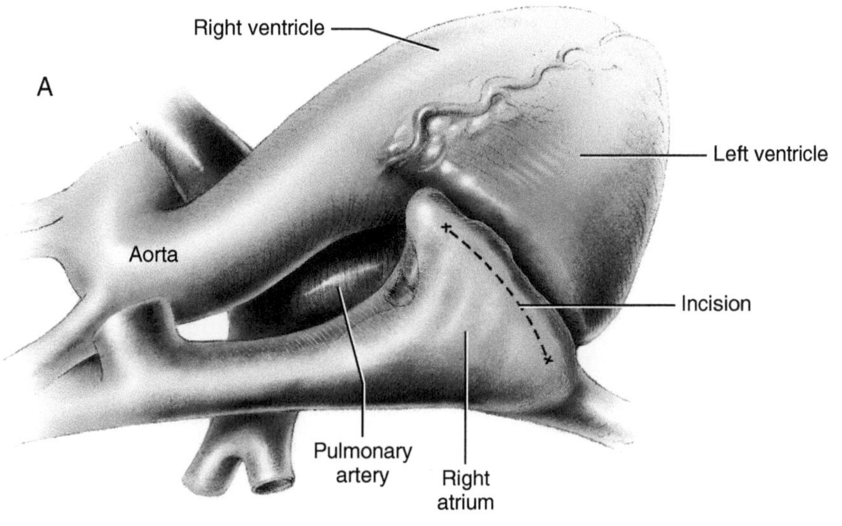

B
Right atrioventricular valve
Primary site of atrioventricular node
Coronary sinus
Secondary site of atrioventricular node

C
Pulmonary valve
Bundle of His
Atrioventricular node
Ventricular septal defect

D
Stitches on left side of septum
Prosthetic patch

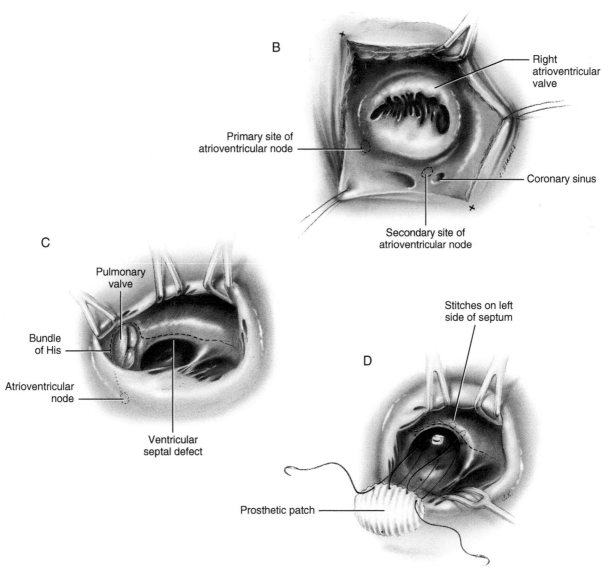

Correction of Pulmonary Outflow Tract Obstruction

Pulmonary outflow tract obstruction in this congenital anomaly may be caused by stenosis of the pulmonic valve cusps, hypoplasia of the pulmonary annulus, or hypertrophy of the subannular myocardium. Commonly, the obstruction is a combination of valvular-annular-subannular stenosis. The significance of the subannular component depends on the amount of myocardium interposed between the pulmonary annulus and the right atrioventricular valve annulus and ventricular septal defect. There is often considerable hypertrophied myocardium in this location, which must be incised or excised. The subendocardial myocardium anterior to the pulmonary annulus contains the bundle of His.

Figure 23-3

A An oblique incision is made in the anterior wall of the pulmonary artery. In the case of significant annular or subannular obstruction, enlargement of the pulmonary outflow tract is required. The incision is extended laterally to the right in a spiral fashion and continued onto the posterior wall of the pulmonary artery. The pulmonary annulus is divided posteriorly, and the incision is extended deep into the subannular obstructing myocardium. The length of the incision into the subannular myocardium depends on the amount of hypertrophied myocardium that separates the pulmonary annulus from the annulus of the atrioventricular valve. The incision may be extended into the ventricular septal defect, but this risks detachment of the left atrioventricular valve. Some of this myocardium may be excised posteriorly without damaging the conduction system. These incisions, combined with incision or excision of any obstructive pulmonary valve tissue, should produce considerable widening of the pulmonary outflow tract. A spiral patch fashioned from a tubular graft of crimped Dacron is used to fill in the defect created by the spiral incision of the outflow tract.

B The Dacron patch is placed in the pulmonary artery across the annulus and into the ventricle. The initial stitches are placed deep in the subannular myocardium via the right atrioventricular valve. A continuous stitch of 4/0 polypropylene is generally used unless the myocardium is unusually soft, in which case pledget-reinforced mattress sutures are used. When the annulus of the pulmonary artery is reached, or if exposure becomes difficult superiorly, the suture ends are passed into the pulmonary artery, and the rest of the repair is exposed from above.

C The pulmonary artery can simply be closed with an outflow patch, leaving the pulmonary valve incompetent, or the pulmonary valve can be replaced. If pulmonary valve replacement is chosen, the prosthetic device is sutured to the natural pulmonary annulus anteriorly and to the prosthetic patch posteriorly at the level of the annulus.

D The rest of the pulmonary artery is sutured to the spiral prosthetic patch to complete the outflow tract enlargement.

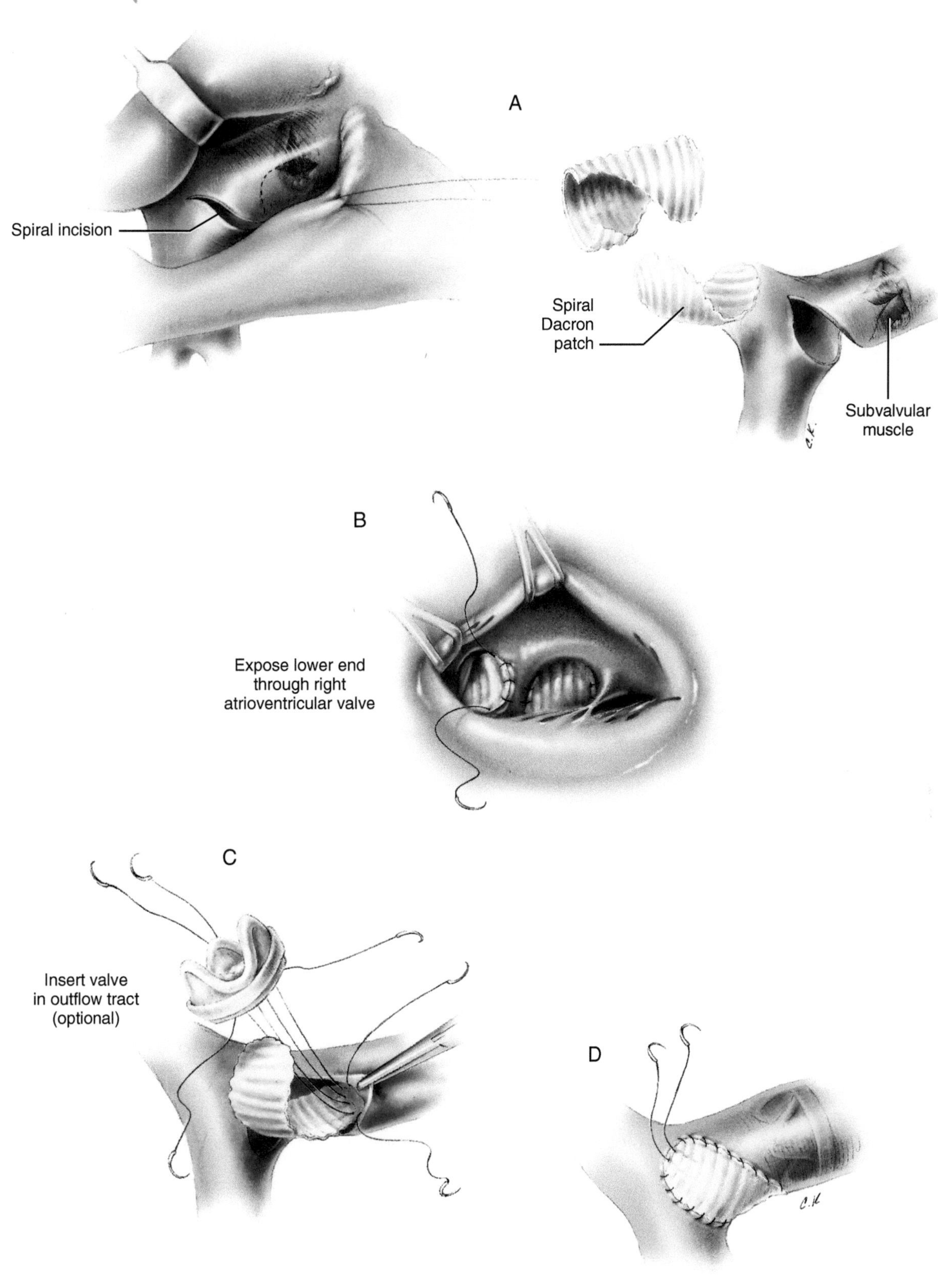
A
Spiral incision
Spiral
Dacron
patch
Subvalvular
muscle
B
Expose lower end
through right
atrioventricular valve
C
Insert valve
in outflow tract
(optional)
D
Completed repair

chapter 24 DOUBLE-OUTLET RIGHT VENTRICLE

Double-outlet right ventricle is defined as an anomaly in which both the aorta and the pulmonary artery originate from the right ventricle. The defect is always associated with a ventricular septal defect. Variations of the anomaly are classified according to the relationship of the ventricular septal defect to the great vessels. By this classification, the ventricular septal defect may be subaortic, subpulmonary, related to both the aorta and the pulmonary artery (doubly committed), or related to neither (noncommitted).

Morphology

Figure 24-1

A Double-outlet right ventricle, subaortic ventricular septal defect, right ventricular view. The heavily trabeculated, hypertrophied right ventricle is opened, and the anterior wall is reflected laterally. The aorta originates from the anterior aspect of the right ventricle. The aorta is identified by the coronary arteries observed in the sinuses of Valsalva of a normal semilunar valve and by the branches of the aortic arch. A normal tricuspid atrioventricular valve occupies the inlet to the right ventricle and is separated from the aortic valve by a conus or infundibular portion of the right ventricle. The conus under the aortic valve obscures the view of the pulmonary valve. There is a defect in the ventricular septum below the aortic valve, separated from the valve by the conus under the aorta.

B Double-outlet right ventricle, subaortic ventricular septal defect, magnified view of aortic outflow tract. Details of the aortic valve, coronary arteries, and tricuspid valve are seen clearly, along with the features of the right ventricular conus leading to the aorta. The ventricular septal defect is located in the perimembranous portion of the ventricular septum and is closely related to the tricuspid valve. There is some distance separating the ventricular septal defect from the aortic valve, even though the defect is directly inferior to the aorta.

C Double-outlet right ventricle, subaortic ventricular septal defect, left ventricular view. The pulmonary trunk is overriding a large perimembranous-type ventricular septal defect with more than 50% of the trunk on the right ventricular side of the septum, thus meeting morphologic criteria for the diagnosis of double-outlet right ventricle. That is, the aorta and pulmonary artery originate entirely or in large part from the right ventricle. There is a much smaller conus or infundibular portion of the right ventricle under the pulmonary artery than was observed under the aorta.

D Double-outlet right ventricle, subaortic ventricular septal defect, magnified left ventricular view. Details of the pulmonary valve, mitral valve, and ventricular septal defect are demonstrated. The mitral valve is not continuous with the pulmonary artery, as it would be in transposition of the great arteries.

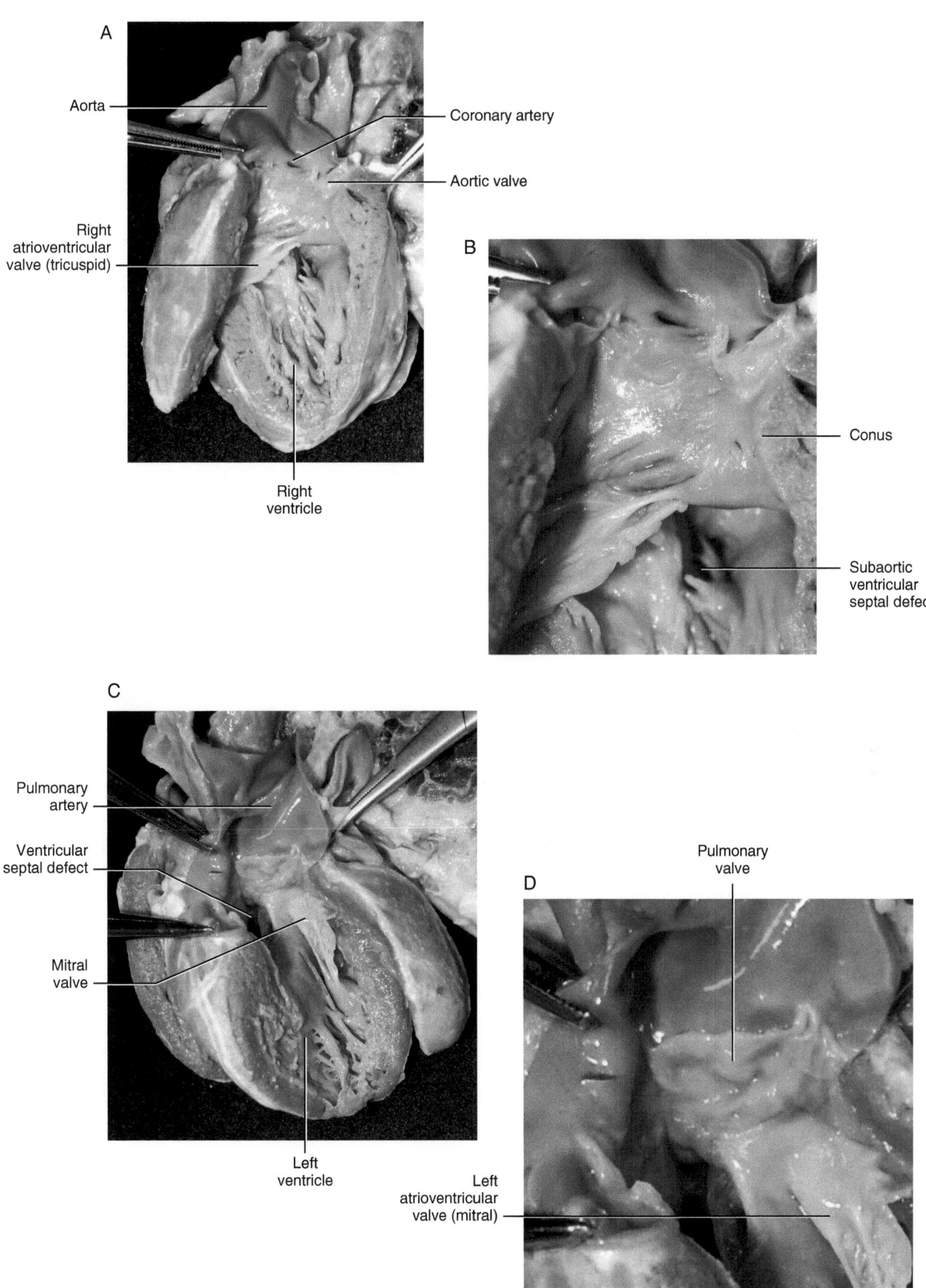
A
Aorta
Coronary artery
Aortic valve
Right atrioventricular valve (tricuspid)
Right ventricle
B
Conus
Subaortic ventricular septal defect
C
Pulmonary artery
Ventricular septal defect
Mitral valve
Left ventricle
D
Pulmonary valve
Left atrioventricular valve (mitral)

Figure 24-1 (continued)

E Double-outlet right ventricle, subaortic ventricular septal defect, operative image. The aorta and pulmonary artery originate from the right ventricle, with the vessels nearly side by side; the aorta is to the right of and only slightly posterior to the pulmonary artery. A double conus on the right ventricle is demonstrated.

F Double-outlet right ventricle, subpulmonary ventricular septal defect, right ventricular view. The right ventricle is opened anteriorly, continuous with the pulmonary artery. The aorta, identified by the branches of the aortic arch, is to the right of the pulmonary artery. The pulmonary trunk is enlarged. There are three normal semilunar leaflets of the pulmonary valve. There is a short conus at the right ventricular outlet to the pulmonary trunk, and there is a defect in the ventricular septum below the pulmonary trunk.

G Double-outlet right ventricle, subpulmonary ventricular septal defect, magnified right ventricular view. Details of the pulmonary valve, conus, and ventricular septal defect are demonstrated. The conus obscures visualization of the aortic outflow tract.

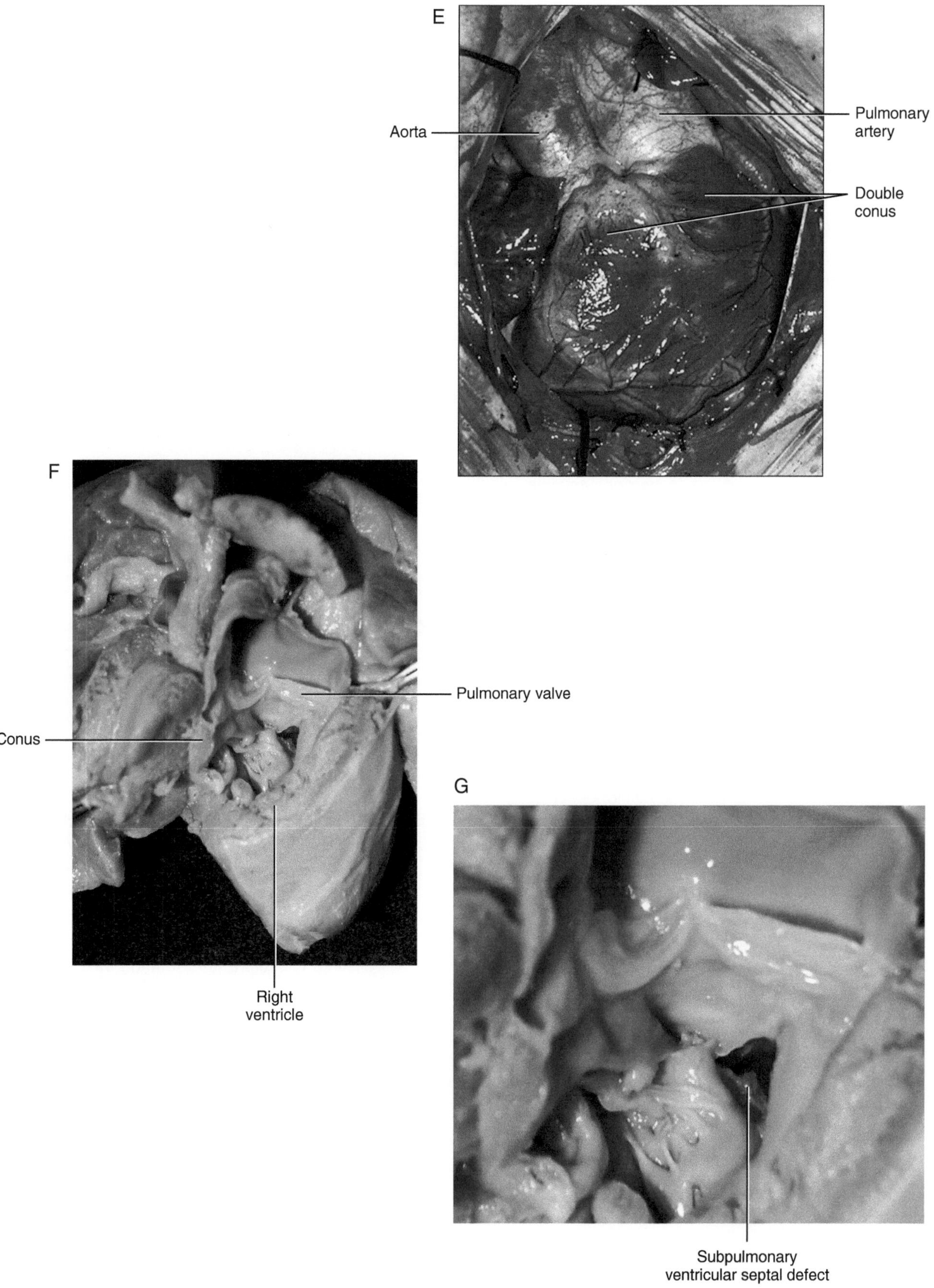
E
Aorta
Pulmonary artery
Double conus
F
Pulmonary valve
Conus
Right ventricle
G
Subpulmonary ventricular septal defect

Subaortic Ventricular Septal Defect

The ventricular septal defect described here—the subaortic type—is the most common of the double-outlet right ventricle varieties. It is sometimes referred to as "simple" double-outlet right ventricle. This defect is identified at operation by the nearly side-by-side position of the aorta and the pulmonary artery. There is often a double conus of infundibular myocardium beneath the great vessels. The aorta assumes a more anterior position than usual because of its origin from the right ventricle.

Figure 24-2

A A transverse incision is made in the right ventricle, which allows ventricular branches of the right coronary artery to be preserved. Traction stitches are placed at the edges of the ventriculotomy to expose the ventricular septal defect and conus myocardium located below the aorta and the pulmonary artery. The configuration of the outflow tract to the aorta and pulmonary artery is studied. The outflow tract of the pulmonary artery must be located in a sufficiently anterior position so that it will not be obstructed by closure of the ventricular septal defect to the aortic outflow tract. When the pulmonary annulus is significantly posterior to the aorta, the ventricular septal defect usually relates more to the pulmonary artery and requires treatment other than simply creating a prosthetic intraventricular conduit from the ventricular septal defect to the aorta. Obstructive myocardium of the infundibular septum should be excised.

B An intraventricular conduit is formed from a tubular graft of crimped, knitted, double-velour polyester. The contours of the graft allow the construction of a conduit to provide an adequate passageway for blood flow from the ventricular septal defect to the aortic annulus. The graft should be oriented to allow the crimped nature of the material to expand in a cephalocaudad dimension, and the graft should be wide enough to create an adequate passageway. The initial stitch in the ventricular septal defect is taken in the right side of the ventricular septum and inferior to the posterior rim of the defect. The second stitch is taken through the septal leaflet of the tricuspid valve to preserve the conduction system.

C The suture line is placed to the right side of the ventricular septum and inferior to the posterior rim of the septal defect, well away from the bundle of His. The patch may be attached to the rim of the ventricular septal defect anterior to the base of the papillary muscle of the conus. The suture line is continued to the subpulmonary conus.

D A continuous mattress stitch is placed along the base of the septal leaflet of the tricuspid valve to attach the patch firmly to leaflet tissue and to avoid injury to the bundle of His as it penetrates the central fibrous body near the posteroinferior rim of the ventricular septal defect. A mattress stitch is used to transition the suture line from the tricuspid anterior leaflet to the myocardium of the subaortic conus.

E The suture line is taken anterior to the subaortic conus, with stitches placed well away from the aortic valve annulus. Adequate patch is retained to ensure a wide completed passageway from the ventricular septal defect to the aortic annulus.

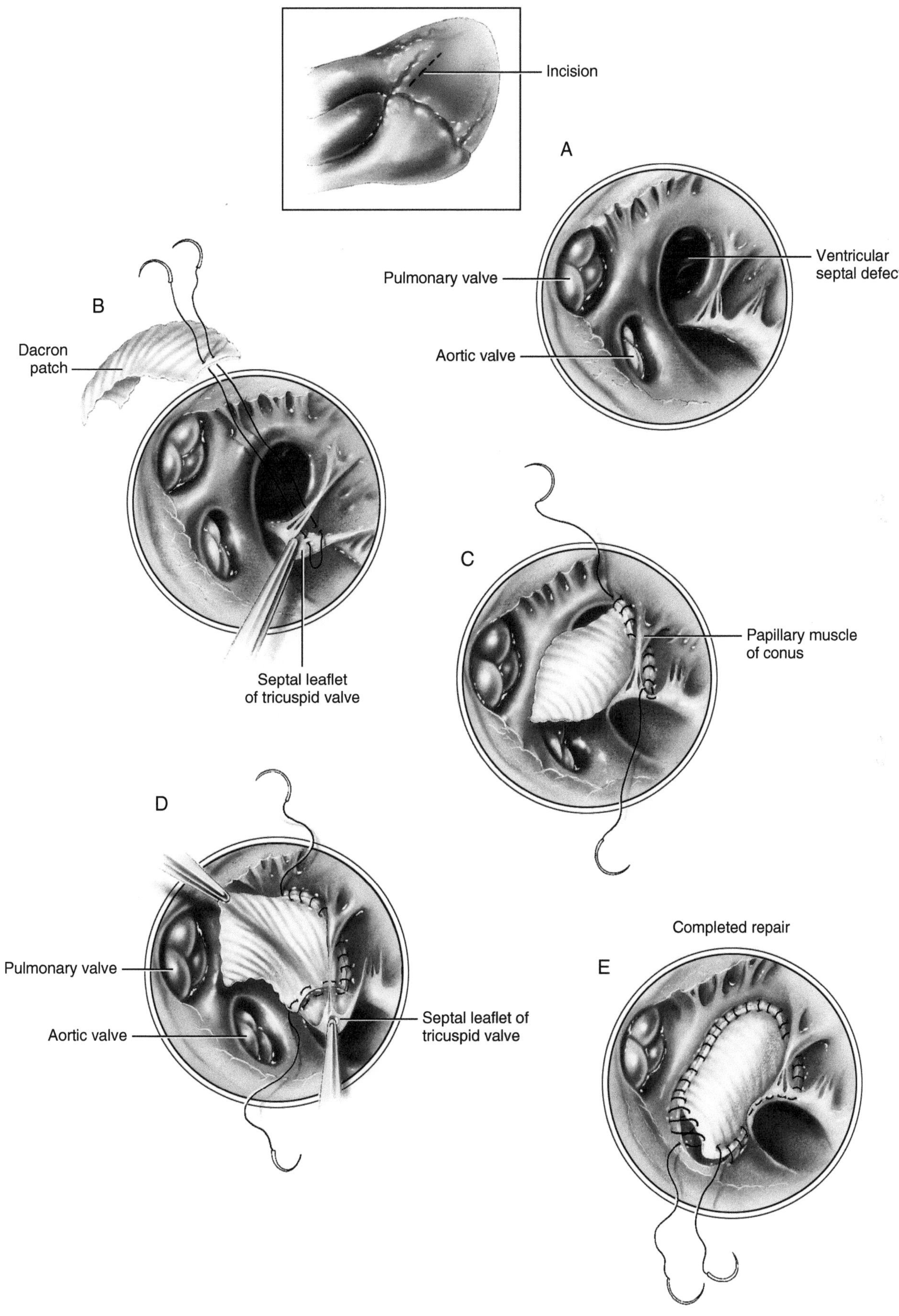
Incision
A
Pulmonary valve
Ventricular septal defect
Aortic valve
B
Dacron patch
Septal leaflet of tricuspid valve
C
Papillary muscle of conus
D
Pulmonary valve
Aortic valve
Septal leaflet of tricuspid valve
Completed repair
E

Subpulmonary Ventricular Septal Defect (Taussig-Bing Malformation)

In this variant of double-outlet right ventricle, the ventricular septal defect is more closely related to the pulmonary artery than to the aorta. Some of the concepts of repair may also apply to those anomalies in which the ventricular septal defect is related to neither the aorta nor the pulmonary artery (noncommitted).

Figure 24-3

A In the Taussig-Bing anomaly, the aorta is usually anterior to and to the right of the pulmonary artery, although sometimes the great vessels are beside each other. The more anterior the aorta is displaced, the more complex the repair becomes. The ventricular septal defect is usually as large as the aortic annulus, but on occasion it may be restrictive. In the Taussig-Bing malformation, the infundibular septum is often large and inserts on the posterior limb of the trabecula septomarginalis, in contrast to an anterior insertion in double-outlet right ventricle with subaortic ventricular septal defect. This large muscle bundle of the infundibular septum effectively obstructs the passageway from the ventricular septal defect to the aorta. The real difficulty in repairing these defects is to establish left ventricle–to–aorta continuity without obstructing the pulmonary outflow tract, which is located quite posteriorly in the right ventricle. Occasionally, it may be impossible to create an unobstructed passageway from the ventricular septal defect to the pulmonary artery.

B A variety of operations can be used to repair Taussig-Bing anomaly. The Damus-Stansel-Kaye operation was suggested independently by three investigators. It uses the pulmonary outflow tract as the passageway from the left ventricle to the aorta. The ventricular septal defect is closed to the pulmonary annulus. The pulmonary artery is divided, and the proximal pulmonary artery is anastomosed to the side of the aorta either directly or with a short tubular prosthesis interposed. An external conduit is created from the right ventricle on the anterior surface to the distal pulmonary artery.

C In the Mustard or Senning procedure, the ventricular septal defect is closed to the pulmonary artery, and an intraatrial venous transposition operation is performed. This operation results in a physiological correction but leaves the right ventricle as the systemic ventricle.

D In most cases, anatomic correction of the defect is possible by the Jatene procedure if the coronary artery anatomy is suitable to allow implantation to the pulmonary artery. The ventricular septal defect is closed to the pulmonary artery. The aorta and the pulmonary artery are divided. The proximal aorta is anastomosed to the distal pulmonary artery, which is brought anterior to the distal aorta (LeCompte maneuver). The distal aorta is anastomosed to the proximal pulmonary artery, along with the coronary arteries.

E If the arrangement of the great vessels is such that the aorta is beside the pulmonary artery, the ventricular septal defect can be closed to the aorta without obstructing the pulmonary outflow tract using the method described by Kawashima. The main obstacle to accomplishing this continuity may be the large, protruding muscle of the infundibular septum. This muscle can be resected to make a passageway from the ventricular septal defect to the aorta. A tunnel is created, using the septum as the posterior wall and a prosthetic patch as the anterior wall. Extreme care must be taken to prevent the patch from entering the pulmonary outflow tract while at the same time creating a tunnel of sufficient diameter to avoid any subaortic obstruction.

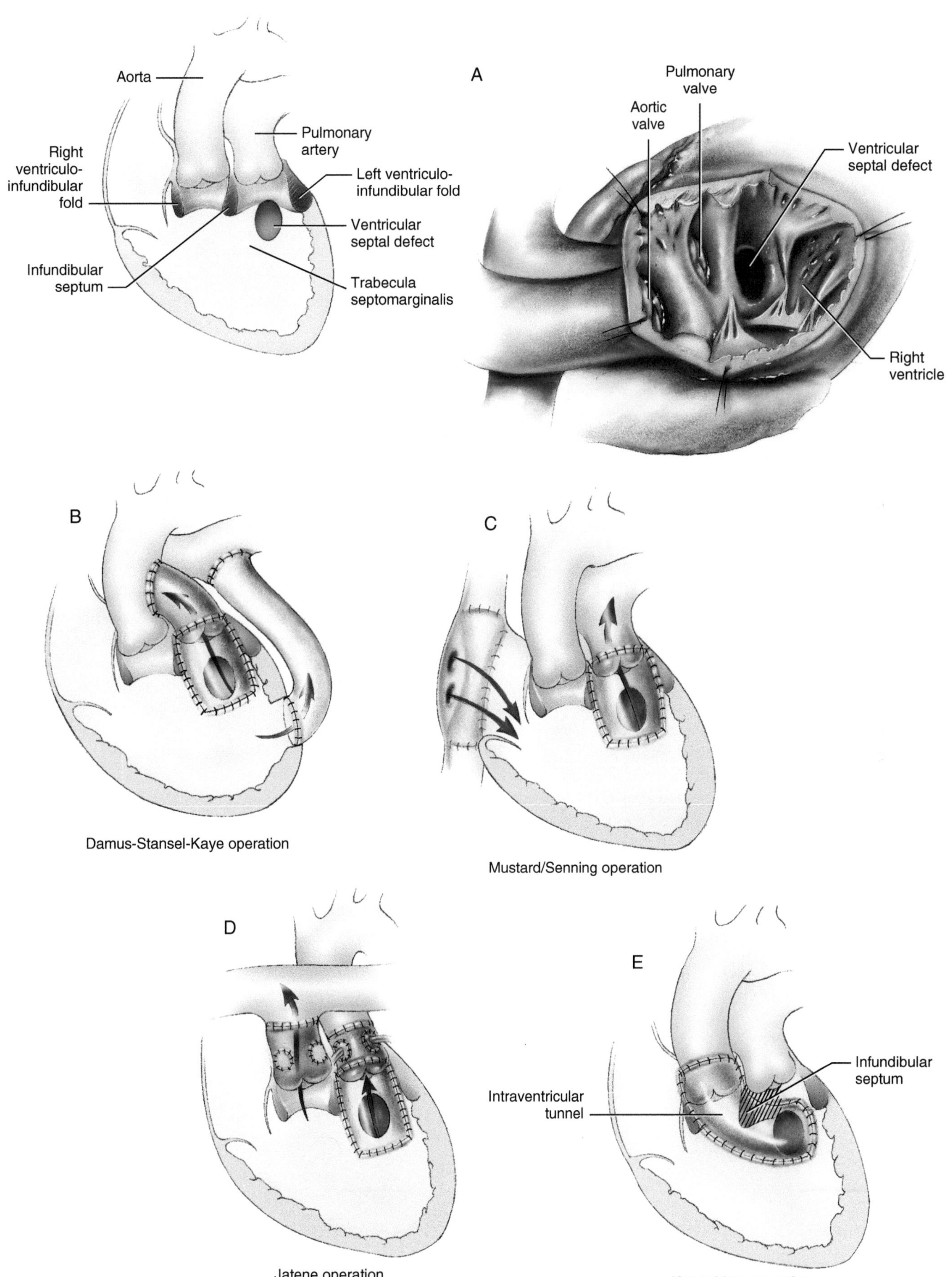
Aorta
Pulmonary artery
Right ventriculo-infundibular fold
Left ventriculo-infundibular fold
Ventricular septal defect
Infundibular septum
Trabecula septomarginalis
A
Pulmonary valve
Aortic valve
Ventricular septal defect
Right ventricle
B
C
Damus-Stansel-Kaye operation
Mustard/Senning operation
D
E
Infundibular septum
Intraventricular tunnel
Jatene operation
Kawashima operation

Figure 24-3 (continued)

F The ventricular septal defect can be connected to the aortic annulus using a tubular prosthesis as an intraventricular conduit (Abe procedure). The connection is simple, but the conduit naturally lies directly across the pulmonary outflow tract. Blood flow from the right ventricle must course around the conduit to reach the pulmonary artery, thus presenting the risk of pulmonary outflow tract obstruction, except in the most ideal of circumstances when the right ventricle is large.

G An interventricular conduit can be used to allow communication between the ventricular septal defect and the aorta. The concept for this operation is the creation of a conduit that consists of a tunnel within the ventricle and a tube within the anterior ventricular wall to bring the ventricular septal defect into continuity with the aorta. The anterior ventricular wall portion also serves as a patch to widen the right ventricular outflow tract.

H A transverse right ventriculotomy is made with reference to the coronary arteries. The anomaly is thoroughly inspected to establish the relationship of the great arteries to the ventricular septal defect, determine the state of the conal muscles, and identify the insertion of the tricuspid papillary muscles. There is usually a free passageway from the ventricular septal defect, along the septum anteriorly, to the free wall of the right ventricle, between the papillary muscle insertions of the tricuspid valve and the subpulmonary infundibulum (trabecula septomarginalis). A tubular polyester prosthesis about the same diameter as the aortic annulus is chosen for the conduit. A sufficiently long bevel is cut from one end of the prosthesis so that the tip approximates the rim of the ventricular septal defect below the tricuspid valve and the heel of the bevel reaches the free wall of the right ventricle at the medial end of the ventriculotomy. The beveled graft is sutured to the ventricular septal defect along the rim superiorly, to the septal leaflet of the tricuspid valve, and to the right ventricular septum 5 mm below the posteroinferior rim to preserve the conduction system.

Continuous stitches of 4/0 polypropylene are used for the repair. The suture line is deviated away from the anterior rim of the ventricular septal defect to create a tunnel along the anterior portion of the septum to the free wall of the right ventricle.

I The anterior end of the tunnel is closed off at the medial end of the right ventriculotomy, thus creating a passageway from the ventricular septal defect exclusively to the prosthetic conduit. The conduit is brought back to the right and shortened with an appropriate bevel to approximate the subaortic conus.

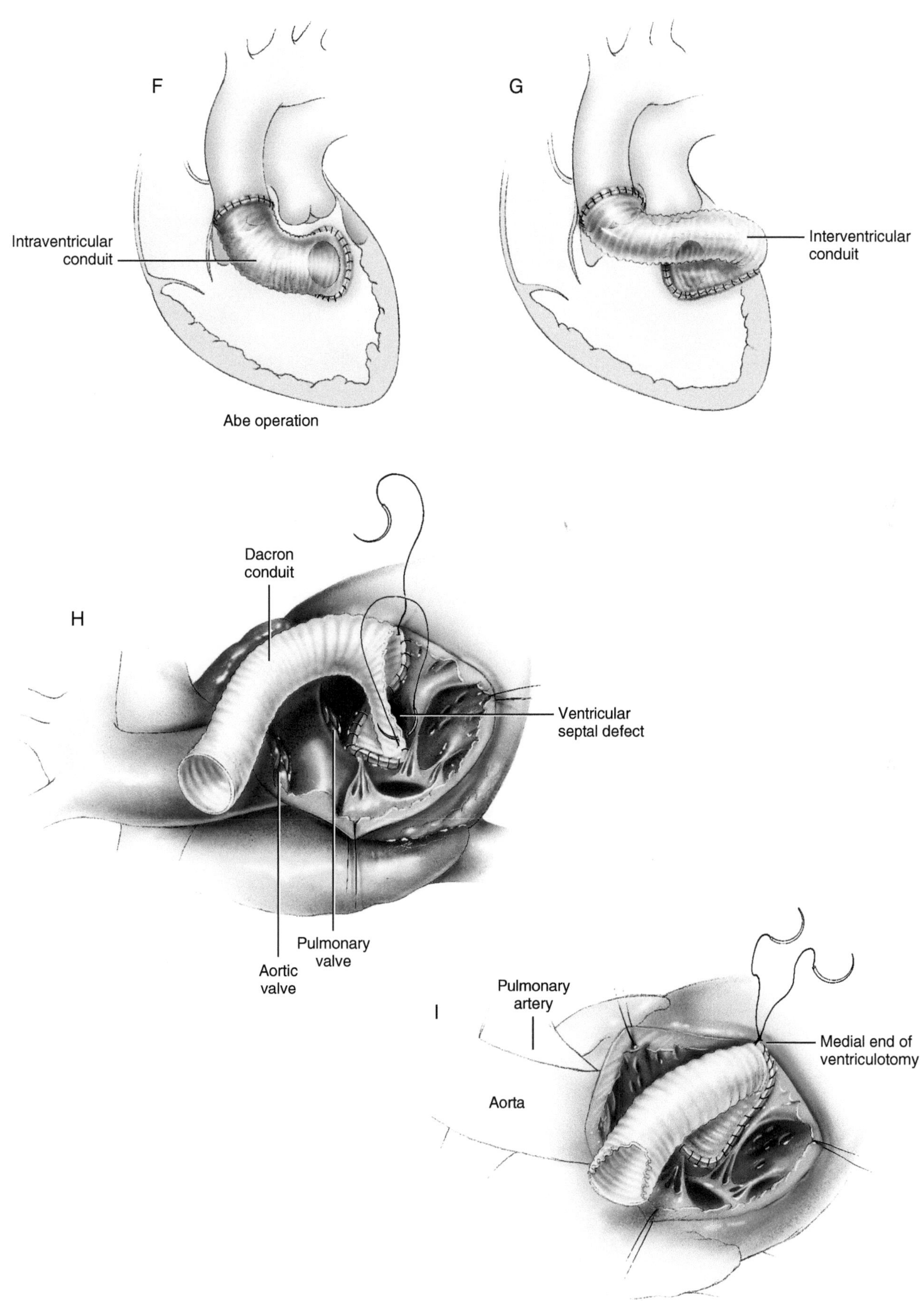
F
G
Intraventricular conduit
Interventricular conduit
Abe operation
Dacron conduit
H
Ventricular septal defect
Pulmonary valve
Aortic valve
I
Pulmonary artery
Medial end of ventriculotomy
Aorta

Figure 24-3 (continued)

J The bevel of the aortic end of the conduit is sutured to the subaortic conus. This muscle consists of the infundibular septum and the ventriculoinfundibular fold. Continuous suture technique is used, with deep bites into the ventricular myocardium.

K Anteriorly, the conduit is attached to either the subaortic conus or a portion of the right ventriculotomy that includes the subaortic conus. The completed conduit thus lies anterior to the pulmonary annulus, leaving a totally unobstructed passageway from the right ventricle to the pulmonary artery. The subaortic conduit should also be completely unobstructed because it is the same diameter as the aortic annulus, but this subaortic passageway is quite long.

L All that remains for completion of the repair is closure of the right ventricle. The conduit is used as an outflow patch to widen the right ventricle and provide a commodious passageway from the right ventricle to the pulmonary artery. Rather than leaving the conduit outside the right ventricle, it is used as a patch to close the ventriculotomy, thus becoming an interventricular conduit. Placing the conduit in the anterior wall of the right ventricle ensures an adequate pulmonary outflow tract as well as secure closure of the right ventricle. Continuous stitches are placed from the right ventricular myocardium, along the ventriculotomy, to the wall of the conduit. About one-third of the circumference of the graft is placed inside the ventriculotomy, and two-thirds of the circumference is actually outside the heart on the anterior surface.

M The repair is completed by approximating both sides of the ventriculotomy to the side of the graft. This places the conduit both within the wall of the heart and on the outside of the ventricle. No valves are required because the aortic valve is retained in its anatomic position.

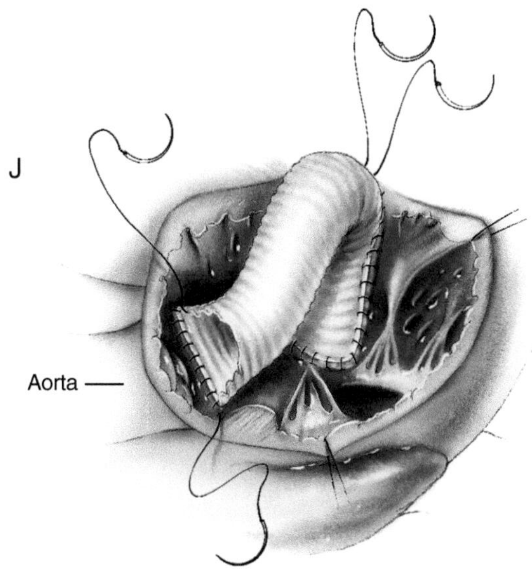

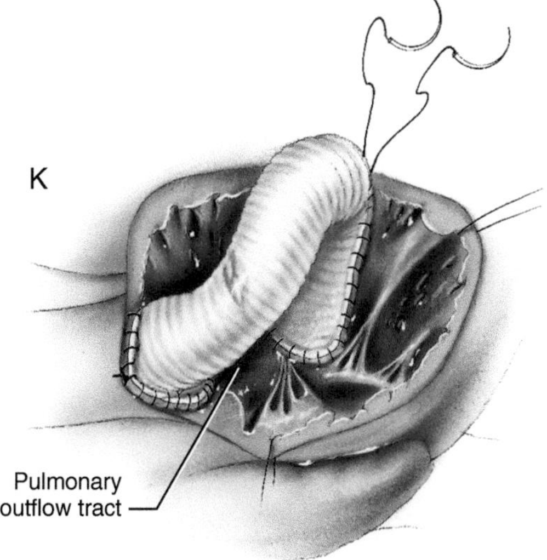

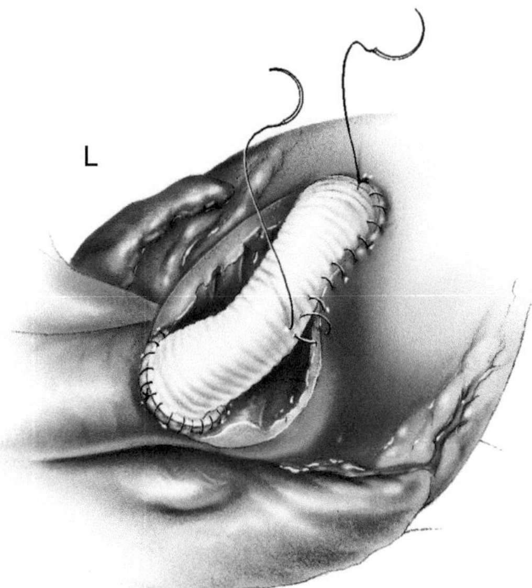

Closing ventriculotomy
to conduit

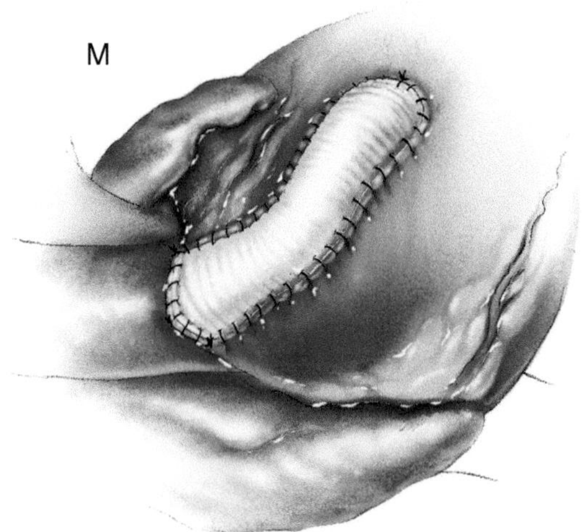

Completed repair

part VIII

Thoracic Arteries and Veins (Congenital)

chapter 25 CORONARY ARTERY ANOMALY

Anomalies of the coronary arteries include anomalous origin of the left or right coronary artery and abnormal course of the coronary arteries from the aorta to the surface of the heart. Here we discuss anomalous origin of the left coronary artery from the pulmonary artery. Congenital coronary arteriovenous fistula is a direct connection of the coronary artery to a cardiac chamber or to one of the major veins of the heart.

Morphology
Figure 25-1

A Anomalous origin of left coronary artery from pulmonary artery. The specimen is opened to the outlet portion of the left ventricle and the aortic root through the noncoronary sinus of Valsalva. The ascending aorta and arch (identified by its aortic branches) and the upper portion of the descending aorta are demonstrated. There is only one coronary artery orifice seen in the aortic root.

B Anomalous origin of left coronary artery from pulmonary artery, magnified view. The single large coronary artery orifice is identified as the right coronary artery. There is no coronary artery orifice in the left coronary sinus. The noncoronary sinus aorta has been divided along with the valve, and there is no identifiable coronary artery in this sinus either.

C Anomalous origin of left coronary artery from pulmonary artery. The right ventricle (RV) is opened anteriorly into the anterior wall of the pulmonary artery. The small left coronary artery orifice is identified on the posterior aspect of the pulmonary artery.

D Anomalous origin of left coronary artery from pulmonary artery, magnified view. The left coronary artery originates from the posterior sinus of Valsalva of the pulmonary artery. The ascending aorta and arch are seen emerging from behind the pulmonary artery. The distance from the origin of the left coronary artery to the ascending aorta can be appreciated by studying the dimensional aspects of this image.

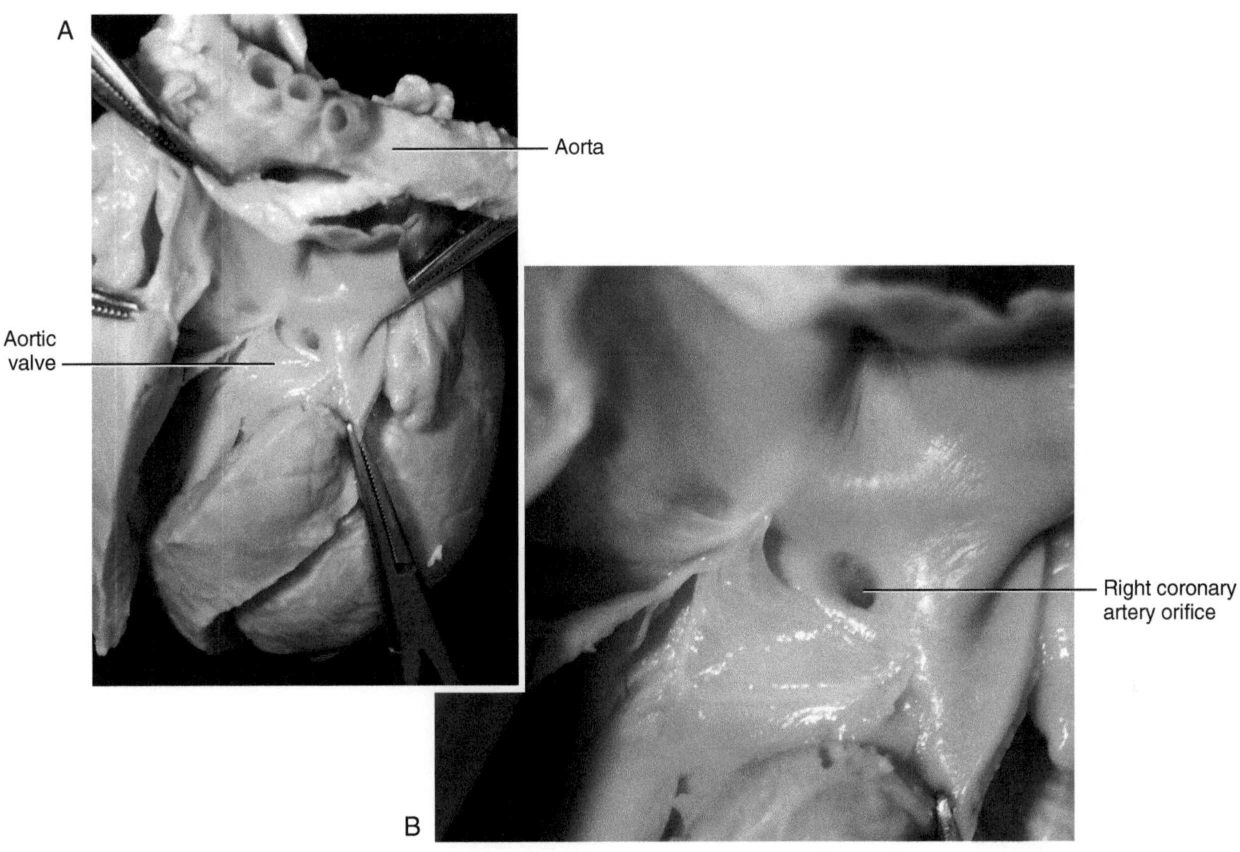
A
Aorta
Aortic valve
Right coronary artery orifice
B

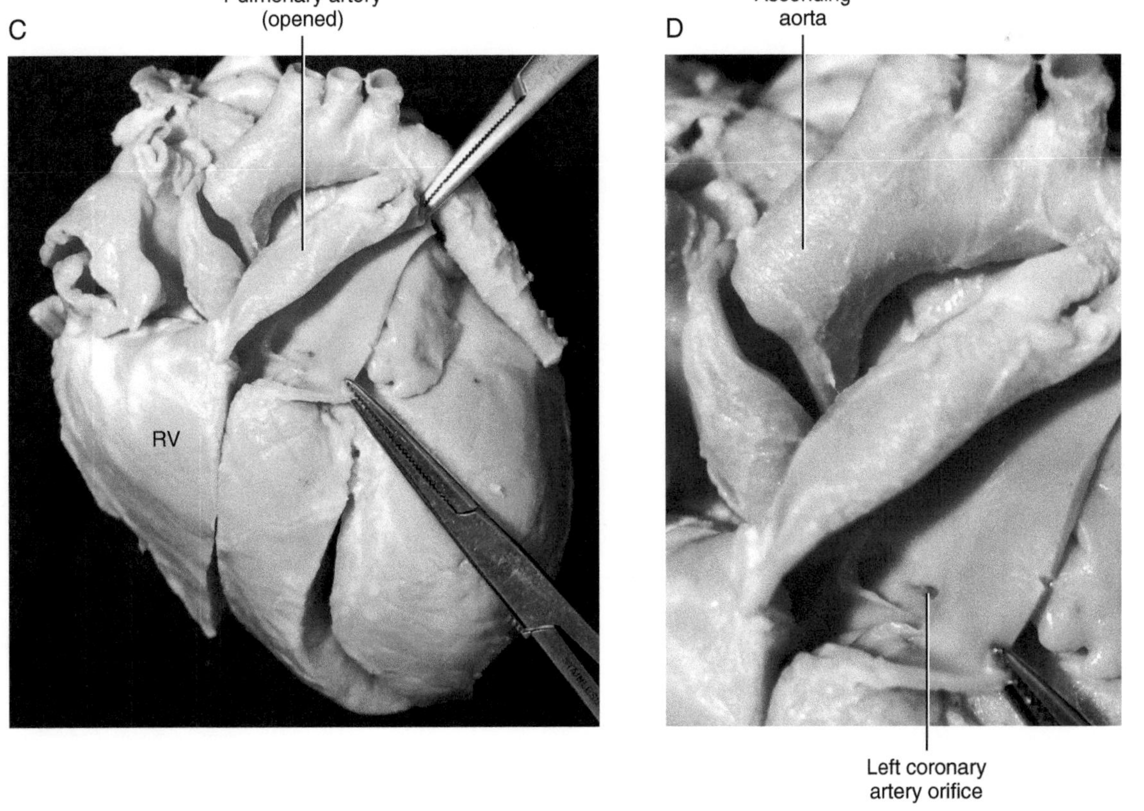
C
Pulmonary artery (opened)
RV
D
Ascending aorta
Left coronary artery orifice

Figure 25-1 (continued)

E Anomalous origin of left coronary artery from pulmonary artery, operative view. This photograph shows dilation of the right coronary artery and dilated branches forming the collateral circulation to the left coronary artery.

F Anomalous origin of left coronary artery from pulmonary artery, operative view. This photograph in another patient shows even more pronounced dilation of the right coronary artery, compensating for the pulmonary artery origin of the left coronary artery.

G Coronary artery–to–cardiac chamber fistula, operative view. This photograph is from a patient with a right coronary artery fistula to the right ventricle. The pronounced dilation of the right coronary artery is comparable to that seen in Figure 25-1, *F*. The difference is that the dilation is confined to the main channel of the right coronary artery; the branch arteries are normal.

H Coronary artery–to–cardiac chamber fistula, operative view. The exposure is through the right atrium. The fistulous opening of the right coronary artery to the right ventricle is located just below the atrioventricular groove and the septal leaflet of the tricuspid valve.

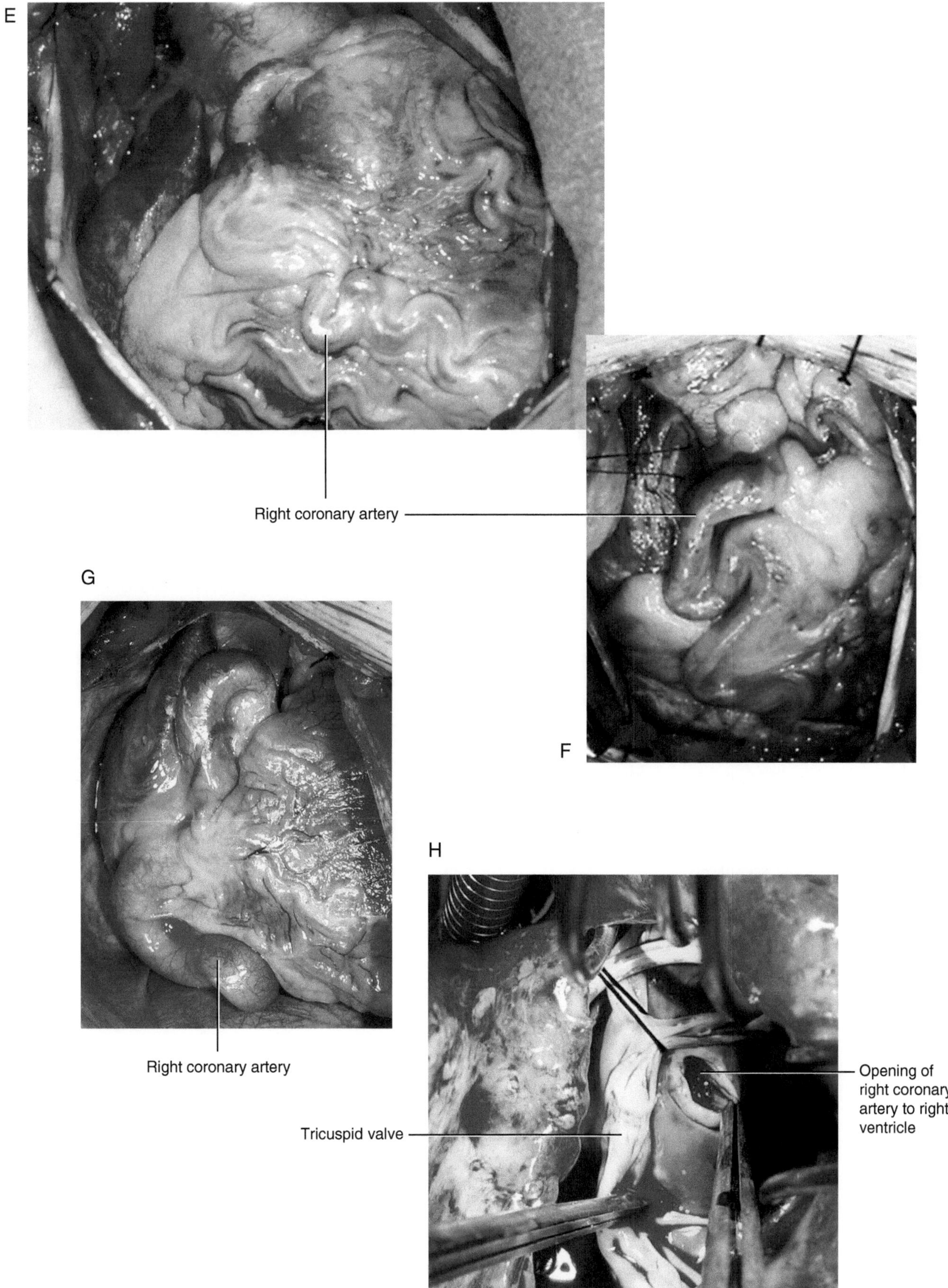
E
F
Right coronary artery
G
Right coronary artery
H
Tricuspid valve
Opening of right coronary artery to right ventricle

Anomalous Origin of Left Coronary Artery: Lateral Approach

Surgical options for anomalous origin of the left coronary artery from the pulmonary artery include ligation of the left coronary artery without reconstruction; saphenous vein or internal mammary artery bypass graft, with ligation or division of the left coronary artery; anastomosis of the left coronary artery to the subclavian artery; and connection of the anomalous left coronary artery to the aorta by either implanting the left coronary artery into the aorta or creating a pathway from the aorta directly to the left coronary artery.

Figure 25-2

A When the heart is not greatly enlarged and the patient's hemodynamic state is reasonably good, it is possible to use a lateral approach to achieve direct implantation of the left coronary artery into the aorta. When the heart is very compromised and enlarged or when the origin of the left coronary artery is suspected to be more lateral than posterior on the pulmonary artery, an anterior approach is used.

An anterolateral thoracotomy incision is made on the left side. Cardiopulmonary bypass is instituted using a single cannula for venous drainage placed in the right atrium, through the appendage, or in the right ventricle; oxygenated blood is returned to the medial wall of the ascending aorta. The repair is accomplished with the aorta occluded under hypothermic cardioplegic conditions.

B The pulmonary artery is retracted anteriorly, and the coronary artery is excised at its anomalous origin from the pulmonary artery, along with a generous (1-cm diameter) button of the wall of the pulmonary sinus of Valsalva. The defect in the pulmonary artery is repaired with a pericardial patch. The main portion of the left coronary artery is mobilized to its bifurcation by sharp dissection. This should provide sufficient length to approximate the origin of the left coronary artery to the left side of the aorta above the sinuses of Valsalva.

C The pulmonary artery is retracted posteriorly, and a longitudinal slit is made in the aorta to allow the introduction of a 4- to 5-mm coronary punch. A circular opening is made in the lateral wall of the aorta.

D An end-to-side anastomosis of the left coronary artery to the aorta is made using continuous stitches of 7/0 polypropylene or polydiaxanone.

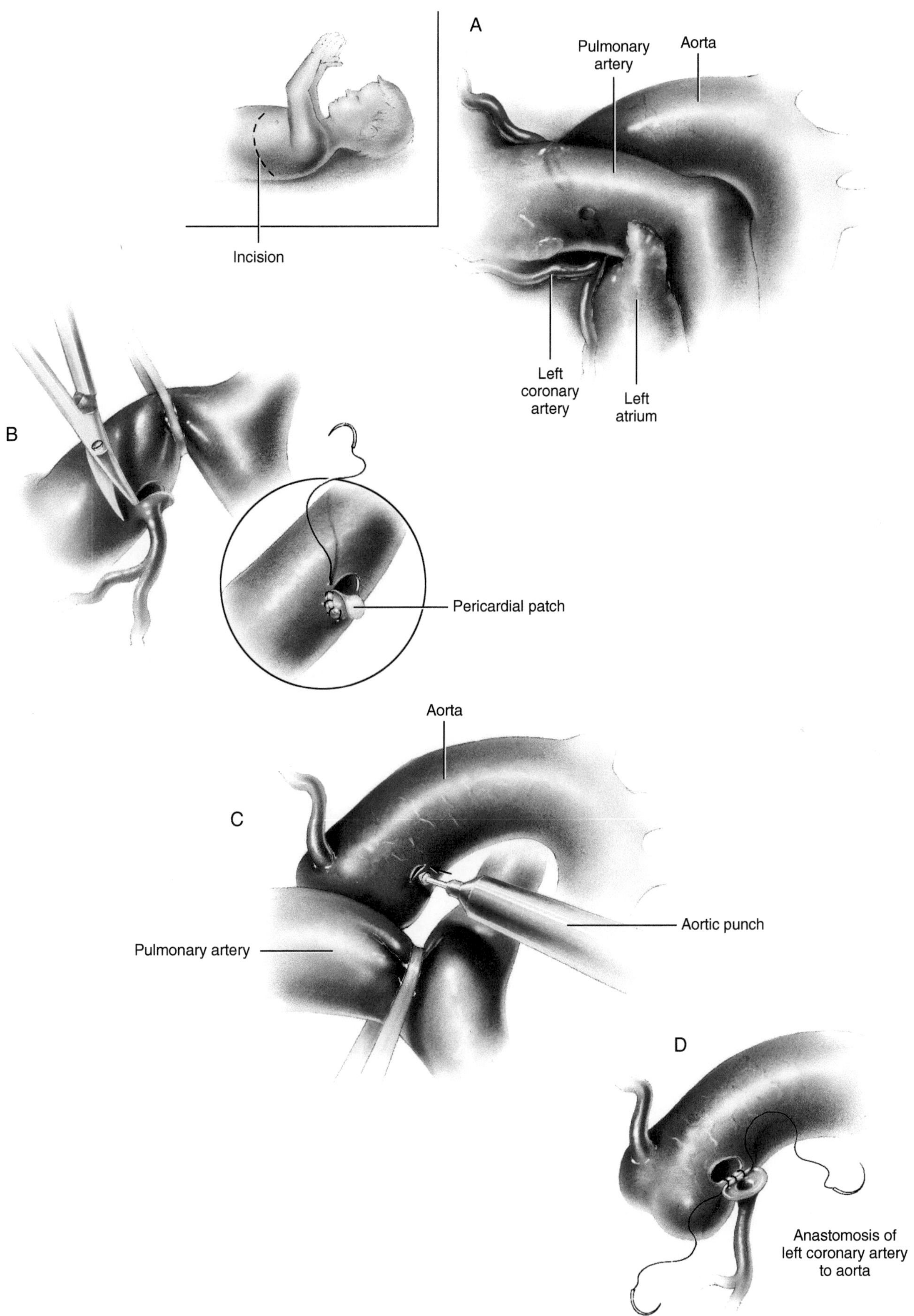
Incision
A
Pulmonary artery
Aorta
Left coronary artery
Left atrium
B
Pericardial patch
Aorta
C
Pulmonary artery
Aortic punch
D
Anastomosis of left coronary artery to aorta

Anomalous Origin of Left Coronary Artery: Anterior Approach (Takeuhi Operation)

Severe ischemia of the myocardium associated with anomalous origin of the left coronary artery from the pulmonary artery may result in gross enlargement of the heart due to a dilated left ventricle, ventricular aneurysm, or mitral valve incompetence. The precarious hemodynamic state, difficult exposure, tension placed on the anomalous left coronary artery by an enlarged heart, and need to perform associated intracardiac procedures dictate an anterior approach rather than anterolateral thoracotomy.

Figure 25-3

A A midsternal incision is made, and cardiopulmonary bypass is instituted in the usual manner using a single venous cannula. A flap of the anterior wall of the pulmonary artery based on its medial wall is created above the sinuses of Valsalva.

B The anomalous origin of the left coronary artery can be seen in the posterior sinus of Valsalva of the pulmonary artery. A circular opening is created at the base of the flap in the pulmonary artery using an aortic punch.

C An opening into the medial wall of the aorta is created exactly opposite the pulmonary artery opening, also using the aortic punch.

D A side-to-side anastomosis of the aorta to the pulmonary artery is performed to create an aortopulmonary window. The anastomosis is constructed using continuous stitches of 7/0 polypropylene. The completed aortopulmonary anastomosis establishes a means by which the left coronary artery can receive aortic blood flow.

E The flap of the anterior wall of the pulmonary artery is displaced posteriorly to cover the back wall of it and create a passageway within the pulmonary artery from the aorta to the left coronary artery. A double-needle suture of 7/0 polypropylene is used. The suture is begun on the left side, with continuous stitches placed inferior to the left coronary orifice in the sinus of Valsalva, where exposure is most difficult. The inferior suture line is continued to the medial wall of the pulmonary artery. The suture line superior to the coronary artery origin is then completed to the medial wall of the pulmonary artery.

F The anterior wall of the pulmonary artery is reconstructed with a patch of crimped polyester or pericardium to complete the repair.

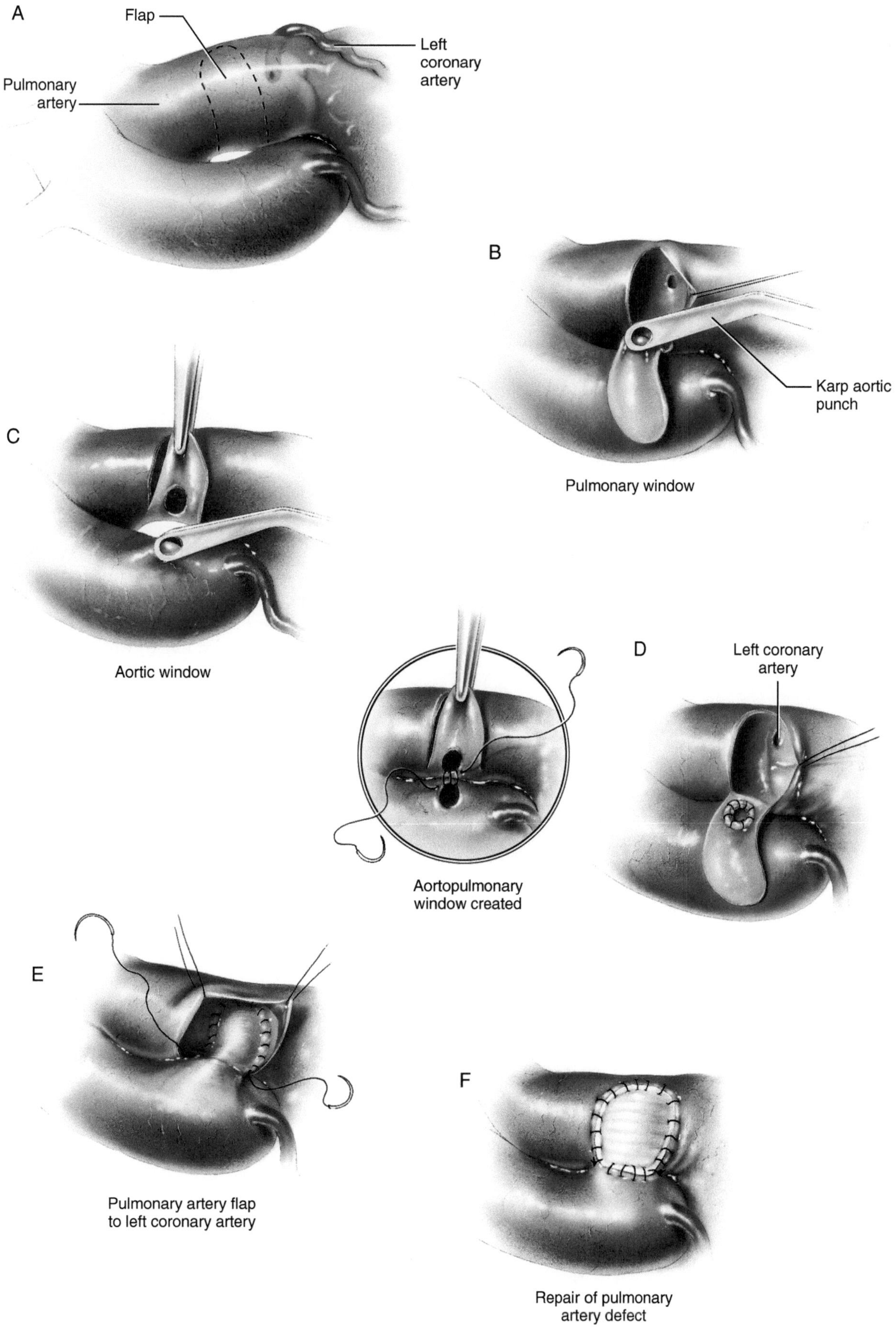
A
Flap
Left coronary artery
Pulmonary artery
B
Karp aortic punch
Pulmonary window
C
Aortic window
Aortopulmonary window created
D
Left coronary artery
E
Pulmonary artery flap to left coronary artery
F
Repair of pulmonary artery defect

Coronary Artery–to–Cardiac Chamber Fistula

A coronary artery may develop fistulous communication with any of the cardiac chambers or large cardiac veins. This unusual congenital deformity most commonly involves communication between the right coronary artery and either the right ventricle or the right atrium. Proximal to the fistula, the coronary artery is dilated and tortuous owing to the large volume of blood carried up to the runoff point. Distal to the fistula, the coronary artery is normal. Closure of the fistula places the coronary artery distribution distal to the fistula at risk of occlusion.

Figure 25-4

A When the surface coronary artery anatomy is well defined and the site of the fistula to the cardiac chamber can be absolutely identified, the fistula can be closed without using a cardiopulmonary bypass. A mattress stitch of 2/0 or 3/0 polypropylene is laced around the site of fistula so that when the suture is tied, only the fistula is occluded and the main coronary artery channel remains undistorted. Closure of the fistula is confirmed by the absence of a continuous thrill over the site.

B When the exact location of the fistula relative to the coronary artery is in question, or when surface ligation may place a branch of the coronary artery at risk of occlusion, the operation is performed with the patient on cardiopulmonary bypass so that the cardiac chamber termination of the fistula can be closed. An example is a right coronary artery-to-right atrium fistula, which may involve the sinus node artery branch. The affected cardiac chamber is opened, and the fistulous site is identified by infusion of cardioplegic solution or removal of the aortic occlusion clamp. The fistula orifice is closed by direct suture.

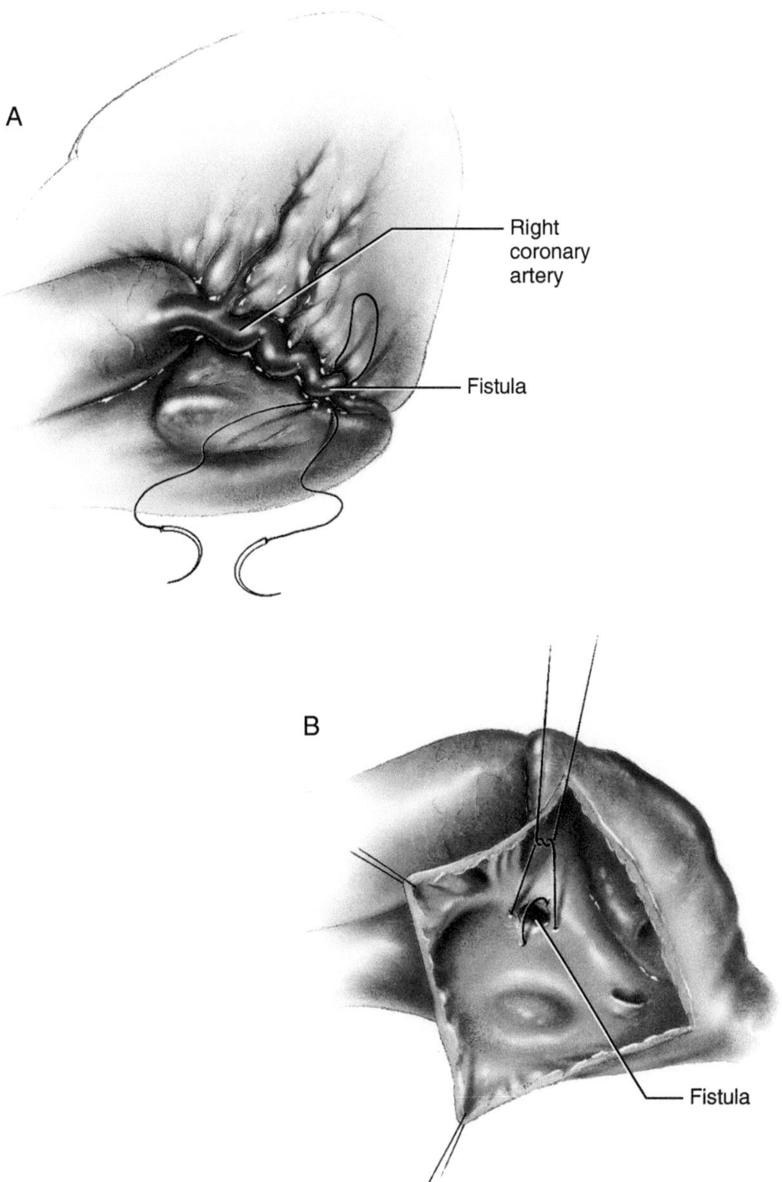
A
Right
coronary
artery
Fistula
B
Fistula

chapter 26 PATENT DUCTUS ARTERIOSUS

The normal function of the ductus arteriosus is to shunt blood from the pulmonary artery to the aorta while the lungs are collapsed during fetal life. Ordinarily, the ductus closes spontaneously shortly after birth when the lungs are inflated and arterial oxygen increases. When the ductus remains patent, a significant shunt from the aorta to the pulmonary artery may occur, as pulmonary vascular resistance falls after birth.

Morphology

Figure 26-1

A Patent ductus arteriosus. The anterior aspect of the cardiac and great vessel specimen is shown. The ductus arteriosus originates from the bifurcation of the pulmonary artery and courses posteriorly to join the aorta just distal to the left subclavian artery.

B Patent ductus arteriosus. Magnified view of the specimen showing details of the origin, course, and junction of the ductus arteriosus with the aorta.

C Patent ductus arteriosus. In this specimen showing the anterior aspect of the heart and great vessels, the main and left pulmonary arteries are opened longitudinally, and the aorta is opened similarly. The ductus arteriosus is opened slightly at its origin from the pulmonary artery bifurcation and joins the pulmonary artery to the aorta distal to the left subclavian artery.

D Patent ductus arteriosus. The ductus arteriosus is demonstrated to be patent by passing a probe from the pulmonary artery through the ductus arteriosus to the aorta.

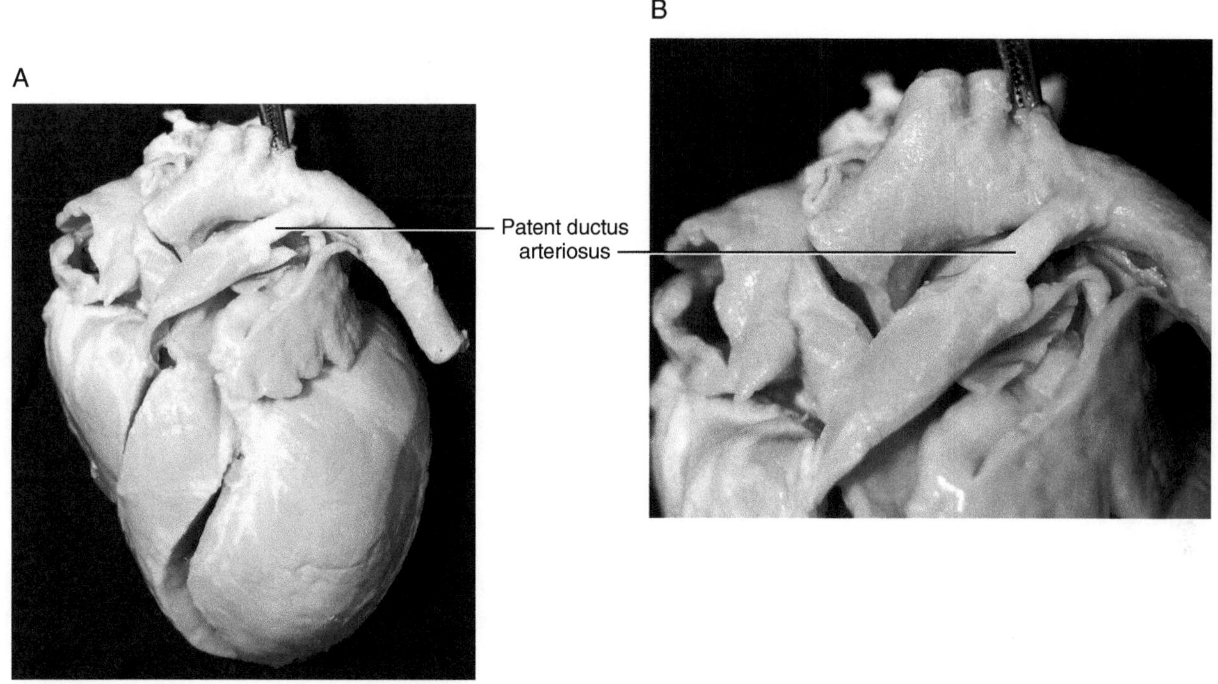
A
B
Patent ductus
arteriosus

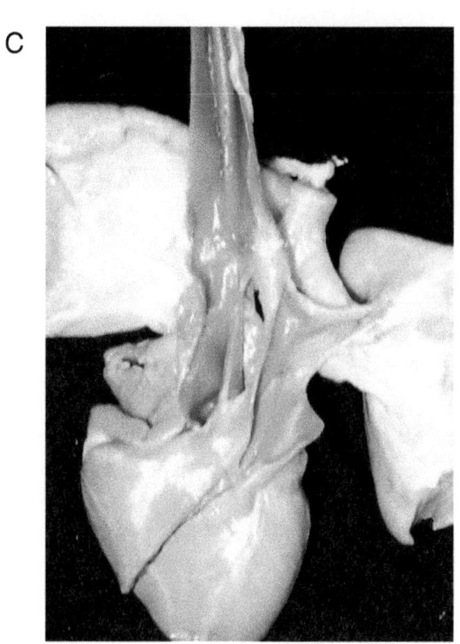
C

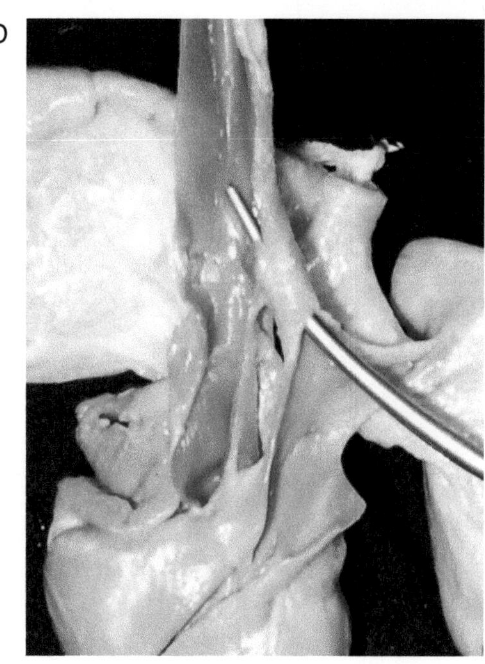
D

Figure 26-2

A A posterolateral thoracotomy is made on the left side. The thorax is entered through the bed of the nonresected fourth rib. The pleura over the upper portion of the descending thoracic aorta is incised. Traction stitches are placed along the anterior edge of the pleural incision, retracting the pleura off the surface of the ductus arteriosus. A moist gauze sponge placed in front of the lung and behind the traction stitches provides continuous exposure without causing trauma to the lung. Connective tissue over the surface of the ductus arteriosus is dissected, beginning on the aorta and continuing toward the pulmonary artery. This allows the vagus nerve and its recurrent branch to reflect anteriorly with the pleural flap.

B A right-angled hemostat is passed beneath the ductus arteriosus from its inferior side. The jaws of the hemostat are separated slightly, and the connective tissue contained between the jaws is grasped with forceps and completely excised (the "ductus maneuver"). This maneuver makes a large opening and completely frees the back wall of the ductus arteriosus.

C A single ligature is passed around the ductus arteriosus. A suture ligature is passed around the ductus arteriosus, taking a few stitches in the adventitia of the aorta to hold this ligature on the surface of the aorta as it is tied down.

D The ductus arteriosus is double ligated, with care taken not to cut the sutures through the delicate tissue. A short segment of the ductus arteriosus should separate the ligatures.

E If the ductus arteriosus is short or calcified, interruption and suture closure may be indicated. A straight Potts clamp is placed across the ductus arteriosus. Anterior retraction on the ductus arteriosus allows an angled Potts clamp to be placed on the aorta.

F The straight clamp is removed from the midportion of the ductus arteriosus, and a second angled clamp is placed at the junction of the ductus arteriosus and the pulmonary artery, aided by posterior retraction of the aortic angled clamp. The ductus arteriosus is divided between the two clamps.

G The aortic end of the ductus arteriosus is closed by direct suture using 5/0 polypropylene. The suture is started at the posterior end of the ductus arteriosus, passing the needle from the superior side of the ductus. A continuous stitch working toward the anterior end of the ductus arteriosus is preferred.

H The suture line is returned to the posterior end of the ductus arteriosus, where it is tied off securely. The pulmonary artery end of the ductus arteriosus is then closed in a similar fashion, working from the posterior end to the anterior end and then returning to the posterior end of the ductus for maximal security. The needle is passed from the inferior side of the pulmonary end of the ductus arteriosus; this allows the needle to pass in its normal curve, without prying on the delicate ductal tissue.

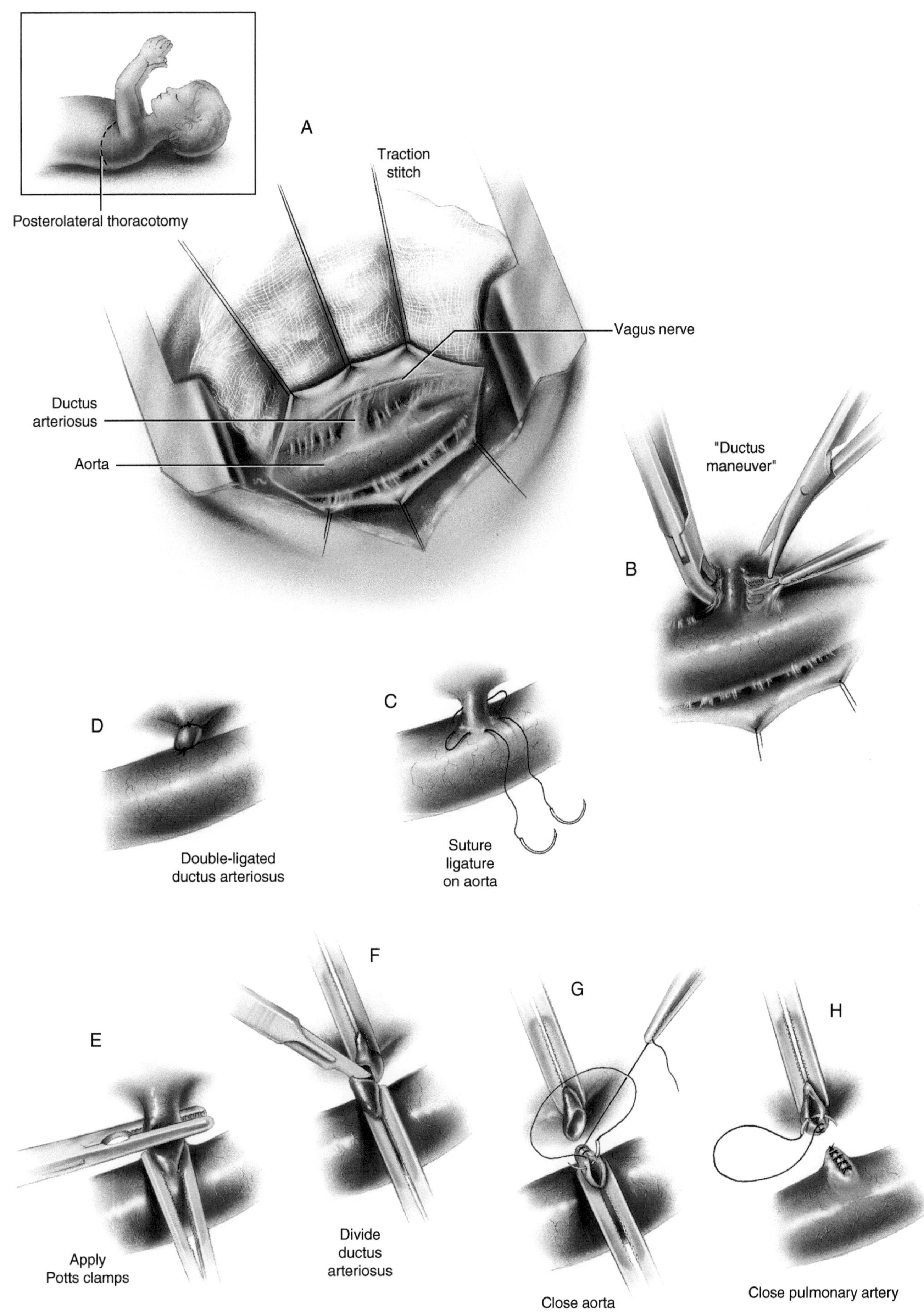
Posterolateral thoracotomy
A
Traction
stitch
Vagus nerve
Ductus
arteriosus
Aorta
"Ductus
maneuver"
B
D
C
Double-ligated
ductus arteriosus
Suture
ligature
on aorta
F
G
H
E
Apply
Potts clamps
Divide
ductus
arteriosus
Close aorta
Close pulmonary artery

chapter 27 COARCTATION OF THE AORTA

Coarctation of the aorta involves localized stenosis of the thoracic aorta, although rare cases are reported to occur in other aortic locations. In other locations the stenosis is usually more diffuse and involves longer segments of the aorta. Most commonly the defect is near the junction of the ductus arteriosus and the aorta. It is probably related to the contractile elements of the ductus arteriosus and is usually a localized morphology. In some cases there is associated hypoplasia of the aortic arch.

Morphology

Figure 27-1

A Coarctation of the aorta. The anterior aspect of the heart and great vessel specimen is shown. Localized stenosis of the aorta begins just distal to the left subclavian artery. The stenosis is opposite or perhaps slightly proximal to the junction of the ductus arteriosus and the aorta. Of note are the four arterial branches of the aorta originating from the arch, with a very short brachiocephalic artery and individual origins of the right subclavian and right common carotid arteries from the aorta.

B Coarctation of the aorta. Magnified view to demonstrate details of the coarctated segment of the aorta.

C Coarctation of the aorta. The coarctated segment of the aorta is located distal to the left subclavian artery and opposite the ductus arteriosus. Enlargement of the upper thoracic intercostal arteries emphasizes the importance of these arteries in collateral circulation to the aorta below the stenosis. Note also the associated aortic dissection.

D Coarctation of the aorta with aortic dissection. A less magnified view shows the extent of associated aortic dissection into the arch and ascending aorta.

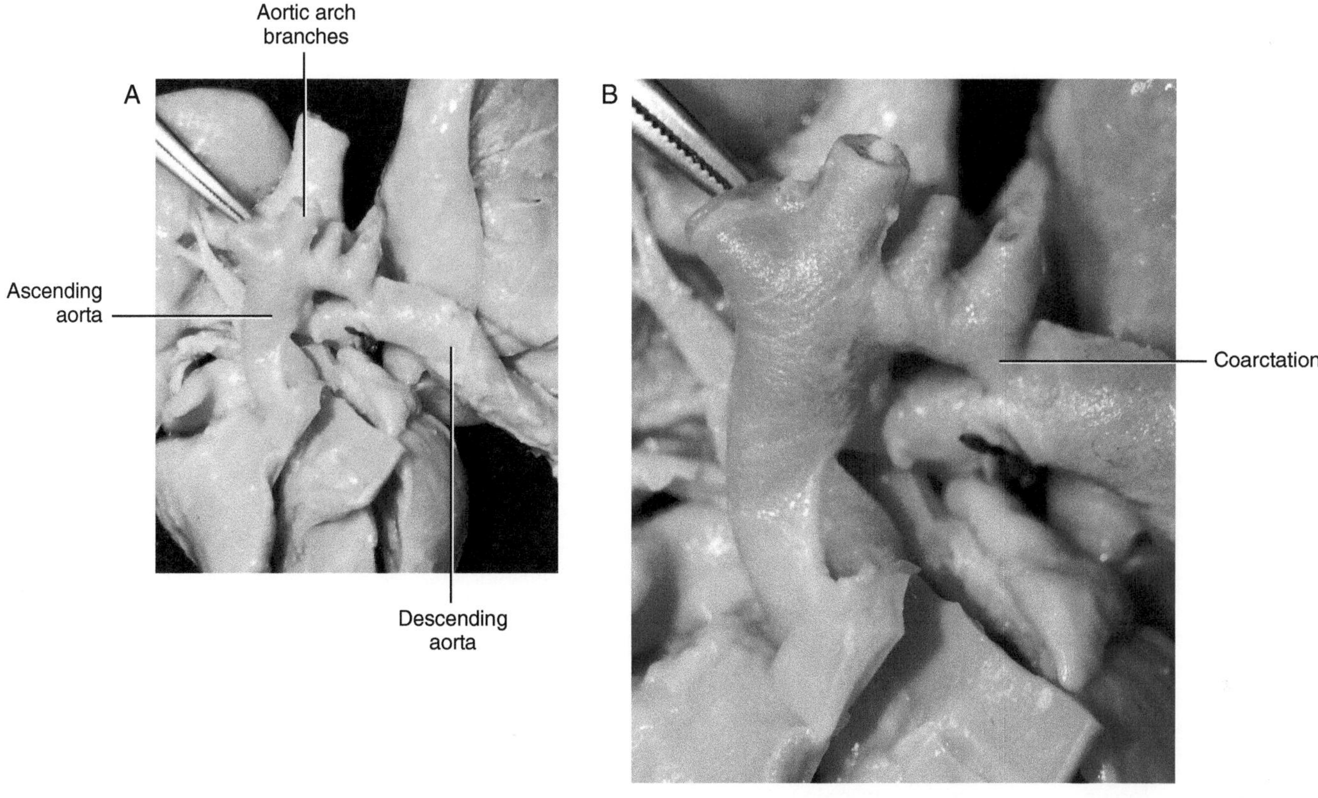
A
B
Aortic arch branches
Ascending aorta
Descending aorta
Coarctation

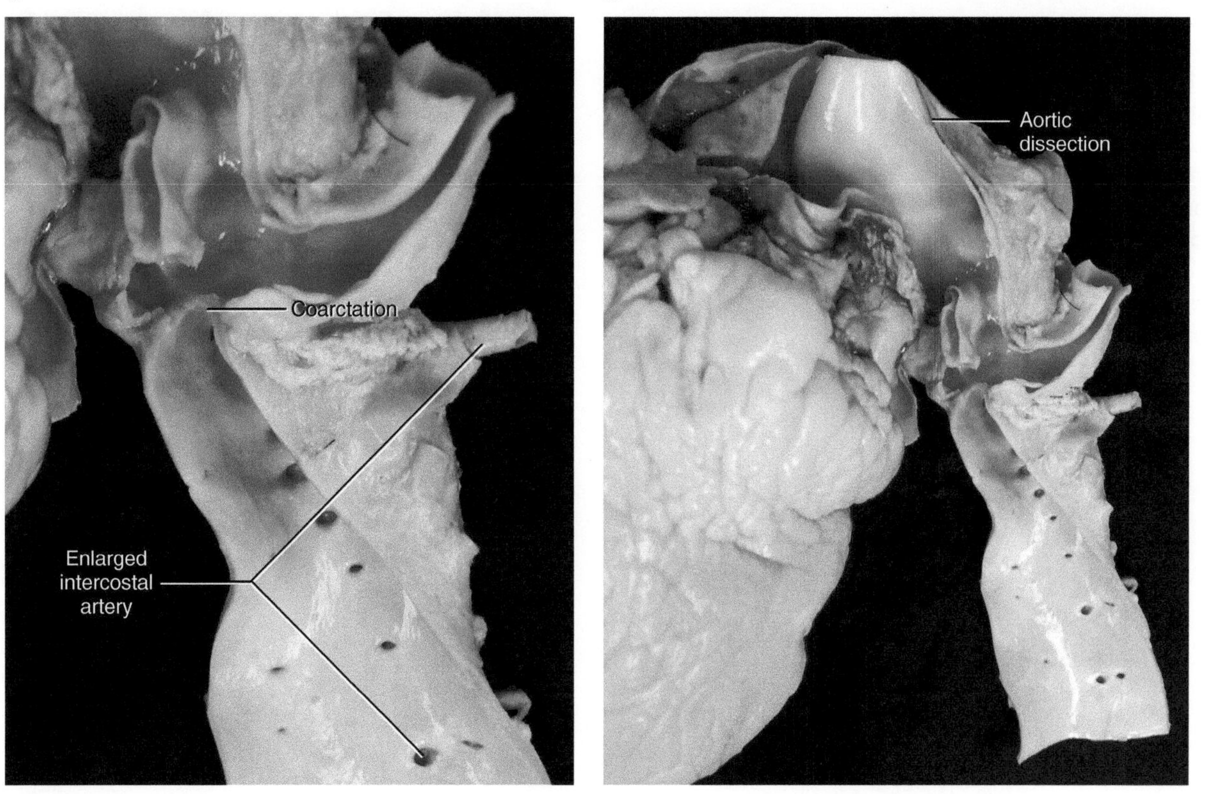
C
D
Coarctation
Enlarged intercostal artery
Aortic dissection

Figure 27-2

A A posterolateral thoracotomy incision is made on the left side. The thorax is entered through the bed of the nonresected fourth rib. The pleura is incised over the upper portion of the descending thoracic aorta, with the incision extending onto the left subclavian artery. Traction stitches are placed in the anterior and posterior edges of the incised pleura to reflect it. This reflection of the pleura contains the lung and provides maximal exposure during the course of dissection. This exposure can be maintained in the event of hemorrhage or other difficulties during the procedure. The connective tissue of the mediastinum is separated from the anterior wall of the upper portion of the descending thoracic aorta, aortic arch, ductus arteriosus, and left subclavian artery. In general, all the dissection is sharp. The tissues are exposed by forceps traction, and the bridging connective tissue fibers are divided by scissors. Blunt dissection is avoided, especially around the enlarged collateral blood vessels.

B The aorta is mobilized in the area of the ligamentum arteriosum or ductus arteriosus and controlled by retraction ligature or umbilical tape above and below the ductus arteriosus. These devices allow strong retraction of the aorta for maximal exposure. The aorta is retracted posteriorly for the initial portion of the dissection of the ductus arteriosus, bronchial and esophageal branches of the upper portion of the descending thoracic aorta, anterior wall of the aortic arch, and left subclavian artery. The aorta is then retracted anteriorly for dissection of the intercostal arteries. Complete mobilization of the intercostal arteries is essential to obtain an adequate length of aorta for anastomosis.

C The distal portion of the aortic arch and the subclavian artery are occluded using the spoon-shaped coarctation vascular clamp. A straight coarctation clamp is used to occlude the upper portion of the descending aorta distal to the coarctated segment. Sufficient length of distal aorta can often be obtained by occlusion proximal to the first intercostal artery branch. If it is necessary to obtain greater length on the upper portion of the descending thoracic aorta, the intercostal arteries may be ligated or temporarily occluded using Dietrich vascular clamps. The ductus arteriosus is ligated and divided.

D The coarctated segment of the aorta is excised close to the aortic arch and base of the left subclavian artery. A diagonal incision is made to excise the coarctated segment in the upper portion of the descending thoracic aorta so as to obtain maximal aortic diameter. The longer dimension of the diagonal is placed posteriorly on the distal end of the aorta.

E The proximal end of the aorta is enlarged by making an incision in the left subclavian artery at its origin from the aorta. This incision not only provides a greater circumference for the anastomosis but also accommodates the diagonal contour of the distal aorta.

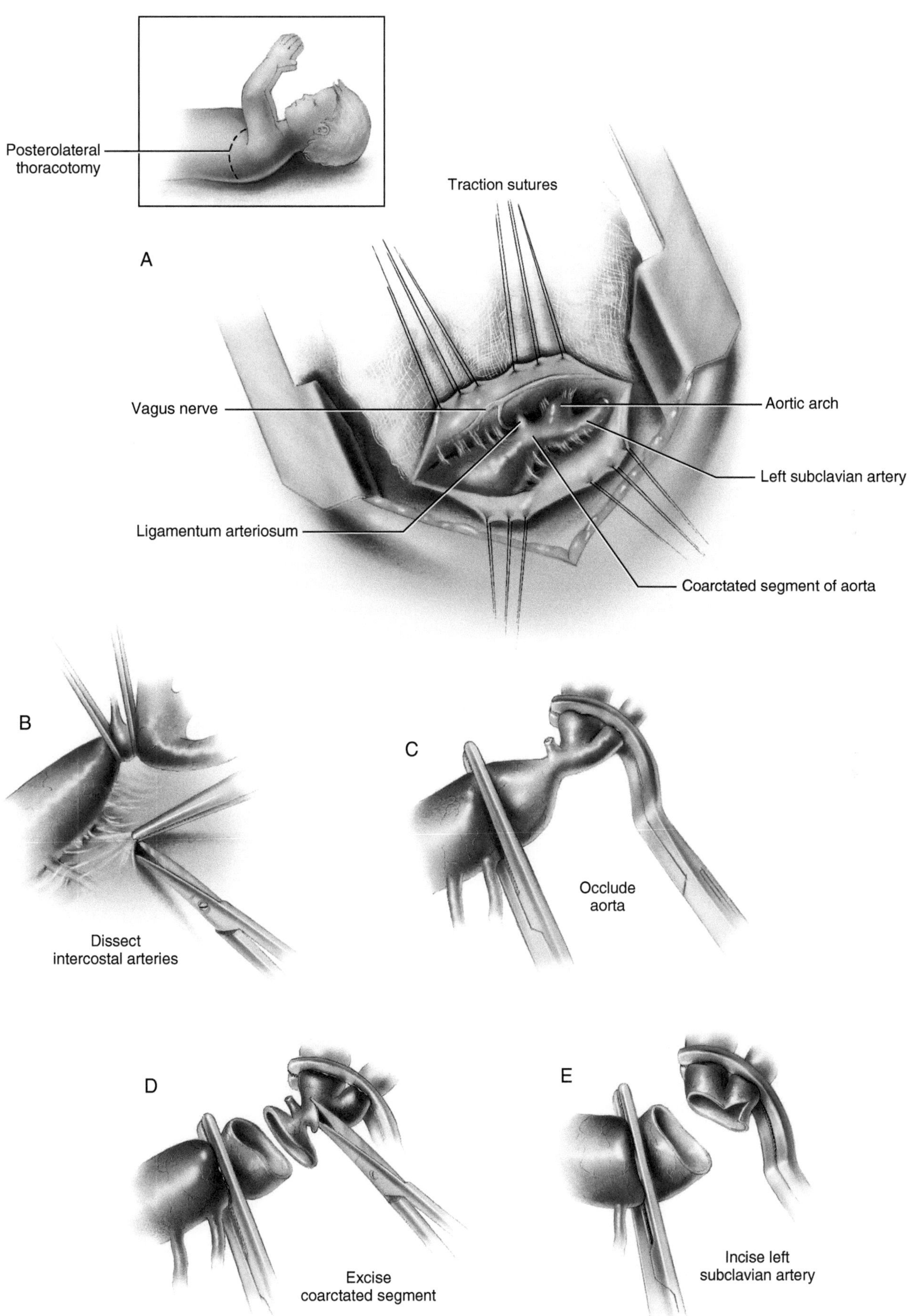
Posterolateral thoracotomy
Traction sutures
A
Vagus nerve
Aortic arch
Left subclavian artery
Ligamentum arteriosum
Coarctated segment of aorta
B
Dissect intercostal arteries
C
Occlude aorta
D
Excise coarctated segment
E
Incise left subclavian artery

Figure 27-2 (continued)

F An end-to-end anastomosis is constructed using a continuous stitch of 5/0 to 7/0 polypropylene, depending on the thickness and quality of the aortic wall. Double-armed suture is used, with the initial stitch placed at the anterior end of the distal aortic segment from inside the aorta. The second stitch is taken through the proximal aortic segment from inside the aorta. This suture is continued into the aorta from the adventitial side on the distal aortic segment.

G This sequence provides placement of a continuous stitch from the intimal surface on the proximal end of the aorta and from the adventitial surface on the distal segment. A nerve hook is used to retract the suture loops to set up the aorta for maximal exposure.

H When all the stitches for the back wall of the anastomosis have been placed, the suture loops are drawn up, and the ends of the aorta are approximated. The nerve hook is used again to adjust suture loop tension.

I The anastomosis is completed, placing several interrupted stitches in the front row. The initial stitches are placed at each end of the anastomosis to tie off the continuous suture. All the interrupted stitches are placed in the front row prior to tying them off; this provides maximal exposure and prevents inadvertent closure of the back wall to the front wall. The completed anastomosis should be larger than the diameter of the descending thoracic aorta because of its oblique nature.

J Infants with coarctation of the aorta often have significant hypoplasia of the aortic arch. Complete mobilization of the aortic arch and the arch branch vessels allows placement of the proximal vascular occlusion clamp across the left carotid artery as well as the aorta and left subclavian artery. The coarctated segment of aorta is excised at the distal portion of the aortic arch. The opening into the aortic arch is enlarged by extending the incision proximally along the inferior aspect of the arch, toward the base of the left carotid artery. The coarctated segment is removed by incising the upper portion of the descending thoracic aorta distal to the narrow point in a diagonal fashion. The long dimension of the diagonal is placed anteriorly to ensure sufficient length to conform to the inferior aspect of the aortic arch for direct anastomosis.

K This technique of incision and control of the aorta provides a very large opening into the aortic arch and a maximal circumference (diameter) for anastomosis to the distal aorta. Although this reconstruction is referred to as an end-to-end anastomosis, it could actually be referred to as an end (aorta)-to-side (aortic arch) anastomosis.

L The posterior row of the anastomosis is created by placing all the suture loops prior to approximation of the proximal and distal aorta. Generally, 7/0 polypropylene suture is chosen, but polydioxanone may be used to allow absorption of the suture and thus reduce the chance of late stenosis. Attention must be given to placement of the stitches at the most proximal point on the aortic arch, where tension is greatest. Substantial tissue bites should be taken, being careful to pull the needle through in its exact arc. The suture loops are drawn tight with the aid of a nerve hook.

M Interrupted stitches in the anterior row complete the repair.

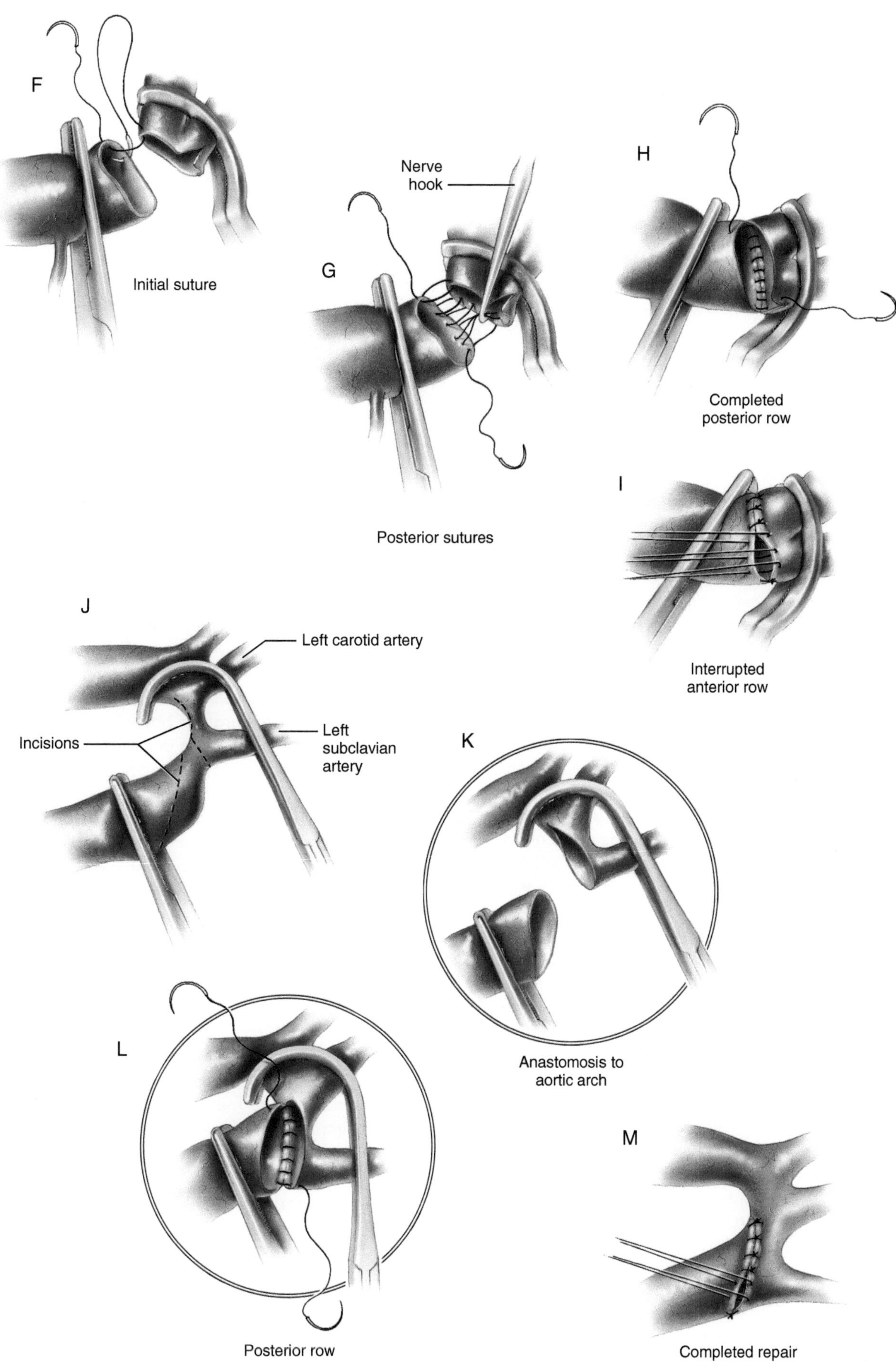
F
Initial suture
Nerve
hook
G
Posterior sutures
H
Completed
posterior row
I
Interrupted
anterior row
J
Left carotid artery
Incisions
Left
subclavian
artery
K
Anastomosis to
aortic arch
L
Posterior row
M
Completed repair

Extraanatomic Bypass for Residual Stenosis Following Repair of Coarctation of the Aorta

Coarctation of the aorta is often associated with bicuspid aortic valve or some other intracardiac anomaly, such as ventricular or atrial septal defect, that may require operative intervention at a later time after repair of the coarctation. Typically, the coarctation is repaired during infancy or childhood, and when the associated intracardiac defect presents for operation years later, residual stenosis of the aorta at the site of the prior coarctation repair is discovered and requires attention. Optimally, incompletely relieved thoracic aortic obstruction is repaired at the time of intracardiac operation by extraanatomic aortic bypass.

Figure 27-3

A Bicuspid aortic valve with dilation of the ascending aorta and associated residual stenosis of the upper portion of the descending thoracic aorta at the site of prior coarctaion repair. Cardiopulmonary bypass is established through a cannula placed in the distal portion of the aortic arch.

B Exposure of the descending thoracic aorta through the posterior pericardium is obtained with the heart arrested and decompressed while circulation to the body is supported on cardiopulmonary bypass. The heart is retracted superiorly for access to the aorta behind the pericardial sac. The pericardial sac is opened over the aorta. Minimal aortic dissection can be accomplished quickly. A partial occlusion clamp is placed on the aorta, and a longitudinal incision is made in the aorta. An end-to-side anastomosis of graft to aorta can be performed quite easily. An externally reinforced polytetrafluoroethylene (PTFE) graft is used for the extraanatomic bypass to avoid graft compression by the heart or surrounding structures. A graft 10 or 12 mm in diameter is sufficient to relieve mild or moderate stenosis of the aorta, based on our knowledge of the diameter required for aortic bypass using axillofemoral extraanatomic grafts. The graft is anastomosed end-to-side to the descending thoracic aorta using continuous stitches of 4/0 or 5/0 polypropylene, depending on the thickness of the aortic wall. It is helpful to use two sutures with double needles so that most if not all of the suture loops are placed before tensioning the suture to approximate the graft to the aorta.

C The shortest route from the ascending aorta to the descending thoracic aorta, and the one least likely to compress the graft, is *posterior* to the inferior vena cava. The location of the great vessels as they penetrate the pericardial sac is shown. There is a nice passageway (*arrow*) behind the inferior vena cava. This passageway is opened by incising the pericardial reflection between the inferior vena cava and the right inferior pulmonary vein. The graft is pulled through the passageway behind the vena cava. The inferior vena cava is less vulnerable to compression if the bypass graft is placed posterior to it.

D The graft is placed in the pericardial sac to the right of the right atrium, passing anterior to the superior vena cava, to approximate the ascending aorta. In this case, the aortic root and ascending aorta have been replaced. The extraanatomic bypass graft is anastomosed to the lateral aspect of the prosthetic ascending aorta in an end-to-side fashion using continuous stitches of 4/0 polypropylene. The location of the bypass graft places it posteriorly in the pericardial sac, protecting it from injury should reentry sternotomy be required at a later time.

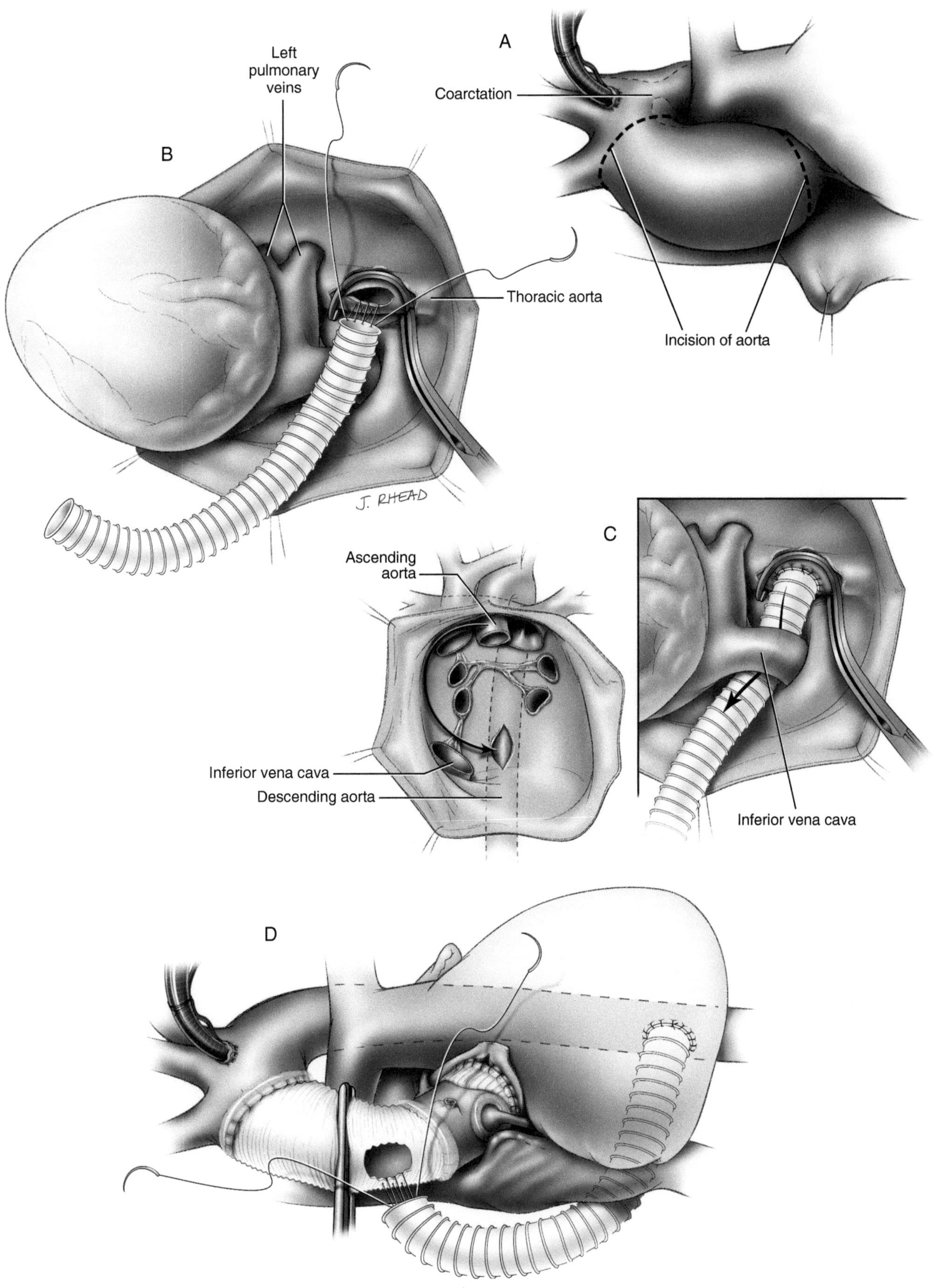
A
Coarctation
Incision of aorta
B
Left pulmonary veins
Thoracic aorta
J. RHEAD
C
Ascending aorta
Inferior vena cava
Descending aorta
Inferior vena cava
D
Completed repair

chapter 28 INTERRUPTED AORTIC ARCH

Interrupted aortic arch is a defect in which the aortic arch is incomplete. The anomaly is classified according to where the arch is separated. Usually the upper compartment arterial circulation is through the ascending aorta, and the lower body receives its blood supply via the ductus arteriosus, which is continuous with the descending thoracic aorta. The size (diameter) of the ascending aorta is correlated with outcome: a small ascending aorta may be associated with atresia of the aortic valve, hypoplastic left ventricle, or both.

Morphology

Classification of interrupted aortic arch is related to the location of the arch separation. Type A refers to separation distal to the left subclavian artery, so that all four arch branches originate from the ascending aorta. Type B is interruption distal to the left carotid artery. Type C is interruption distal to the brachiocephalic (innominate) artery or the right common carotid artery.

Figure 28-1

A Interrupted aortic arch, type C. The heart and great vessels are viewed laterally, with the left ventricle opened. A large main pulmonary artery originates from the right ventricle and is overlying the ascending aorta. Two branches are seen above the main pulmonary artery—the right subclavian and right common carotid arteries. The pulmonary artery gives origin to the ductus arteriosus, which continues as the descending thoracic aorta. The left subclavian artery originates at the junction of the ductus arteriosus and the descending thoracic aorta. The left common carotid artery has been cut flush with the aorta and is barely visible as a little stump. A large ventricular septal defect is associated with the interrupted arch.

B Interrupted aortic arch. This magnified view demonstrates the details described above.

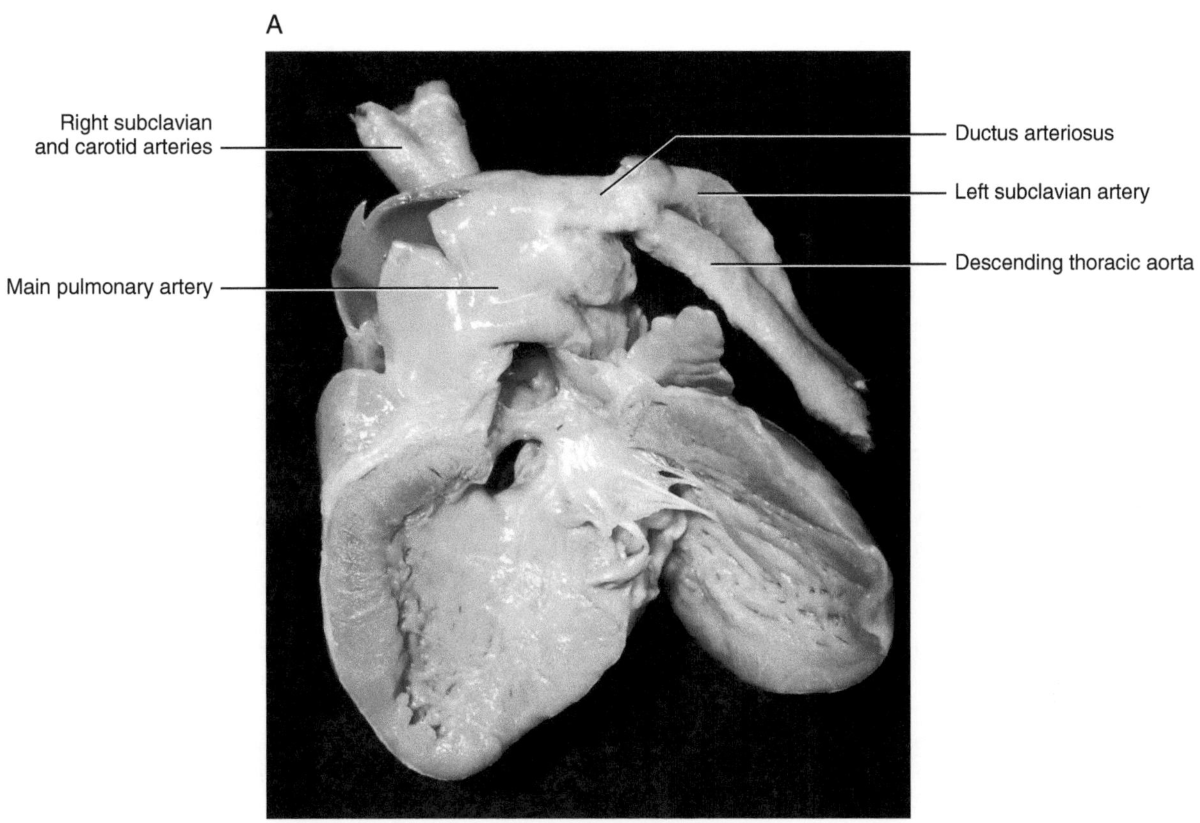
A
Right subclavian and carotid arteries
Main pulmonary artery
Ductus arteriosus
Left subclavian artery
Descending thoracic aorta

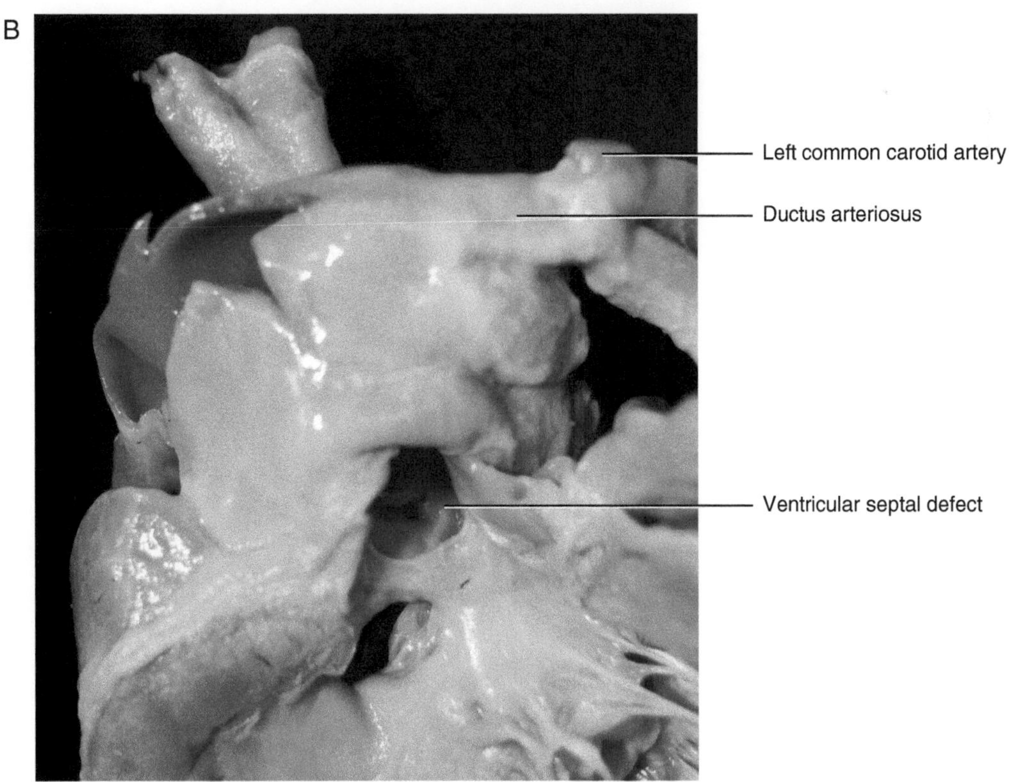
B
Left common carotid artery
Ductus arteriosus
Ventricular septal defect

Figure 28-2

A Cardiopulmonary bypass is complicated in these patients, and the method depends on where the arch is interrupted. Single venous cannulation is usually performed, and the repair is made using deep hypothermia and circulatory arrest. Monitoring of the temperature in the upper and lower compartments is essential so that uniform cooling of the vital organs is ensured. It may be necessary to perfuse both the aorta and the pulmonary artery, but usually one or the other is sufficient to cool the entire body.

B While cooling is proceeding, the descending thoracic aorta is completely mobilized. Some intercostal arteries may have to be divided, but extensive mobilization of these arteries usually allows the aorta to be sufficiently lengthened to reach the ascending aorta. When circulatory arrest is established, the ductus arteriosus is divided.

C The proximal end of the ductus arteriosus is oversewn with 5/0 or 6/0 polypropylene suture.

D An end-to-side anastomosis of the descending thoracic aorta to the ascending aorta is constructed with 6/0 or 7/0 polypropylene or polydioxanone suture material. Complete mobilization of the descending aorta allows this anastomosis to be made without tension.

E There are usually associated ventricular and atrial septal defects. These lesions are repaired by the transatrial approach in the usual fashion. A Dacron patch is placed into the ventricular septal defect, and the atrial septal defect is closed by direct suture. Rewarming of the patient is accomplished by perfusing the reconstructed aorta.

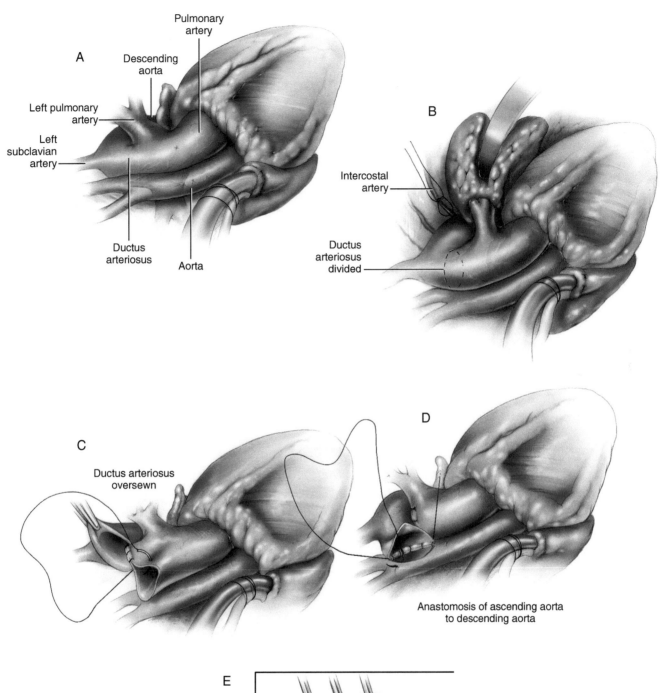

A
Pulmonary artery
Descending aorta
Left pulmonary artery
Left subclavian artery
Ductus arteriosus
Aorta

B
Intercostal artery
Ductus arteriosus divided

C
Ductus arteriosus oversewn

D
Anastomosis of ascending aorta to descending aorta

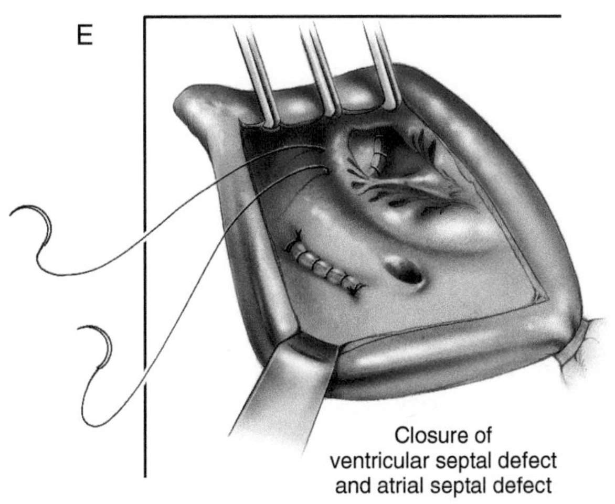

Closure of ventricular septal defect and atrial septal defect

chapter 29 VASCULAR RING AND SLING

Abnormal development of the aortic arch may result in vascular abnormalities that compress the trachea and esophagus. These anomalies, commonly known as vascular rings, cause airway obstruction, dysphagia, or both. The diagnosis is made by clinical symptoms confirmed by barium esophagram, which shows posterior compression of the esophagus by the abnormal aortic arch of the branch artery as it courses behind the esophagus and trachea. Computed tomography or magnetic resonance imaging can also be used to delineate the arterial anomaly. The operative approach in nearly every case is a left posterolateral thoracotomy through the bed of the nonresected fourth rib.

Anomalous origin of the left pulmonary artery from the right pulmonary artery outside the pericardial sac and coursing to the left, posterior to the tracheal bifurcation and anterior to the esophagus, to reach the hilum of the left lung forms a vascular sling around the trachea. The operative approach to this vascular anomaly is through a midline sternotomy incision while the patient is on cardiopulmonary bypass.

Morphology

Double aortic arch is the classic vascular ring. The ascending aorta separates into right- and left-sided arches that course to the sides of the trachea and esophagus and then rejoin behind the esophagus as the descending thoracic aorta. Another common type of complete vascular ring is a right aortic arch with a retroesophageal left subclavian artery. The left ligamentum arteriosum completes the ring. A left aortic arch with a retroesophageal right subclavian artery originating as the fourth branch of the aortic arch (aberrant right subclavian artery) is an incomplete vascular ring. Although technically not a vascular ring, tracheal compression by the innominate artery, which may be associated with rotation of the aortic arch or heart, is included in this discussion.

Figure 29-1

A Right aortic arch with retroesophageal left subclavian artery and left ligamentum arteriosum, anterior view. The specimen is viewed on the anterior aspect of the great vessels, with the forceps on a partially opened main pulmonary artery (PA). The right aortic arch (Ao) is seen as it emerges from behind the forceps. Three arterial branches of the arch are present. The ligamentum arteriosum takes its origin from the bifurcation of the pulmonary artery. The left pulmonary artery (LPA) is clearly visible below the ligamentum arteriosum. The origin of the left subclavian artery is not seen because it is behind the trachea (T) and esophagus.

B Right aortic arch with retroesophageal left subclavian artery and left ligamentum arteriosum, trachea, and esophagus reflected anteriorly. The ligamentum arteriosum is seen joining the descending aorta (Ao) to complete the vascular ring surrounding the trachea (T) and esophagus (E). The left subclavian artery stump originating from the aortic diverticulum is not well visualized.

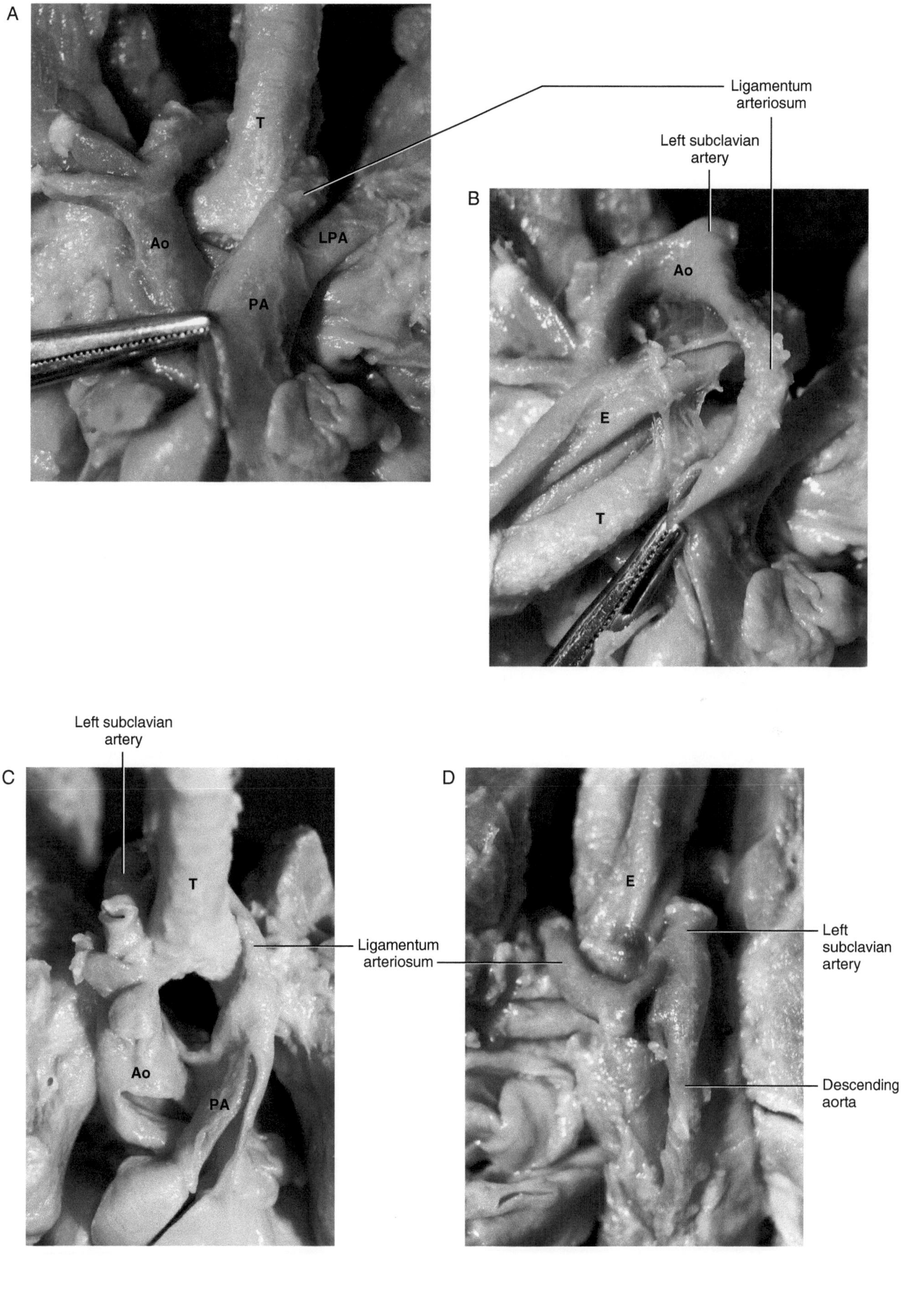

A
T
Ligamentum arteriosum
Ao
LPA
PA

B
Left subclavian artery
Ligamentum arteriosum
Ao
E
T

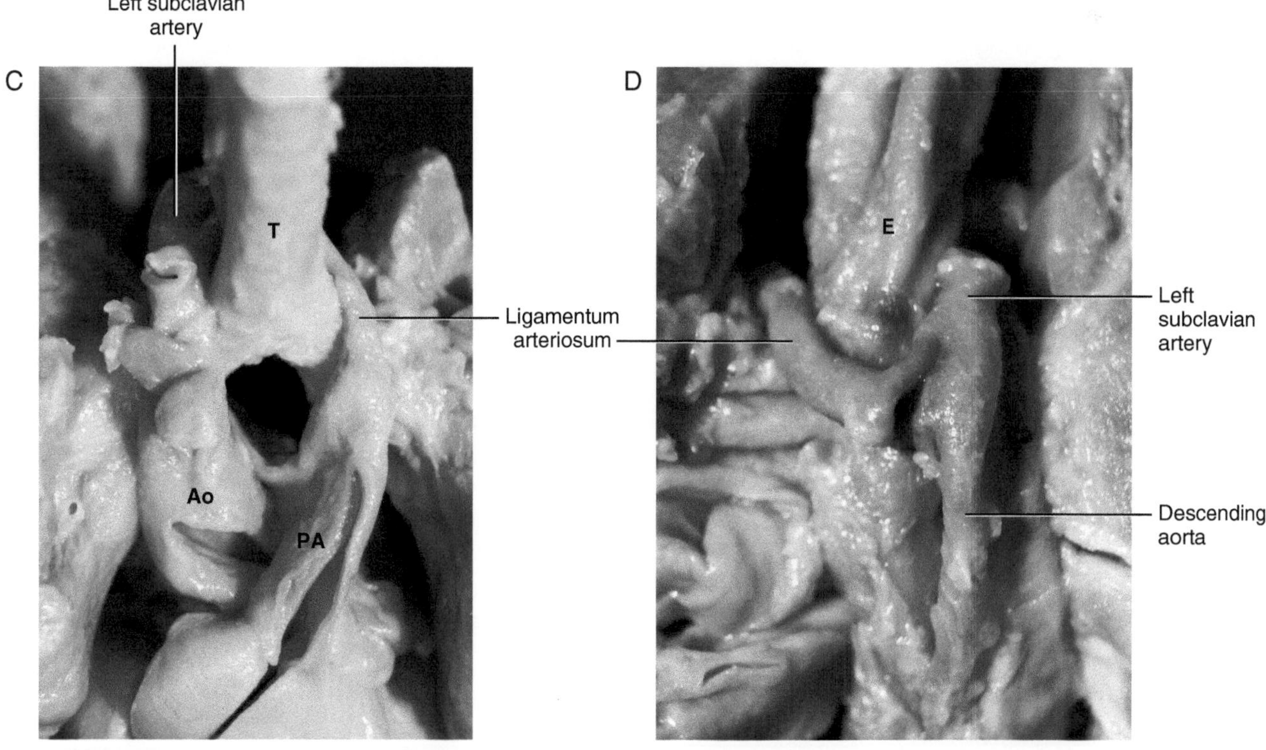

Figure 29-1 (continued)

C Right aortic arch with retroesophageal left subclavian artery and left ligamentum arteriosum, superior view. This view from above demonstrates the complete ring. The partially opened ascending aorta (Ao) and the right aortic arch with its branches wrap around the right side of the trachea (T). The left subclavian artery is in the shadow of the trachea, coming from the aortic diverticulum. The ligamentum arteriosum originates from the partially opened pulmonary artery (PA) and wraps around the left side of the trachea.

D Right aortic arch with retroesophageal left subclavian artery and left ligamentum arteriosum, posterior view. The vascular ring is shown compressing the posterior aspect of the esophagus (E) in this view from behind the trachea and esophagus.

Double Aortic Arch
Figure 29-2

A Double aortic arch is the classic form of vascular ring. Either the left or the right arch may be dominant. Dominant left arch is seen in about 50% of patients. The anterior perspective shows the larger left arch passing in front of the trachea. The posterior perspective shows the smaller right arch passing behind the trachea and esophagus to join the left-sided descending aorta and complete the ring. The superior view shows the left subclavian and common carotid arteries originating from the larger left arch and the right common carotid and subclavian arteries originating from the smaller, posteriorly placed right aortic arch.

Dominant right arch is found in about 25% of patients. The anterior perspective shows the smaller left arch in front of the trachea and the larger right arch passing to the right of the trachea. The posterior perspective shows the larger right arch behind the trachea and esophagus. The superior perspective demonstrates that the arrangement of the arch vessels is similar to that in the case of a dominant left arch, with the left common carotid and subclavian arteries coming off the smaller, anteriorly placed left aortic arch and the right common carotid and subclavian arteries originating from the right arch. A balanced pattern of the two arches is seen in the remaining 25% of patients.

B The vascular ring is approached through a left-sided thoracotomy. The pleura over the upper portion of the thoracic aorta and left subclavian artery is opened with dissection over the adventitia of the aortic arches and branches, so that the vagus nerve is mobilized anteriorly with the pleural flap. The left aortic arch and the left carotid and left subclavian arteries are mobilized up to the junction with the ascending aorta. The retroesophageal left arch is completely mobilized away from the esophagus and trachea. During the course of the retroesophageal dissection, the right carotid and right subclavian arteries should be identified. Dissection of the left arch should be complete to the ascending aorta. Absolute identification of the aortic arch branch arteries is required. The vascular ring is opened by dividing the narrowest point on the aortic arch. This figure shows a common point of division of the vascular ring on the left (anterior) arch, between the left common carotid artery and the left subclavian artery.

C The left aortic arch is divided between vascular clamps, and the ends are oversewn with 5/0 polypropylene. The distal stump suture line, which is often proximal to the left subclavian artery, is attached by suture to the prevertebral fascia to completely open the space lateral to the trachea and esophagus. The ligamentum arteriosum is divided.

A

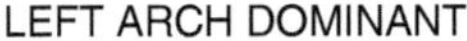
LEFT ARCH DOMINANT

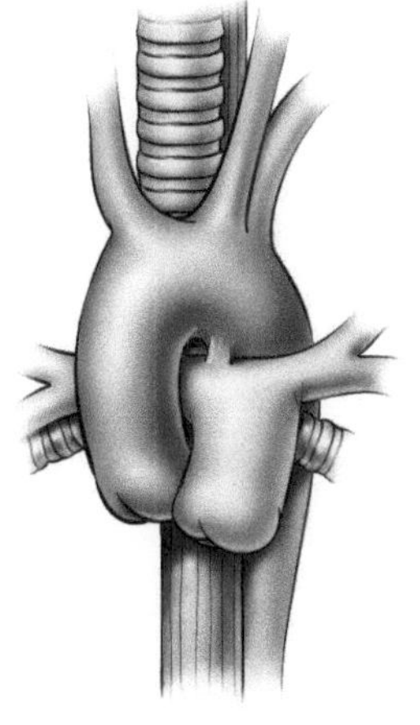
Anterior view

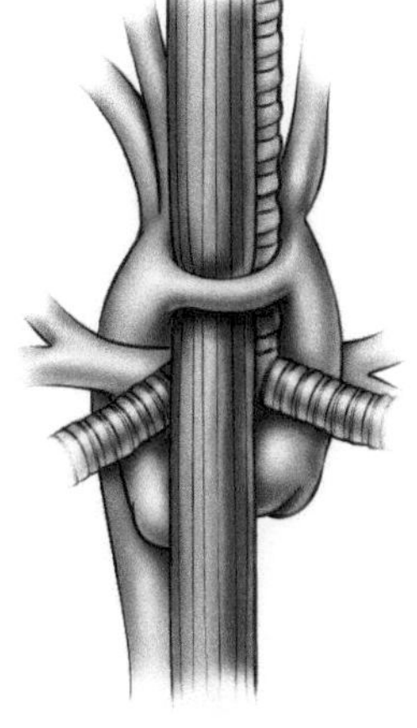
Posterior view

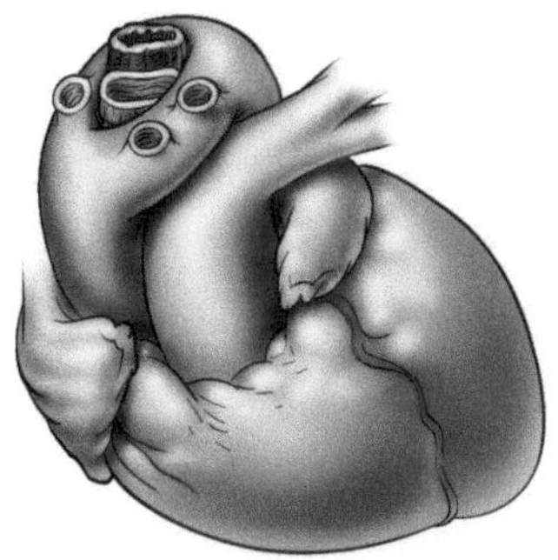
Superior view

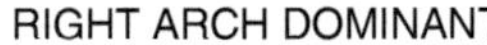
RIGHT ARCH DOMINANT

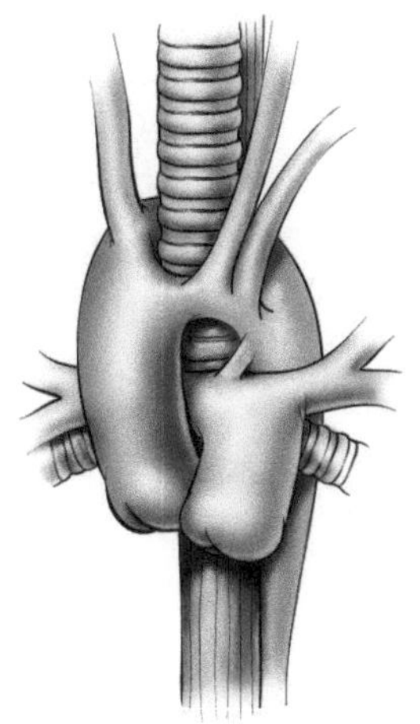
Anterior view

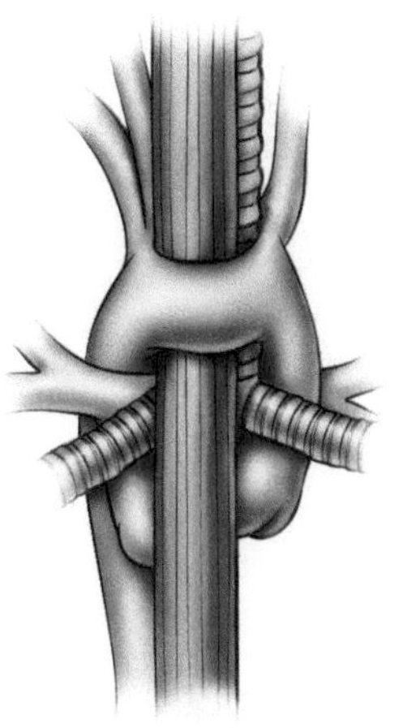
Posterior view

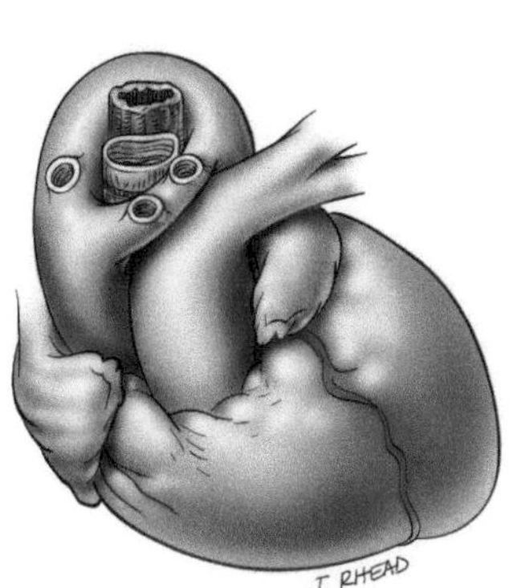

Superior view

B

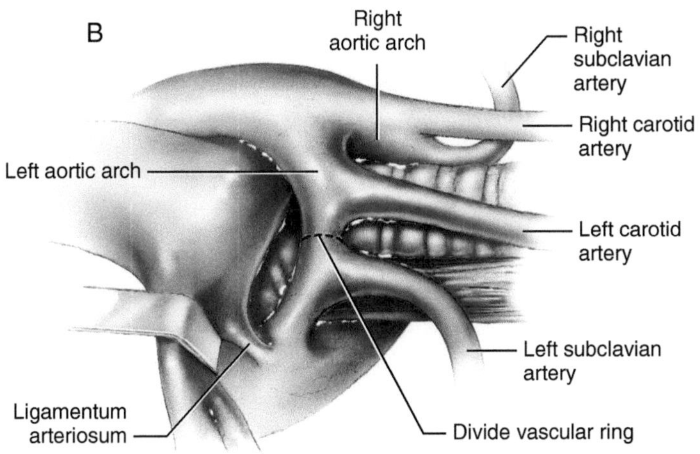

C

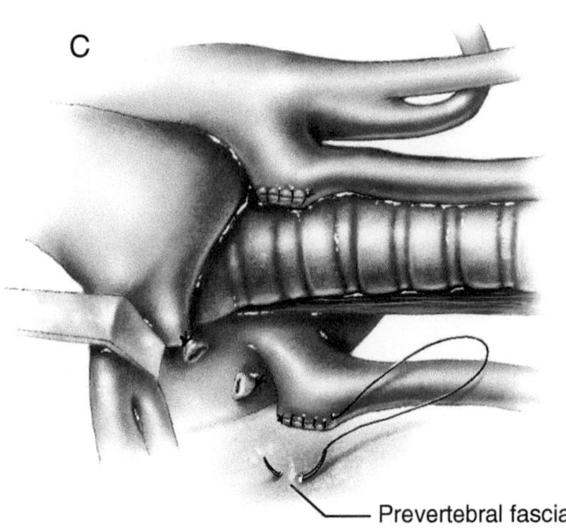

Right Aortic Arch with Retroesophageal Left Subclavian Artery and Left Ligamentum Arteriosum
Figure 29-3

A The inset diagram shows the aortic arch on the right side, along with the descending thoracic aorta. The left subclavian artery originates from the distal right aortic arch behind the esophagus. The vascular ring is completed by the left-sided ligamentum arteriosum, which extends from the upper descending aorta near the left subclavian artery behind the esophagus to the left main pulmonary artery. The vascular ring is approached through a left-sided thoracotomy. The surgeon's view corresponds to the anatomy described in the inset. The pleura lateral to the esophagus and left subclavian artery is opened. All the arch branches should be identified and dissected.

B The ligamentum arteriosum and the left subclavian artery are completely mobilized. The ligamentum arteriosum is ligated and divided. The left subclavian artery is completely freed from the posterior surface of the esophagus back to its origin from the thoracic aorta.

A

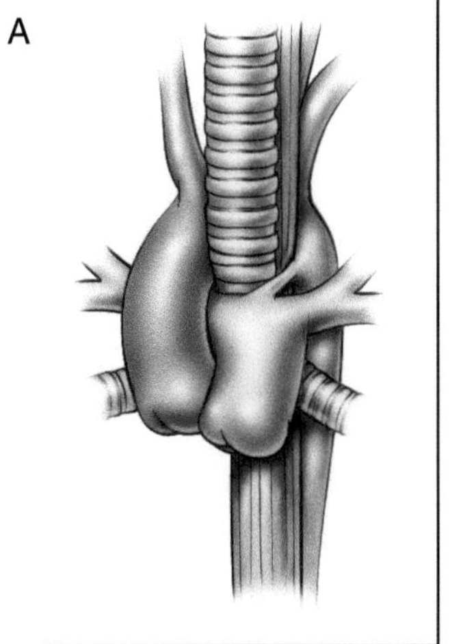

Right aortic arch with retroesophageal left subclavian artery and left ligamentum arteriosum

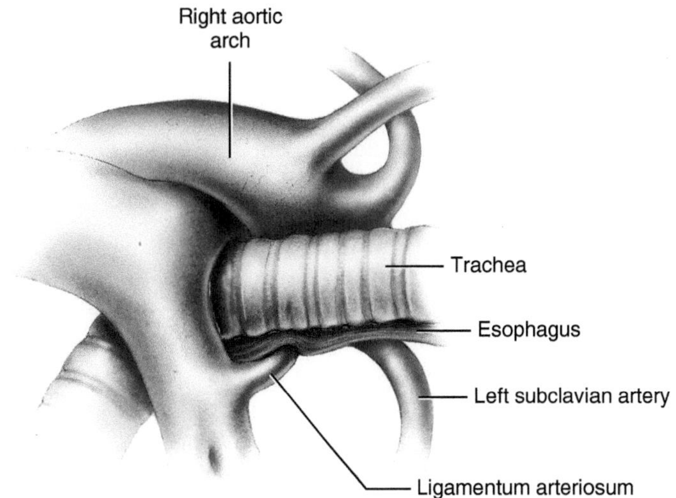

B

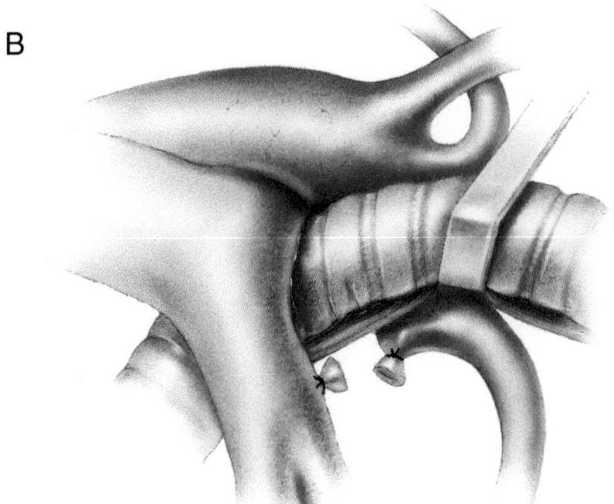

Divided ligamentum arteriosum

Left Aortic Arch with Retroesophageal Right Subclavian Artery Originating as Fourth Branch of the Arch
Figure 29-4

A This anomaly is an incomplete vascular ring because there is no vascular structure to the right side of the trachea. The inset diagram shows the right subclavian artery passing behind the esophagus from its origin as a fourth branch of the arch (aberrant). The aortic arch is on the left side. The surgeon's view when the approach is through a left-sided thoracotomy shows the esophagus compressed from behind by the right subclavian artery. Symptoms such as difficulty swallowing generally do not appear until later in life, when there is some ectasia of the subclavian artery (dysphagia lusoria). Aneurysmal dilation of the subclavian artery on the right side beyond the point of compression with the esophagus dictates that the lesion be approached from the right, so that reconstruction of the subclavian artery by anastomosis to the right carotid artery can be accomplished.

B For children, only simple mobilization and division of the retroesophageal right subclavian artery are required. The pleura over the aorta and left subclavian artery is opened. The right subclavian artery is identified and dissected from its origin behind the esophagus and to the right as far as possible. The right subclavian artery is ligated and divided. The distal end is allowed to retract to the right from behind the esophagus.

A

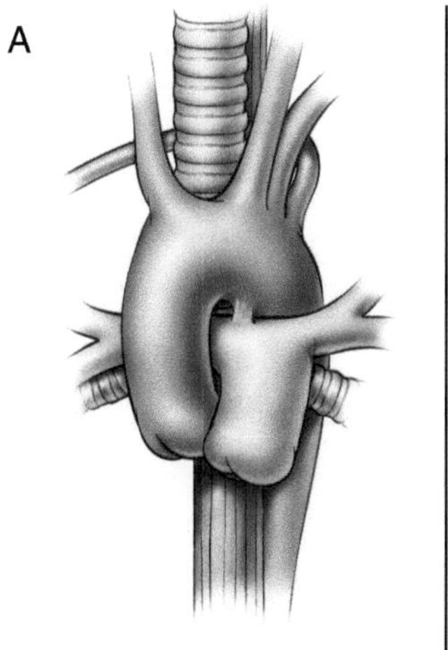

Left aortic arch with retroesophageal right subclavian artery originating as fourth branch of aorta

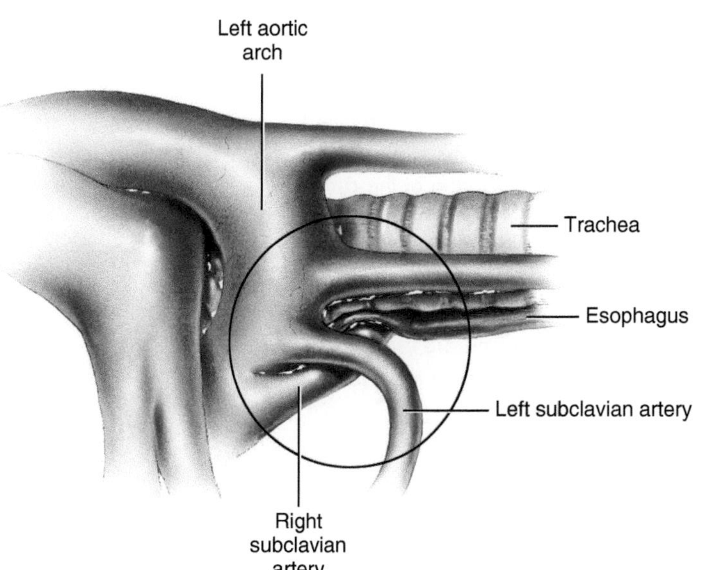

B

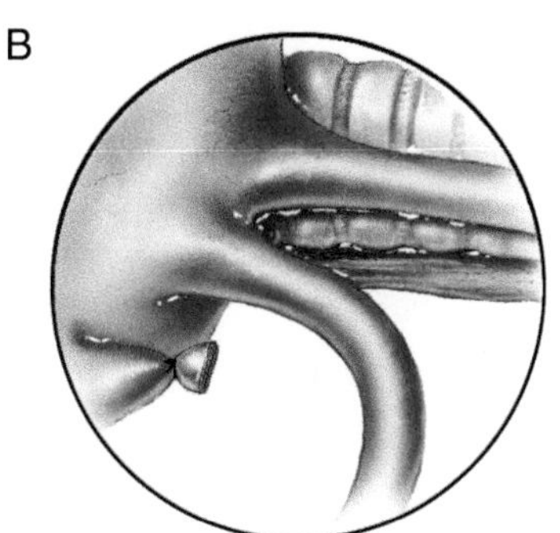

Divided right subclavian artery

Tracheal Compression by Innominate Artery
Figure 29-5

A Tracheal compression by the innominate artery is not a vascular ring but is grouped here because the associated symptoms of respiratory distress due to tracheal obstruction are similar to those of vascular ring. These lateral diagrams show the trachea compressed by the innominate artery anteriorly as it crosses the trachea abnormally owing to a more distal origin from the aortic arch than usual or rotation of the arch to the left. An anterior thoracotomy is used to completely mobilize the innominate artery away from the trachea, from its origin on the arch to well above tracheal contact. Interrupted, pledget-reinforced mattress stitches of 3/0 or 4/0 polypropylene are used to attach the innominate artery to the posterior table of the sternum, suspending it away from the trachea. The stitches are passed through the adventitia of the artery and the periosteum of the sternum.

B An alternative method described by Hawkins is preferred because it addresses more directly the morphology of the displaced, more distal origin of the innominate artery on the aortic arch. An anterior thoracotomy is performed. The aortic arch and innominate artery are thoroughly mobilized. The origin of the artery is isolated by partial occlusion of the aortic arch by a vascular clamp. The artery is divided at its origin, and the aortic arch is closed by continuous stitches of 5/0 or 6/0 polypropylene. A longitudinal incision is made more proximally in the aorta. The innominate artery is anastomosed to the aorta using continuous stitches of 5/0 or 6/0 polypropylene at the new, more proximal location.

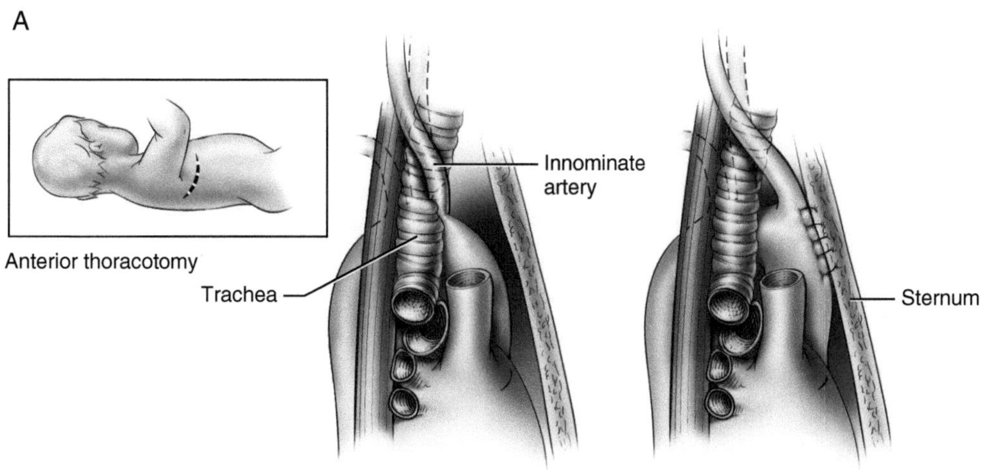
A
Anterior thoracotomy
Trachea
Innominate
artery
Sternum

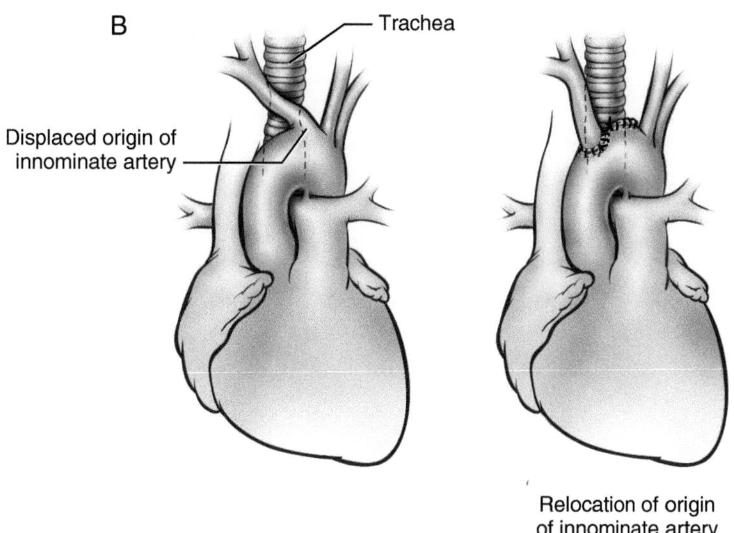
B
Trachea
Displaced origin of
innominate artery
Relocation of origin
of innominate artery

Vascular Sling

Anomalous origin of the left pulmonary artery from the right pulmonary artery outside the pericardial sac is the cause of vascular sling. The left pulmonary artery passes between the trachea and the esophagus to the hilum of the left lung. This creates a tight sling around the trachea, causing compression and stenosis of the trachea at or just above the bifurcation. Tracheal cartilages may become complete stenotic rings with the absence of the membranous portion of the trachea. Pulmonary artery sling is a rare condition.

Figure 29-6

A Superior view of the origin of the left pulmonary artery from the right pulmonary artery. The course of the left pulmonary artery between the trachea and esophagus to the hilum of the left lung is also shown. The distal trachea is caught in the vascular sling created by the abnormal course of the left pulmonary artery.

B This anomaly is repaired through a midline sternotomy. The pericardial sac is opened, and the aorta and right and left pulmonary arteries are mobilized and separated. Cardiopulmonary bypass is established.

C The left pulmonary artery is divided at its origin from the right pulmonary artery and extracted from between the trachea and esophagus. The condition of the trachea can be assessed at this point, and a decision can be made regarding the need for tracheoplasty or resection and reanastomosis of the trachea. The vascular anomaly is corrected by anastomosis of the left pulmonary artery to a longitudinal incision in the main pulmonary artery anterior to the trachea. The anastomosis is created using continuous stitches of 6/0 polypropylene. Postoperative care may be complicated by tracheal stenosis, which tends to worsen in the days after operation due to tissue edema. Because this edema occurs at or near the tracheal bifurcation, below the position of the tip of the endotracheal tube, respiratory support is difficult, especially during the expiratory phase of the pulmonary cycle.

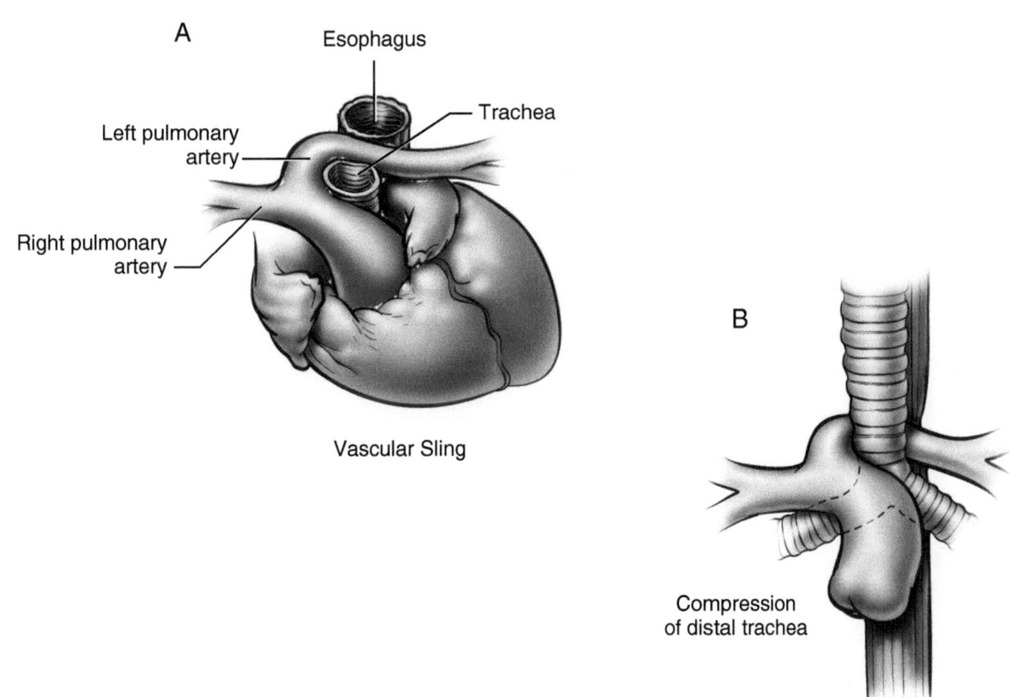
A
Esophagus
Trachea
Left pulmonary artery
Right pulmonary artery
Vascular Sling
B
Compression of distal trachea

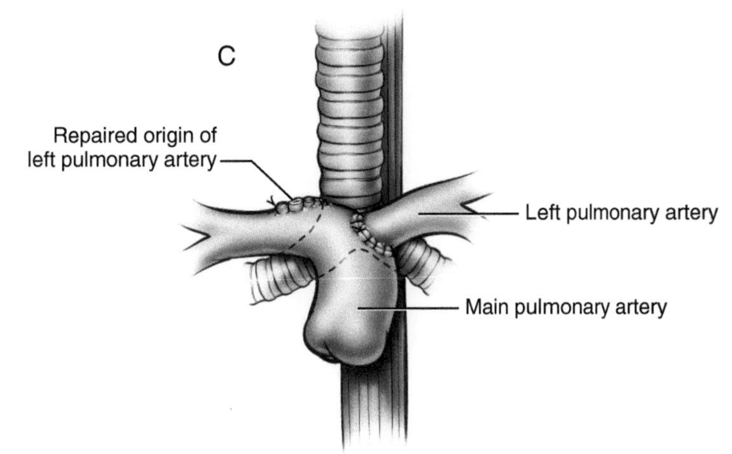
C
Repaired origin of left pulmonary artery
Left pulmonary artery
Main pulmonary artery

chapter 30 PALLIATIVE OPERATIONS

Operations have been devised to improve hemodynamics and balance blood flow in complex congenital cardiac anomalies. These operations are performed in a staged manner, to allow intervention for complete repair at a later time when the patient's age and size and the clinical situation are more conducive to a successful outcome.

Subclavian Artery–Pulmonary Artery Anastomosis

Prior to the landmark work of Alfred Blalock, MD, surgery for "blue" babies was not performed. The feasibility of anastomosis of a systemic artery to a pulmonary artery was demonstrated experimentally and carried to the operating room by Blalock and associates in 1944. The initial operation in a 15-month-old girl weighing 4 kg involved anastomosis of the left subclavian artery to the left pulmonary artery. The right innominate or subclavian artery was used for anastomosis in subsequent operations.

Figure 30-1

Blalock-Taussig Shunt

A Right subclavian artery–right pulmonary artery anastomosis (Blalock-Taussig shunt). This specimen demonstrates a perfectly executed Blalock-Taussig shunt. The aorta enters the middle of the image from below. The three arch branches are demonstrated; the brachiocephalic or innominate artery is the first branch and is intact. The left carotid and left subclavian arteries have been divided. The hemostat is on the right carotid artery. The right subclavian artery has been divided after ligating its side branches with hemoclips. The right subclavian artery is turned down to the right pulmonary artery, where anastomosis has been performed with interrupted stitches of fine polypropylene.

B A posterolateral thoracotomy incision is made on the side opposite the aortic arch. In most cases the incision is a right thoracotomy. The thorax is entered through the bed of the nonresected fourth rib. The mediastinal pleura is opened from the pulmonary artery parallel to the superior vena cava and over the right subclavian artery. The azygos vein is mobilized, ligated, and divided. The distal ligature on the doubly ligated superior vena cava side of the azygos vein may be used as a traction suture for the vena cava to retract it medially and anteriorly. The right pulmonary artery is completely mobilized, and double-loop tourniquet ligatures are placed on the apical anterior segmental branch and the pars intermedius of the pulmonary artery. The right pulmonary artery is mobilized as far medially as possible. The pericardium is dissected off the right pulmonary artery, preserving the integrity of the pericardial sac.

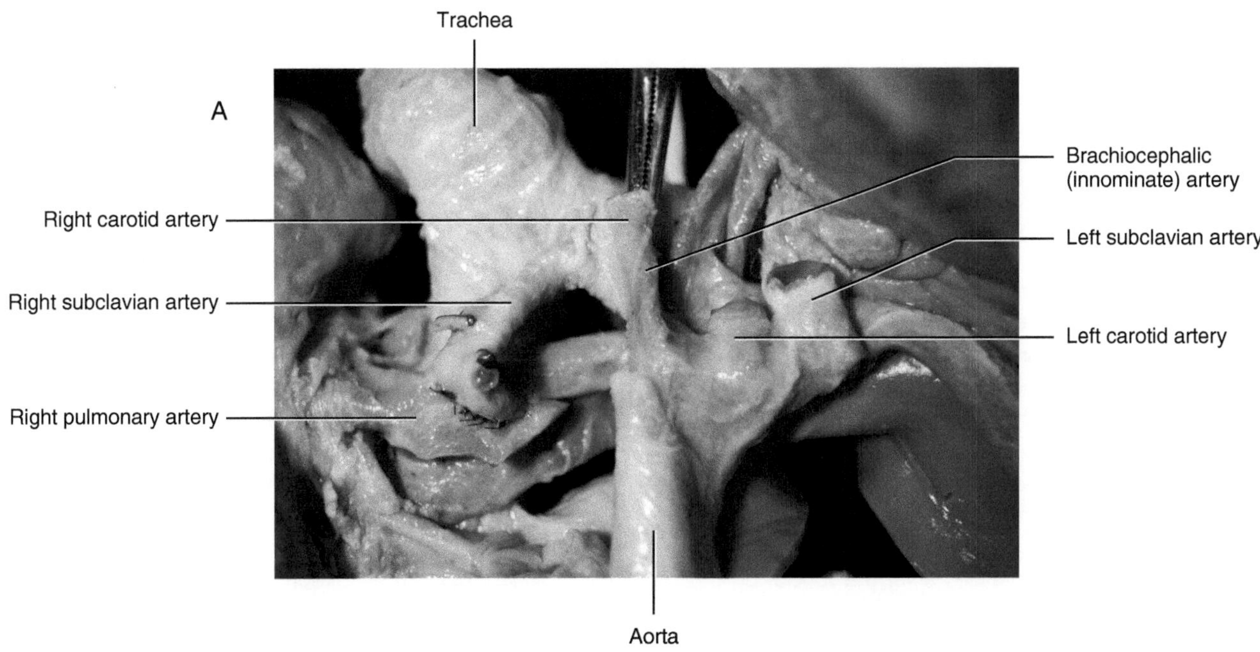
A
Trachea
Right carotid artery
Right subclavian artery
Right pulmonary artery
Brachiocephalic (innominate) artery
Left subclavian artery
Left carotid artery
Aorta

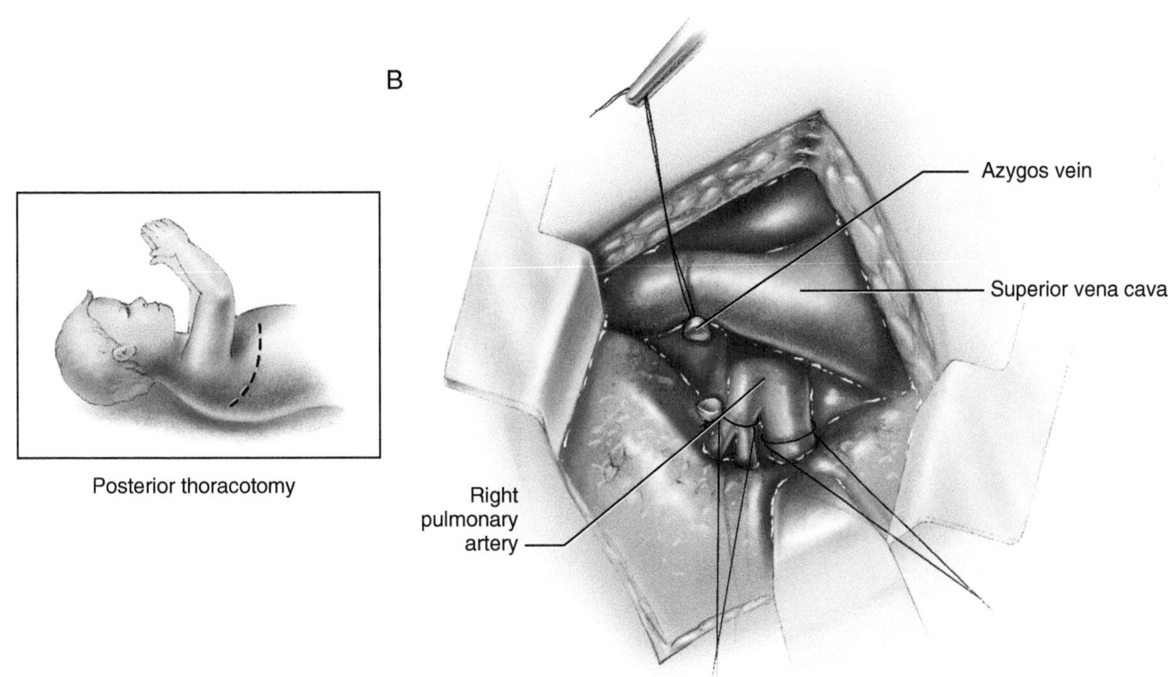
B
Posterior thoracotomy
Azygos vein
Superior vena cava
Right pulmonary artery

Figure 30-1 (continued)

C The right subclavian artery is identified and mobilized. Heparin 100 U/kg is administered intravenously to prevent fibrin formation within the subclavian artery during dissection. A rubber band or vessel loop is passed around the right subclavian artery for atraumatic retraction. The branches in the subclavian artery are ligated and divided. The vagus nerve is identified. A small right-angled clamp is passed beneath the vagus nerve, and the anterior surface of the subclavian artery is mobilized from beneath the nerve. The subclavian artery is ligated. A Cooley vascular clamp is passed beneath the vagus nerve and used to occlude the subclavian artery distally at the ligature. The subclavian artery is divided, and the Cooley clamp is withdrawn from beneath the vagus nerve to remove the subclavian artery from the loop formed by the vagus nerve and its recurrent branch.

D With the Cooley clamp on the distal end of the subclavian artery for retraction, the carotid and innominate arteries are completely mobilized from the connective tissue of the mediastinum. Dissection should be taken as far as possible on the carotid artery and as far medially on the innominate artery as possible to obtain maximal mobilization and length of the subclavian artery for approximation to the right pulmonary artery.

E A Dietrich vascular clamp is placed on the subclavian artery at its takeoff from the innominate artery. A Blalock vascular clamp is placed across the right pulmonary artery, and tourniquet ligatures on the distal branches of the right pulmonary artery are secured. Using a No. 11 scalpel, an incision is made halfway across the subclavian artery proximal to the occlusion clamp, preserving the appropriate length to reach the right pulmonary artery incision; at the same time, the incision is made as far proximal in the subclavian artery as possible to obtain maximal diameter.

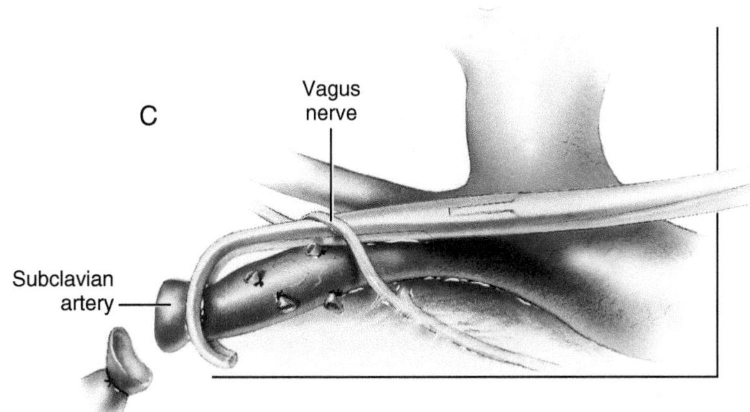
C
Vagus nerve
Subclavian artery

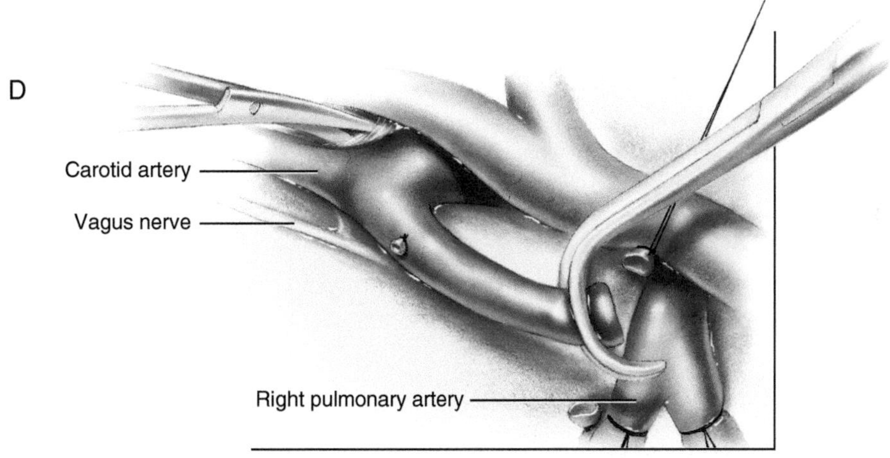
D
Carotid artery
Vagus nerve
Right pulmonary artery

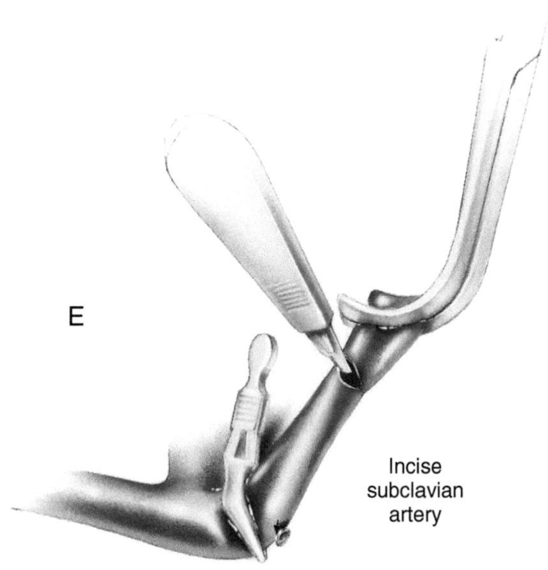
E
Incise subclavian artery

Figure 30-1 (continued)

F A longitudinal incision is made in the anterior and superior aspects of the right pulmonary artery. The length of the incision should approximate the diameter of the subclavian artery, recognizing that the pulmonary artery incision always enlarges during the course of the anastomosis.

G Continuous stitches of 7/0 polypropylene are used to construct a back row in the anastomosis. All the suture loops are placed for this back row before the arteries are approximated. The needle is passed from the lumen or intimal surface out of the subclavian artery and then passed from the adventitial surface of the pulmonary artery into its lumen. The end of the subclavian artery is excised, and an appropriate bevel is fashioned. This step must be performed carefully to preserve length on the anterior surface of the subclavian artery.

H The suture loops are then pulled up to approximate the subclavian artery to the pulmonary artery.

I The front row of the anastomosis is completed using interrupted stitches. Two stitches are placed initially at each end of the anastomosis to secure the continuous stitch. All interrupted stitches of the front row are placed before any are tied; this ensures the accuracy of the anastomosis and prevents picking up the back row of the anastomosis.

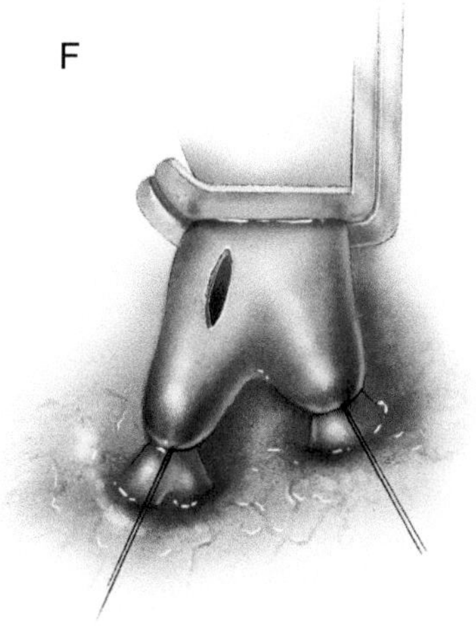

Incise pulmonary artery

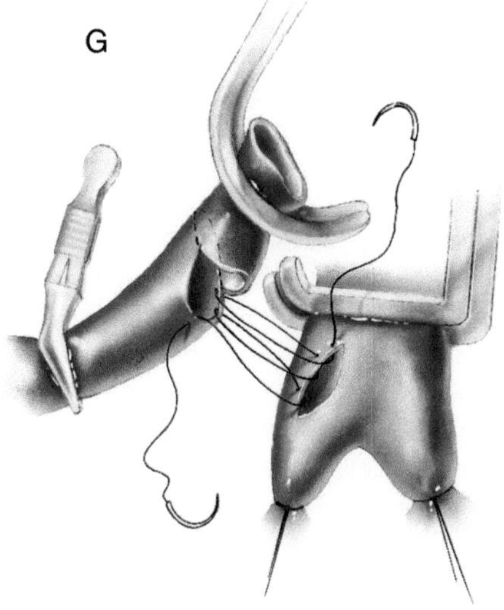

Place stitches in back row; then shorten and bevel artery

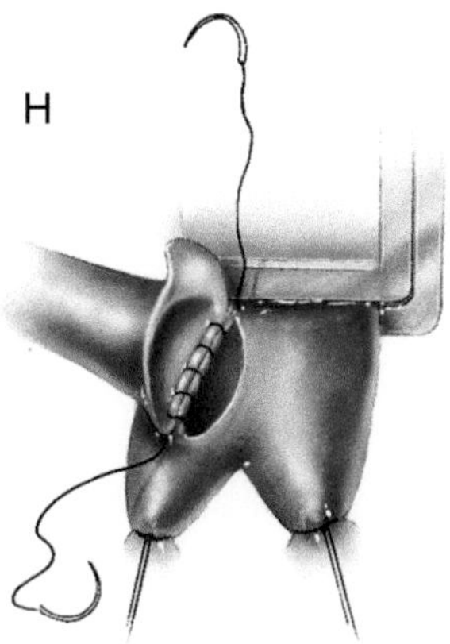

Pull up suture loops

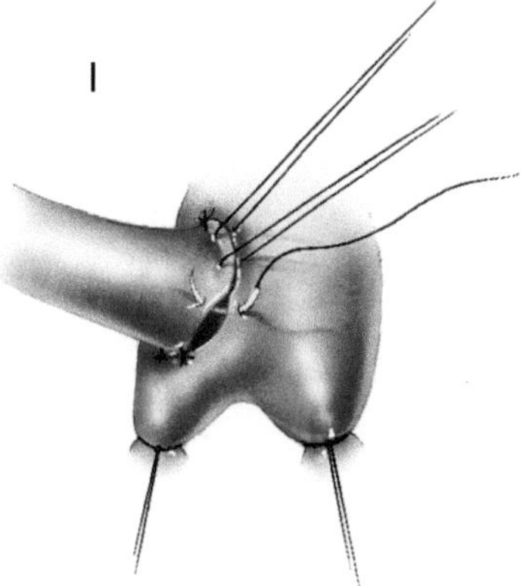

Interrupted front row

Figure 30-1 (continued)

Laks-Castaneda Modification

J When it is necessary to use the subclavian artery on the same side as the aortic arch, the Laks-Castaneda subclavian aortoplasty may be used to prevent kinking of the subclavian artery over the aortic arch. After complete mobilization of the subclavian artery and the distal portion of the aortic arch, the subclavian artery is ligated and divided. A partial-occlusion vascular clamp is placed on the distal aortic arch to exclude the base of the subclavian artery. An incision is made in the base of the subclavian artery, extending distally on the artery and into the aortic arch, opposite the base of the artery. This longitudinal incision is closed in a transverse fashion using fine polypropylene suture in continuous stitches. This suture line transplants the subclavian orifice onto the anterior wall of the aortic arch so that the subclavian artery is directed toward the pulmonary artery without distortion or kinking.

K The anastomosis of the distal end of the subclavian artery to the pulmonary artery is constructed by partial exclusion of the pulmonary artery using a technique similar to that described for the standard Blalock-Taussig shunt.

Modified Blalock-Taussig Shunt

L A modification of the Blalock-Taussig shunt principle, in which a prosthetic graft is interposed between the subclavian and pulmonary arteries, combines simplicity of performance, favorable blood flow characteristics controlled by the size of the subclavian artery, lack of distortion of the pulmonary artery, and preservation of subclavian artery blood flow. The operation may not be perfect for long-term palliation, but it is satisfactory when palliation for less than 2 years is required.

The shunt is performed on the same side as the aortic arch, in most instances through a posterolateral thoracotomy. For patients with the usual left arch anatomy, the left subclavian artery and the proximal portion of the left pulmonary artery are mobilized. A small, curved vascular clamp is used to isolate the left subclavian artery just distal to its origin. A 4- or 5-mm polytetrafluoroethylene (PTFE) graft is beveled to fit the side of the subclavian artery and is directed toward the proximal pulmonary artery. An end-to-side anastomosis of the graft to the subclavian artery is constructed by continuous stitches with 6/0 or 7/0 polypropylene.

M The vascular clamp is used to isolate a portion of the left pulmonary artery. The graft is then beveled appropriately to approximate the pulmonary artery. An end-to-side anastomosis of the graft to the pulmonary artery is constructed by continuous stitches using fine polypropylene suture.

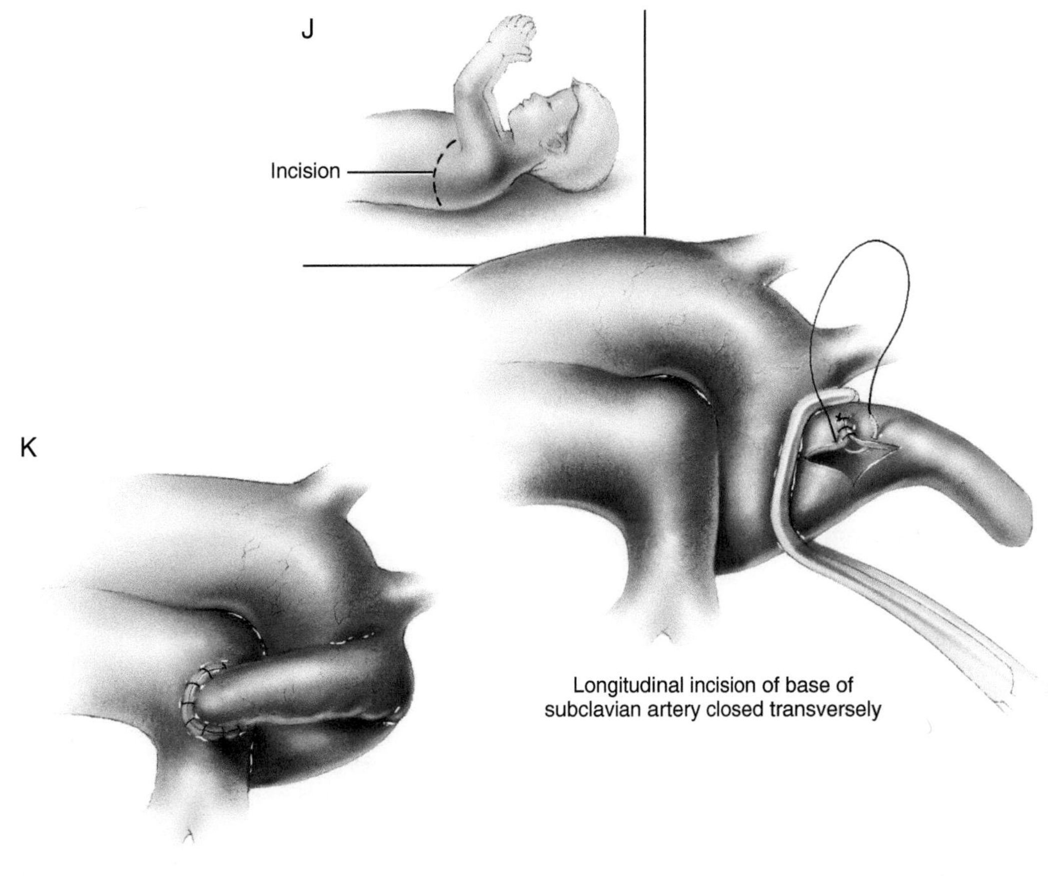
J
Incision
K
Longitudinal incision of base of subclavian artery closed transversely
Completed anastomosis

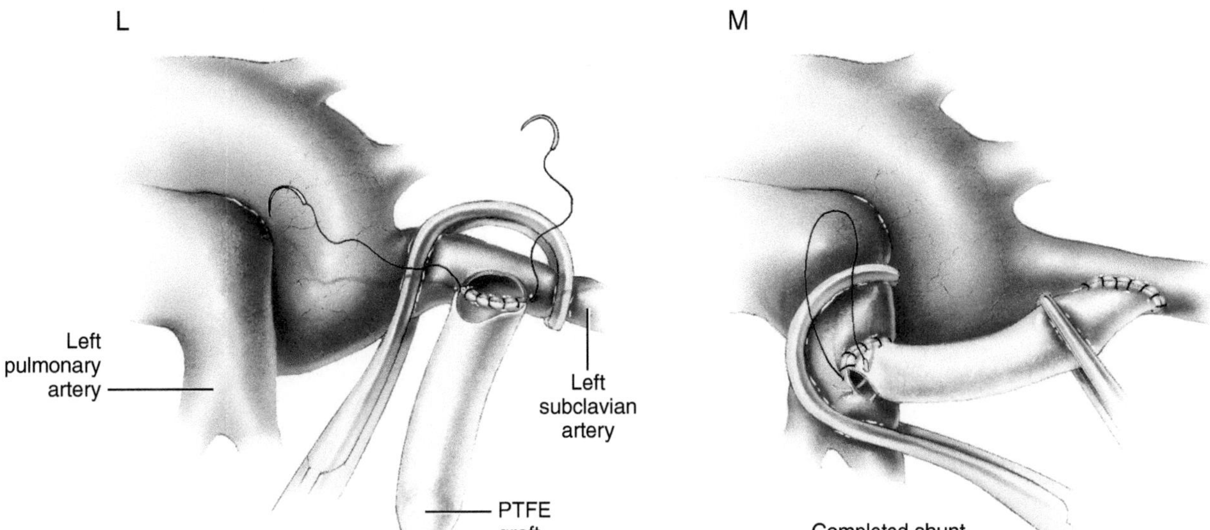
L
M
Left pulmonary artery
Left subclavian artery
PTFE graft
Completed shunt

Ascending Aorta–Right Pulmonary Artery Anastomosis

Direct anastomosis of the ascending aorta to the right pulmonary artery was once a frequently used shunt technique. However, because stenosis of the right pulmonary artery often occurred postoperatively, this shunt is seldom performed today.

Figure 30-2

Waterston-Cooley Shunt

A A posterolateral thoracotomy incision is made on the right side. The azygos vein is mobilized and divided. The pericardium is entered over the right pulmonary artery. The right pulmonary artery is completely mobilized, and tourniquet ligatures are placed around the apical anterior segmental branch and the pars intermedius portion of the pulmonary artery. The pericardium is mobilized off the ascending aorta. A partial-occlusion vascular clamp is placed on the right pulmonary artery and the ascending aorta, including both vessels between the jaws of the clamp. As the clamp is applied, the aorta is rotated anterior and to the left to bring the posterior wall of the aorta into the occlusion clamp in approximation to the anterior wall of the right pulmonary artery. Tourniquet ligatures on the branches of the pulmonary artery are secured. Parallel incisions are made in the aorta and the right pulmonary artery. The length of the incisions is accurately calibrated using cornea calipers to measure 3.0 to 4.0 mm, depending on the age and weight of the child.

B A side-to-side anastomosis of the aorta to the right pulmonary artery is constructed with a running stitch of 7/0 polypropylene. The initial stitches are placed at the superior apex of each of the aortic and pulmonary incisions, working from the intimal surface out. The needle from the aortic end is then brought from the adventitial surface into the lumen of the pulmonary artery. A retraction stitch placed anteriorly on the aorta exposes the anastomosis site.

C Sutures are placed across the back row of the anastomosis, working from the intimal surface of the aorta. Care must be taken to include only the anterior wall of the pulmonary artery.

D The anastomosis is completed anteriorly.

A

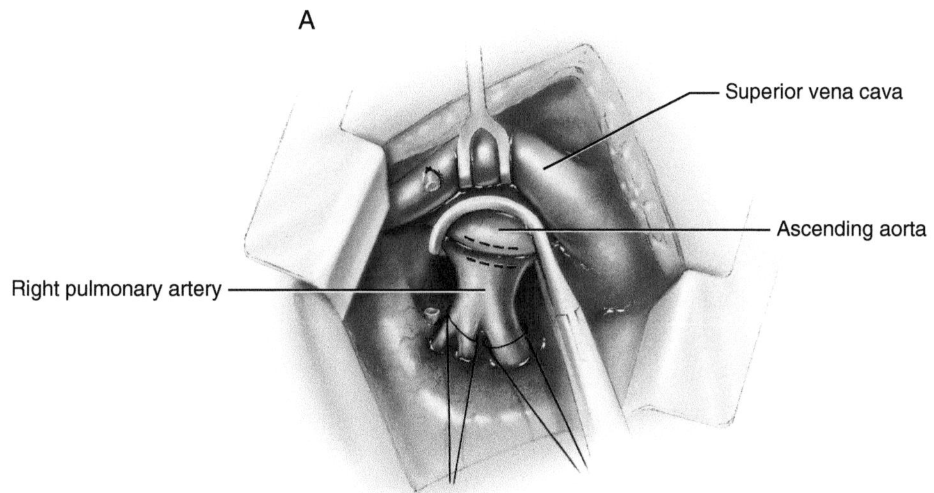

B

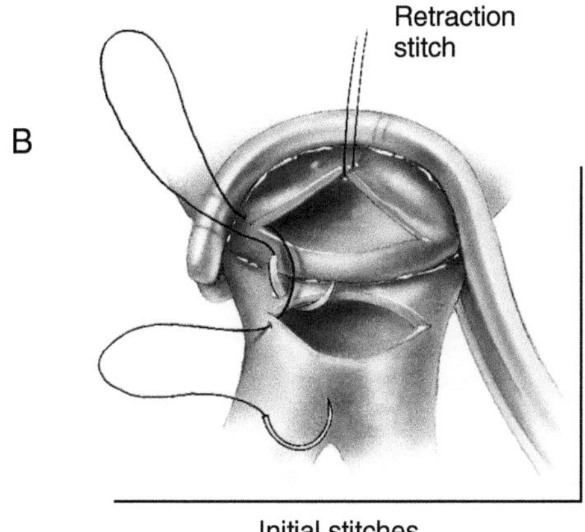

Initial stitches

C

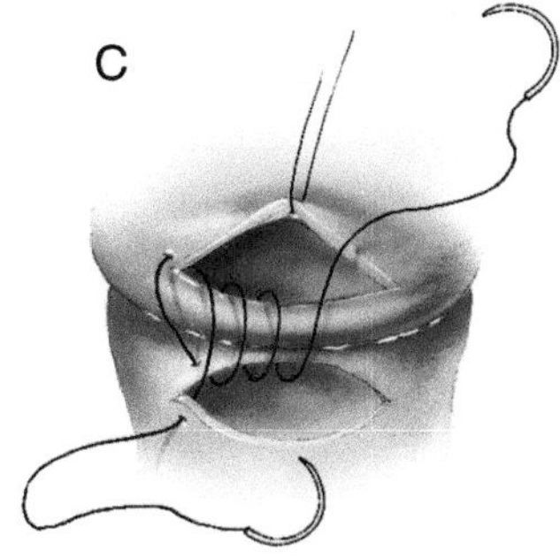

Anastomosis of back wall

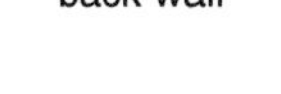

D

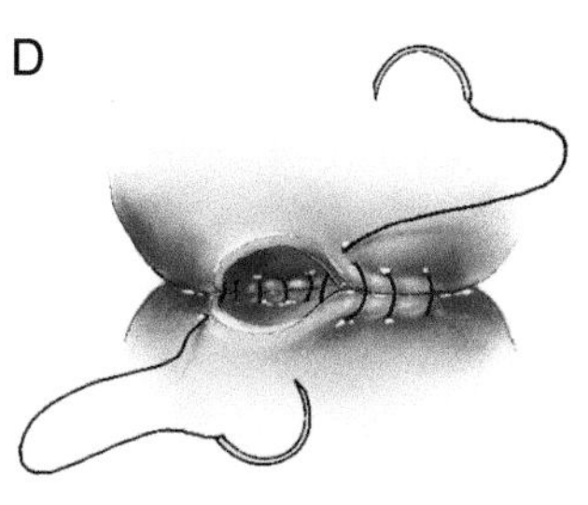

Completed shunt

Superior Vena Cava–Right Pulmonary Artery Anastomosis

Anastomosis of the superior vena cava to the right pulmonary artery (Glenn shunt) has application in certain patients with tricuspid atresia and other univentricular heart anomalies. The procedure has certain advantages, in that the pulmonary venous return to the ventricle is not increased, and the total volume load presented to the single ventricle is less than that resulting from systemic artery-to-pulmonary artery shunts.

Figure 30-3

Glenn Shunt

A The superior vena cava is mobilized; the azygos vein is ligated and divided; and the right pulmonary artery is mobilized, and its branches are controlled with tourniquet ligatures. The pulmonary artery is ligated as centrally as possible and then divided.

B A portion of the superior vena cava just above the right atrial junction is isolated by partial occlusion with a vascular clamp. A longitudinal incision approximately the same length as the diameter of the pulmonary artery is made in the superior vena cava, exactly opposite the pulmonary artery. An end (pulmonary artery)-to-side (vena cava) anastomosis is constructed by continuous stitches using 6/0 or 7/0 polypropylene. The initial stitch of a double-needle suture is placed from the intimal surface out on the pulmonary artery. The opposite needle is passed from inside and out at the superior apex of the superior vena cava incision.

C This needle is through the pulmonary artery from the adventitial surface to the inside, so that the back-row stitches of the anastomosis can be constructed from the intimal surfaces.

D The front wall of the anastomosis is completed by continuous suture.

E The vascular clamp and tourniquet ligatures are removed to establish blood flow through the anastomosis. A purse-string stitch of 3/0 polypropylene is placed around the superior vena cava just inferior to the anastomosis and above the right atrial junction.

F Ligation of the superior vena cava diverts all the upper compartment venous return to the right pulmonary artery. In effect, an end-to-end connection is established by closure of the vena cava.

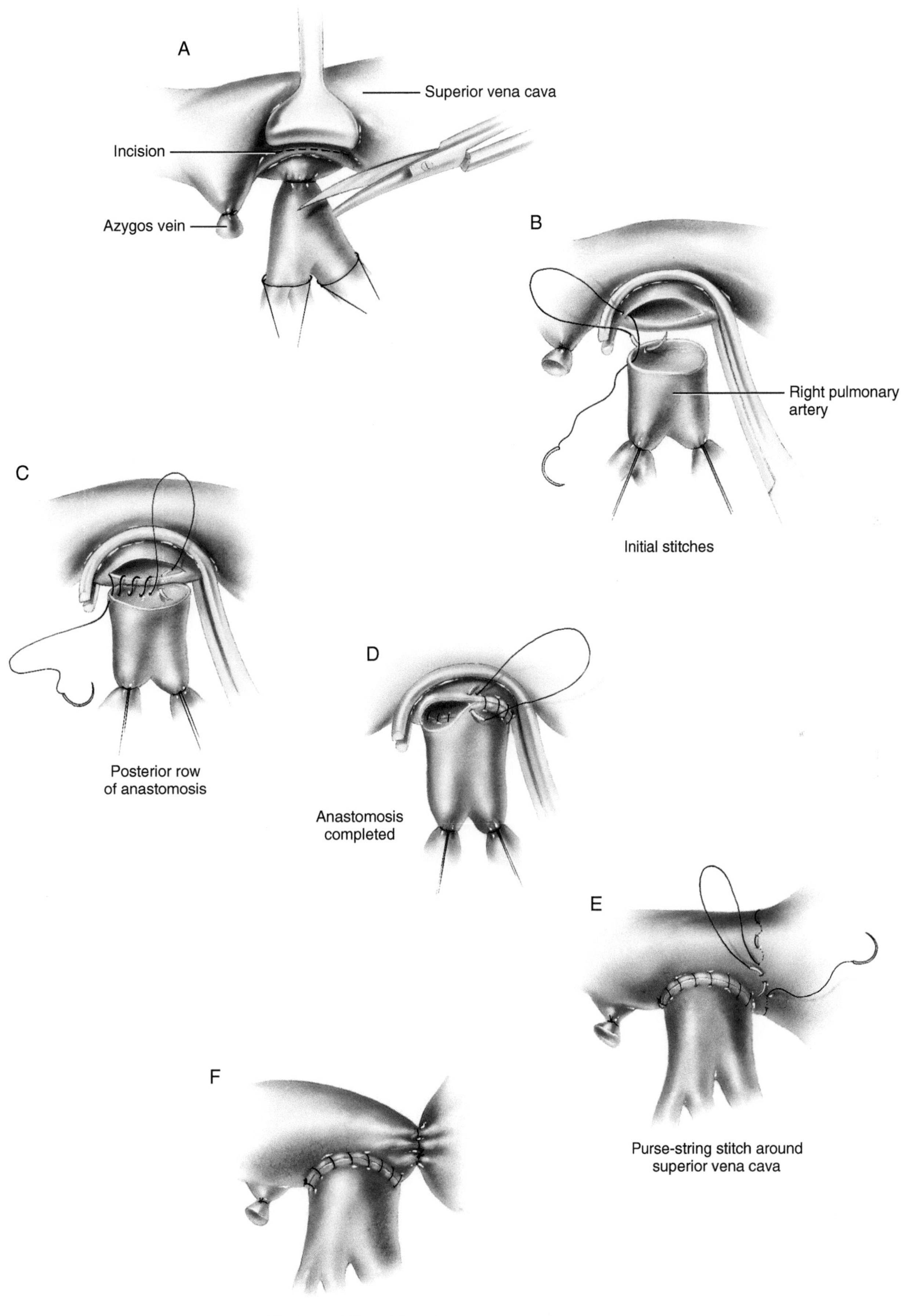
A
Superior vena cava
Incision
Azygos vein
B
Right pulmonary artery
Initial stitches
C
Posterior row of anastomosis
D
Anastomosis completed
E
Purse-string stitch around superior vena cava
F
Ligate superior vena cava

Figure 30-3 (continued)

Bidirectional Glenn Shunt

G If flow to both the right and left pulmonary arteries is desired, the superior vena cava–right pulmonary artery anastomosis is constructed differently. The superior vena cava is divided at the level of the right pulmonary artery.

H Incisions are made in the superior and inferior aspects of the right pulmonary artery. The upper end of the superior vena cava is anastomosed to the superior incision in the pulmonary artery using 6/0 polypropylene or polydioxanone suture. Similarly, the lower end of the superior vena cava is anastomosed to the inferior aspect of the right pulmonary artery. This anastomotic arrangement allows blood to flow from the cava to the right pulmonary artery and also across the pulmonary bifurcation to the left pulmonary artery.

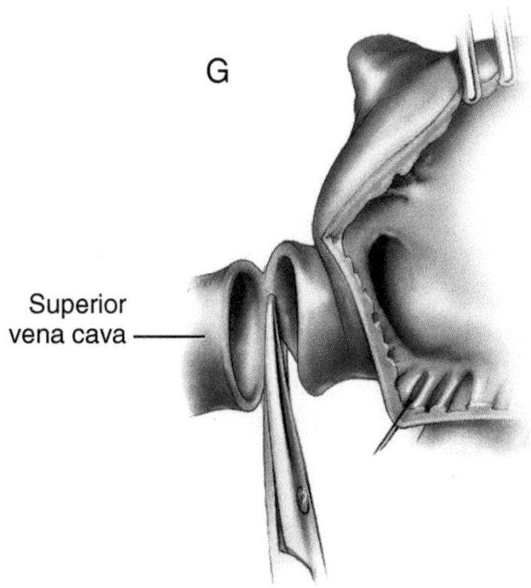
G
Superior vena cava

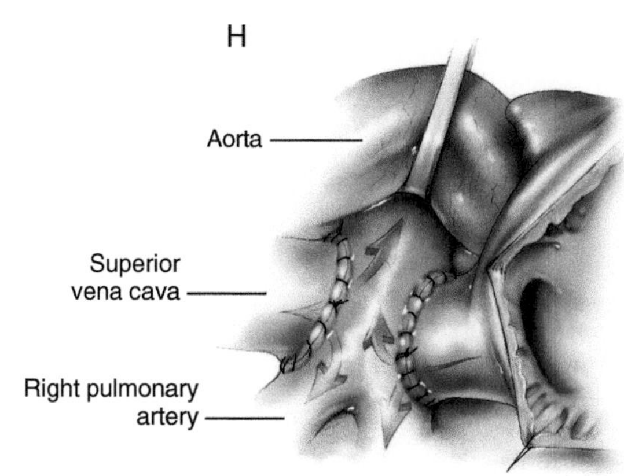
H
Aorta
Superior vena cava
Right pulmonary artery

Atrial Septectomy

Excision of the atrial septum allows the mixing of blood between the right and left atria. This procedure is useful in transposition anomalies.

Figure 30-4

Blalock-Hanlon Operation

A A posterolateral thoracotomy is made on the right side. The chest is entered through the bed of the nonresected fifth rib. The pericardium is incised posterior to the phrenic nerve. The right pulmonary artery and the right superior and inferior pulmonary veins are mobilized and controlled with tourniquet ligatures. An opening should be made between the right pulmonary artery and the right superior pulmonary vein to allow a clamp to pass posterior to both pulmonary veins into the created opening.

B Tourniquet ligatures are tightened around the right pulmonary artery and the pulmonary veins. In addition to controlling blood flow through these vessels, the ligatures retract the lung for maximal exposure. A partial-occlusion vascular clamp is placed on the right and left atria posterior to the right pulmonary veins, thereby excluding a portion of the interatrial groove. Parallel incisions are made in the right atrium just anterior to the interatrial groove and in the left atrium just posterior to the interatrial groove. The white, shiny endocardium of the atria should be clearly visualized while making these incisions.

C The atrial septum at the interatrial groove is grasped with forceps, and a septal incision is made at each end of the atriotomy. The length of the septal incision should be clearly limited; it should not be too close to the occlusion clamp or beyond the limit of the pulmonary veins.

D The partial-occlusion clamp is opened briefly to release the septum. Strong lateral traction with the forceps delivers the lateral portion of the atrial septum into the operative field. The partial-occlusion vascular clamp is closed again to secure hemostasis. The lateral portion of the atrial septum can then be excised through the foramen ovale. The vascular clamp is opened to release the cut edge of the atrial septum and reclosed for hemostasis.

E The anterior edge of the right atriotomy is then sutured to the posterior edge of the left atriotomy by a running stitch of 4/0 or 5/0 polypropylene. The suture line is taken from the inferior apex to the superior apex to complete the anastomosis.

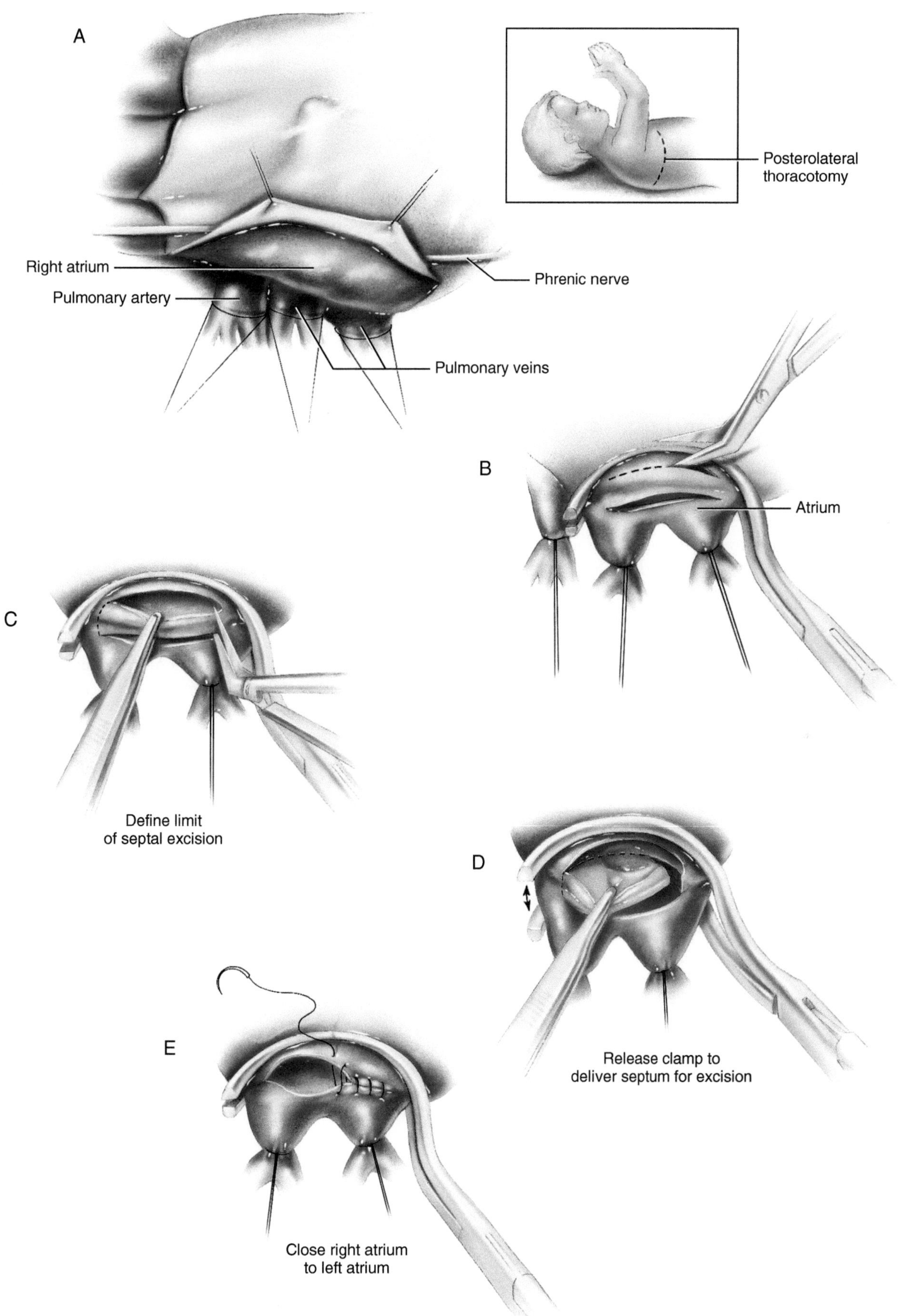
A
Posterolateral thoracotomy
Right atrium
Pulmonary artery
Phrenic nerve
Pulmonary veins
B
Atrium
C
Define limit of septal excision
D
Release clamp to deliver septum for excision
E
Close right atrium to left atrium

Banding of Pulmonary Artery

A stenosis of the pulmonary artery is created by placing a band around the artery to reduce pulmonary blood flow when such flow is excessive.

Figure 30-5

Muller-Dammann Operation

A An anterolateral thoracotomy incision is made on the left side. The chest is entered through the bed of the nonresected fourth rib. The pericardium is incised anterior to the phrenic nerve. Traction stitches are placed along the margins of the pericardium to expose the great vessels and to retract the lung. A small polyvinyl catheter is placed into the left atrium through the left superior pulmonary vein or the left atrial appendage to monitor left atrial pressure. A catheter is inserted into the distal pulmonary artery at the pericardial reflection through a purse-string stitch to monitor pulmonary artery pressure distal to the pulmonary band. A small catheter should have already been placed in a peripheral artery after induction of anesthesia to monitor intraarterial pressure.

B The fascial plane between the aorta (Ao) and the pulmonary artery (PA) is opened. Dissection is continued in this plane close to the aorta to completely encircle it. A right-angled clamp is placed around the aorta, and a piece of Teflon or Dacron tape is pulled around the aorta into the plane between the aorta and the pulmonary artery.

C The right-angled vascular clamp is then placed through the transverse sinus, and the end of the band to the right of the aorta is grasped and pulled back through the transverse sinus to bring the band around the pulmonary artery.

D As the systemic artery, pulmonary artery, and left atrial pressures are simultaneously monitored, the band is tightened around the main portion of the pulmonary artery to lower the pulmonary artery pressure distal to the band to approximately 50% of systemic arterial pressure. Left atrial pressure should be reduced by the maneuver as pulmonary blood flow is reduced, resulting in less filling pressure to the left atrium. A hemoclip in the open position is placed over the ends of the band and moved toward the pulmonary artery, thus tightening the band until the desired hemodynamic state is achieved. When the hemodynamic state is optimal, the hemoclip is closed to secure the band. The hemoclip technique has the advantages of ease and control of application, narrow width, and ease of removal should the band be too tight when initially applied. A second or third hemoclip can easily be applied to finely control the degree of narrowing of the pulmonary artery.

E After an appropriate period of monitoring the patient to ensure that the hemodynamic state continues to be optimal, the band is further secured by interrupted mattress stitches of 4/0 silk, leaving the hemoclip in place and placing the stitches in the band distal to the hemoclip.

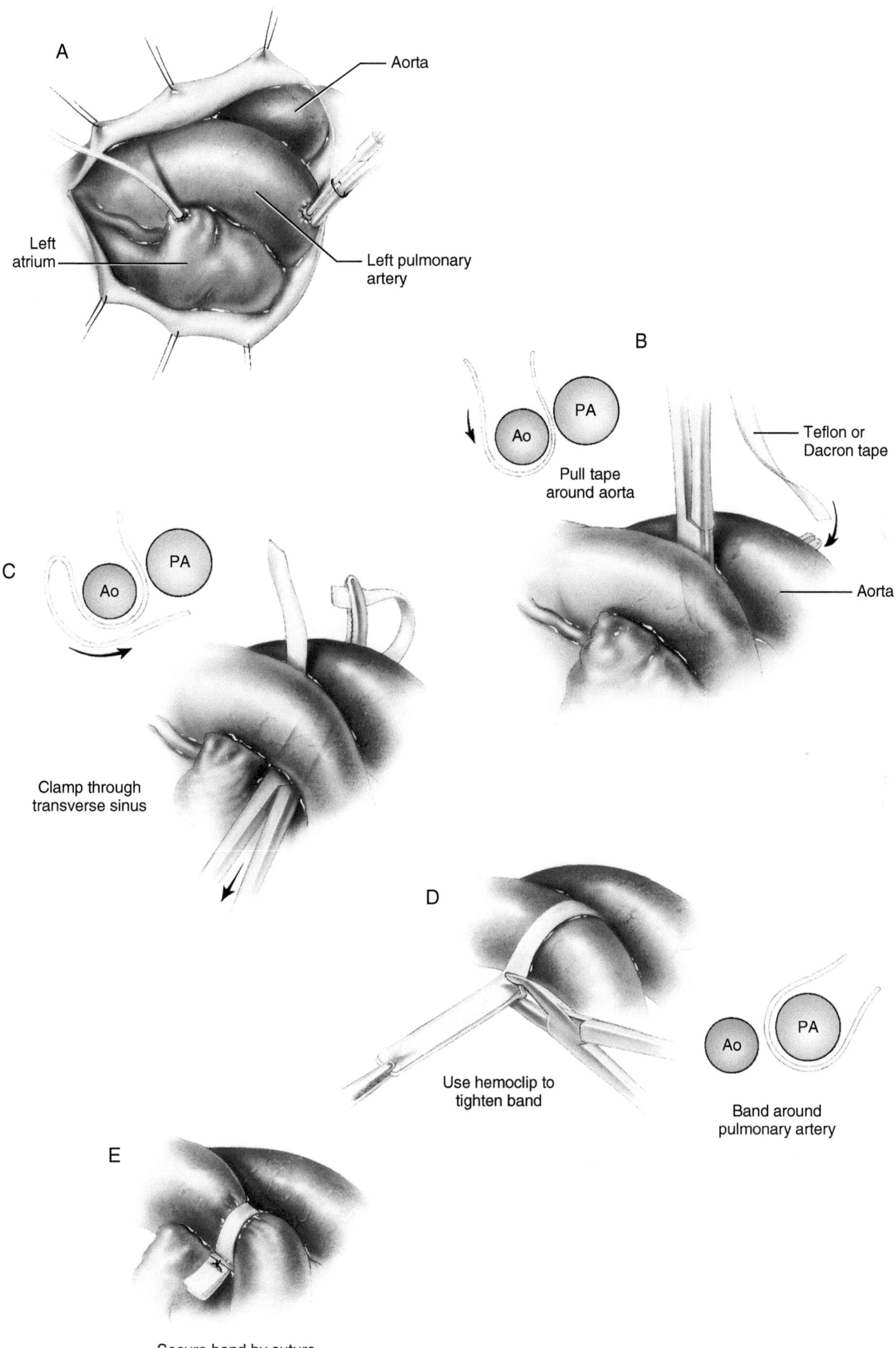
A
Aorta
Left atrium
Left pulmonary artery
B
PA
Ao
Pull tape around aorta
Teflon or Dacron tape
Aorta
C
PA
Ao
Clamp through transverse sinus
D
Use hemoclip to tighten band
Ao
PA
Band around pulmonary artery
E
Secure band by suture

Removal of Pulmonary Artery Band

The band must be removed from the pulmonary artery at the time of definitive repair of the cardiac anomaly.

Figure 30-6

A The fabric of the band is exposed for a short distance. The band is divided. Traction on the band usually causes it to separate from the pulmonary artery, allowing it to be removed.

B Banding of the pulmonary artery always leaves a permanent stenotic defect; repair of the pulmonary artery deformity is required. The repair technique depends on where the band was located. If the band was correctly placed in the midportion of the main pulmonary artery, the area of scarring can be excised.

C After the scarred portion is removed, the pulmonary artery is usually quite pliable. The artery proximal and distal to the area of the band has a good-sized diameter, which allows end-to-end anastomosis. The anastomosis is constructed with continuous stitches of 5/0 polypropylene or polydioxanone suture.

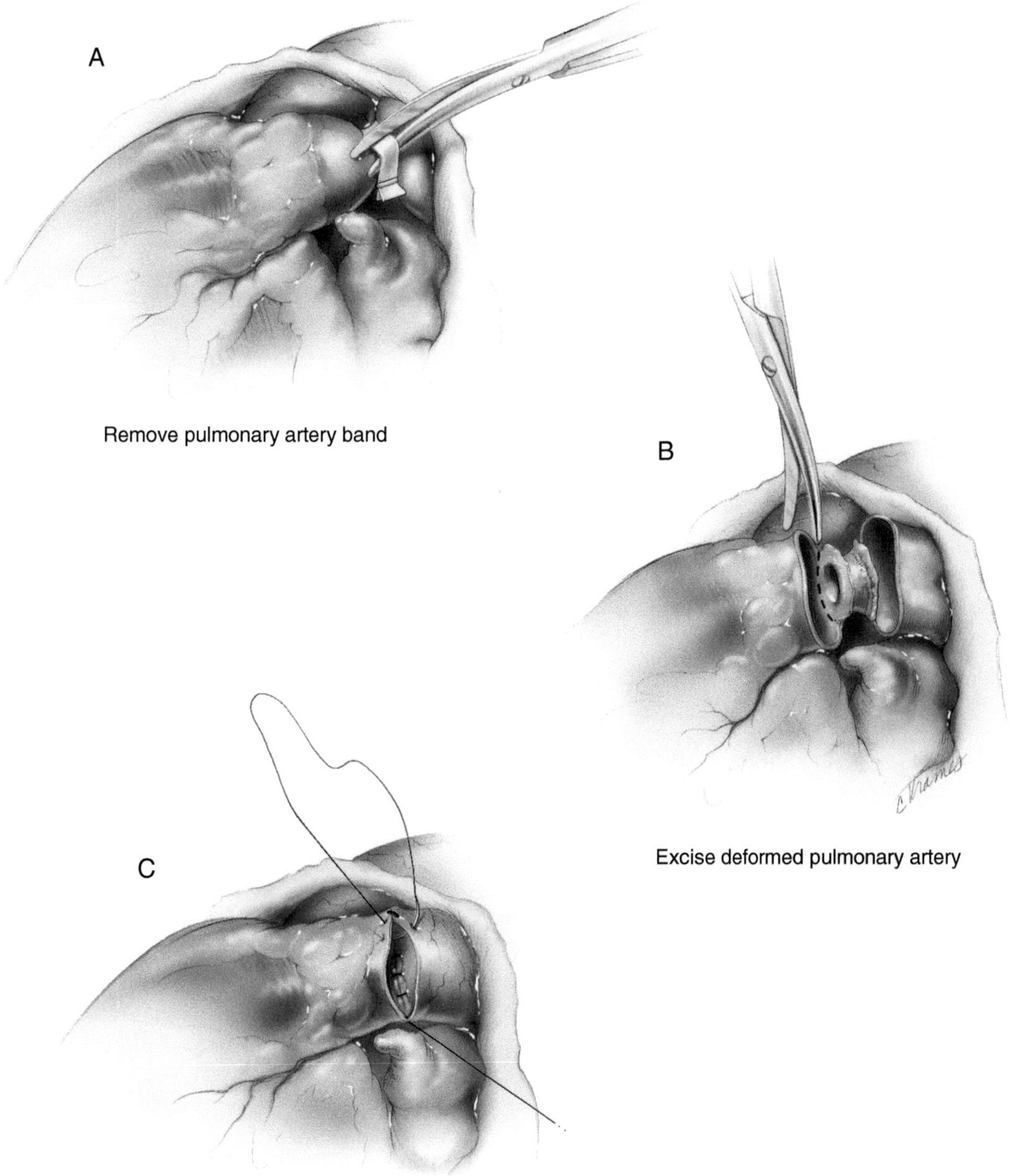

Remove pulmonary artery band

Excise deformed pulmonary artery

End-to-end anastomosis

Figure 30-6 (continued)

D The pulmonary artery band commonly slips distally, so the pulmonary artery bifurcation is deformed, narrowed, and scarred. It is not possible to simply remove the band and resect the scarred portion of the artery because the origins of the right and left pulmonary artery branches are involved. Reconstruction of the pulmonary artery bifurcation is required.

E In the main pulmonary artery a longitudinal incision is made that crosses the band and extends into the pulmonary artery branches beyond the area of scarring and stenosis. Usually both the right and left pulmonary arteries must be incised. The fabric of the band is removed.

F To remodel the bifurcation, a prosthetic (PTFE or Dacron) or pericardial patch that extends into both the right and left pulmonary arteries is fashioned. The patch is attached to the pulmonary artery with 5/0 polypropylene suture by continuous stitches.

G Occasionally the band slips proximally, narrowing the sinus rim of the pulmonary artery or even distorting the sinus of Valsalva of the pulmonary valve. The pulmonary valve becomes secondarily involved by the supravalvular stenosis. The commissures of the valve are drawn too close to each other at the sinus rim, producing buckling of the free edge of the valve cusps. In this situation the pulmonary valve must be reconstructed, in addition to widening the pulmonary artery.

H An incision is made in the main pulmonary artery and extended proximally to cross the band. There is usually a commissure of the pulmonary valve located anteriorly. The incision is extended across the sinus rim into the sinus of Valsalva on each side of the anterior commissure. This incision relieves the supravalvular stenosis and allows anterior displacement of the anterior commissure, which lengthens the two adjacent cusps of the pulmonary valve. This should restore the valve configuration. Some tissue may have to be resected posteriorly to improve posterior cusp length.

I A prosthetic or pericardial patch is tailored to an appropriate configuration to rebuild the sinuses and suspend the anterior commissure. The patch is fashioned much like that used for supravalvular aortic stenosis. The patch is sutured to the pulmonary artery with continuous stitches of 5/0 polypropylene.

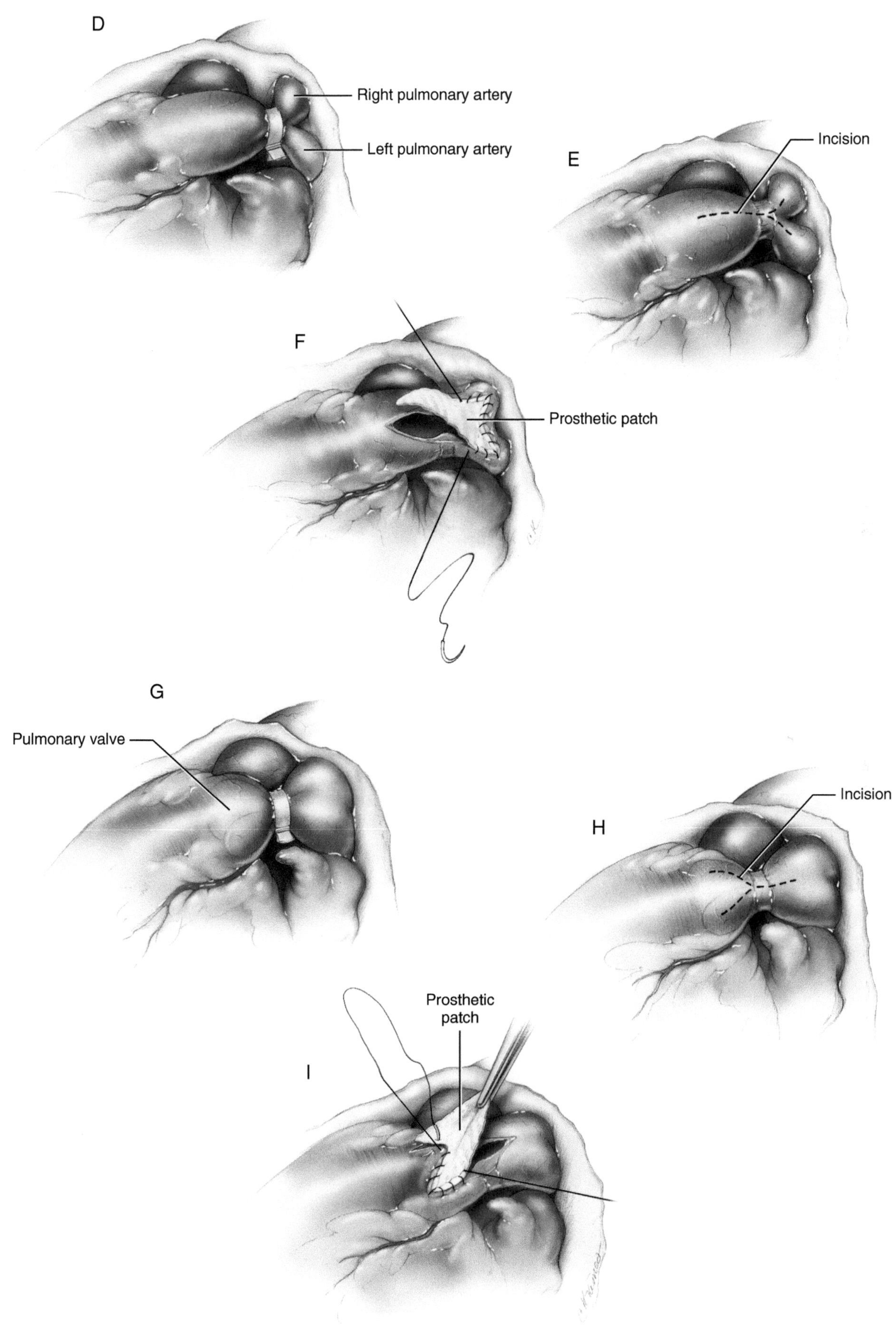
D
Right pulmonary artery
Left pulmonary artery
E
Incision
F
Prosthetic patch
G
Pulmonary valve
H
Incision
I
Prosthetic patch

part IX

Valve Lesions (Acquired)

chapter 31 AORTIC VALVE REPLACEMENT

Aortic valve replacement is usually required when operative intervention is performed for aortic valve stenosis or incompetence in older patients. Several replacement devices are available, but all operations share a common approach and principles.

Morphology

Figure 31-1

A Operative image of aortic valve stenosis, degenerative type. Normal three-leaflet architecture is maintained. Commissures are not fused. Leaflets are held in a closed position due to diffuse, nodular calcific deposits. Calcification, often described as "eggshell," may involve the sinuses of Valsalva. This morphology is presumed to be atheromatous.

B Operative image of aortic valve stenosis, degenerative type. There are three leaflets and no commissural fusion. The degeneration is advanced, with marked nodular calcification. As aortic valve degeneration progresses, the aortic valve area decreases at a rate of 0.12 cm^2/year.

C Operative image of aortic valve stenosis, congenital type. The valve is bicuspid, with fusion of the commissure between the left and right coronary leaflets. There is heavy dystrophic calcification of the leaflets. The valve orifice is eccentric and slit-like.

D Operative image of aortic valve stenosis, congenital type. There is only one open commissure, that between the left and noncoronary leaflets. The other two commissures are completely fused. This may be called a unicuspid valve. Calcification is not as severe as in Part *C*.

E Operative image of the ascending aorta in aortic valve stenosis. The aorta is frequently abnormal in patients with bicuspid aortic valve. This image shows dilation of the ascending aorta.

F Aortic valve stenosis and regurgitation, rheumatic type, in an excised valve specimen. Normal three-leaflet structure is retained. There is scarring and shortening of the leaflets with rolling of the free edges, resulting in central regurgitation due to a lack of leaflet coaptation. The thickened leaflets also obstruct left ventricular outflow (aortic valve stenosis).

G Operative image of aortic valve regurgitation. The noncoronary leaflet of the aortic valve is redundant and prolapsed. Many cases of aortic valve regurgitation are caused by an abnormality of the aorta, primarily dilation, producing secondary changes in otherwise near-normal aortic valve leaflets. These cases are often amenable to repair by correcting the aortic morphology.

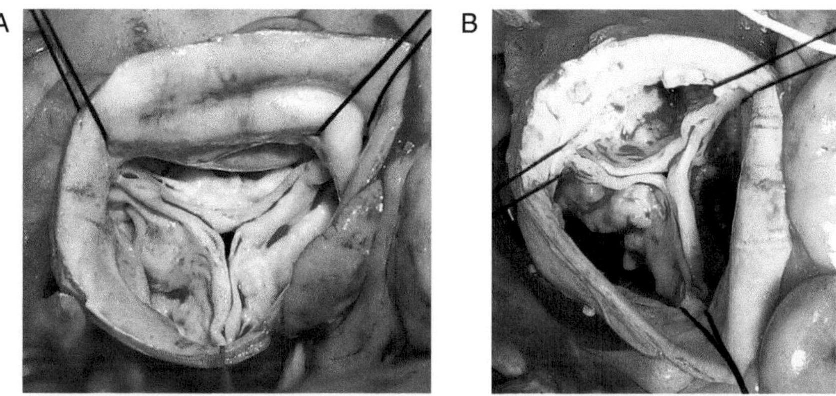

Aortic valve stenosis, degenerative type

C

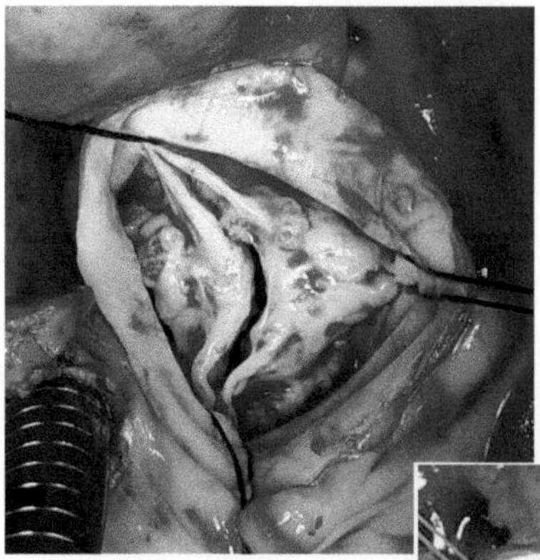

Aortic valve stenosis, congenital type

D

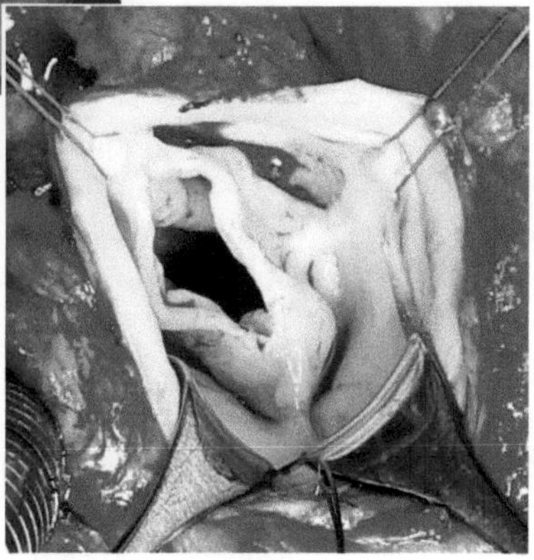

E

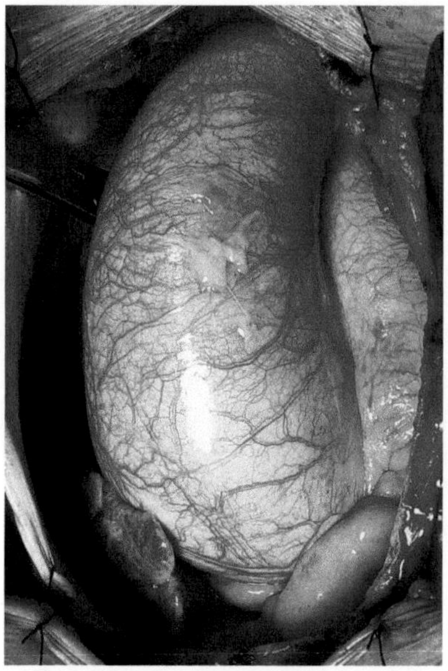

Ascending aorta in aortic valve stenosis

F

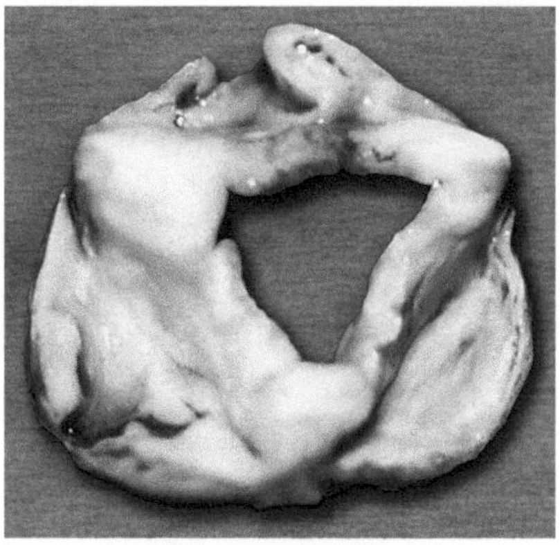

Aortic valve stenosis and regurgitation, rheumatic type

G

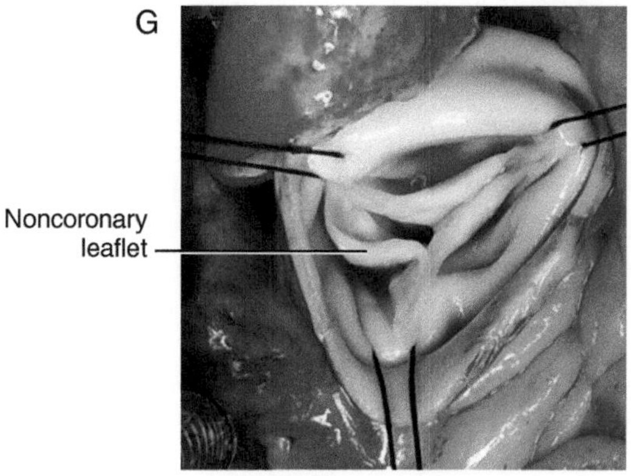

Noncoronary leaflet

Aortic valve regurgitation

Valve Excision and Débridement
Figure 31-2

A The operation is performed with the patient on cardiopulmonary bypass using a single venous cannula (two stages), with oxygenated blood returned to the ascending aorta. A vent catheter is inserted by way of the right superior pulmonary vein to the left atrium and left ventricle. The aorta is occluded, and hypothermic cardioplegic solution is administered to ensure total electromechanical arrest and to protect the myocardium from ischemic injury. Retrograde perfusion of the myocardium via a catheter in the coronary sinus is the preferred method because of its effectiveness, even with aortic valve incompetence, its simplicity, and the absence of cannulae in the aortic root. The coronary arteries can also be perfused in an antegrade fashion through a cannula in the wall of the aorta to perfuse the aortic root or, if there is aortic valve regurgitation, directly in the coronary ostia using coronary perfusion cannulae. A transverse incision is made in the ascending aorta and extended into the noncoronary sinus of Valsalva. This is the classic incision for operations on the aortic valve. An alternative incision (inset) makes implantation of aortic valve bioprostheses or aortic homografts easier and more anatomic in the aortic root. The aorta is completely divided above the sinotubular junction, leaving the noncoronary sinus intact. Exposure of the intact aortic root is enhanced by traction sutures placed at the apex of each aortic valve commissure or the remnant thereof. Traction sutures rotate the aortic root inferiorly, achieving the excellent views demonstrated in Figure 31-1, *A–D* and *G*. This approach requires anastomosis of the aorta following aortic valve replacement, but this suture line is actually more secure than incisions deep into the noncoronary sinus, which may lead to troublesome bleeding from the apex of the incision as pressure is restored to the aorta.

B Excision of the aortic valve is begun at the commissure between the right and noncoronary sinuses, where there is little danger of extending the incision outside the heart. The commissure is excised from the aortic wall, and the right coronary cusp is excised at the annulus. Careful and deliberate excision of the valve cusp, with attention to removing as much of the annular calcification as possible, hastens the procedure. Curved Mayo scissors are ideal for excision of the valve; their relatively blunt tips and strong blades allow the calcium deposits to be squeezed away from the annulus and aortic sinuses, with little risk of aortic perforation.

C The commissure between the left and right coronary cusps is removed from the aortic wall, and the left coronary cusp is excised.

D The noncoronary cusp is excised toward the commissure between the left and noncoronary cusps, completing the excision posteriorly. Extreme caution must be used during excision of the aortic valve in the area of the commissure between the left and noncoronary cusps and in the left cusp because the risk of extending the incision outside the heart is greatest in this area.

E Any remaining nidus of calcium is removed from the aortic annulus. A vascular forceps is used to grasp and remove the pieces of calcium with a twisting motion. This technique preserves all the connective tissue of the aortic annulus, preventing overexcision and perforation of the aorta. The forceps technique is gentler and more controlled, making it preferable to other techniques. Rongeurs or other instruments that cut the tissues must be used with caution. During this portion of the procedure a small bit of gauze should be placed in the left ventricular outflow tract below the aortic valve annulus to catch any bits of calcium that fall away as the débridement proceeds. With patience and attention to detail, essentially all the calcium deposits can be removed from the aortic annulus to allow better seating and healing of the valve prosthesis.

F Traction stitches are placed at the sinotubular junction (sinus rim) above each of the commissures. These stitches are pulled up tightly to provide maximal exposure of the aortic annulus. The annulus is calibrated, and an appropriately sized prosthesis is selected for replacement of the aortic valve. There is no advantage in choosing an oversized prosthesis, which risks mechanical malfunction. If the aortic annulus is too small to accommodate a prosthesis that will provide adequate hemodynamic performance, the annulus should be enlarged.

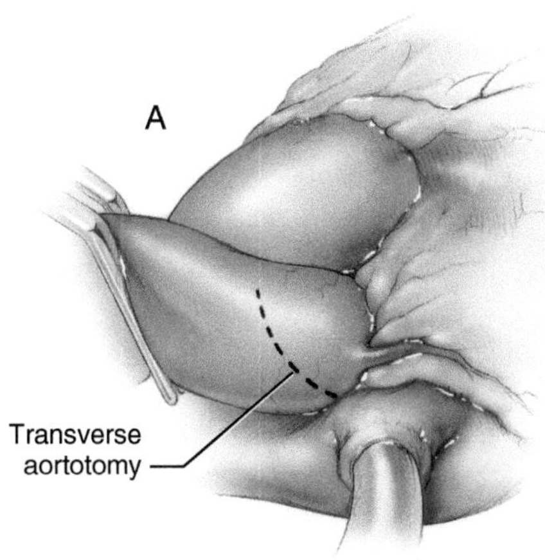

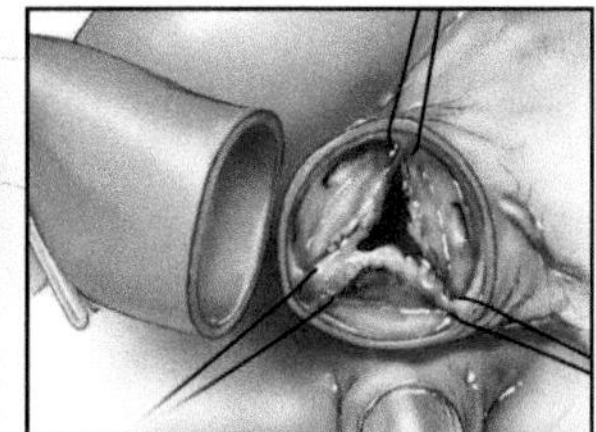

Alternative incision

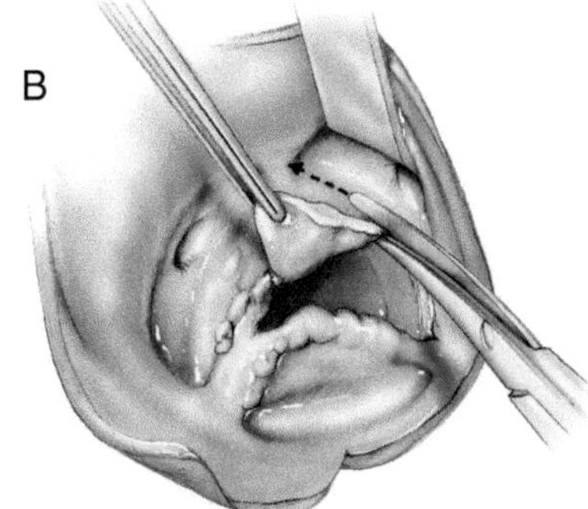

Excise valve, right sinus

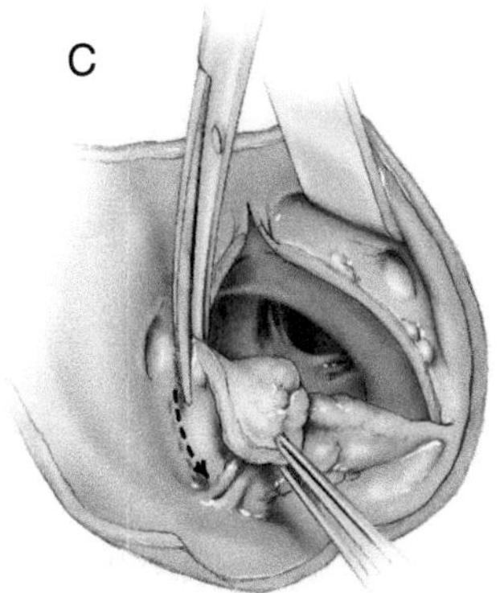

Excise valve, left sinus

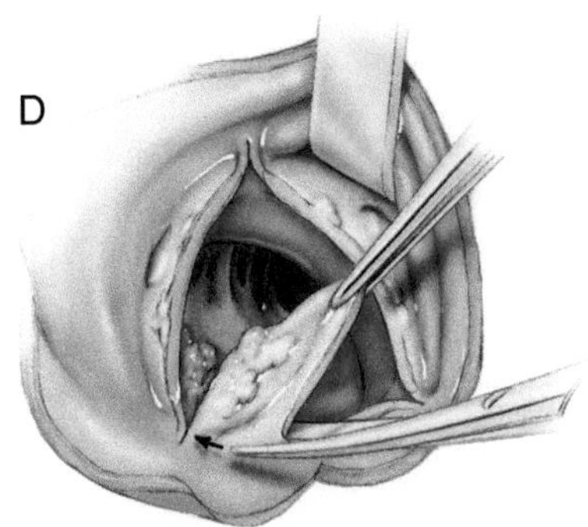

Complete excision,
noncoronary sinus

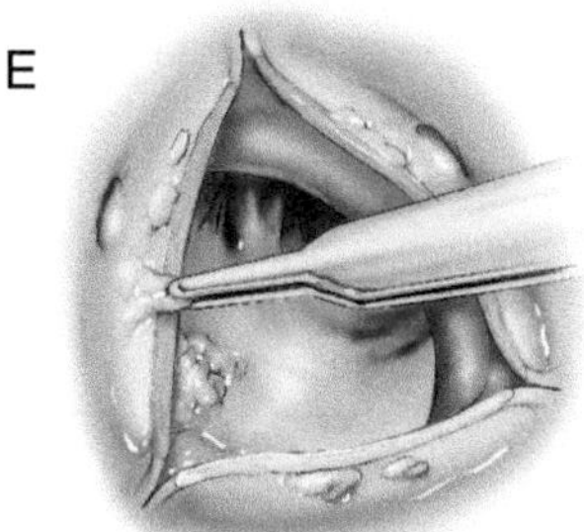

Débridement
of calcium

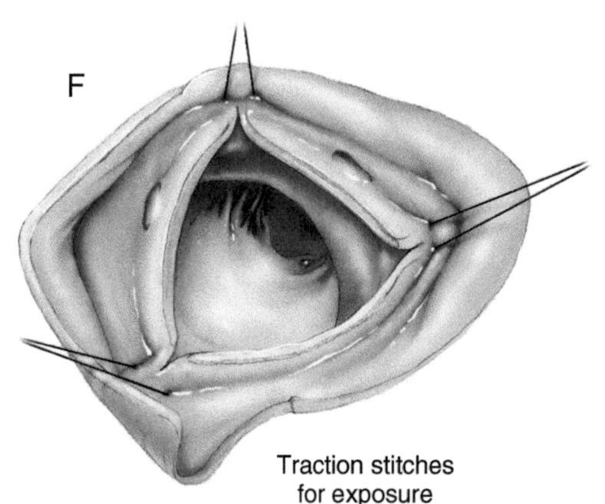

Traction stitches
for exposure

Continuous Suture Technique

Continuous suture technique for aortic valve replacement has some distinct advantages over the more standard pledget-reinforced mattress suture technique. A larger prosthesis can be accommodated in the aortic outflow tract with the continuous suture technique because the tissues are not compressed, as they are with the mattress suture technique. The tension on each suture can also be adjusted and made uniform with the continuous suture technique. In addition, there are fewer knots, which can act as potential nidi for clot formation.

Figure 31-3

A Retraction stitches are placed just above the commissures. The aortic annulus is divided into three segments by the commissures. During the valve replacement procedure the annulus is subdivided at the midpoint on the annulus between the commissures to create six subsegments. A double-needle 2/0 polypropylene suture with a compressed Teflon pledget in the center of the suture is used. An initial mattress stitch is placed at the center of the sinus of Valsalva, through the aortic annulus, and brought through the sewing ring of the prosthesis. The prosthetic valve is held away from the annulus and positioned and retracted for added exposure. Exactly three stitches are placed between the initial pledget-reinforced stitch and the commissure on each side of the sinus. The final stitch at each end is secured to the wound drapes by a hemostat. A loop of 0 silk suture is placed around the polypropylene suture as the first suture loop is completed through the prosthesis in each subsegment. This silk loop is held by a hemostat and is later used to adjust tension on the suture line.

B Sutures in the right coronary annulus are placed from the center toward the commissures in the first and second subsegments. The initial stitch in the left coronary sinus passes through the sewing ring of the prosthesis, opposite the last stitch of the second subsegment. Working from the center to the commissures in the left coronary sinus, the surgeon attaches the third and fourth subsegments to the prosthesis. Last, sutures are placed in the fifth and sixth subsegments in the noncoronary sinus.

C Traction is placed on the six 0 silk loop sutures to pull the prosthesis into the annulus of the aortic valve. The pledget must be tightly approximated because this is the lowest point in the annulus and has the most tension when drawn up to the prosthesis. This is accomplished by pulling up on the loop sutures adjacent to the pledget to seat it firmly. Care must be taken not to draw the pledget beneath the prosthesis.

D The silk traction suture loops are removed sequentially, and the ends of the polypropylene suture are pulled up tightly to approximate the sewing ring of the prosthesis precisely to the annulus of the aortic valve. The occluder of the prosthesis is opened, and the surgeon checks to ensure that there are no loose suture loops beneath the aortic prosthesis in the outflow tract of the left ventricle. This traction suture loop technique, which was devised by Dr. Russell M. Nelson, makes it easy to pull the prosthesis into the annulus of the aortic valve and tighten the continuous sutures.

E A final check is performed to verify approximation of the sewing ring of the aortic prosthesis to the annulus of the aortic valve. Special attention is paid to accurate placement of the pledget, which should be above the annulus at the point of maximal stress, deep in the center of the sinus of Valsalva. The suture ends are then joined by a knot at the three commissures.

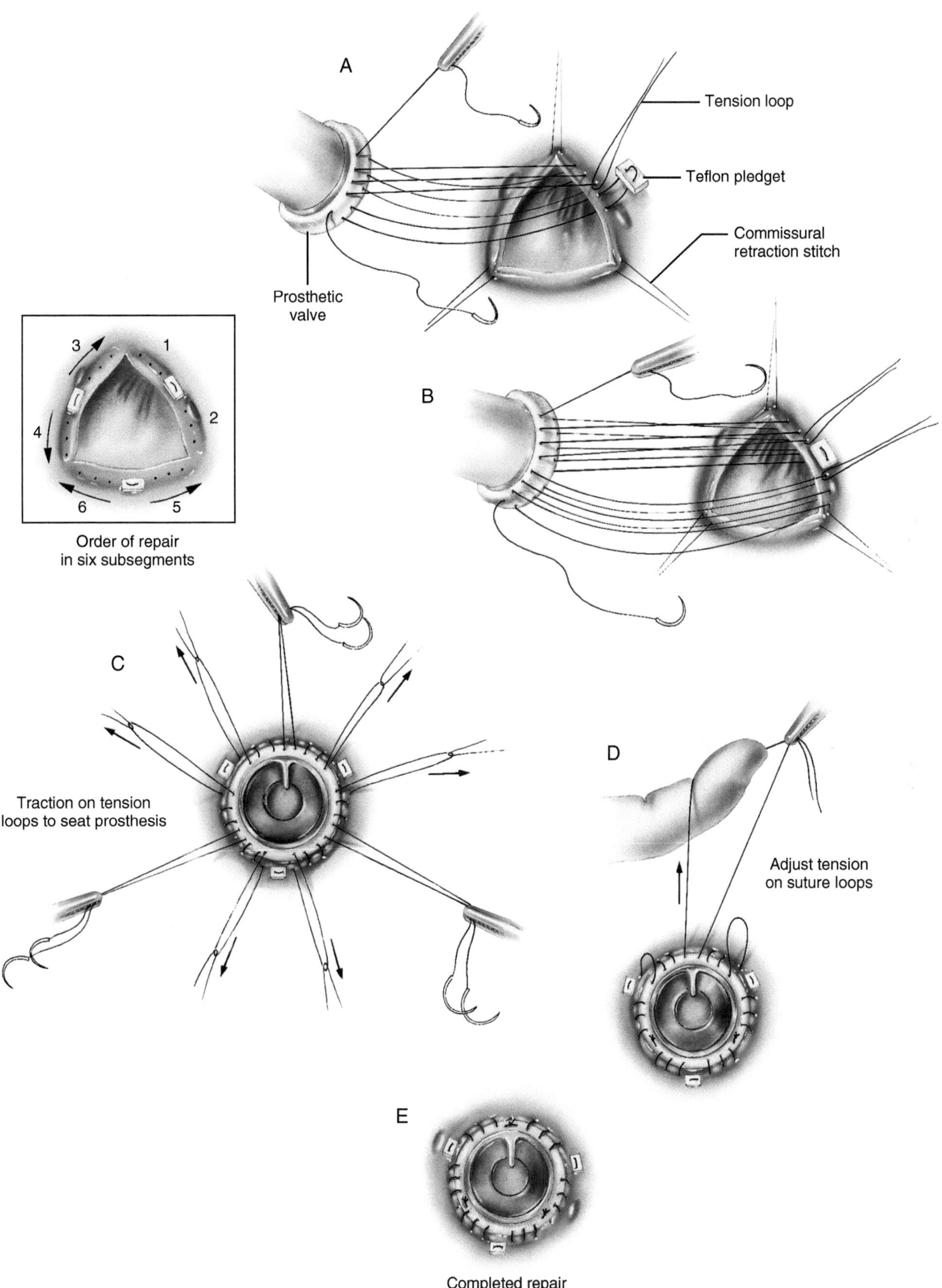
A
Tension loop
Teflon pledget
Commissural retraction stitch
Prosthetic valve
3
1
2
4
6
5
Order of repair in six subsegments
B
C
Traction on tension loops to seat prosthesis
D
Adjust tension on suture loops
E
Completed repair

Interrupted Suture Technique

Interrupted suture technique is standard for replacement of the aortic valve. This method offers maximal strength of prosthetic attachment and has the lowest incidence of perivalvular leak.

Figure 31-4

A A double-needle suture of synthetic material with a centrally placed, compressed Teflon pledget is used for the repair. Using sutures of two different colors (green or blue and white) simplifies intraoperative identification of the suture pairs. In this way, the sutures from each annulus repair beneath each sinus of Valsalva can be held together as a group. Mattress stitches are taken through the annulus of the aortic valve, beginning at the commissure between the left and right coronary cusps. Stitches are placed in the right coronary annulus in a clockwise fashion, working toward the commissure between the right and noncoronary sinuses. Separate stitches are placed close to one another, and the space along the aortic annulus is taken beneath the pledget of the mattress stitch. The prosthesis is held away from the aortic annulus until all stitches have been placed.

B The annulus of the left coronary sinus of Valsalva is then approximated to the sewing ring of the aortic valve prosthesis. The sutures are placed in a counterclockwise fashion, beginning at the commissure between the left and right coronary cusps.

C The annulus of the noncoronary sinus of Valsalva is approximated to the valve prosthesis, working in a clockwise fashion from the commissure between the right and noncoronary cusps toward the commissure between the left and noncoronary cusps. The needles are passed through the annulus in a backhand fashion. The three groups of sutures are then strongly retracted so that the prosthesis can be slid over the suture loops into the aortic annulus. The position of the occluder mechanism can be adjusted before the valve holder is removed.

D The sutures are sorted and tied down in a specific order. First the sutures in the noncoronary sinus are tied down in a counterclockwise fashion. The first suture in the left coronary sinus closest to the commissure between the left and right coronary cusps is tied directly across the annulus from those sutures already tied in the noncoronary sinus, to ensure that the prosthesis is securely seated. The sutures of the left coronary sinus are then tied down in a counterclockwise fashion. To complete the repair, the sutures are tied in the right sinus in a clockwise fashion. If a portion of the valve prostheses projects below the sewing ring and is thus positioned partially below the annulus in the left ventricular outflow tract, the order of suture tying is altered so that those portions of the prosthesis below the annulus are secured first.

E An alternative technique for placement of the pledget-reinforced stitches is used in cases of a small aortic annulus. The pledgets are placed below the annulus in the left ventricular outflow tract by placing a mattress stitch with a center pledget via a double-needle suture; the suture is passed from below the annulus and up through the prosthesis. A larger prosthesis is thereby secured above the annulus as the annulus is compressed between the sutures and the device.

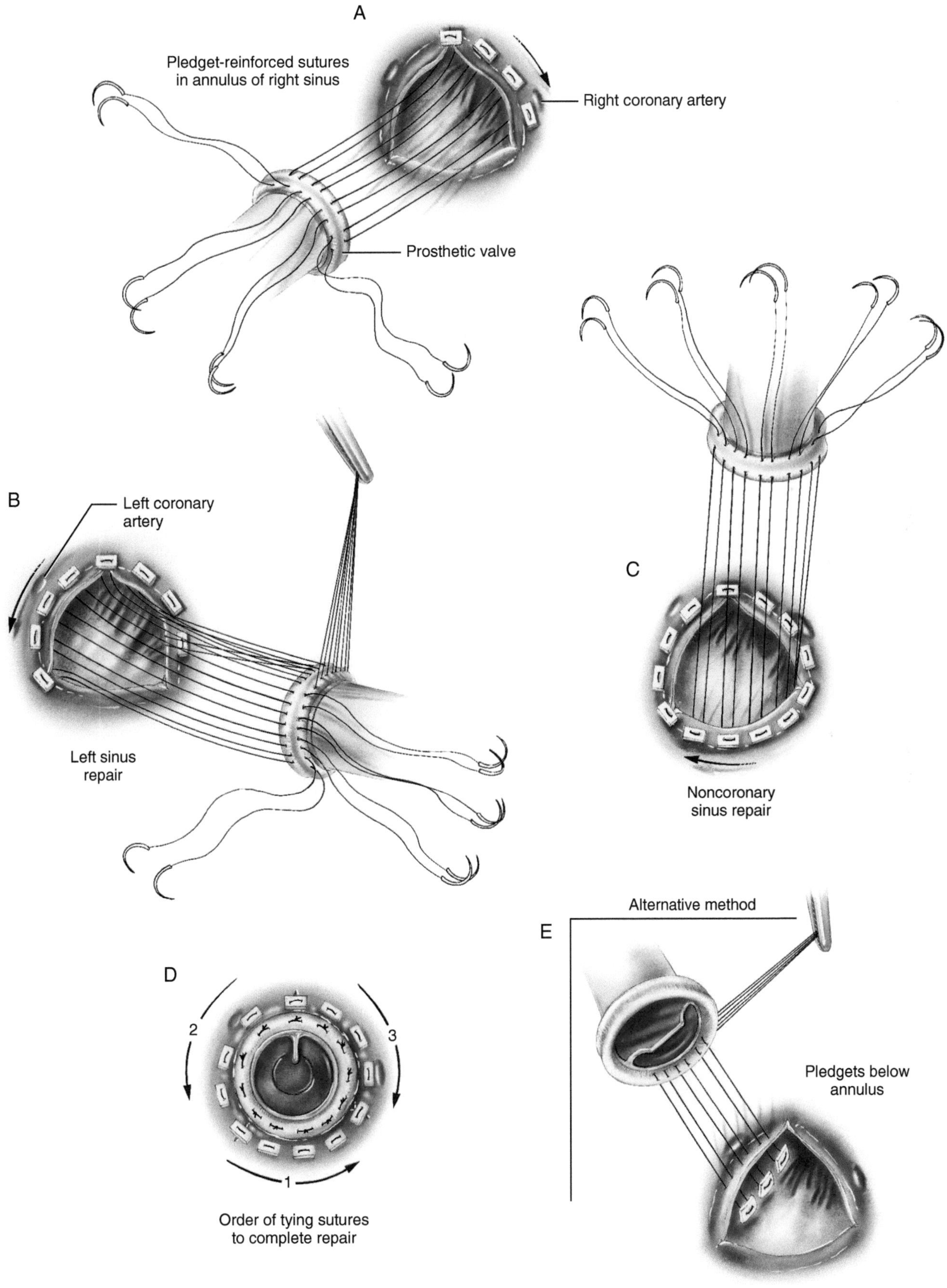
A
Pledget-reinforced sutures in annulus of right sinus
Right coronary artery
Prosthetic valve
B
Left coronary artery
Left sinus repair
C
Noncoronary sinus repair
D
2
3
1
Order of tying sutures to complete repair
E
Alternative method
Pledgets below annulus

Aortic Allograft: Kirklin/ Barrett-Boyes 120-Degree Rotation Technique

Transplantation of human aortic valves has become possible because of cryopreservation techniques and tissue banking, resulting in the availability of valves of various sizes for aortic surgery. Experience has shown that aortic allograft valves are durable, and their hemodynamic performance is superior to that of any other replacement device currently available. The virtual absence of embolism without the need for anticoagulation makes aortic allografts very attractive, especially in young patients and in those in whom anticoagulants are contraindicated. A clear understanding of the anatomy and geometry of the aortic root is essential because the aortic allograft depends on the host aortic tissues for support. Major deformity of the aortic sinuses should be appreciated and corrected, or the procedure should be abandoned in favor of a conventional valve replacement. The 120-degree rotation technique assumes that there are three symmetrically placed commissures in the host aorta that will support the aortic allograft valve. If there is abnormal commissure formation, asymmetric commissure placement, or sinus abnormality, it is preferable to use another method of allograft implantation that uses more graft aortic wall in the repair to compensate for deficiencies in the host.

Figure 31-5

A A transverse aortotomy is made, with the incision extended into the noncoronary sinus of Valsalva midway between the commissures. Alternatively, the aorta can be divided above the sinotubular junction.

B The aortic valve is carefully inspected to determine which reconstructive procedures are possible. When a decision is made to replace the aortic valve, it is excised by the usual techniques. The entire valve must be removed, and the annulus must be completely débrided of calcium deposits.

C The diameter of the aortic root at the level of valve cusp attachment (annulus) is determined using standard sizing devices. This dimension must be accurately measured and clearly visualized. The aortic homograft valve that will be placed inside the aortic root will consume space simply because of the thickness of its wall. Therefore, the aortic homograft valve chosen for replacement must be 1 to 2 mm smaller in internal diameter than the measured aortic annulus. Experience has shown that this amount of downsizing is just about right to account for the anticipated minor shrinkage of the graft cusp tissues and for absorption of the septal myocardium. Greater downsizing risks aortic valve incompetence 3 or 4 months after the operation.

D The aortic homograft is removed from the liquid nitrogen freezer used at the valve bank and thawed according to protocol. The septal muscle is excised with a finger placed inside the aorta to stabilize the graft and gauge the thickness of the trimmed graft.

E Excess aorta is trimmed away from the valve cusps, leaving a 3- to 4-mm rim of aorta beyond the attachment of the cusps. Most of the aortic sinus (sinus aortae) is removed. The aorta is shortened until it is approximately the same distance above the top of the commissural attachment. The graft is rotated 120 degrees counterclockwise from its anatomic position to place the portion of the valve below the right coronary sinus into the host aorta below the left coronary sinus. The purpose of this maneuver is to place the thick septal muscle contained on the graft opposite the flat portion of the outflow tract above the mitral valve.

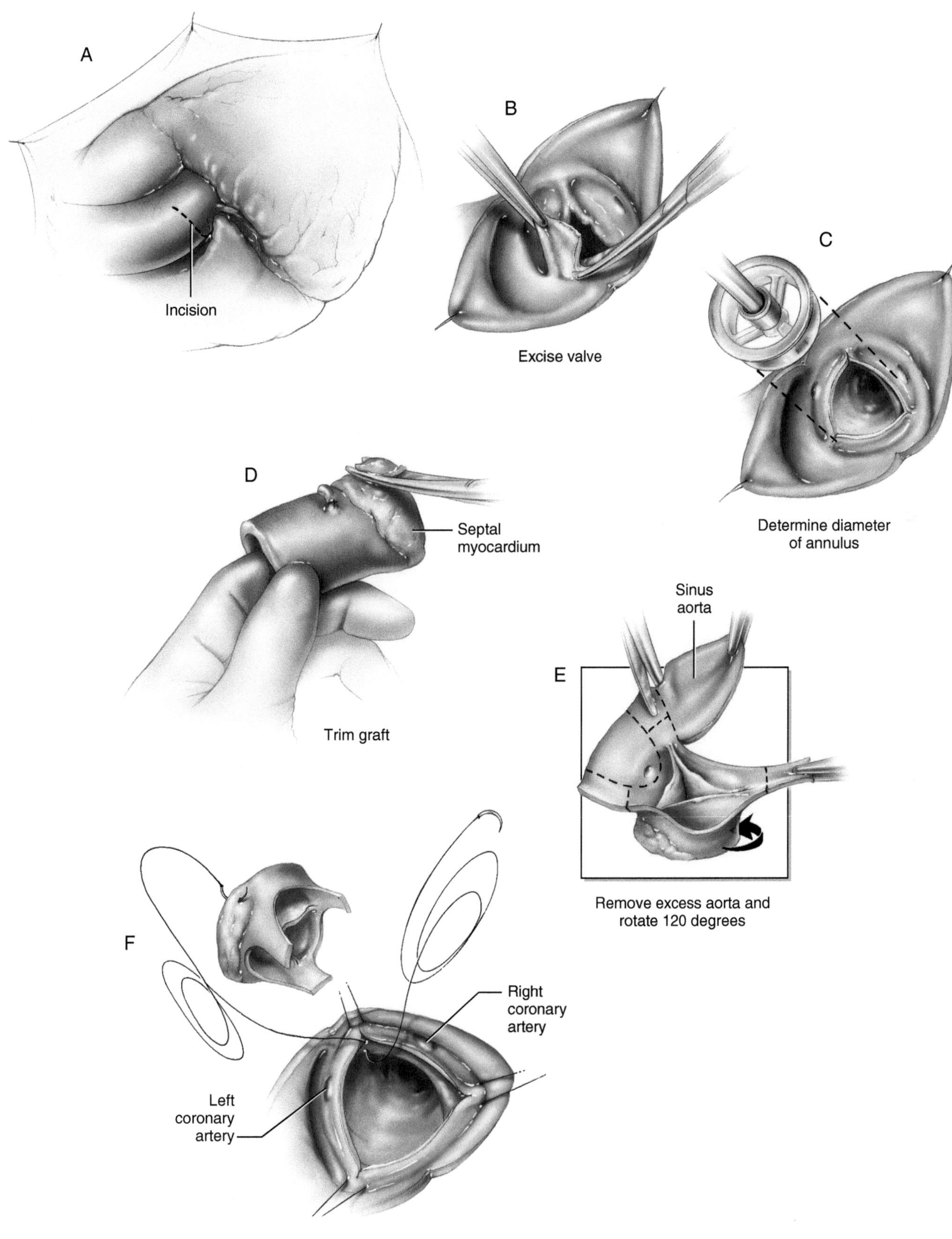
A
Incision
B
Excise valve
C
Determine diameter
of annulus
D
Septal
myocardium
Trim graft
Sinus
aorta
E
Remove excess aorta and
rotate 120 degrees
F
Right
coronary
artery
Left
coronary
artery
Attach graft to outflow tract

Figure 31-5 (continued)

F Three stitches are used to attach the valve to the outflow tract. The first is a double-needle suture of 3/0 polypropylene using two small, strong needles. This monofilament suture is chosen because of the needle strength and because the suture loops slide easily without a tendency to cut through the allograft tissue, especially in the region of the septal myocardium. This suture is placed through the graft septal muscle below the appropriate commissure and then through the host aortic outflow tract below the medial commissure between the right and left coronary sinuses. The stitch is placed below the annulus of the host aortic valve. To aid in aligning the allograft with the aortic root, two sutures of 4/0 polypropylene are placed; these stitches will be removed later because the primary suture line involves their position. These stitches are placed beneath the appropriate commissure of the graft and directly below the anterior and posterior commissures of the host aorta.

G The allograft valve is lowered into position in the aortic root, guided by the alignment sutures. The commissures of the graft are inverted through its annulus into the left ventricle of the host to expose the subvalvular edge of the graft. A knot is placed in the primary suture, and the stay sutures are tightened to align the graft with the aortic outflow tract.

H Stitches are placed between the graft and the aortic outflow tract below the level of the annulus. Because the aortic annulus is not actually annular but is, in fact, crescent-shaped (semilunar), the stitches will be below the fibrous "annulus" in the subcommissural region (interleaflet triangle), and they will come through this fibrous tissue at the midpoint of the aortic sinus. A real effort should be made to keep the plane of the suture line at an even level in the outflow tract. The stitches below the left coronary sinus are placed first. The suture line is taken to a point below the posterior commissure.

I With the opposite needle, the stitches between the graft and the aortic outflow tract are placed below the right coronary sinus and completed below the noncoronary sinus.

J The commissures of the aortic homograft are pulled out of the left ventricle so that the valve assumes its normal position and configuration. The commissures of the homograft are attached to the host aorta by continuous sutures of 4/0 polypropylene. Separate stitches are used for each aortic sinus. The first stitch is taken horizontally through the aortic sinus, slightly above the aortic annulus, and then passed through the graft.

K The initial stitches should be placed deep in the sinus of the host to preserve function of the sinus of Valsalva. As the suturing proceeds up the commissure, the stitches in the host aorta should be placed away from the actual fibrous commissure in the tissue of the aortic sinus so that the graft commissure is placed flat against the host aortic wall. The final stitches securely fasten the commissure of the graft to the aortic wall.

L Suturing proceeds in each aortic sinus until the graft is completely attached. In general, suturing of the right coronary sinus is completed first, sewing from the center point of the sinus to each of the commissures using opposite ends of the suture. Suturing of the left sinus follows, and the repair is completed with suturing of the noncoronary sinus.

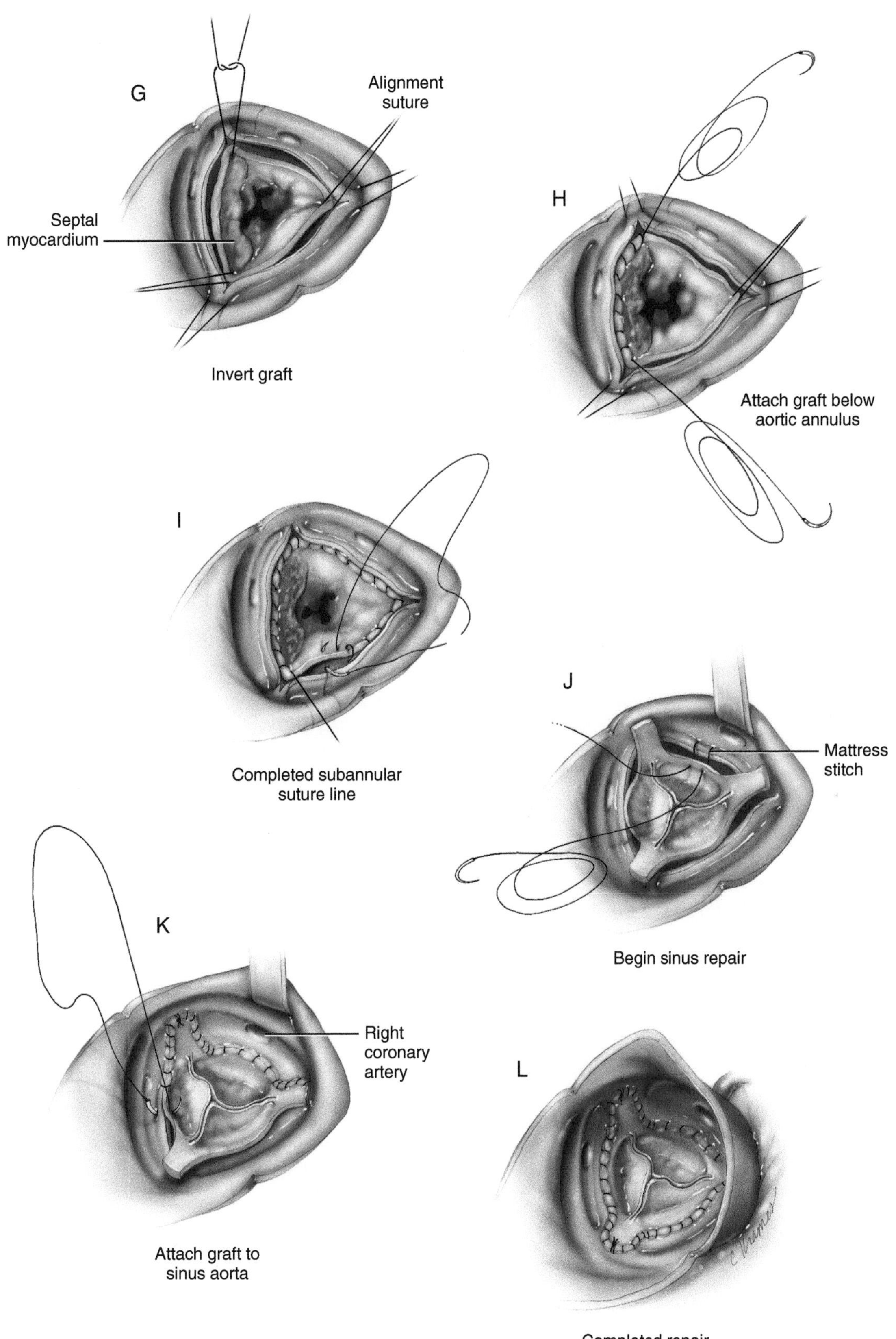
G
Alignment suture
Septal myocardium
Invert graft
H
Attach graft below aortic annulus
I
Completed subannular suture line
J
Mattress stitch
Begin sinus repair
K
Right coronary artery
Attach graft to sinus aorta
L
Completed repair

Aortic Allograft: Ross Intact Noncoronary Sinus Technique

This technique is probably the most useful and reproducible method for replacing the aortic valve with an aortic allograft valve by the "freehand" technique. It is particularly useful in patients with aortic valve incompetence due to leaflet prolapse because this condition is usually caused by deformity and enlargement of the noncoronary sinus of Valsalva. The noncoronary sinus of the graft is not disturbed, so it serves as a substitute for the deformed sinus of the host. Because the sinotubular junction (sinus rim) of the noncoronary sinus of the graft remains intact, two of the commissures of the graft remain in a fixed position. The need to properly position only one commissure of the graft simplifies valve implantation and makes graft valve competence more likely.

Figure 31-6

A The principles of aortic root anatomic assessment, valve excision, annular sizing, choice of allograft size, and method of trimming are exactly as described for the 120-degree rotation technique (see Figure 31-5, *A-D*), except that the noncoronary sinus of the graft remains intact and is not trimmed. A significant length of graft aorta is left above the sinus rim. This will be trimmed later during closure of the aorta. Transecting the aorta rather than using an oblique incision is probably preferable for the reasons explained earlier.

B The graft is attached to the aortic outflow tract exactly as shown in Figure 31-5, *F*. Only one alignment suture is shown here. The actual suture used for the repair is placed below the medial commissure.

C The graft is lowered into the aortic outflow tract, and the aortic tissue is inverted to expose the lower edge of the graft. The lower suture line proceeds as demonstrated in Figure 31-5, *H* and *I*. Shown here are the final stitches taken in the noncoronary sinus. An effort is made to keep the lower suture line in a level plane. Maintaining a level suture line is not possible in the segment of the right coronary sinus occupied by the conduction system; there, sutures must be placed through the fibrous annulus. Because many patients have deformed nonconorary sinuses that are much deeper than the other sinuses, it may be necessary to adjust the position of the lower suture line in this segment. In some cases it is actually more desirable to bring the lower suture line above the annulus into the aortic sinus to compensate for the deformity, rather than distorting the graft by attempting to pull it down to achieve a subannular suture line, as described for the 120-degree rotation technique.

D The sinus aorta of the graft is attached to the sinus aorta of the host using continuous stitches of 4/0 polypropylene. The suture line is started deep in the sinus at the midpoint with a horizontal stitch, as described in Figure 31-5, *J*. The initial stitches the are placed deep in the sinus aorta to preserve sinus of Valsalva function. Suturing begins in the right coronary sinus and proceeds to the top of each adjacent commissure of the graft. Repair of the left coronary sinus follows.

E Noncoronary sinus repair is accomplished by one of two methods. In one method, the aorta is closed over the graft if the noncoronary sinus of the host is enlarged and the graft will not be compressed or distorted by the repair. Continuous 4/0 polypropylene suture is used to close the aorta to a point above the sinus rim. The graft aorta is excised above the sinus rim. The aorta of the graft is closed to the host aorta just above the sinus rim by continuous sutures.

F In the second method, if the noncoronary sinus of the host will not accommodate the graft without distortion, the edges of the aortotomy are left open to allow the graft sinus to expand without restriction. The edges of the aortotomy are loosely attached to the adventitia of the graft at an appropriate point. The graft is tapered and worked into the aortotomy closure above the sinus rim.

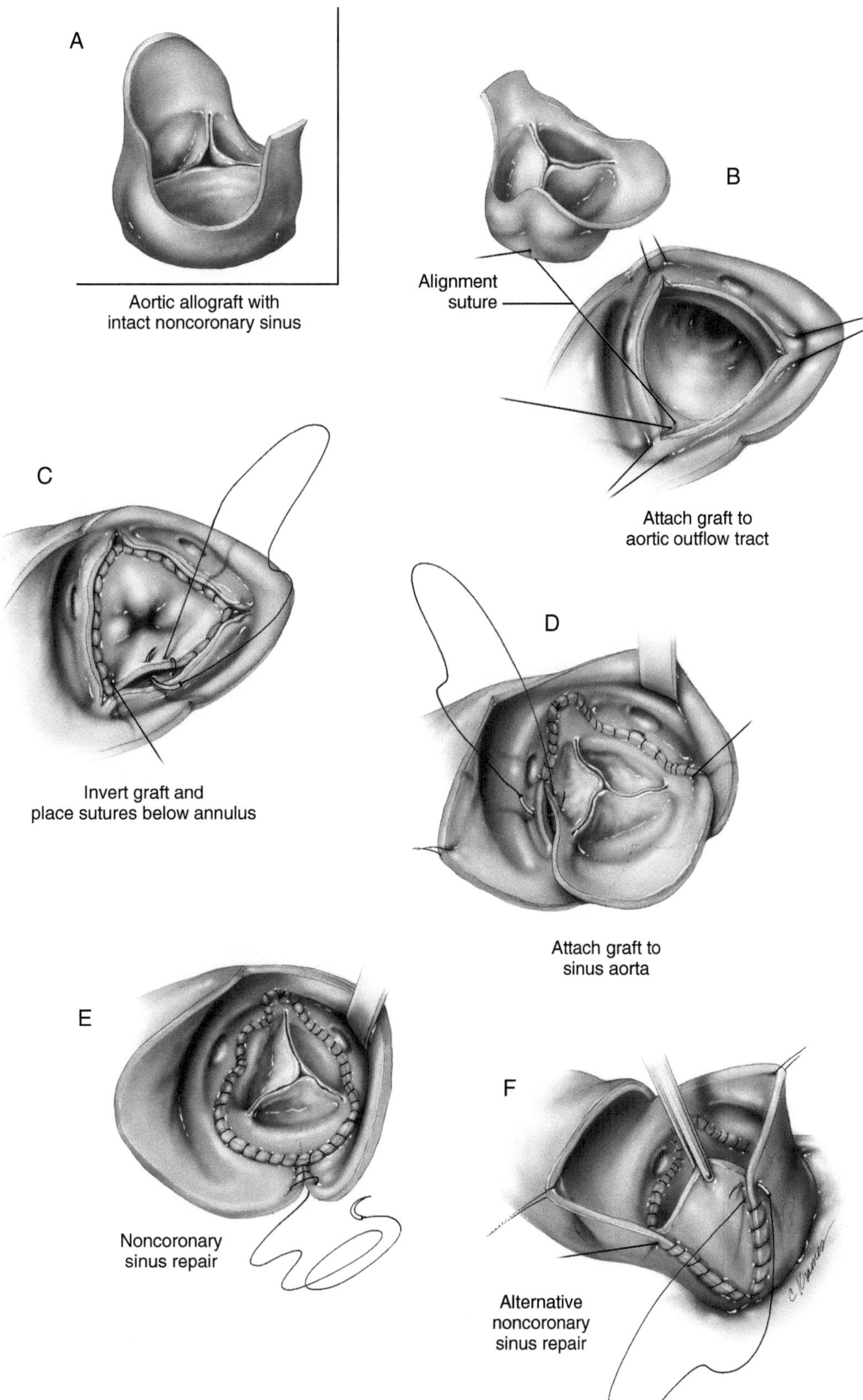
A
Aortic allograft with intact noncoronary sinus
B
Alignment suture
Attach graft to aortic outflow tract
C
Invert graft and place sutures below annulus
D
Attach graft to sinus aorta
E
Noncoronary sinus repair
F
Alternative noncoronary sinus repair

Aortic Allograft: Aortic Root Enlargement Technique

An aortic allograft may be used for valve replacement as part of a root-enlarging operation. This procedure is a modification of the Ross intact noncoronary sinus method. The intact graft aorta in the noncoronary sinus allows the placement of an oversized graft that can expand laterally through the noncoronary sinus and above the left atrium.

Figure 31-7

A A transverse incision is made in the aorta. The incision is extended to the posterior aspect of the aorta and into the posterior commissure between the left and noncoronary sinuses.

B An incision into the triangular space below the commissure (interleaflet triangle) between the fibrous attachments of the natural aortic valve opens into the aortic root, where there is little fibrous support. The edges of the aortotomy separate widely as the interleaflet triangle is opened. To achieve the desired separation of the edges of the incision, it is extended to the upper edge of the anterior leaflet of the mitral valve, but it need not enter the leaflet tissue. Part or all of the noncoronary sinus aortae and fibrous annulus can also be excised to gain more space. The increased diameter of the aortic root is measured, and an appropriately sized aortic allograft is chosen. The aortic allograft is trimmed, leaving the noncoronary sinus intact. The aortic sinus of the graft is removed from the left and right sinuses, leaving a few millimeters of tissue attached to the fibrous support of the cusps.

C The allograft is attached to the rim of the anterior leaflet of the mitral valve and to the superior aspect of the left atrium with interrupted stitches of 3/0 or 4/0 polypropylene. The stitches are placed in the corresponding mitral valve and left atrium of the noncoronary sinus of the allograft. A Teflon felt strip is fashioned, slightly longer than the length of the unsupported area of the separated aortotomy.

D The sutures of the noncoronary sinus are tied down over the Teflon felt strip. Note that the sutures are not passed through the prosthetic felt but are simply tied over the material so that it is incorporated and thus fills in any potential defects in the suture line (Ross method).

E The commissures of the valve are inverted to the outflow tract of the left ventricle. The lower suture line is constructed by continuous suture of 3/0 polypropylene, as described for routine freehand aortic allograft valve replacement (see Figure 31-5, *H* and *I*). The stitches are placed below the aortic valve annulus except at the midportion of the sinus, where the stitches are approximated to the annulus.

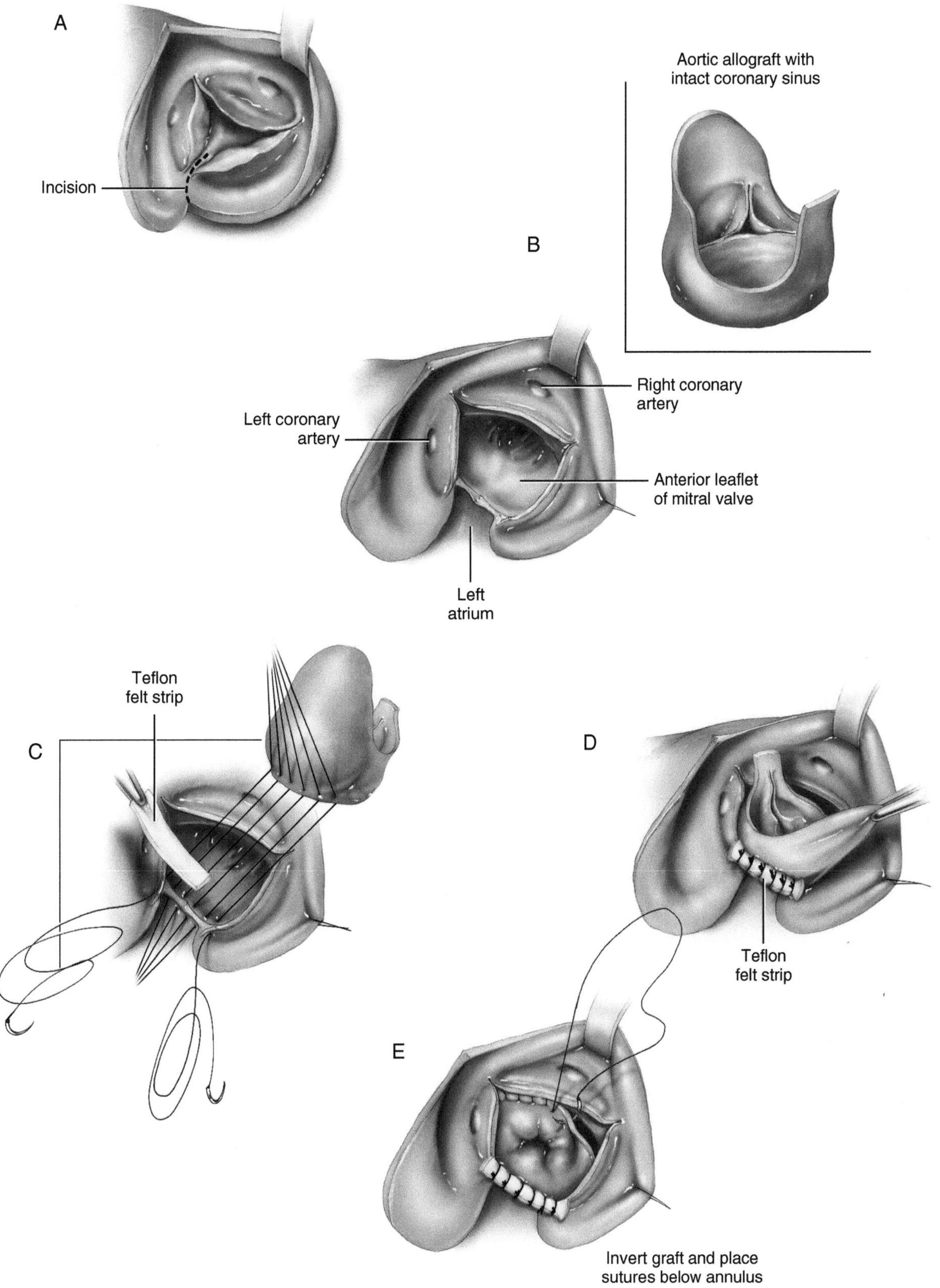
A
Incision
B
Aortic allograft with
intact coronary sinus
Right coronary
artery
Left coronary
artery
Anterior leaflet
of mitral valve
Left
atrium
C
Teflon
felt strip
D
Teflon
felt strip
E
Invert graft and place
sutures below annulus

Figure 31-7 (continued)

F The sinus aorta (aortic sinus) of the allograft is attached to the host aorta. The commissures are pulled up into the aortic root. The stitches are placed exactly as described previously, making sure that the commissures are elevated well up onto the aortic wall.

G The suture line is continued as a transition from the sinus aorta to the edges of the aortotomy.

The intact noncoronary sinus of the allograft is used to close the aortotomy and widen the aortic root.

H The aortotomy is completely closed, incorporating the aortic allograft.

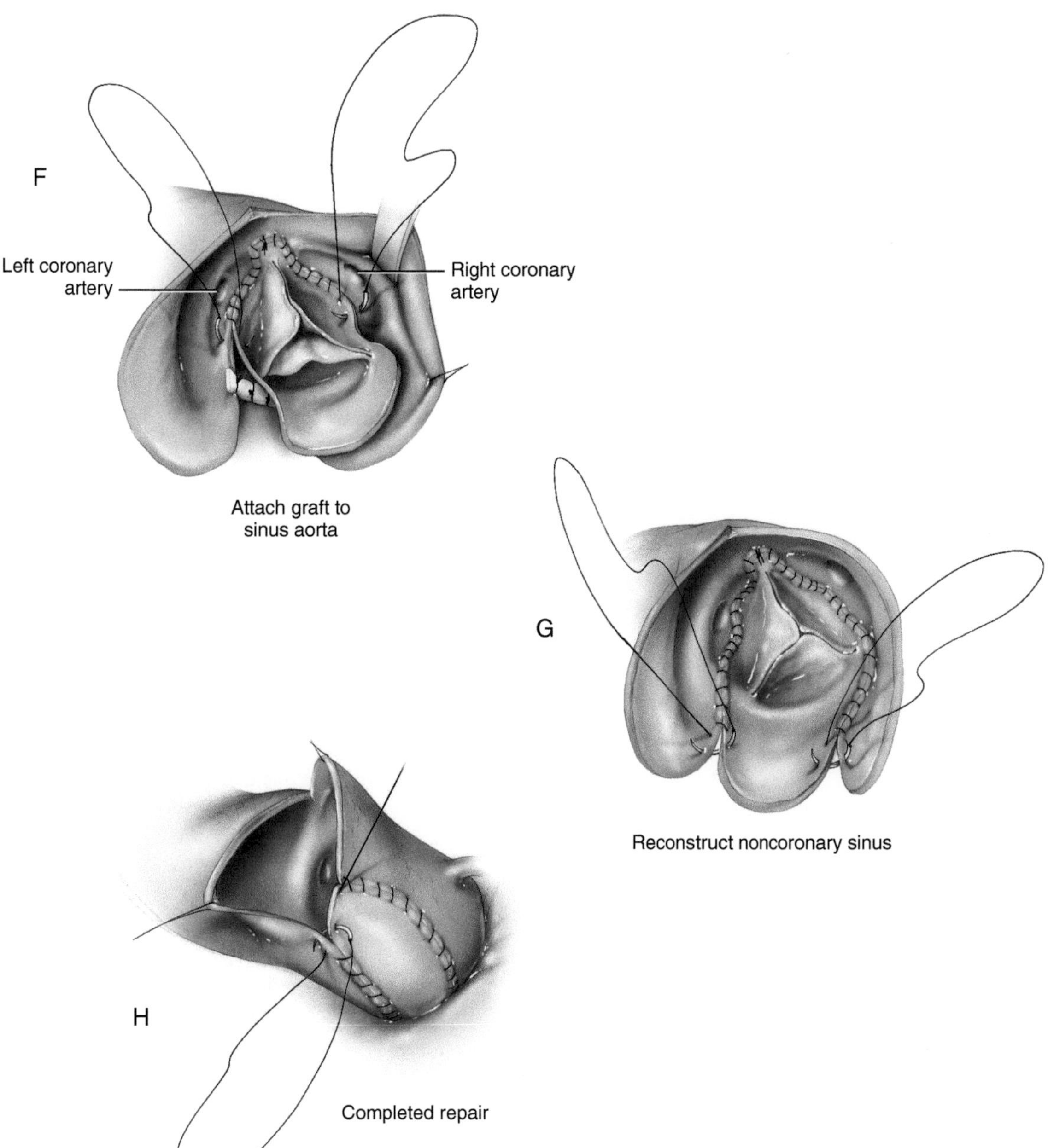
F
Left coronary artery
Right coronary artery
Attach graft to sinus aorta
G
Reconstruct noncoronary sinus
H
Completed repair

Aortic Allograft: Aortic Root Enlargement with Mitral Valve

Aortic allografts are usually processed with the anterior leaflet of the mitral valve attached in an anatomic position. This mitral tissue can be used to enlarge the aortic root when there is associated subvalvular aortic stenosis. The anterior leaflet of the graft mitral valve can also be used to repair defects or even replace most of the natural anterior mitral leaflet.

Figure 31-8

A The aortic valve is excised as usual. When inspection of the aortic root discloses a significant subvalvular component to the left ventricular outflow tract obstruction, the incision is deviated posteriorly to the commissure between the left and noncoronary cusps of the aortic valve. The incision is taken into the interleaflet triangle between the fibrous attachments of the aortic valve at the commissure.

B The incision is extended through the stenotic region below the aortic valve, onto the anterior leaflet of the mitral valve at its midpoint. The roof of the left atrium is also entered.

C An aortic allograft of the appropriate size for the enlarged aortic root is selected and trimmed, leaving the noncoronary sinus intact and leaving a sufficient amount of the mitral valve's anterior leaflet attached to widen the outflow tract. The anterior leaflet tissue of the graft is attached to the defect in the anterior leaflet of the host using interrupted stitches of 3/0 braided suture material or 4/0 Cardionyl. Although it may be tempting to use continuous suture technique for the valve repair, this method should be avoided because interrupted suture technique results in a stronger repair.

D The aortic allograft is attached to the aortic root exactly as described for the intact noncoronary sinus technique: continuous stitches of 3/0 polypropylene are used for the inflow suture line, and the aortic sinus of the graft is attached to the aortic sinus of the host using continuous 4/0 polypropylene. The defect in the roof of the left atrium is closed with an appropriately sized patch of graft aorta fashioned from what was trimmed away. The patch is attached to the left atrial remnant of the graft and to the edges of the left atrial defect with continuous stitches of 4/0 polypropylene.

E In some cases the anterior leaflet of the mitral valve is deficient due to scarring or perforation. The anterior leaflet can be preserved and replaced with graft tissue if the chordae tendineae that support it are normal. In these cases the abnormal portion of the anterior leaflet is cut away. This abnormal tissue may account for nearly the entire anterior leaflet; thus, only the edge supported by chordae is spared.

F The aortic allograft is prepared, leaving the entire anterior leaflet of the mitral valve attached. This tissue is attached to the edge of the host mitral valve using interrupted stitches of 3/0 braided suture or 4/0 Cardionyl.

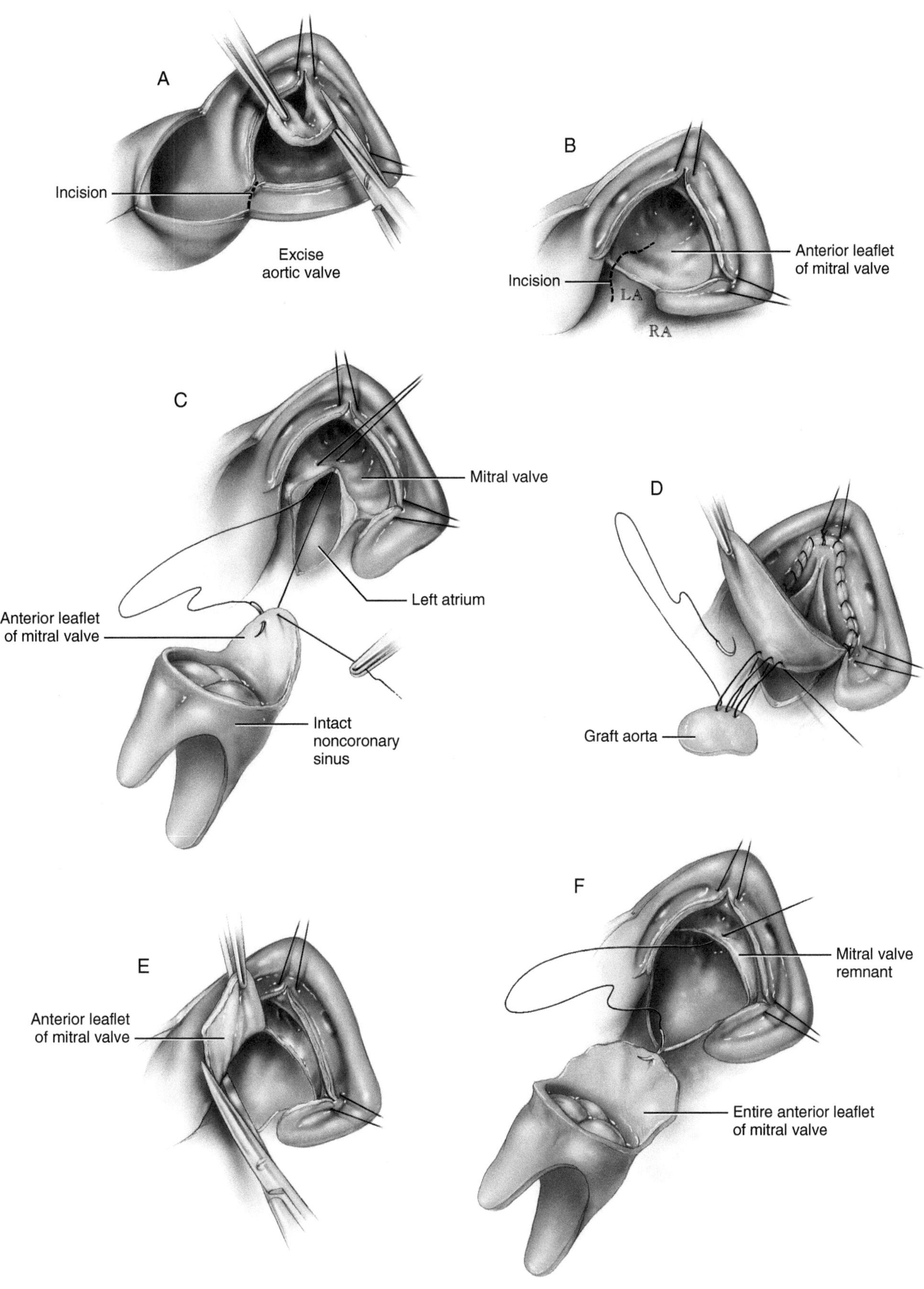
A
Incision
Excise
aortic valve
B
Incision
LA
RA
Anterior leaflet
of mitral valve
C
Mitral valve
Left atrium
Anterior leaflet
of mitral valve
Intact
noncoronary
sinus
D
Graft aorta
E
Anterior leaflet
of mitral valve
F
Mitral valve
remnant
Entire anterior leaflet
of mitral valve

Aortic Allograft: Miniroot (Inclusion) Technique

The aortic allograft can be used to replace the aortic valve by keeping the graft aortic root intact and simply inserting the cylinder of the graft within the host aortic root. This technique has the advantage of a high probability of early graft valve competence because the graft aortic root remains largely unaltered. It has the disadvantage of placing a considerable amount of graft aorta, which could calcify and harden, inside the host aortic root.

Figure 31-9

A The usual transverse incision is made to expose the aortic valve. The valve is excised, and the annulus is measured in the usual fashion. An aortic allograft with an inside diameter 1 to 2 mm smaller than that of the aortic root is chosen, thawed, and trimmed of excess septal myocardium. The excess aorta is trimmed from the graft just above the sinotubular junction. The lower end of the graft is attached to the left ventricular outflow tract with interrupted stitches of 3/0 polypropylene. The fibrous hinge point of the aortic valve (annulus) is used when possible, keeping the lower suture line in a level plane. Continuous suture technique can also be used.

B The lower suture line can be supported by a Teflon felt or pericardial strip placed within the suture loops as the proximal suture line is secured. The proximal suture line can also be left unsupported because the graft root is contained entirely within the host aorta.

C The graft coronary arteries are removed flush with the aorta to create generous coronary openings. The left and right coronary arteries are anastomosed to the graft by continuous stitches of 3/0 polypropylene. The stitches are placed deeply into the intact tissues surrounding the coronary ostia and completely through the graft. Special care must be taken with these suture lines because even the slightest leak can cause a false passage, which could distort the graft or lead to paravalvular leak.

D The upper end of the graft is anastomosed to the host aorta at or above the sinotubular junction. Again, the sutures should be placed deeply and securely into the intact host aorta posteriorly; any deficiency in the suture line predisposes to paravalvular leak. Continuous stitches of 3/0 polypropylene are employed. The host aorta is closed to approximate the upper edge of the graft.

E The upper edge of the graft can be incorporated into the aortotomy closure if it is appropriately placed and convenient to do so. One of the pitfalls of this procedure is the possible mismatch of the diameters of the upper end of the graft and the host aorta, which may be dilated. Excess tension on the suture line attaching the graft to the aorta to make up for a size discrepancy also may lead to dehiscence and paravalvular leak.

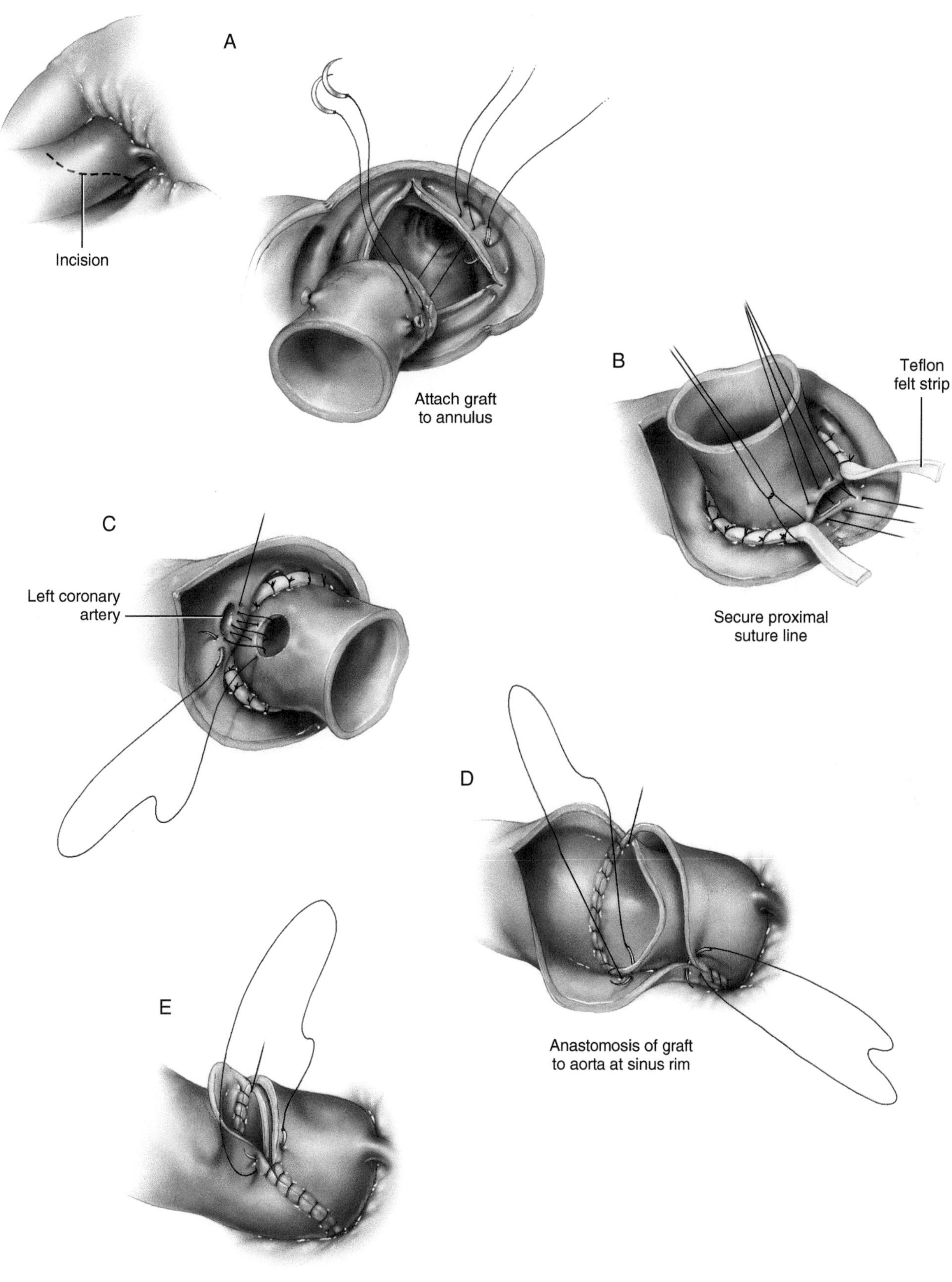
A
Incision
Attach graft
to annulus
B
Teflon
felt strip
Secure proximal
suture line
C
Left coronary
artery
D
Anastomosis of graft
to aorta at sinus rim
E
Close aorta, including graft

Aortic Allograft: Complete Root (Freestanding) Technique

An aortic homograft can be used to completely replace the aortic root when there is gross deformity caused by infection or congenital anomaly. It can also be used for an aortic root–enlarging procedure. This technique, as utilized by Donald Ross, has been only slightly modified.

Figure 31-10

A The usual transverse incision is made. In this procedure, however, the aorta is always divided. The coronary arteries are minimally mobilized by incising the sinus aorta surrounding the coronary ostia. The rest of the sinus aorta is excised, leaving only fibrous aortic valve attachments that are normal and uninvolved by the disease process being treated.

B An appropriately sized aortic allograft is selected. Sizing of the graft is less important here than in freehand valve replacement or the miniroot technique because the graft is freestanding and not enclosed by host aorta. The graft is used intact and in a natural orientation, with only the excess septal myocardium and the anterior leaflet of the mitral valve removed. Before removing the mitral valve tissue, however, the pathologic defect should be evaluated to determine whether the graft mitral valve will be of use in the reconstruction of the aortic root. The allograft is attached to the left ventricular outflow tract by simple interrupted stitches of 3/0 polypropylene. In many cases the stitches are placed through the septal myocardium, the unsupported anterior leaflet of the mitral valve, and the roof of the left atrium because the annular connective tissue has been removed or destroyed by the disease process.

C The Ross technique employs a Teflon felt collar to ensure a hemostatic proximal suture line. This collar also supports the proximal suture line and prevents dilation of the aortic allograft root. The felt is cut into a strip approximately 5 mm wide and long enough to exceed the circumference of the aortic allograft. The felt strip will shorten as the sutures are tied over it and it is compressed between the graft and the host aorta.

D The allograft is slipped over the sutures into the outflow tract in the desired position. The sutures are then tied down, incorporating the felt strip within the suture loops. This technique effectively seals any potential leak points. Use of an autogenous pericardial strip or a continuous suture line sealed with BioGlue is preferred in cases of aortic root replacement for infection.

E The coronary ostia of the graft are anastomosed to the sinus aorta surrounding the coronary arteries of the host using continuous stitches of 3/0 or 4/0 polypropylene. Shown here is the right coronary artery anastomosis, which in practice is performed after completing the left coronary anastomosis.

F The repair is completed by end-to-end anastomosis of the distal end of the allograft to the host aorta. Continuous stitches of 3/0 or 4/0 polypropylene are used. Division of the natural aorta allows the posterior suture line to be constructed in the most secure fashion. Suturing to the intact posterior wall of the aorta and use of the aorta to cover the repair are not recommended.

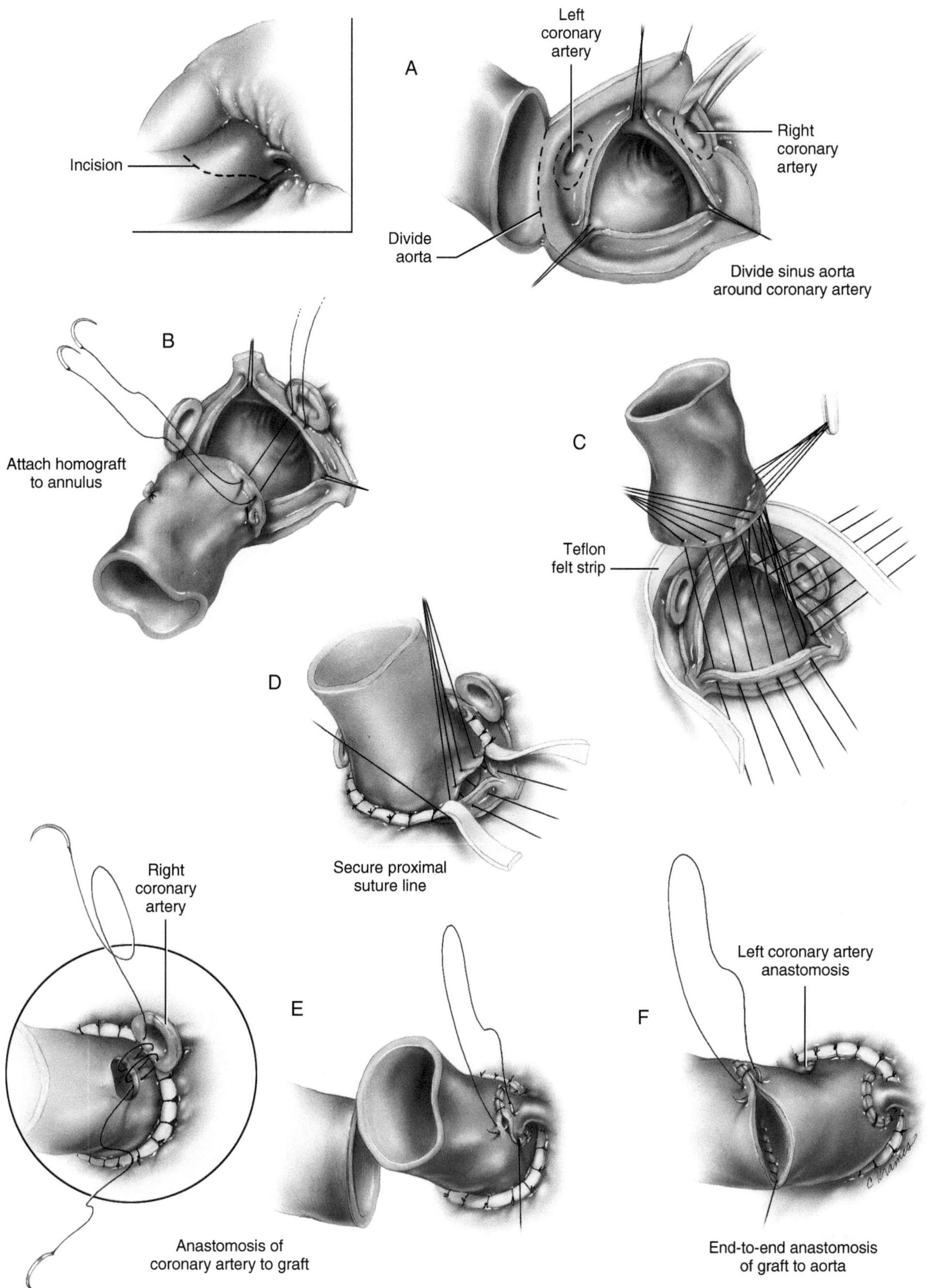
Incision
A
Left
coronary
artery
Right
coronary
artery
Divide
aorta
Divide sinus aorta
around coronary artery
B
Attach homograft
to annulus
C
Teflon
felt strip
D
Secure proximal
suture line
Right
coronary
artery
E
Anastomosis of
coronary artery to graft
F
Left coronary artery
anastomosis
End-to-end anastomosis
of graft to aorta

Stentless Porcine Xenograft: Subcoronary Valve Replacement

Glutaraldehyde-preserved porcine xenograft aortic valves are frequently used for aortic valve replacement. These xenograft valves may be supported by a stent frame and implanted as an aortic valve prosthesis using standard continuous or interrupted suture technique, or they may be constructed without a stent, using the patient's aortic root for support. Stentless xenografts have a significant hemodynamic advantage over stented valves, especially in cases of small valve diameters. Because the patient's aorta is used to support the valve, there is more flexibility, which may translate into longer durability.

Figure 31-11

A There are several manufacturers of stentless porcine xenograft aortic valves. Grafts that use the entire untrimmed aortic root appear to offer the most flexibility and utility (Freestyle, Medtronic Inc., Minneapolis, MN). The implant technique is very similar to that of aortic valve replacement with aortic allograft using the intact noncoronary sinus technique (freehand) or complete root replacement (freestanding). The device comes with sizers to guide selection of the proper valve. In this respect, it is similar to choosing a prosthetic valve, and downsizing is not required. The sinus aorta is removed from the graft in the right and left sinuses of Valsalva. The lower edge of the aortic root of the graft is covered with Dacron fabric to aid implantation and to prevent graft shrinkage when the graft septal myocardium is absorbed. This cloth limits how deeply the sinus aorta can be excised, especially in the right coronary sinus. Care should be taken not to disrupt the cloth covering.

B The aortic valve is excised in the usual fashion, and all calcareous deposits are removed from the aortic annulus. Exposure is enhanced by placing traction sutures at the sinus rim above each of the commissures. Markings on the cloth covering the lower edge of the graft correspond to each commissure. Continuous stitches of double-needle 3/0 polypropylene are used to attach the lower edge of the graft to the aortic annulus. A small needle with a taper-cut design is best to easily penetrate the Dacron fabric. The suture line is started in the interleaflet triangle below the commissure between the left and right sinuses.

C The valve is held away from the annulus as the suture loops are placed. A heavy silk suture (0 or 2/0) is passed around every third suture loop to act as a tension-adjusting loop suture. These tension loops are secured by small hemostats. Suturing proceeds from below the right sinus to the commissure below the right and noncoronary sinuses.

D Suturing continues from below the left coronary sinus of Valsalva to below the commissure between the left and noncoronary sinuses. Tension loops are placed at every third stitch. The valve is seated in the aortic root by sequentially pulling up on the tension loops to approximate the fabric of the valve to the aortic annulus.

E The tension loops are removed sequentially after final adjustment of the proximal suture line below the left and right coronary sinuses.

F The noncoronary sinus repair follows. The xenograft prosthesis is sufficiently flexible to allow good exposure in this area simply by lifting the fabric of the prosthesis away from the aortic annulus as the suturing proceeds. Three stitches taken from each end usually suffice to join the prosthesis to the aortic annulus in the noncoronary sinus and still allow one to adjust tension on the suture line by pulling up on the suture loops.

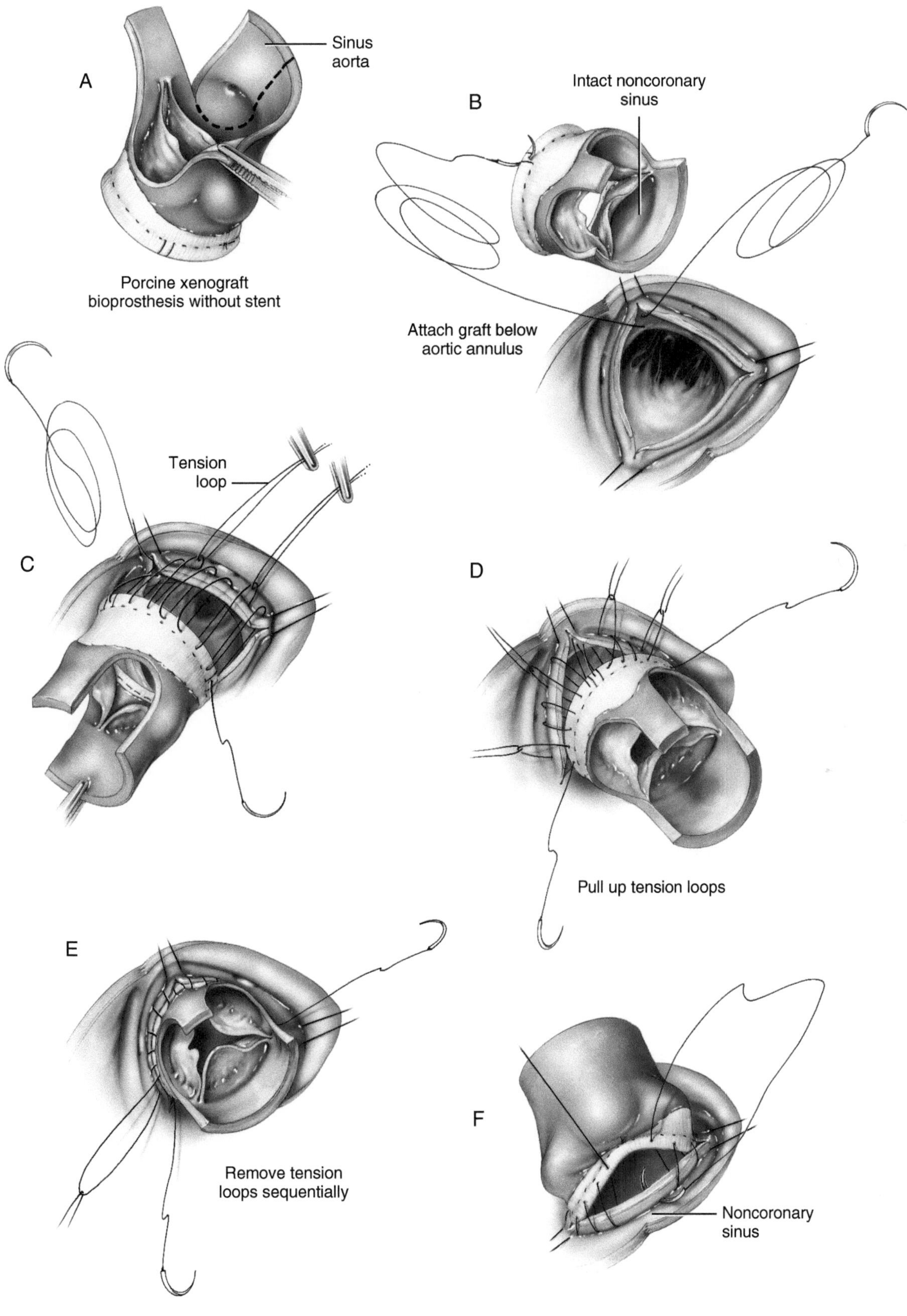
A
Sinus aorta
Porcine xenograft bioprosthesis without stent
B
Intact noncoronary sinus
Attach graft below aortic annulus
C
Tension loop
D
Pull up tension loops
E
Remove tension loops sequentially
F
Noncoronary sinus

Figure 31-11 (continued)

G The sinus aorta of the graft is attached to the sinus aorta of the patient by continuous stitches of 4/0 polypropylene. A mattress stitch is taken in the host sinus aorta just below the coronary ostia. Here the repair differs from the aortic allograft technique because xenograft aortic tissue, being glutaraldehyde preserved, is stiff and holds its shape and must be approximated to the host aorta without distorting that shape. Allograft tissue, in contrast, can be folded to conform. The suture line comes very close to the coronary ostia to achieve a proper fit of the xenograft tissues to the sinus aorta of the patient. This is especially true for the right coronary sinus of the graft, which is covered with cloth quite high on its external surface. Because the cloth cannot be removed, the suture line must come close to the coronary ostia. The commissure between the right and left sinuses of the graft must be carefully located so as not to distort the graft. Suturing continues to the top of the other two commissures, leaving the intact noncoronary sinus of the graft to be repaired later.

H The closeness of the suture line to the right coronary ostium, which is unique to the stentless xenograft technique, can be appreciated in this figure. The noncoronary sinus can be repaired by direct closure of the host aortotomy if there is sufficient space in the sinus to accommodate the graft without distortion. This is usually the situation when intervention has been for aortic valve incompetence and the aortic root is enlarged. In these cases, the graft is trimmed just above the sinotubular junction and attached securely to the intact aorta of the patient.

I An alternative noncoronary sinus repair is used if there is even the slightest chance of distortion of the noncoronary sinus of the graft, such as when the aortic root is normal or small, as it might be in patients with aortic valve stenosis. A double-needle 4/0 polypropylene suture is started at the apex of the aortotomy. Each side of the aortotomy is attached to the adventitia of the graft at a comfortable position to allow the noncoronary sinus of the graft to bulge between the edges of the aortotomy. The graft aorta is tapered and worked into the aortotomy above the sinotubular junction.

J Operative photograph of a completed subcoronary aortic valve replacement with a porcine xenograft. After considerable experience, it became apparent that the preferred approach to the aortic valve was through the divided aorta and the intact aortic root. This provides excellent exposure while leaving the noncoronary sinus intact. The xenograft fits into the intact aortic root in nearly all cases. This allows the noncoronary sinus aorta to be trimmed at the level of the host aorta in the noncoronary sinus for direct approximation by continuous suture at the edges. The aortic anastomosis is secure and oversews the noncoronary sinus repair.

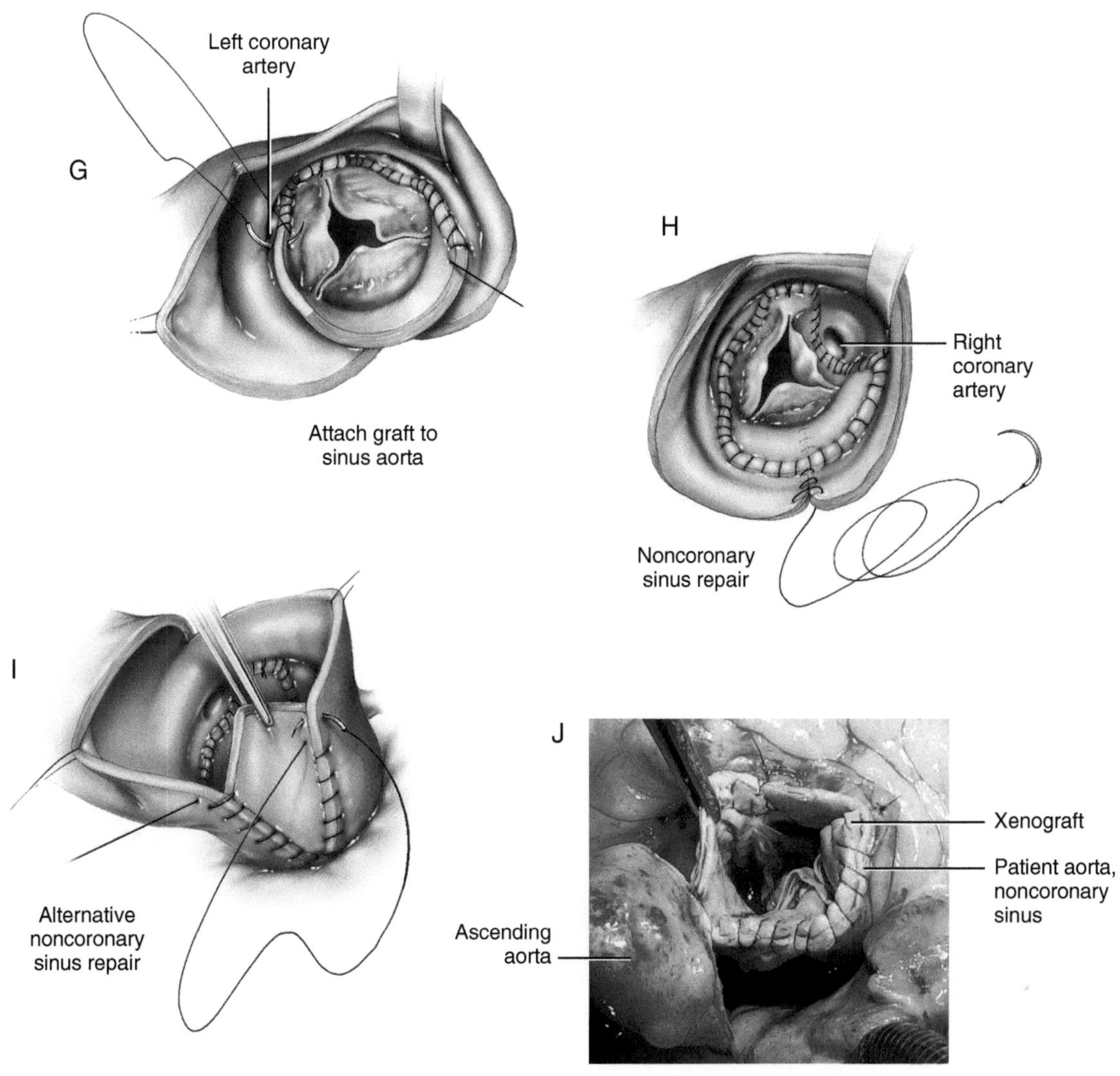
G
Left coronary artery
Attach graft to sinus aorta
H
Right coronary artery
Noncoronary sinus repair
I
Alternative noncoronary sinus repair
J
Xenograft
Patient aorta, noncoronary sinus
Ascending aorta
Divided aorta repair

Stentless Equine Xenograft: Subcoronary Aortic Valve Replacement

Implantation of a stentless bioprosthesis is preferred to obtain optimal hemodynamics. For individuals with isolated aortic valve disease without associated root pathology, such as a small aortic root, the equine stentless xenograft can be utilized without the need for formal root replacement. To use this bioprosthesis, the diameters of the annulus and the sinotubular junction cannot differ by more than 3 to 4 mm.

K The aorta is transected 2 cm above the sinotubular junction. This ensures that the commissural tabs of the bioprosthesis can be safely attached well below the aortotomy. Retention sutures are placed at the top of each native commissure to expose the valve.

L After removal of the diseased native valve, the annulus is sized. The sizer has guiding slots for proper orientation. The bottom slots are positioned at the nadir of each commissure of the native valve. The lower portions of the top slots correlate to the midpoint of each commissural tab of the bioprosthesis. The upper portions of the top slots correspond to the top of each commissural tab.

M The sizer is positioned at the level of the aortic annulus. The bottom slots are aligned with the nadir of the native commissures. The aorta is gently pulled upward to approximate a normal contour. Three reference marks are made on the inside of the aorta at the level of the top slots to guide later placement of the commissural tabs at exactly 120 degrees.

N The bioprosthesis is attached to the annulus using simple interrupted 2/0 braided sutures. Alternatively, three continuous 3/0 polypropylene sutures can be used for the annular suture line. The bioprosthesis is lowered into position, and the sutures are secured.

O The three commissural tabs are attached to the aortic wall at the previously marked sites, maintaining the 120-degree alignment. Three 4/0 polypropylene sutures are used for each tab. The needles are placed through the tab, through the aorta, and through a corresponding pledget on the outside of the aorta. One suture is placed horizontally across the top of the tab, and two sutures are placed vertically. The sutures are tied on the outside of the aorta, and the aortotomy is closed with continuous 4/0 polypropylene suture.

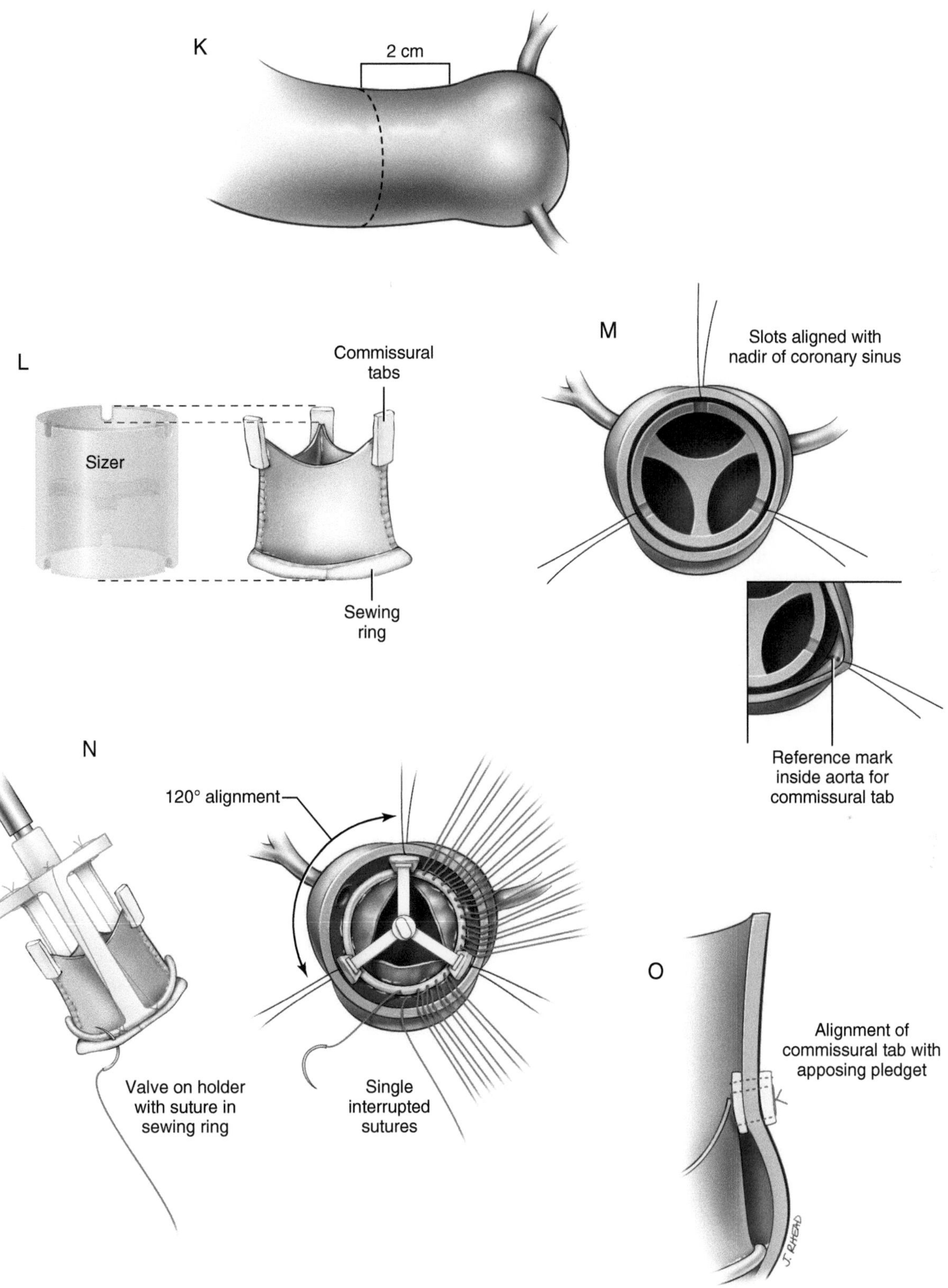
K
2 cm
L
Commissural tabs
Sizer
Sewing ring
M
Slots aligned with nadir of coronary sinus
Reference mark inside aorta for commissural tab
N
120° alignment
Valve on holder with suture in sewing ring
Single interrupted sutures
O
Alignment of commissural tab with apposing pledget
J. RHEAD

Stentless Porcine Xenograft: Aortic Root Replacement

This technique employs the glutaraldehyde-preserved porcine aortic root. The valve leaflets are unlikely to be distorted because they are supported by the intact graft aortic root. Aortic valve competence is ensured.

Figure 31-12

A The aorta is divided above the sinotubular junction. Traction stitches are placed above each commissure for optimal exposure of the aortic valve. The aortic valve is excised. The coronary arteries are separated from the aorta, retaining a generous button of aortic sinus around the orifice. The noncoronary sinus is removed. The diameter of the aorta at the level of the aortic valve is measured, and an appropriately sized aortic root bioprosthesis is selected. The diameter of the bioprosthesis may be the same size as or 2 mm larger than the diameter of the aortic annulus.

B Continuous stitches of 3/0 polypropylene are used to attach the inflow suture cuff of the bioprosthesis to the fibrous tissues at the aortic valve hinge point. A small taper-cut needle makes perforation of the sewing cuff easier. Suturing begins at the commissure between the left and right coronary sinuses of Valsalva, using the markers on the sewing cuff to line up the bioprosthesis in an anatomic position relative to the coronary ostia. The stitches are placed around the hinge point of the excised aortic valve and passed through the Dacron sewing cuff of the bioprosthesis below the marker indicating the level of the porcine xenograft valve. A loop suture of 0 silk is placed around every third suture loop to allow tension adjustment later. The bioprosthesis is held away from the annulus during suturing. Suturing continues in the right coronary sinus to the midpoint of the noncoronary sinus. Returning to the starting point, the opposite end of the suture is used, proceeding counterclockwise below the left sinus to completion at the midpoint of the noncoronary sinus. The bioprosthesis is seated in the aortic root by pulling up on the silk tension sutures sequentially.

C The left coronary artery of the porcine bioprosthesis always lines up with the left coronary artery of the patient. The porcine left coronary artery is removed from the bioprosthesis to create a generous opening. Continuous stitches of 5/0 polypropylene are used to anastomose the left coronary artery to the graft.

D Operative photograph of aortic root replacement with a porcine xenograft. The porcine aortic root has been attached to the aortic annulus. The right coronary artery may not approximate the position of the porcine right coronary artery on the bioprosthesis.

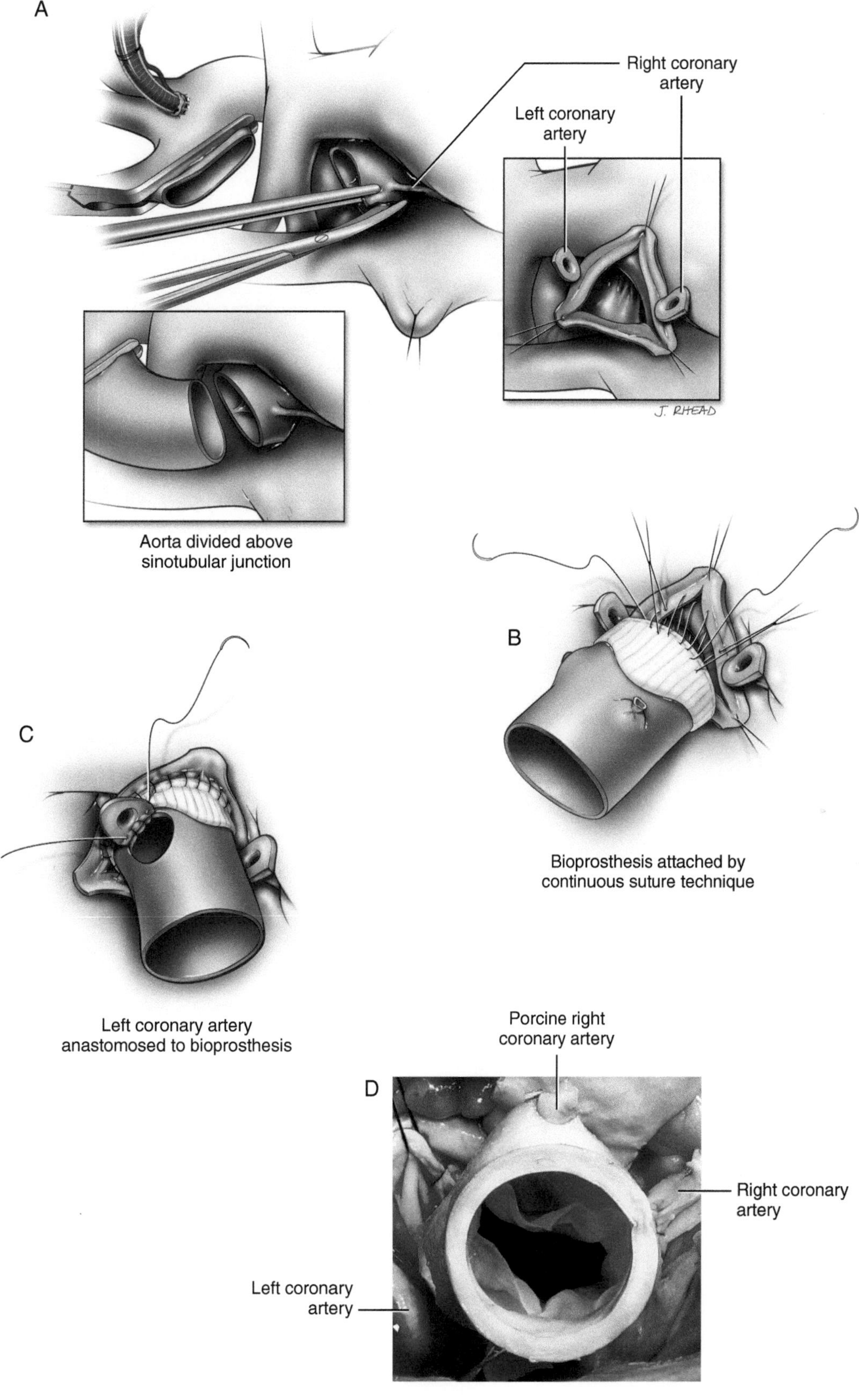
A
Right coronary artery
Left coronary artery
J. RHEAD
Aorta divided above sinotubular junction
B
Bioprosthesis attached by continuous suture technique
C
Left coronary artery anastomosed to bioprosthesis
D
Porcine right coronary artery
Right coronary artery
Left coronary artery

Figure 31-12 (continued)

E The right coronary artery of the porcine aortic root is often too far left of the patient's right coronary artery for proper anastomosis. Filling the right ventricle by temporarily occluding the venous uptake catheter raises the right coronary artery toward the bioprosthesis so that the exact location for anastomosis can be determined. A generous opening into the graft is made at that point. The right coronary artery is anastomosed to the graft using 5/0 polypropylene. The inset shows sealing of the coronary artery anastomosis with BioGlue. Sealant is placed on both coronary artery anastomoses and on the graft–to–aortic root suture line.

F The aorta is restored by end-to-end anastomosis of graft to aorta. A cuff of tubular Dacron graft is placed over the aorta before constructing the anastomosis.

G The Dacron cuff is slid down over the anastomosis to seal it. BioGlue is applied beneath the Dacron cuff to seal it to the anastomosis.

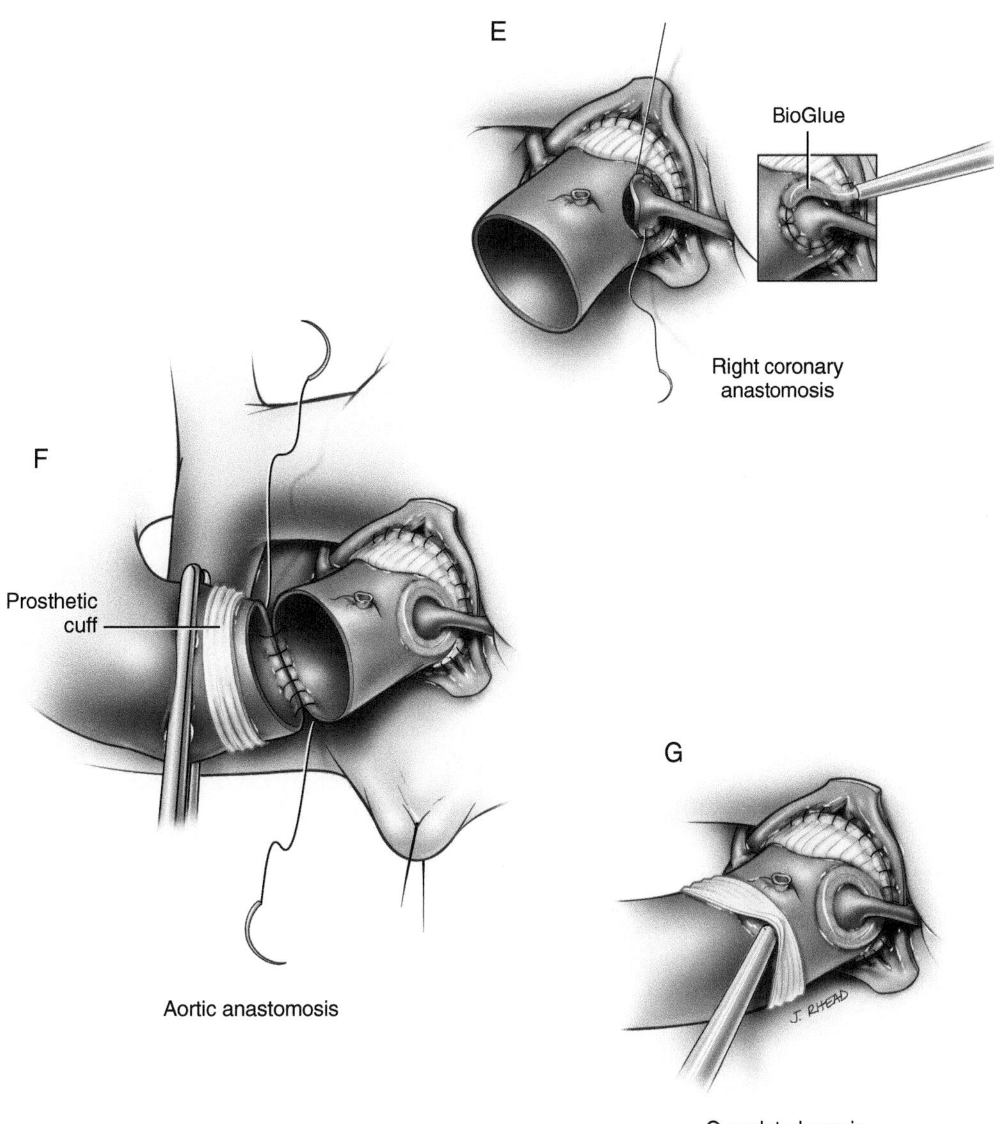
E
BioGlue
Right coronary anastomosis
F
Prosthetic cuff
Aortic anastomosis
G
J. RHEAD
Completed repair with BioGlue application

Pulmonary Autograft (Ross Procedure)

The aortic valve can be replaced with the patient's own pulmonary valve (pulmonary autograft), and a pulmonary allograft can be used to replace the pulmonary valve. This operation was devised by Donald Ross and appropriately carries his name. The operation has the advantage of placing autogenous tissue in the high-pressure aortic valve position, where at least in theory, it should last indefinitely, assuming the operation is technically correct. The allograft tissue is placed in the low-pressure pulmonary position, where, even if it fails, the valve incompetence or mild to moderate stenosis should be well tolerated for a long time.

Figure 31-13

A Pulmonary trunk, operative photograph. The pulmonary trunk is ideal for replacement of the aortic valve because, being the patient's own normal structure, it is exactly the right size for the purpose. In nearly all respects the pulmonary trunk has the same anatomic structure as the aortic root, but without coronary arteries attached.

B Key to performing the Ross procedure is an understanding of the anatomy of the left coronary artery and its relationship to the aortic root and the right ventricular outflow tract. Specifically, the first septal branch of the left anterior descending coronary artery originates behind the medial posterior commissure of the pulmonary valve. It courses across the pulmonary valve hinge point and into the infundibular septum toward the papillary muscle of the conus (see Figure 1-3, *B* and *C*, for more detail).

C Cardiopulmonary bypass is established using two cannulae for venous drainage. A right-angled cannula is placed directly into the superior vena cava at the pericardial reflection; the other cannula is placed in the inferior vena cava via the right atrium at the diaphragm. Oxygenated blood is returned to the ascending aorta. The usual transverse incision is made. The aortic valve is removed, and the aortic root is explored. Once the decision is made to proceed with the pulmonary autograft operation, the ascending aorta is divided, and all of the sinus aorta is removed except for a generous rim around the coronary ostia. A traction stitch on the aorta above the right coronary artery is helpful. Only the fibrous connection of the aortic cusps remains for attachment of the pulmonary autograft. Traction stitches are placed above each commissure.

D The pulmonary artery is separated from the aorta up to the bifurcation. Dissection between the medial commissure of the aorta and the pulmonary artery is extended down onto the muscle of the right ventricular outflow tract. Thorough dissection between the aorta and the pulmonary artery, especially low onto the right ventricle, makes removing the pulmonary trunk much easier later. The pulmonary artery is divided at the bifurcation, taking care not to shorten the right pulmonary artery.

E The pulmonary valve is inspected from above. The anterior interleaflet triangle is identified as a reference point for opening the right ventricular outflow tract. A small right-angled clamp is placed precisely in the anterior interleaflet triangle and pushed through the anterior wall of the right ventricle. The small opening created is thus carefully enlarged.

F While separating the pulmonary trunk from the right ventricle, the surgeon looks inside frequently to ensure that the appropriate length of right ventricle below the pulmonary valve is maintained.

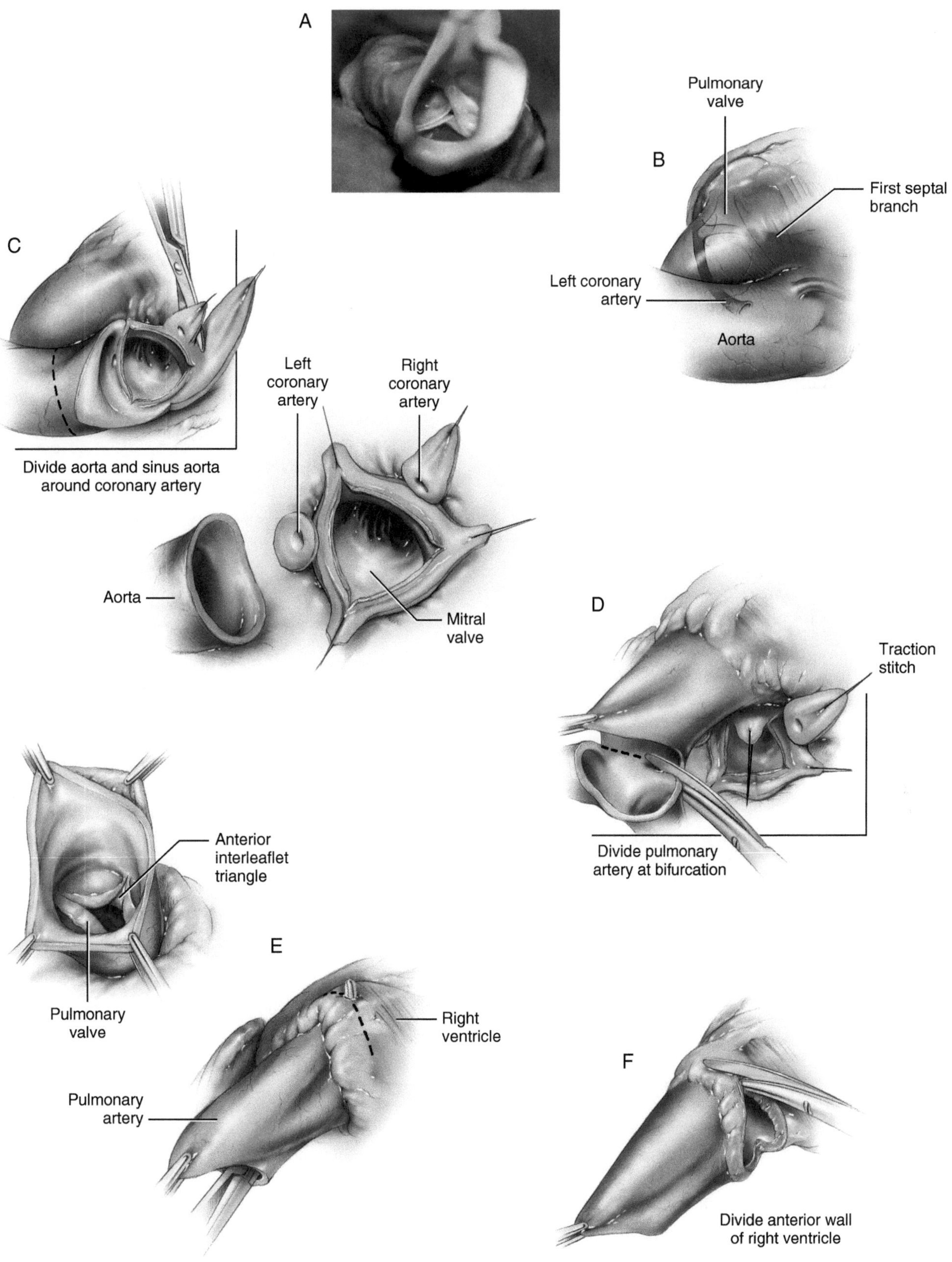
A
B
Pulmonary valve
First septal branch
Left coronary artery
Aorta
C
Divide aorta and sinus aorta around coronary artery
Left coronary artery
Right coronary artery
Aorta
Mitral valve
D
Traction stitch
Divide pulmonary artery at bifurcation
Anterior interleaflet triangle
Pulmonary valve
E
Right ventricle
Pulmonary artery
F
Divide anterior wall of right ventricle

Figure 31-13 (continued)

G The critical and unique part of the Ross procedure is separation of the pulmonary trunk from the right ventricular outflow tract above the infundibular septum. Correct performance of this part of the operation allows the rest of it to proceed safely. Injury to the underlying first septal branch of the anterior descending coronary artery is the major source of morbidity in this operation.

A shallow incision is made in the endocardial surface to join both ends of the partly excised pulmonary trunk. The incision extends completely across the remaining undivided right ventricular outflow tract. The angle of the scalpel is immediately changed to shave off the ventricular myocardium almost parallel to the endocardial surface. The inset diagram shows the shallow incision and the angle of the cut to shave off the pulmonary trunk without injuring the underlying first septal branch. This part of the operation should be performed deliberately and under precise control. The septal excision eventually separates the pulmonary trunk completely, leaving the left main coronary artery and the first septal branch behind and protected by a generous layer of tissue. To prevent tissue loss or inadvertently confusing the separated pulmonary trunk with the allograft, the separated pulmonary trunk is not removed from the operating field but is placed in the pericardial sac for immediate use. At this point it is convenient to measure the dimensions of the right ventricular outflow tract using standard prosthetic valve sizers and then to choose a pulmonary allograft for preparation and later use.

H The pulmonary autograft is attached to the left ventricular outflow tract using interrupted stitches of 3/0 polypropylene. The graft is marked below each of the commissures for orientation. The suturing proceeds below each sinus, separating the stitches into three groups. Stitches are placed through the strong fibrous tissue of the aortic annulus, keeping the plane of the repair as level as possible.

I A strip of Teflon felt or autogenous pericardium about 5 mm wide is used to fix the diameter of the proximal suture line and to ensure hemostasis between the sutures. A "supported" repair is favored to prevent dilation of the pulmonary autograft at the proximal suture line. Some surgeons prefer a continuous suture line without prosthetic material. However, the accuracy of carefully spaced individual stitches and supported fixation of the annulus are best. The pulmonary autograft is inverted partially into the outflow tract. The felt strip is placed within the suture loops so that it is incorporated as the sutures are tied down, taking care to ensure direct tissue approximation without interposed felt.

J An alternative method of constructing the proximal suture line begins with a purse-string stitch using double-needle 2/0 polypropylene to fix the diameter of the aortic outflow tract (Elkins method). The initial stitch is placed from outside the aorta into the fibrous hinge point of the aortic valve at the middle of the noncoronary sinus. Stitches are placed in a clockwise fashion in a level plane below the left coronary sinus, continuing around to the right coronary sinus, coming through the fibrous hinge point at the midpoint, staying in the fibrous tissue until past the commissure between the right and noncoronary sinuses where the bundle of His is located, and continuing to the midpoint of the noncoronary sinus, where the suture is brought to the outside of the aorta. The opposite needle is brought into the aorta and used to place a second row of stitches in a level plane slightly above the first row, continuing the stitches around the aortic outflow tract to the midpoint of the noncoronary sinus, where the suture is brought to the outside of the aorta. A chart (CryoLife Inc.) relating the diameter of the normal aortic valve to body surface area and gender is used to determine the optimal aortic outflow tract diameter (mean plus standard deviation). An appropriately sized Hegar dilator is placed through the aortic outflow tract as the purse-string stitch is tied down to fix the diameter optimally.

K Interrupted stitches are placed around the purse-string stitch to attach the pulmonary autograft to the aortic outflow tract. The pulmonary autograft is partially inverted into the outflow tract as the sutures are tied down to ensure tissue-to-tissue approximation.

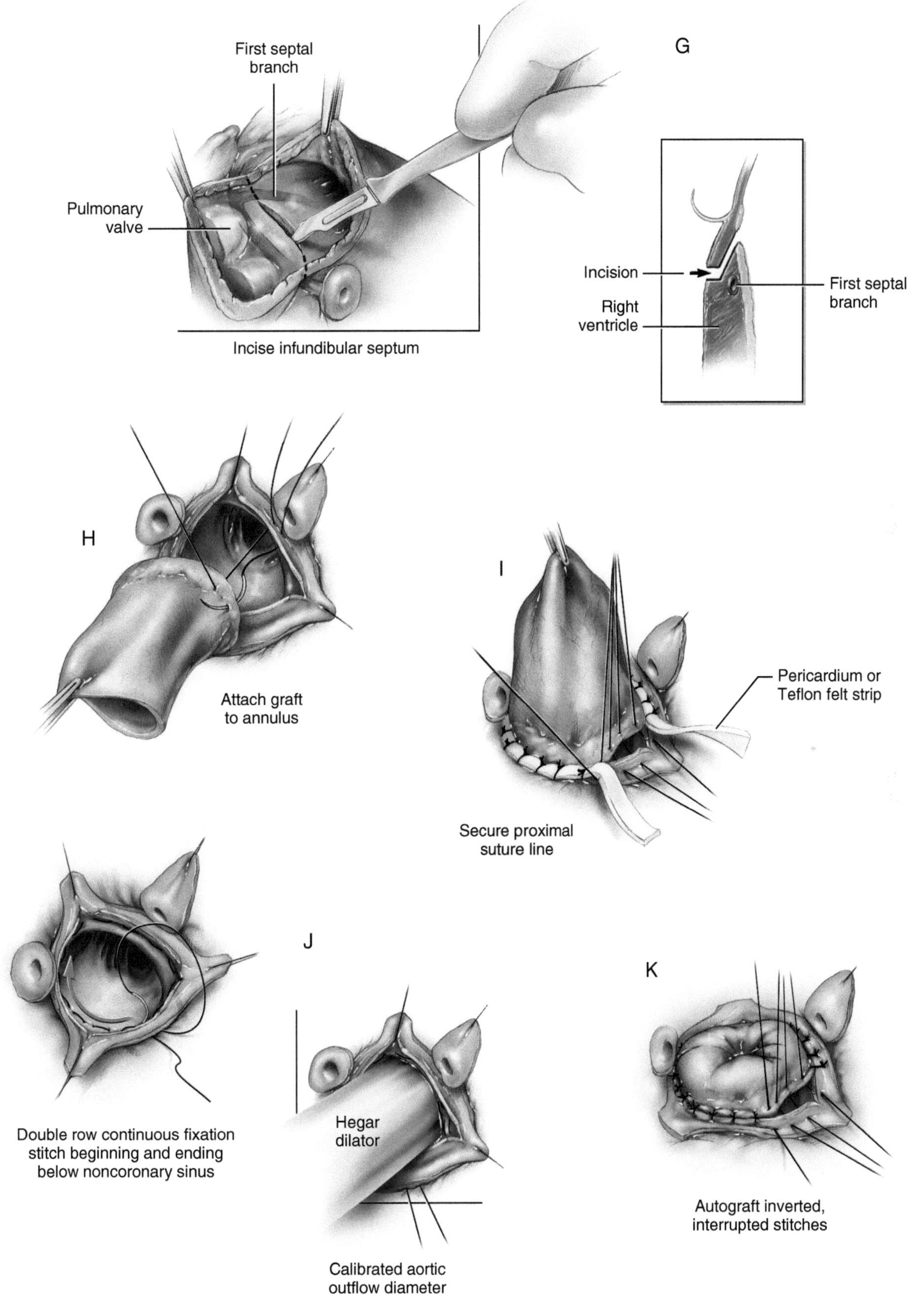
First septal branch
Pulmonary valve
Incise infundibular septum
G
Incision
Right ventricle
First septal branch
H
Attach graft to annulus
I
Pericardium or Teflon felt strip
Secure proximal suture line
J
Double row continuous fixation stitch beginning and ending below noncoronary sinus
Hegar dilator
Calibrated aortic outflow diameter
K
Autograft inverted, interrupted stitches

Figure 31-13 (continued)

L An opening is made into the left coronary sinus of the autograft using a scalpel. Only a minimal strip of sinus tissue is excised from one side of the opening because the delicate pulmonary artery dilates and separates readily. The sinotubular junction of the graft is preserved to maintain the proper relationships of the commissures and leaflets. The left coronary artery anastomosis proceeds, working on the outside of the pulmonary graft. Continuous stitches of 5/0 polypropylene are employed. For convenience, this diagram shows only the right coronary artery anastomosis, but as a practical matter, it is best to perform the right coronary artery anastomosis after completing the aortic anastomosis so that the pulmonary trunk can be temporarily distended by removing the aortic cross-clamp. The right coronary artery anastomosis typically fits above the sinotubular junction on the anterior wall of the pulmonary trunk rather than in the anterior sinus.

M The sinotubular junction of the pulmonary autograft is fixed with a collar of tubular Dacron graft that is the same diameter as the left ventricular outflow tract diameter determined from the CryoLife chart. Three mattress stitches of 5/0 polypropylene are passed from inside the pulmonary trunk to outside of it at the tip of each valve commissure (indicated by the *broken line*). These stitches are passed through the collar at three equidistant points. The collar is then secured to the outside of the pulmonary autograft.

N An end-to-end anastomosis of the pulmonary autograft to the ascending aorta is performed. As mentioned earlier, it is best to perform the aortic anastomosis before the right coronary artery anastomosis so that the proper location of the latter can be determined with the aorta distended. It may also be advisable to anastomose the pulmonary allograft to the bifurcation of the pulmonary artery before the aortic anastomosis is performed if there is any chance that the medial aspect of the pulmonary anastomosis will be obscured by the overlying aorta. Often the diameter of the aorta is larger than that of the pulmonary trunk, but the pulmonary trunk is usually long enough that a bevel can be created to take up any size discrepancy.

In situations with gross aortic enlargement or aneurysm, the entire ascending aorta can be removed and the pulmonary trunk extended with a prosthetic graft, or the aorta can be tailored and wrapped with a prosthesis.

O The cryopreserved pulmonary allograft is trimmed minimally. An end-to-end anastomosis of the pulmonary allograft to the pulmonary artery bifurcation is performed using continuous stitches of 4/0 polypropylene. It is usually preferable to perform this anastomosis before constructing the aortic anastomosis.

P The proximal end of the pulmonary allograft trunk is anastomosed to the right ventricular outflow tract. Continuous stitches of 3/0 polypropylene are used. The inset diagram demonstrates that the needle must penetrate only a partial thickness of the infundibular septum to avoid injuring the underlying first septal branch of the left anterior descending coronary artery. A potentially weak point of the anastomosis at the transition from the infundibular septum to the medial aspect of the right ventricular free wall can be reinforced with a Teflon pledget worked into the suture line.

Q The completed repair produces a remarkably normal anatomic appearance. This series of illustrations has shown the essential steps of the operation, but there are a number of choices when performing the individual components. A useful order of operation is as follows: (1) anastomose the pulmonary autograft to the aortic annulus, (2) connect the left coronary artery to the pulmonary autograft, (3) anastomose the pulmonary allograft to the distal pulmonary artery, (4) anastomose the pulmonary autograft to the ascending aorta, (5) temporarily distend the aorta to determine the proper location for the anastomosis of the right coronary artery to the pulmonary autograft, (6) anastomose the right coronary artery to the pulmonary autograft, (7) connect the proximal end of the pulmonary allograft to the right ventricular outflow tract. Data show that fixation of the diameter of the aortic annulus and fixation of the diameter of the sinotubular junction achieve better long-term competence of the "aortic" valve.

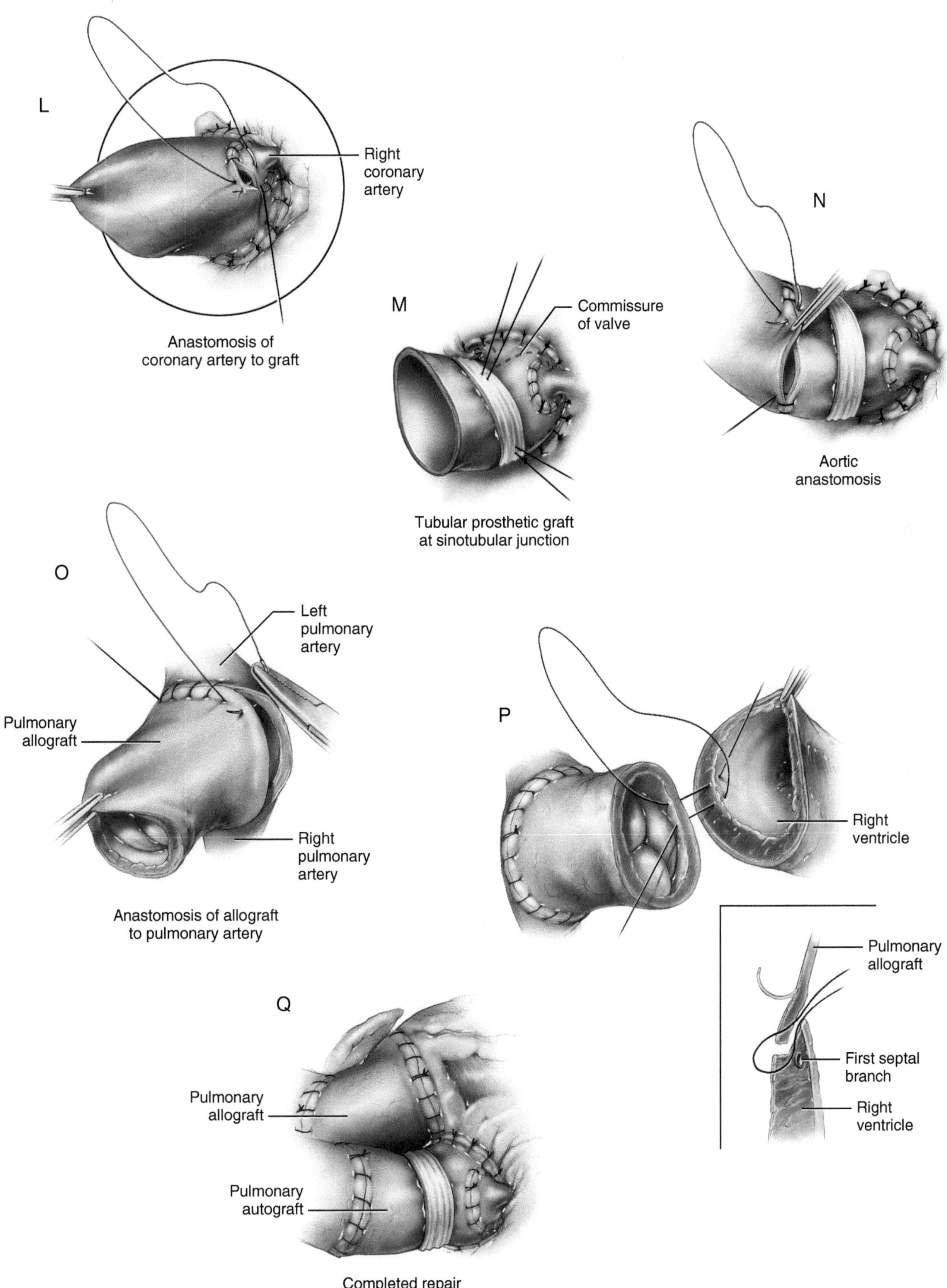
L
Right
coronary
artery
Anastomosis of
coronary artery to graft
M
Commissure
of valve
Tubular prosthetic graft
at sinotubular junction
N
Aortic
anastomosis
O
Left
pulmonary
artery
Pulmonary
allograft
Right
pulmonary
artery
Anastomosis of allograft
to pulmonary artery
P
Right
ventricle
Pulmonary
allograft
First septal
branch
Right
ventricle
Q
Pulmonary
allograft
Pulmonary
autograft
Completed repair

Pulmonary Autograft: Dilated Aortic Annulus

Enlargement of the aortic annulus can present a significant technical challenge when performing aortic valve replacement with pulmonary autograft. The diameter of the pulmonary valve is naturally about 2 mm larger than that of the aortic valve at the annulus. This is usually sufficient to accommodate minor aortic annular dilation. If the aortic annulus exceeds the measured diameter of the pulmonary annulus by 2 mm or more, a tailoring annular reduction is done.

Figure 31-14

A When the diameter of the aortic annulus is 2 to 3 mm greater than that of the pulmonary trunk, an aortic "annuloplasty" is performed. This procedure can correct most cases of variance in annular diameters. It is done by placing a double purse-string suture just below the aortic annulus to fix the diameter of the aortic outflow tract, as described in Figure 31-13, *J*. Another simple method, shown in the inset, is to place interrupted mattress stitches of 2/0 braided suture reinforced with Teflon pledgets through the fibrous tissue that supports the aortic leaflets alongside each of the commissures. The stitches are placed across the interleaflet triangle so that the triangle is obliterated when the sutures are tied down. As described earlier, a chart is used to determine the optimal aortic diameter, and an appropriately sized Hegar dilator is placed in the aortic outflow tract to limit the reduction to the desired aortic diameter as the purse-string or interleaflet triangle sutures are tied.

B The Ross procedure proceeds as usual with suture placement to symmetrically align the aortic annulus and the cuff of the right ventricular outflow tract on the pulmonary autograft.

C The suture line can be supported with a Teflon felt or pericardial strip placed within the suture loops to further control the diameter of the graft and the aorta at the annulus.

D The sutures are tied down over the annular support strip, which fixes the diameter of the aorta and helps prevent dilation of the pulmonary autograft in the aortic position. The coronary arteries are anastomosed to the pulmonary trunk in the usual fashion, beginning with the left coronary artery. The right coronary artery is usually connected to the pulmonary trunk after the aortic anastomosis to ensure proper positioning.

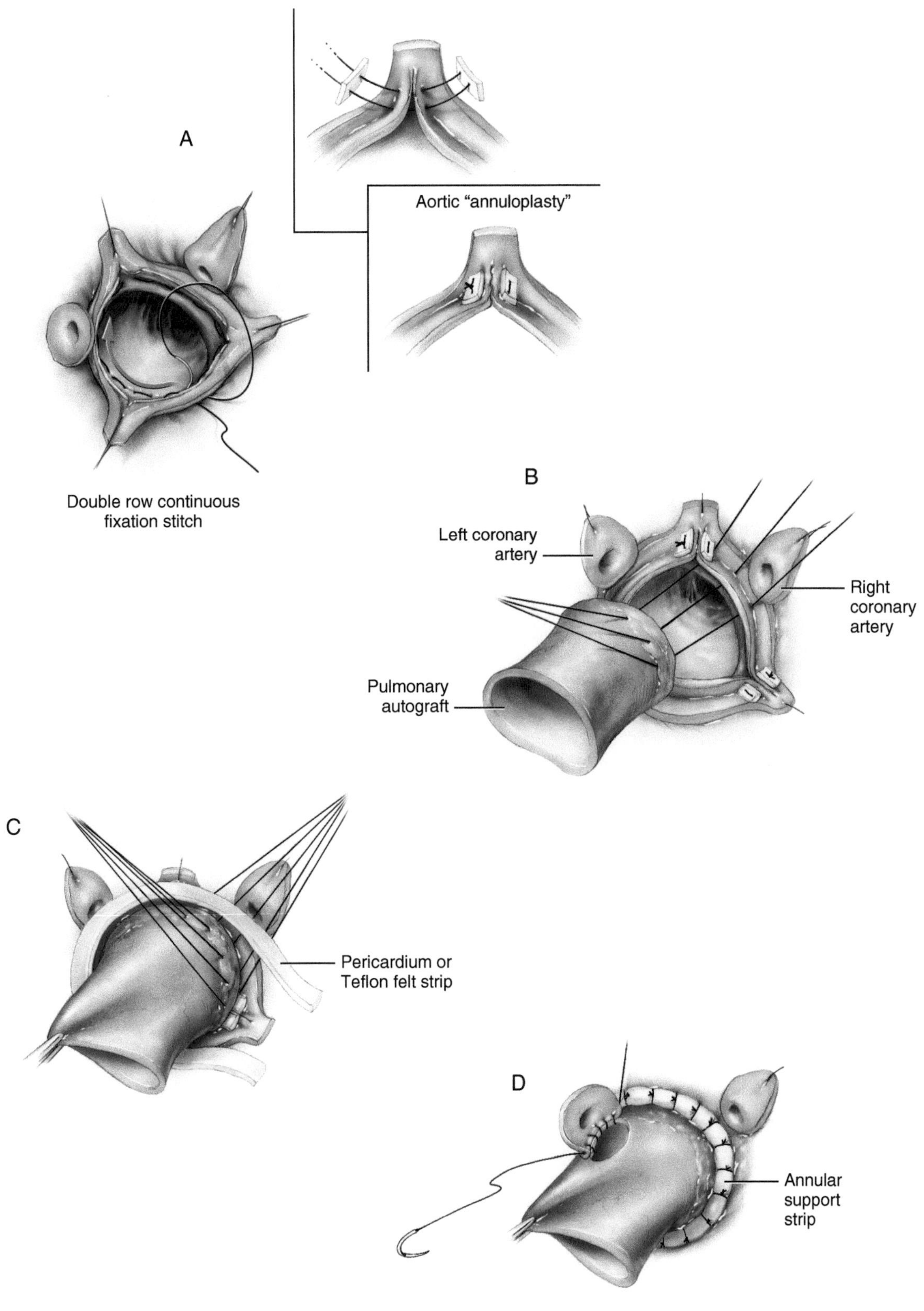
A
Aortic "annuloplasty"
Double row continuous fixation stitch
B
Left coronary artery
Right coronary artery
Pulmonary autograft
C
Pericardium or Teflon felt strip
D
Annular support strip

Pulmonary Autograft: Dilation or Aneurysm of the Ascending Aorta

Matching the distal end of the pulmonary autograft to a dilated or aneurysmal ascending aorta is a common technical problem. The options for repair in this situation include remodeling (reduction) aortoplasty or replacement of the ascending aorta with a prosthetic graft.

Figure 31-15

A A remodeling (reduction) annuloplasty is performed to correct a mild to moderate discrepancy between a dilated ascending aorta and a pulmonary autograft that has been transferred to the aortic position. Tailoring of the pulmonary autograft is not recommended. A wedge excision of the anterior wall of the ascending aorta is performed. Sufficient aorta is removed so that the circumference of the proximal end of the ascending aorta equals the circumference of the distal end of the pulmonary autograft.

B Remodeling of the ascending aorta is accomplished by closing the edges of the aorta anteriorly with 4/0 or 3/0 polypropylene suture, depending on the aorta's thickness. The size of the aorta at the proximal end is reduced to approximate the distal end of the pulmonary autograft. An end-to-end anastomosis of the aorta to the pulmonary autograft can then be performed using continuous stitches of 4/0 polypropylene.

C Patients presenting with a bicuspid aortic valve and dilation or aneurysm of the ascending aorta require special consideration because of the high probability of intrinsic weakness of the aorta. The external surface of the repaired aorta is reinforced with polyester fabric to protect the suture line and to prevent subsequent dilation of the aorta. The fabric is sutured tightly around the aorta with continuous stitches of 3/0 polypropylene.

D Aneurysm of the ascending aorta precludes repair; the aorta should be replaced. A tubular prosthesis of collagen-impregnated, double-velour, knitted Dacron, with a diameter matching that of the distal end of the pulmonary autograft, is selected for replacement of the ascending aorta. The ascending aorta is resected, including all abnormal aorta. An end-to-end anastomosis is constructed to attach the prosthetic graft to the ascending aorta or arch beyond the extent of the aneurysm. An end-to-end anastomosis, using continuous stitches of 4/0 polypropylene, attaches the graft to the pulmonary autograft.

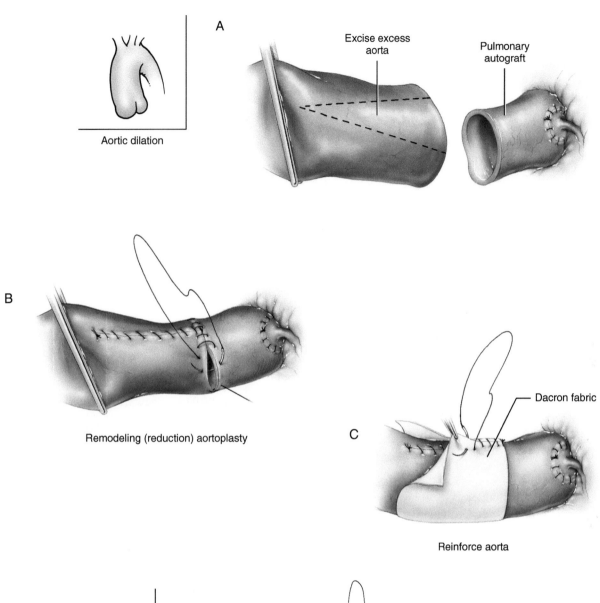

A

Aortic dilation

Excise excess aorta

Pulmonary autograft

B

Remodeling (reduction) aortoplasty

C

Dacron fabric

Reinforce aorta

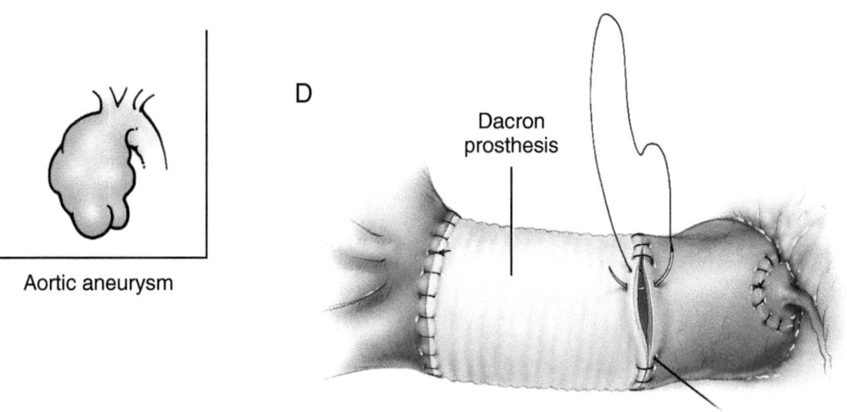

Replace ascending aorta with prosthesis

Pulmonary Autograft: Small Aortic Root (Ross-Konno Procedure)

Aortic root enlargement procedures allow the aortic valve to be replaced with pulmonary autograft in patients with hypoplasia of the left ventricular outflow tract. Enlargement of the aortic root is preferable to forcing the pulmonary autograft into a root that is too small to accommodate it. Enlargement procedures may be required for patients with subvalvular components of left ventricular outflow tract obstruction.

Figure 31-16

A The dashed lines in this illustration show the location of incisions to separate the pulmonary autograft from the right ventricular outflow tract. The usual incision is used when the pulmonary trunk will be implanted in the aortic root at the level of the aortic annulus. An incision that includes more of the anterior wall of the right ventricle may be used when the aortic root–enlarging procedure extends into the ventricular septum.

B The aortic valve is excised in the usual fashion. All of the aortic sinus is removed except for a generous button around the coronary ostia.

C The commissures between the left and right coronary cusps and between the left and noncoronary cusps are excised through the interleaflet triangle. Posteriorly, the excision is above the hinge point of the mitral valve. Entering the interleaflet triangle where the connective tissues are less dense often allows the aortic root diameter to expand sufficiently to accommodate the pulmonary autograft.

D This figure shows the relation of the aortic root to the right ventricular outflow tract after excision of the pulmonary autograft. The relation of the aortic root to the infundibular septum is also readily appreciated. These structures are in close proximity. There is no other operation that demonstrates these relationships so clearly. Additional enlargement of the left ventricular outflow tract is accomplished by incision of the ventricular septum.

E An incision into the ventricular septum greatly widens the left ventricular outflow tract. The increase in diameter of the left ventricular outflow tract is proportional to the length of the septal incision. Deep incision into the ventricular septum is usually not required. The incision is placed through the interleaflet triangle below the right and left coronary leaflets of the aortic valve.

F A longer portion of the anterior wall of the right ventricle is retained on the pulmonary autograft when it is separated from the right ventricular outflow tract. This extra length allows the pulmonary autograft to fill the defect created in the ventricular septum as the proximal suture line attaches the autograft to the left ventricular outflow tract. The pulmonary valve is thereby maintained in an anatomic position at the level of the aortic annulus.

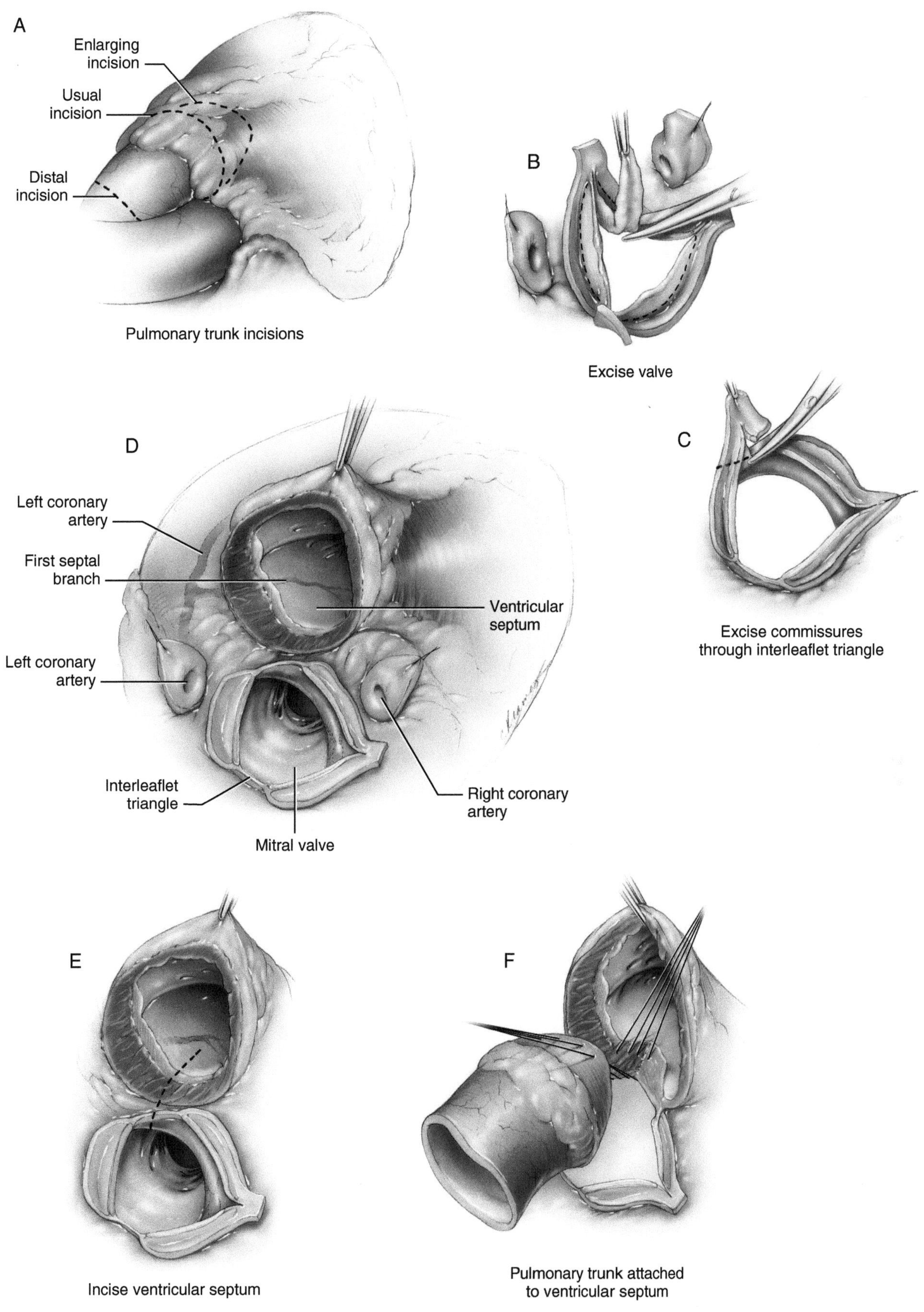

A
Enlarging incision
Usual incision
Distal incision
Pulmonary trunk incisions
B
Excise valve
C
Excise commissures through interleaflet triangle
D
Left coronary artery
First septal branch
Ventricular septum
Left coronary artery
Interleaflet triangle
Mitral valve
Right coronary artery
E
Incise ventricular septum
F
Pulmonary trunk attached to ventricular septum

Apical-Aortic Conduit

Certain patients with aortic stenosis may be unsuitable candidates for traditional open aortic valve replacement due to the hostile anatomy of the aortic root. This may include a porcelain aorta, multiple prior cardiac operations, or various conditions that preclude the use of cardiopulmonary bypass with myocardial arrest. In these individuals, placement of a valved conduit between the left ventricular apex and the descending thoracic aorta relieves the obstruction from aortic stenosis without replacing the aortic valve.

Figure 31-17

A A left thoracotomy is performed to expose both the left ventricular apex and the descending thoracic aorta. The inferior pulmonary ligament is divided to retract the lung superiorly. A retraction suture in the diaphragm is useful for additional exposure. The pericardium is opened in a cruciate fashion, and retention sutures are placed to elevate and stabilize the left ventricular apex.

B The conduit is constructed by attaching a stentless porcine bioprosthetic root in an end-to-end fashion to a Dacron prosthetic graft. Continuous 4/0 polypropylene suture is used for the anastomosis. The porcine root is attached in a similar fashion to the apical connector for later insertion into the left ventricular apex.

C A partial-occlusion clamp is placed on the descending thoracic aorta, and the distal end of the conduit is attached in an end-to-side fashion using continuous 4/0 polypropylene suture. The partial-occlusion clamp is removed to flush air and debris from the conduit.

D Pledgeted, horizontal, braided 0 mattress sutures are placed in a circumferential fashion around the left ventricular apex. A stab wound is made in the apex, and a balloon catheter is inserted into the left ventricular chamber. An appropriately sized coring device is placed over the balloon catheter. Rapid ventricular pacing is used to prevent ejection while the coring device is inserted to remove a section of the apical muscle. The balloon catheter is inflated and gently drawn back to occlude the apical hole.

E The mattress sutures are placed through the sewing ring of the apical connector. The balloon catheter is removed, and the conduit is carefully positioned within the left ventricle by securing the mattress sutures.

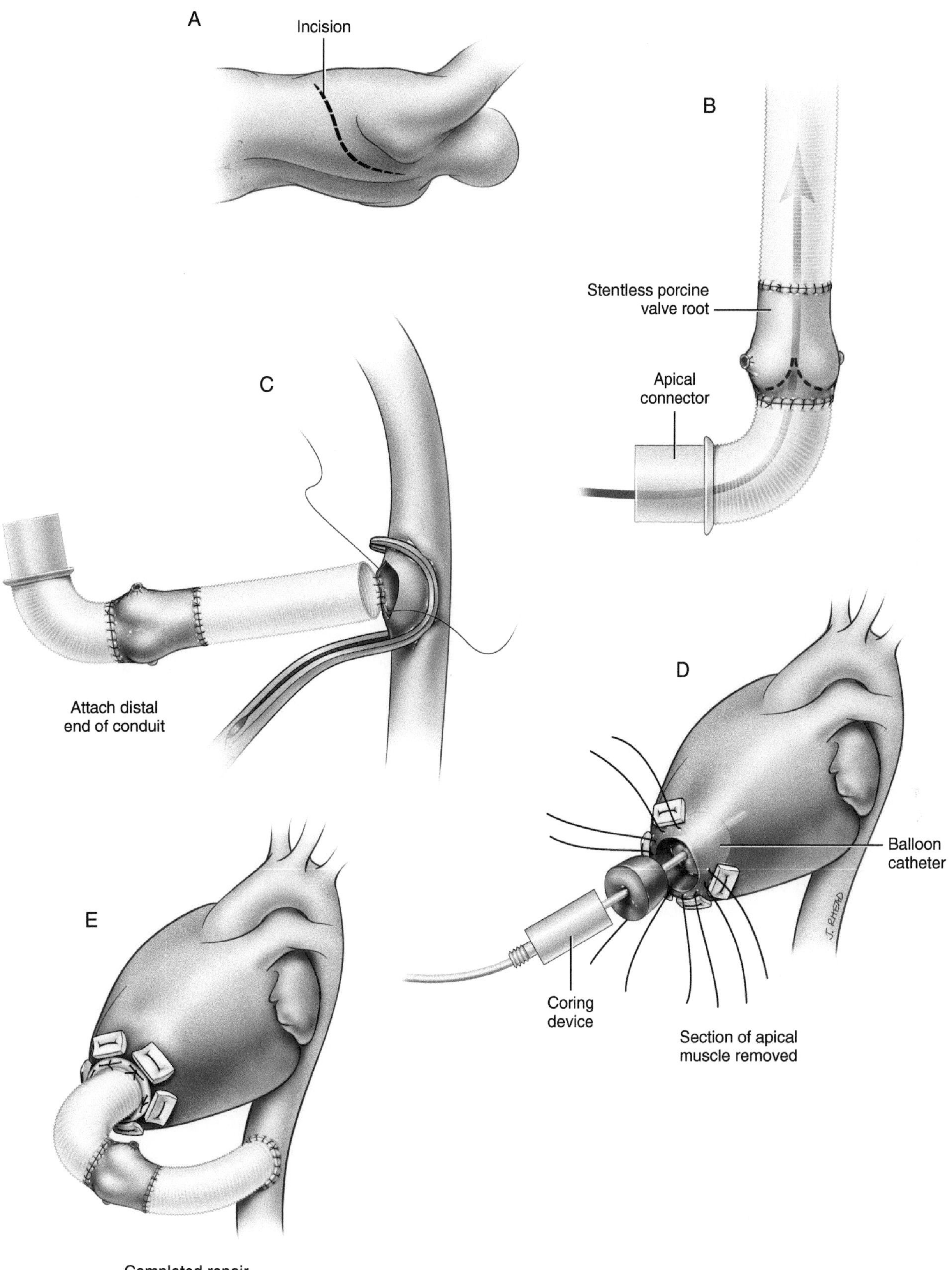
A
Incision
B
Stentless porcine valve root
Apical connector
C
Attach distal end of conduit
D
Balloon catheter
Coring device
Section of apical muscle removed
J. RHEAD
E
Completed repair

Transcatheter Aortic Valve Implantation

Certain patients may be at substantial risk if they undergo standard aortic valve replacement. Catheter-based valve technologies have been developed as a potential solution for these undefined patient populations. The native aortic valve is not excised; rather, the delivery system implants a prosthetic valve within the native valve. These procedures require combined fluoroscopic and echocardiographic guidance and are best performed in a setting where both optimal imaging and operative sterility can be assured.

The suitability of the femoral vessels is critical to the operative approach. If the femoral vessels are of adequate diameter and relatively free of atherosclerotic disease, the transfemoral approach is preferred. The transapical approach is selected for patients with diminutive or heavily diseased femoral vessels.

Figure 31-18

A The common femoral artery is exposed and controlled with vascular snares. Imaging catheters are inserted through the contralateral femoral artery. Fluoroscopic guidance is used to position the stiff guidewire for the valve delivery catheter across the native aortic valve and into the left ventricle. Temporary pacing wires are placed in the right heart for eventual rapid ventricular pacing.

B Balloon aortic valvuloplasty is performed to prepare the annulus. Rapid ventricular pacing is used for precise positioning of the balloon during inflation.

C The valve delivery system is inserted over the stiff guidewire and positioned within the left ventricle. Care is taken to align the valve in exact orientation to avoid tilting or malpositioning.

D Rapid ventricular pacing is again initiated, and the valve is rapidly deployed to seat it within the native aortic annulus. The catheter delivery system is removed.

E The balloon catheter is reinserted and positioned within the prosthetic valve. The balloon is inflated during rapid ventricular pacing to completely expand the prosthetic valve within the annulus.

F Angiography and echocardiography are used to confirm proper valve position, measure transvalvular gradients, and assess valve competence. The femoral artery is repaired in standard fashion.

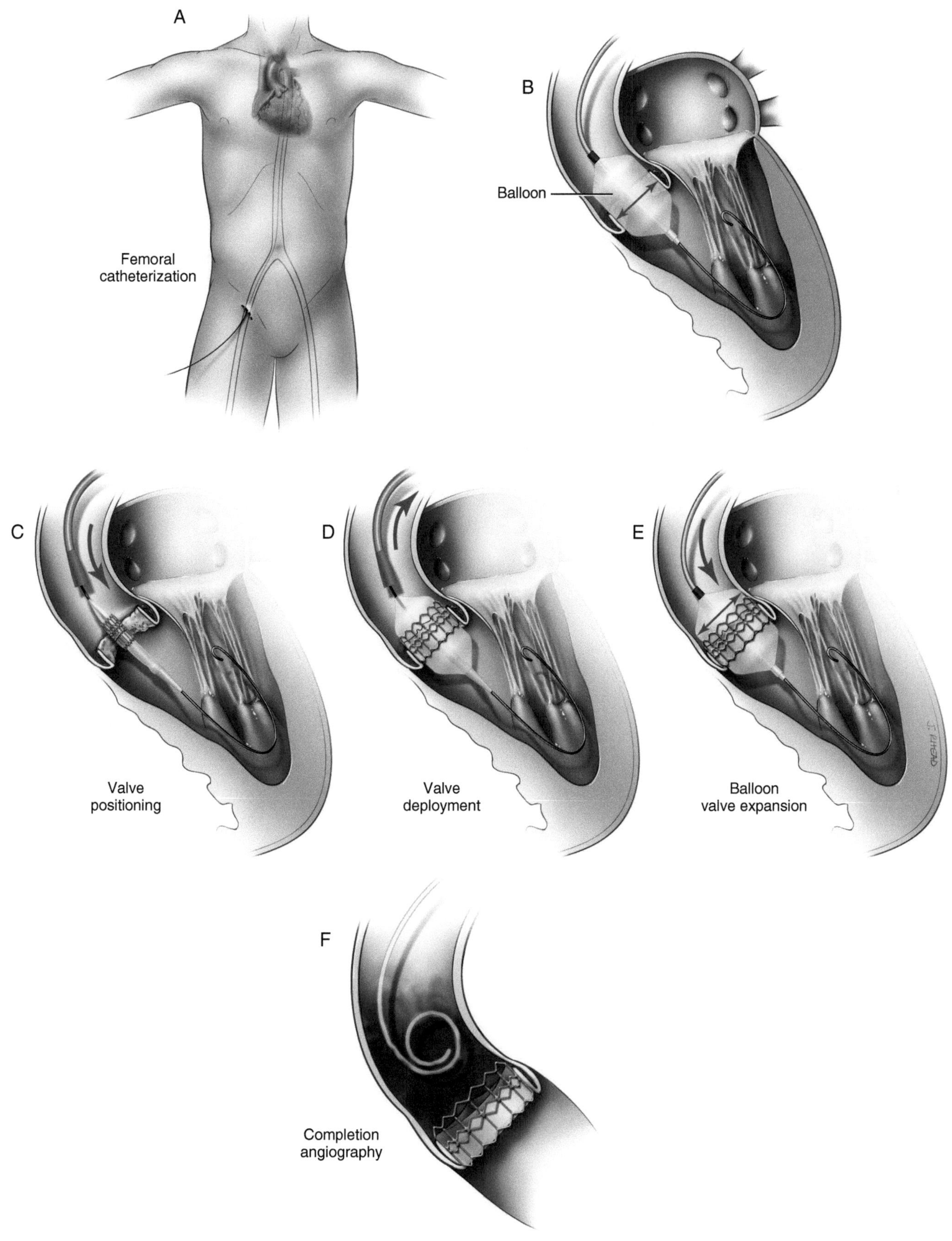
A
Femoral
catheterization
B
Balloon
C
Valve
positioning
D
Valve
deployment
E
Balloon
valve expansion
F
Completion
angiography

Figure 31-18 (continued)

G The transapical approach is selected for patients with hostile femoral anatomy or prior cardiac surgery. An anterior thoracotomy is performed to expose the left ventricular apex. Fluoroscopy and echocardiography are used to determine the ideal location of the incision so that insertion of the transapical delivery system can follow a direct perpendicular line from the apex to the aortic annulus.

H Braided sutures with pledgets are placed in mattress fashion around the left ventricular apex. The apex is punctured with a needle, and a guidewire is inserted through the apex and across the aortic annulus. Successive dilations are performed to accommodate the valve delivery sheath.

I Aortic valvuloplasty is performed by successive balloon inflation during rapid ventricular pacing to prepare the aortic annulus. The balloon catheter is removed.

J The valve delivery system is inserted over the guidewire and positioned within the aortic annulus. Care is taken to align the valve in the exact orientation and avoid excessive torque at the apex, which can result in tearing of the ventricular muscle.

K Rapid ventricular pacing is again initiated, and the valve is rapidly deployed to seat it within the native aortic annulus. The catheter delivery system is removed.

L The balloon catheter is reinserted and positioned within the prosthetic valve. The balloon is inflated during rapid ventricular pacing to completely expand the prosthetic valve within the annulus.

M Angiography and echocardiography are used to confirm proper valve position, measure transvalvular gradients, and assess valve competence. The left ventricular apex is closed by securing the mattress sutures, and a small drain is placed in the left pleural space.

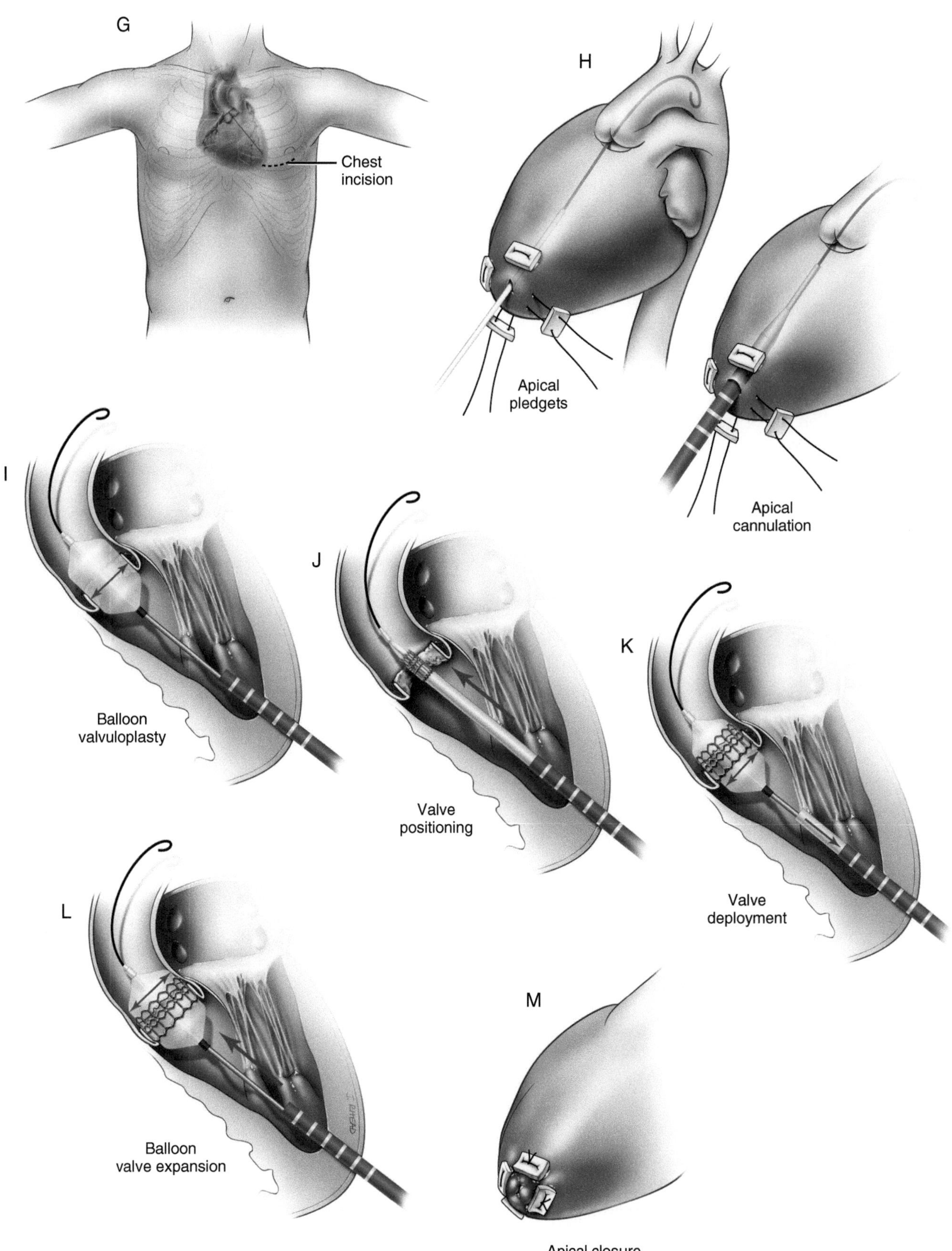
G
Chest incision
H
Apical pledgets
Apical cannulation
I
Balloon valvuloplasty
J
Valve positioning
K
Valve deployment
L
Balloon valve expansion
M
Apical closure

chapter 32 MITRAL VALVE RECONSTRUCTION

Mitral valve reconstruction is desirable for patients with normal sinus rhythm because there is no need for anticoagulation, and hemodynamic performance is enhanced after surgery.

Morphology

Figure 32-1

A Myxomatous degeneration of the mitral valve, autopsy specimen. Leaflets are of variable thickness but are generally thin, with typical "hoods" or bulging.

B Myxomatous degeneration of the mitral valve, magnified. Hooding of leaflet tissue is seen clearly. Chordae tendineae are thin and of normal length in this specimen, but they may be elongated or ruptured.

C Myxomatous degeneration of the mitral valve, showing the leaflet position in systole. An irregular coaptation surface at multiple locations causes valve regurgitation.

D Severe myxomatous degeneration of a surgically excised mitral valve specimen, showing the atrial surface. A reconstructive operation is not feasible due to the extent of disease, extensive hooding, and inadequate approximation of valve leaflets in more than one area.

E Severe myxomatous degeneration of a surgically excised mitral valve, showing the ventricular surface. Note the thick and thin chordae, elongation, and rupture of chordae tendineae.

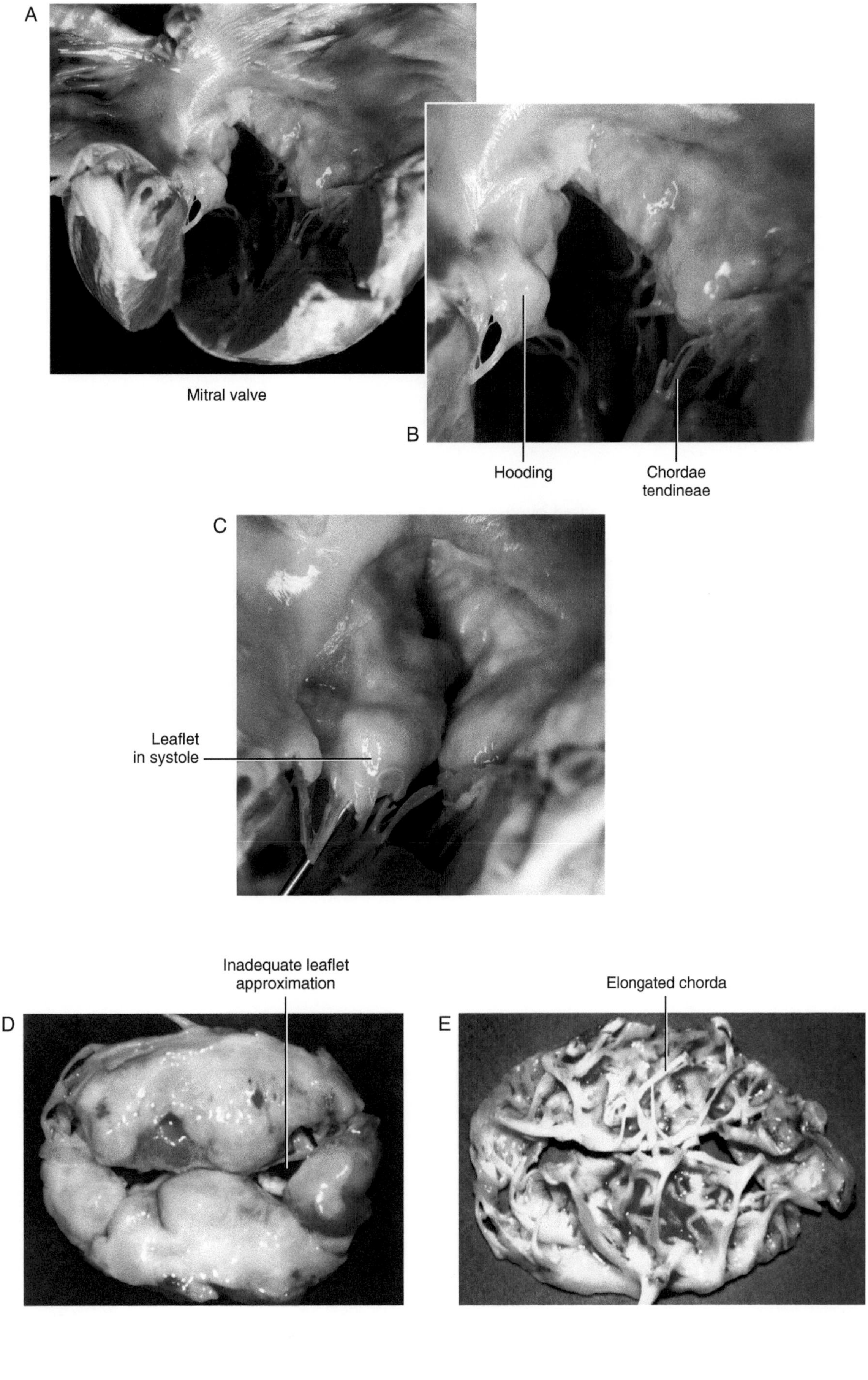

A

Mitral valve

B

Hooding

Chordae tendineae

C

Leaflet in systole

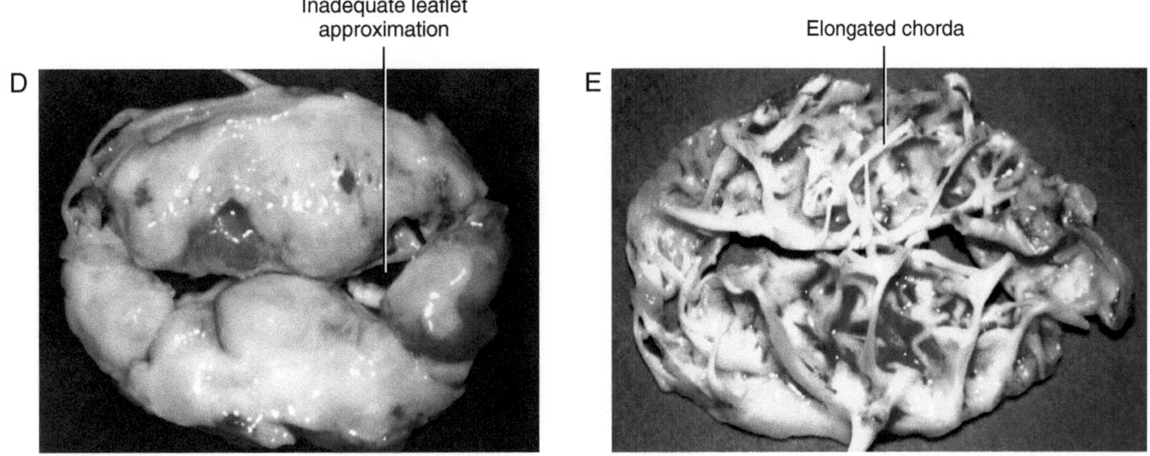

Introduction to Mitral Valve Reconstructive Techniques
Figure 32-2

A The incision is made in the left atrium just posterior to the interatrial groove on the right side. The space between the right inferior pulmonary vein and the inferior vena cava is opened to allow extension of the incision posterior to the vena cava. The decision to perform a superior incision must be weighed carefully against the risk of possible abnormal rhythm after operation.

B In patients with mitral valve stenosis caused by commissural fusion and with reasonably normal subvalvular supporting structures, the commissures of the mitral valve can be divided to relieve the stenosis. The anterior leaflet of the mitral valve must be mobile and long enough to approximate the posterior leaflet. Reasonable mobility and adequate length of the posterior leaflet are also required. The atrial septum is retracted anteriorly to expose the mitral valve. A forceps is used to grasp the anterior and posterior leaflets of the mitral valve opposite the fused commissure. A No. 15 scalpel is used to accurately incise the commissure. A forceps is then used to position the commissure and, with traction, assist in teasing the commissure open accurately. Incision of the mitral valve commissure should be anatomic and as close to the mitral valve annulus as possible without exceeding the anatomic limits of the commissure.

C If necessary, the chordae tendineae and papillary muscles of the mitral valve can be lengthened somewhat by incising the papillary muscle precisely between the chordae tendineae.

D When redundant leaflet tissue appears to be located in a segment of the mitral valve adjacent to a commissure, the mitral valve annulus can be narrowed by placing interrupted pledget-reinforced mattress stitches through the annulus at the commissure and drawing the redundant valve tissue into the mattress stitch at the annulus. This repair is the least controllable and least symmetric and must be done judiciously. In all cases mitral valve competence should be tested by distending the ventricle with isotonic electrolyte solution using a Robinson catheter placed through the valve. This demonstrates any areas of residual leakage, which can be repaired with additional sutures.

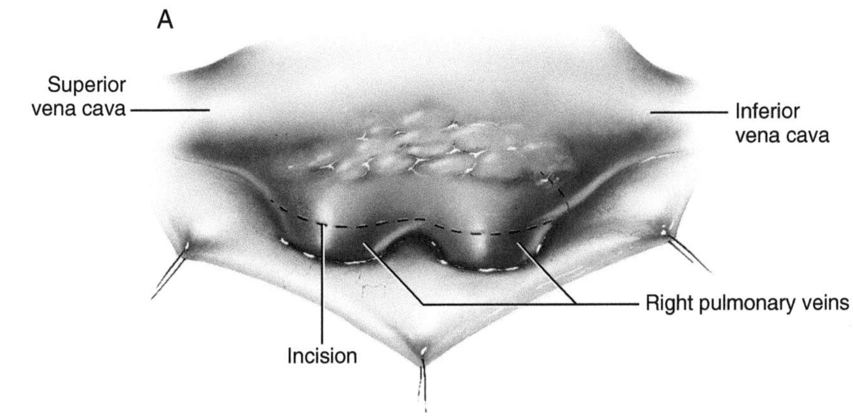

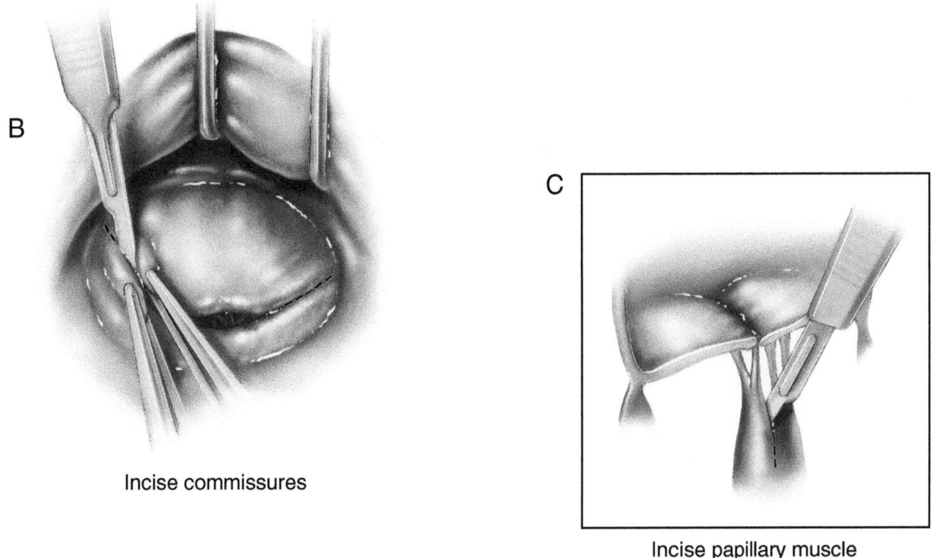

Incise commissures

Incise papillary muscle (chordal lengthening)

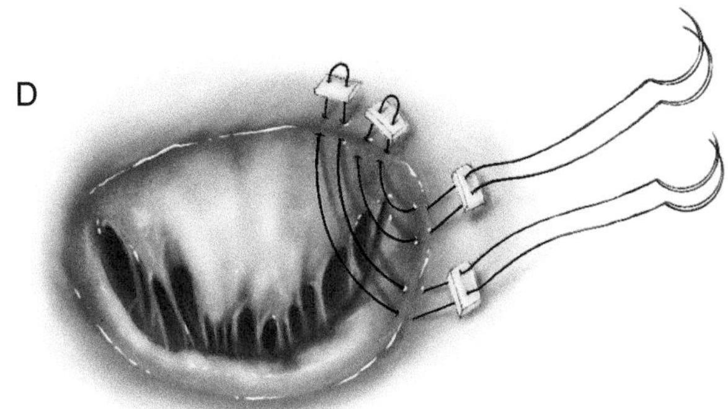

Segmental annuloplasty

Annuloplasty Techniques

Prosthetic devices can be used in repairs of the mitral valve to reduce annular diameter, remodel the shape of the annulus, and support the annulus and stabilize the repair.

Posterior Leaflet Excision and Repair, with or without Annular Support

Figure 32-3

A When major chordae tendineae become detached from the leading edge of the posterior leaflet of the mitral valve, leaflet support is lost, and lengthening of the leaflet in the affected area occurs due to prolapse and valve insufficiency.

B Ruptured chordae tendineae to the posterior leaflet of the mitral valve can be repaired by quadrangular excision of the unsupported, redundant, and prolapsed portion of the mitral valve.

C The defect in the posterior leaflet is repaired by approximation of the annulus with a double-loop stitch of 2/0 braided suture that brings the leaflet edges together.

D The leaflet edges are approximated using interrupted stitches of 4/0 Cardionyl suture. A continuous stitch technique should be avoided because of the risk of dehiscence of the repair. Pledget-reinforced stitches provide maximal strength, but the bulk of the felt interferes with leaflet motion.

E The repair is supported with a segmental annuloplasty. The support is provided by a portion of a flexible annuloplasty ring. Alternative materials such as pericardium, Teflon felt, or braided Dacron tape can be used.

F For cases of ruptured chordae to the posterior leaflet without extensive leaflet redundancy, the unsupported leaflet can be excised in a triangular fashion back to the annulus.

G The defect in the posterior leaflet is repaired by accurate edge-to-edge approximation of the leaflet with interrupted stitches of 4/0 Cardionyl suture.

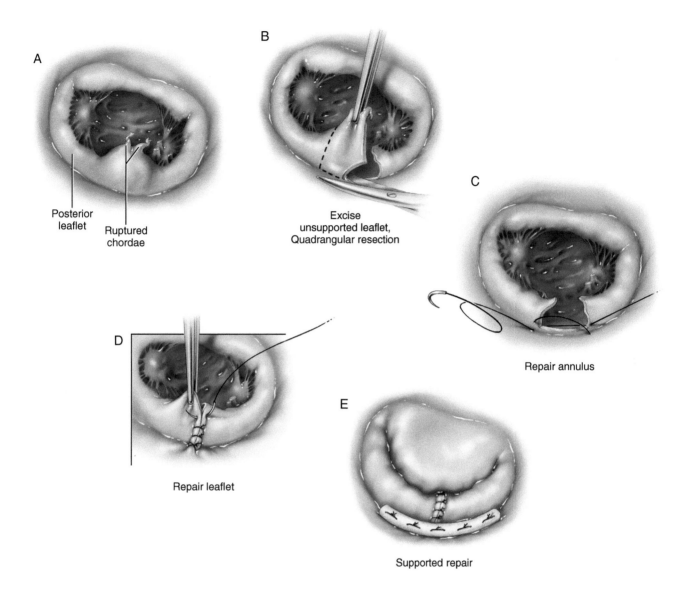

A

Posterior leaflet

Ruptured chordae

B

Excise unsupported leaflet, Quadrangular resection

C

Repair annulus

D

Repair leaflet

E

Supported repair

F

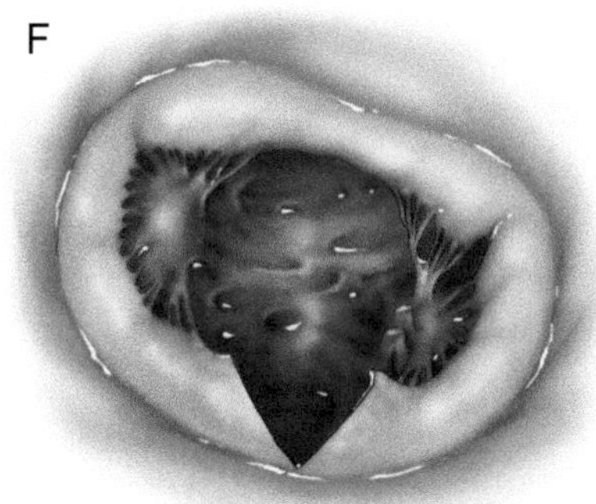

Triangular resection

G

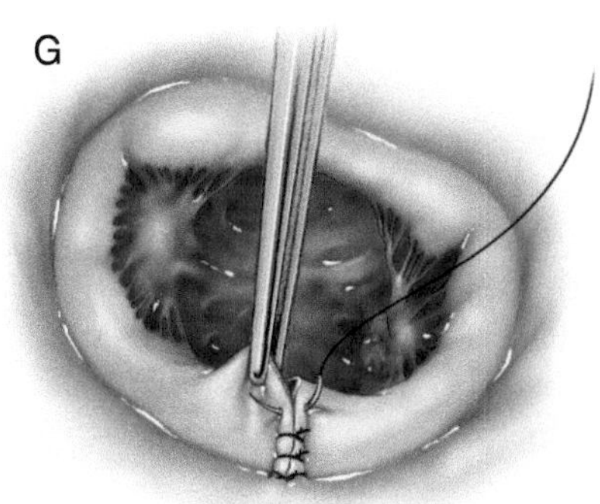

Repair leaflet

Ring Annuloplasty

Prosthetic ring annuloplasty can be used to reduce annular diameter, reshape the annulus, and strengthen the annular support of a valve leaflet repair. The prosthetic device may be a true circumferential ring or a partial ring designed to reduce only the annulus supporting the posterior leaflet. Prosthetic rings may be rigid or semi-rigid, designed to remodel the shape of the annulus of the mitral valve. Prosthetic ring size can be determined by a variety of methods, depending on the prosthetic device chosen for the repair. Methods of sizing are based on the length of the septal (anterior) leaflet at its annular connection because this dimension remains relatively unchanged during annular dilatation, which occurs almost exclusively in the annulus supporting the posterior leaflet at the free wall of the left ventricle. Sizing devices use the commissures of the mitral valve or the fibrous trigones as reference points. The surface area of the anterior leaflet should also be considered.

Figure 32-4

Reduction Annuloplasty

A Mitral valve incompetence may be the result of annular dilatation. Valve leaflet tissue is often nearly normal. Annular reduction by ring annuloplasty produces the most symmetric reconstruction.

B Interrupted sutures of 2/0 braided synthetic material with double-end needles are used. The stitches are placed into fibrous trigones and along the fibrous tissue of the annulus. Large bites of the annulus are taken, and the needles are passed close together through the partial ring prosthesis.

C As the sutures are tied down to approximate the prosthetic ring to the mitral valve annulus, the annular diameter is reduced and its contour is improved. The anterior leaflet is drawn posteriorly into approximation with the posterior leaflet. The repair allows the leaflet tissue to approximate in an anatomic fashion. This type of repair preserves much of the annular flexibility. The competence of the repair is tested by injecting electrolyte solution through a catheter into the left ventricle.

Remodeling Annuloplasty

D Rigid or semirigid (Carpentier) rings have been designed to reshape the annulus of the mitral valve to achieve competent valve function. These devices produce predictable results because the principle of repair is based on actually changing the shape of the annulus (remodeling). Being rigid, these devices change the shape of the tissues rather than conforming to existing tissue conditions or the tension applied on the sutures used to attach the device to the annulus. The size of the prosthesis is determined by device-specific sizers that measure the distance between the commissures anteriorly, allowing this distance to be compared to the surface area of the anterior leaflet. The ring is attached to the mitral annulus with double-needle 2/0 braided suture. The suture is passed through the fibrous tissue of the annulus, taking up more tissue than annuloplasty ring as the needles are passed through the device. Marks on the device correspond to the position of the commissures for proper orientation.

E The device is slid down over the sutures to the annulus, and the sutures are tied firmly, attaching the device to the annulus. The device completely remodels the shape of the mitral annulus, forcing the posterior leaflet forward to approximate the anterior leaflet of the mitral valve.

Remodeling Annuloplasty for Ischemic Mitral Valve Regurgitation

F Studies have shown that saddle-shaped remodeling annuloplasty rings can reproduce normal mitral annular geometry and reduce leaflet stress and chordal strain. This results in longer durability of mitral valve repair, especially in cases of mitral valve regurgitation due to myocardial ischemia. Three-dimensional (3-D) rings are attached using accurately placed mattress stitches of 2/0 braided polyester. Reference markers on the 3-D ring are guides to the location of the mitral valve commissures and the midposition on the posterior leaflet.

G The completed repair shows that the 3-D ring not only reshapes the orifice but also elevates the position of the anterior annulus somewhat higher than the rise in the posterior annulus.

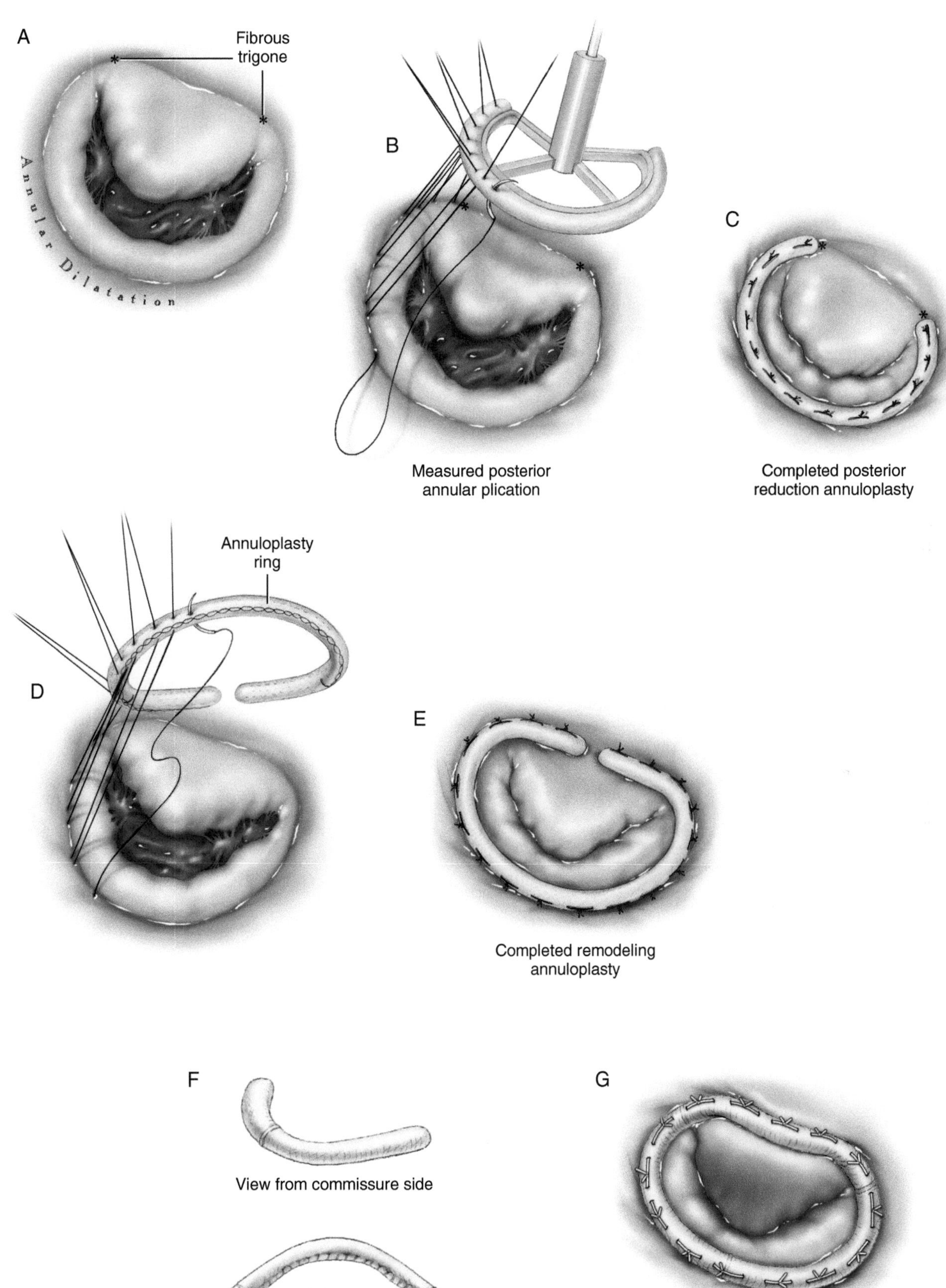
A
Fibrous
trigone
Annular Dilatation
B
Measured posterior
annular plication
C
Completed posterior
reduction annuloplasty
D
Annuloplasty
ring
E
Completed remodeling
annuloplasty
F
View from commissure side
View from posterior leaflet side
G
Completed 3-D
remodeling annuloplasty

Sliding Valvuloplasty with Remodeling Annuloplasty
Figure 32-5

A Repair of the mitral valve in patients with advanced myxomatous degeneration and excessive leaflet tissue (Barlow's syndrome) requires special attention. The usual remodeling annuloplasty techniques may result in systolic anterior motion and left ventricular outflow tract obstruction. Excessive posterior leaflet tissue should be removed to avoid this complication. The condition is recognized by noting that the posterior leaflet is too wide as well as too long. The central portion of the posterior leaflet is resected, along with a curving wedge resection of the annulus on each side involving about half the posterior leaflet or all the widened portion of the valve (indicated by the *broken line* in the figure).

B The repair is facilitated by the placement of annuloplasty stitches for attachment of the annuloplasty ring. Interrupted mattress stitches of 2/0 polyester are placed at the hinge point of the valve leaflet and the annulus, passing the needles from the ventricular side into the atrium. With the valve leaflet detached, exposure is enhanced for accurate suture placement.

C The sutures are divided into two groups at the midpoint of the posterior annulus. Traction placed on the sutures reduces the size of the annulus, making it easy to approximate the cut ends of the valve leaflet. It also provides excellent exposure for the valve repair.

D The cut edges of the posterior leaflet are reattached to the posterior annulus by continuous stitches of 4/0 Cardionyl. The posterior leaflet is advanced along the annulus (sliding valvuloplasty) to the midpoint posteriorly, where the edges of the valve should meet.

E The edges of the posterior leaflet are repaired with interrupted stitches of 4/0 Cardionyl.

F The repair is supported and the annulus is remodeled with a rigid or semirigid annuloplasty ring attached to the annulus with interrupted mattress stitches of 2/0 braided suture.

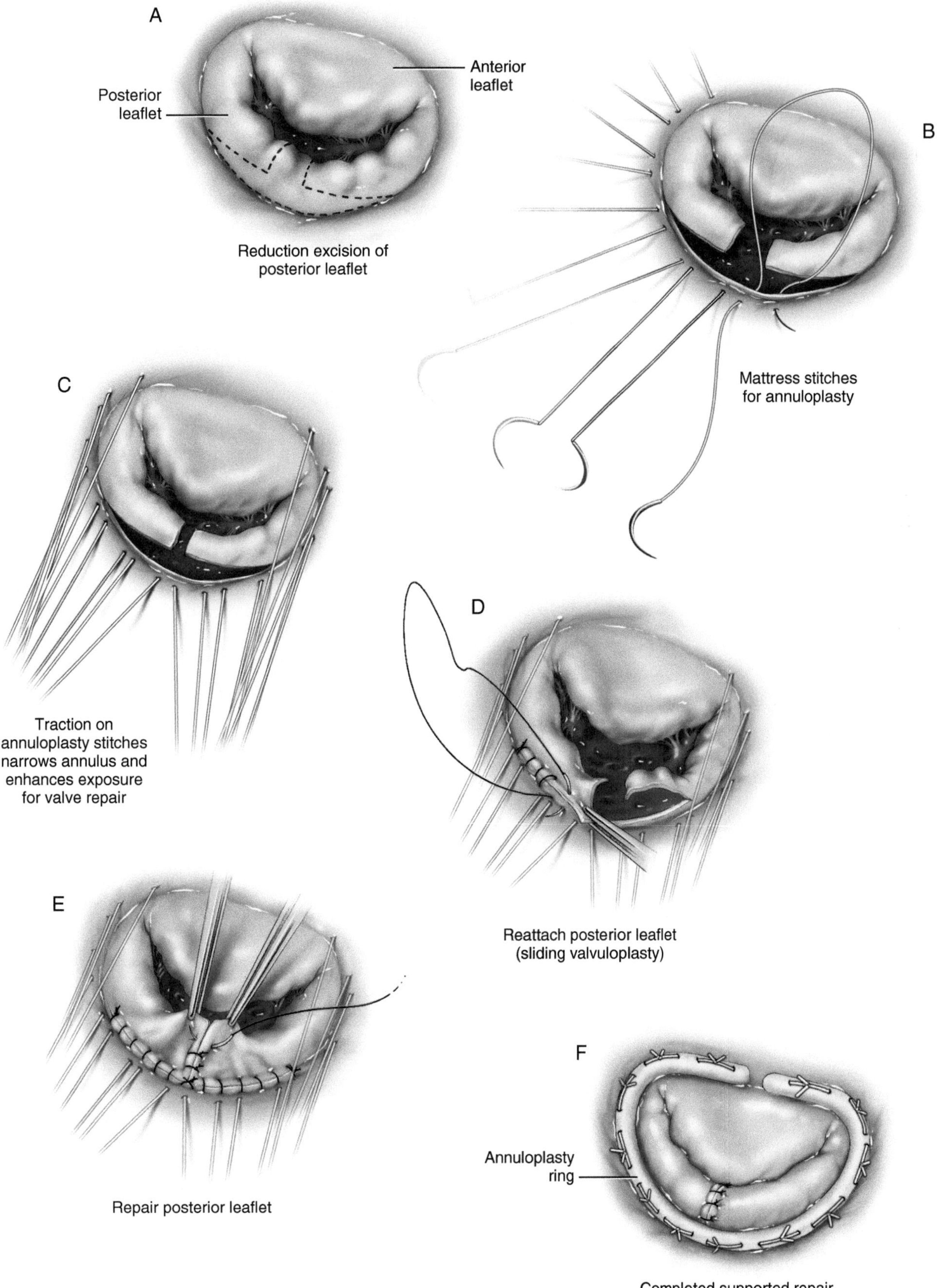
A
Posterior leaflet
Anterior leaflet
Reduction excision of posterior leaflet
B
Mattress stitches for annuloplasty
C
Traction on annuloplasty stitches narrows annulus and enhances exposure for valve repair
D
Reattach posterior leaflet (sliding valvuloplasty)
E
Repair posterior leaflet
F
Annuloplasty ring
Completed supported repair

Anterior Leaflet Augmentation

The mitral valve may be damaged by rheumatic disease, phentermine and fenfluramine (phen-fen) toxicity, or previous operation for partial atrioventricular septal defect, resulting in insufficient width of the anterior leaflet or scarring of the posterior leaflet, such that there is inadequate valve tissue for coaptation of the leaflets. The chordae tendineae supporting the anterior leaflet may be normal or nearly normal. Anterior leaflet augmentation provides a means of restoring mitral valve function in these cases by creating sufficient width of the anterior leaflet to approximate the posterior leaflet. Note that this morphology is the opposite of Barlow's valve, in which there is excessive posterior leaflet tissue.

Figure 32-6

A The anterior leaflet of the mitral valve demonstrates scarring at the A2 segment and along the free edge. The posterior leaflet is scarred in the P2 segment. Scar contraction has resulted in inadequate approximation of the leaflets, with central mitral valve regurgitation. The broken line defines the area for posterior leaflet resection.

B Part of the P2 segment of the posterior leaflet has been removed. Mattress stitches of 2/0 braided suture are placed in the annulus of the mitral valve. The broken line demonstrates the incision to be made in the anterior leaflet.

C All the annuloplasty stitches are in place. Traction on these stitches reduces the diameter of the mitral annulus. The anterior leaflet has been incised, and the edges of the incision separate. The defect in the posterior leaflet is brought together by tension on adjacent annuloplasty stitches. The posterior leaflet is repaired by interrupted stitches of 4/0 Cardionyl and reinforced by a double-loop stitch of 2/0 braided suture at the annulus.

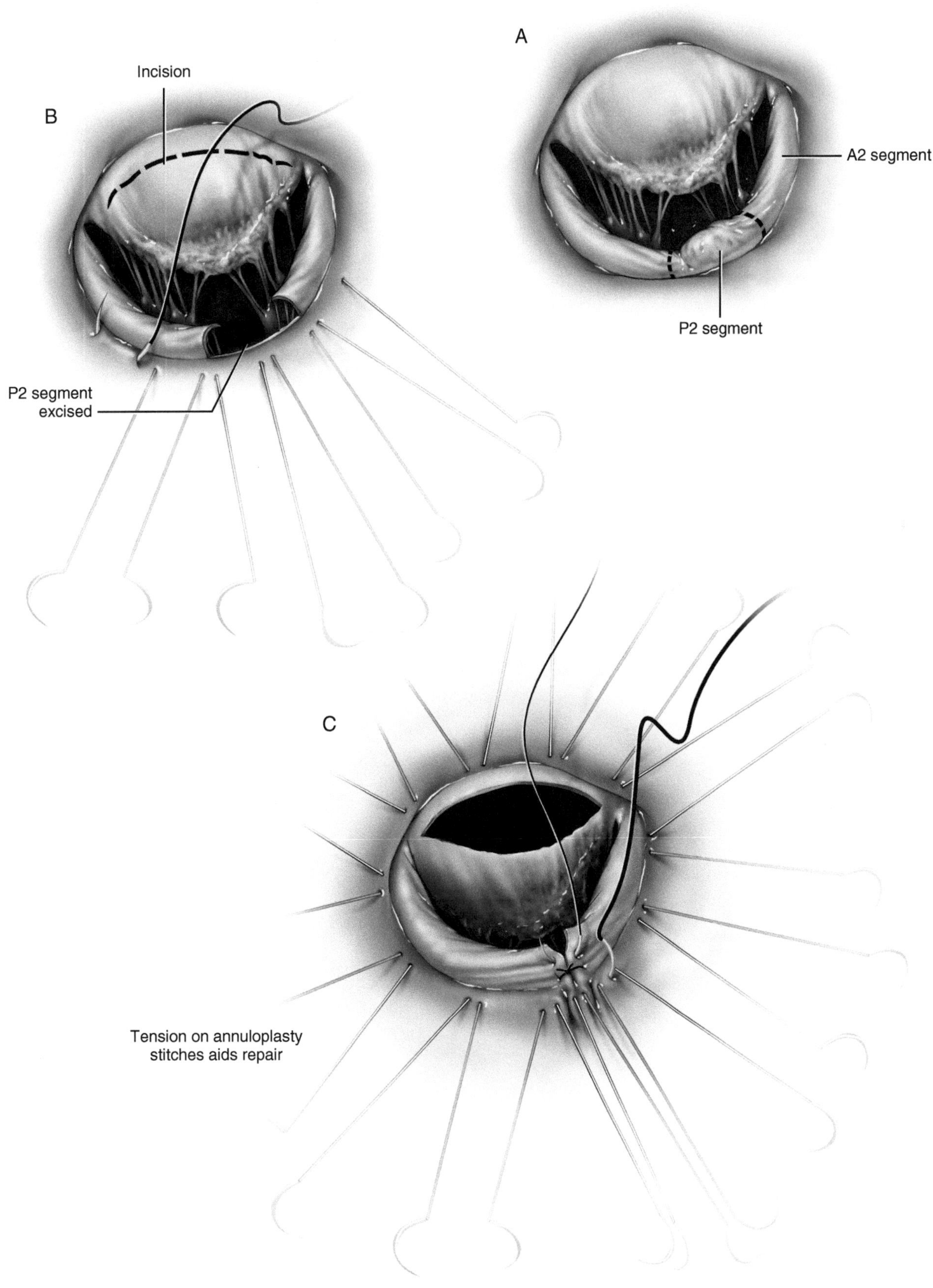
A
A2 segment
P2 segment
B
Incision
P2 segment excised
C
Tension on annuloplasty stitches aids repair

Figure 32-6 (continued)

D A patch of autogenous pericardium taken from the anterior pericardial sac is soaked in glutaraldehyde solution. The patch is used to repair the defect created in the anterior leaflet. A continuous stitch of 4/0 Cardionyl is used for the repair. This augmentation of the anterior leaflet has the effect of widening it so that it can appose the posterior leaflet. It also increases the leaflet's flexibility.

E Annuloplasty stitches are placed through a complete annuloplasty ring to remodel the annulus and reduce it to the proper dimensions. The completed repair is illustrated.

F Operative photograph of anterior leaflet augmentation and incision of the anterior leaflet, as described in **C**.

G Operative photograph of completed anterior leaflet augmentation repair. There is ample anterior leaflet to appose the posterior leaflet and achieve valve competence.

D

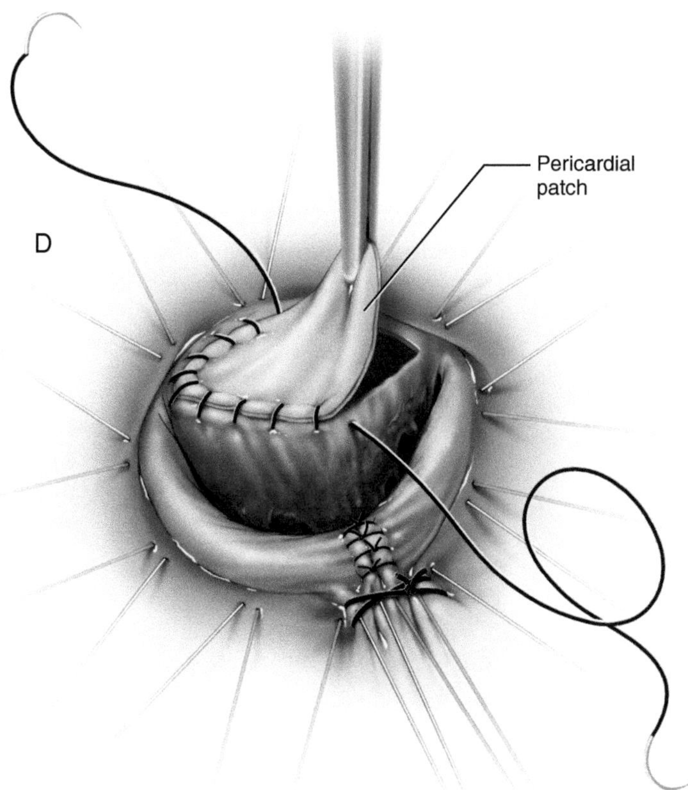

E

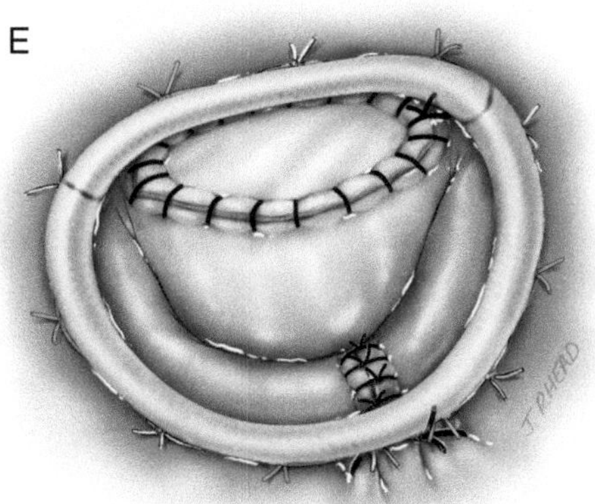

Completed anterior leaflet augmentation

F

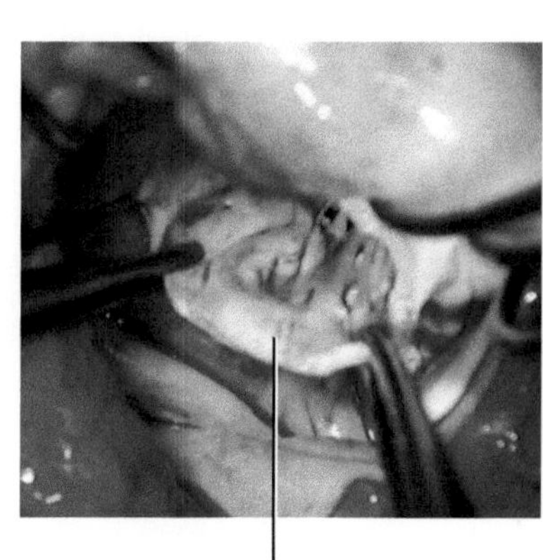

G

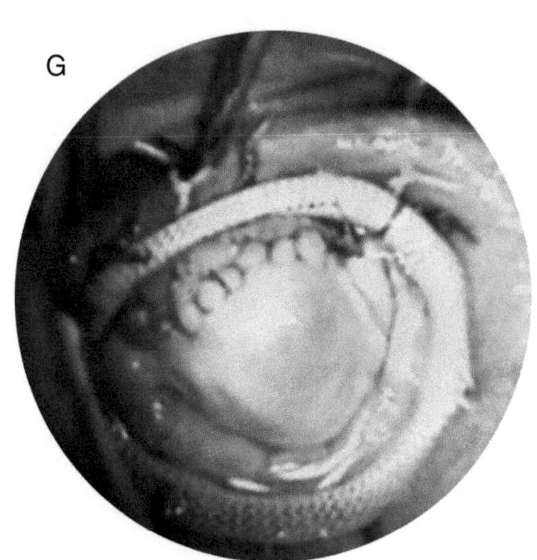

Completed repair

Repair of Elongated or Ruptured Chordae Tendineae

Prolapsed leaflets may be associated with elongated, redundant chordae tendineae or ruptured chordae tendineae. Chordal shortening techniques have largely been replaced by the use of artificial chordae tendineae.

Chordae Tendineae Replacement and Chordal Transfer Techniques

Figure 32-7

A Elongated or ruptured chordae are resected. Chordal replacement is performed using double-needle 5/0 PTFE suture.

B A figure-eight stitch (double loop) is placed through tough fibrous tissue at the tip of the appropriate papillary muscle. The needles are then passed through the leading edge of the prolapsed leaflet more than once to reef up the valve tissue back to the apposing edge of the leaflet. Several artificial chordae may be required to support the leaflet tissue.

C After all the stitches are in place, a valve hook or guyline stitch is used to elevate the apposing edge of the leaflet to the level of the apposing, nonprolapsed leaflet to determine the appropriate length of the artificial chordae. While maintaining the position of the hook, the chordal replacement stitches are tied. Tying PTFE accurately without slippage is the most difficult and uncontrollable step of the procedure. Various techniques have been suggested, including temporarily placing a hemoclip on the suture to secure the length of the suture loop while multiple knots are applied and then removing the clip. Other methods involve using measured, preformed PTFE loops and attaching them individually; although this technique may be more reproducible, it seems more difficult and time-consuming.

D Repairing the ruptured chordae to the anterior leaflet by resecting the unsupported leaflet may substantially reduce the area of the anterior leaflet.

E One method of replacing the anterior leaflet tissue lost during resection of the unsupported leaflet is to mobilize the apposing posterior leaflet and transfer it to the space occupied by the resected anterior leaflet. The resected edges of the anterior leaflet are marked with fine polypropylene suture for reference.

F The posterior leaflet to be transferred anteriorly is retained with fine polypropylene suture. The posterior leaflet tissue is rotated anteriorly with the supporting chordae attached.

G The transposed posterior leaflet tissue is used to repair the defect in the anterior leaflet. The edges of the leaflets are joined using interrupted stitches of 4/0 Cardionyl. Pledgets are not used. A double-loop stitch of 2/0 braided suture is placed to shorten the annulus posteriorly and bring the edges of the posterior leaflet together.

H The repair is completed by approximating the edges of the posterior leaflet with 4/0 Cardionyl suture. The repair is supported by an annuloplasty ring, which fixes the size of the annulus for long-term valve competence and reduces tension on the repair.

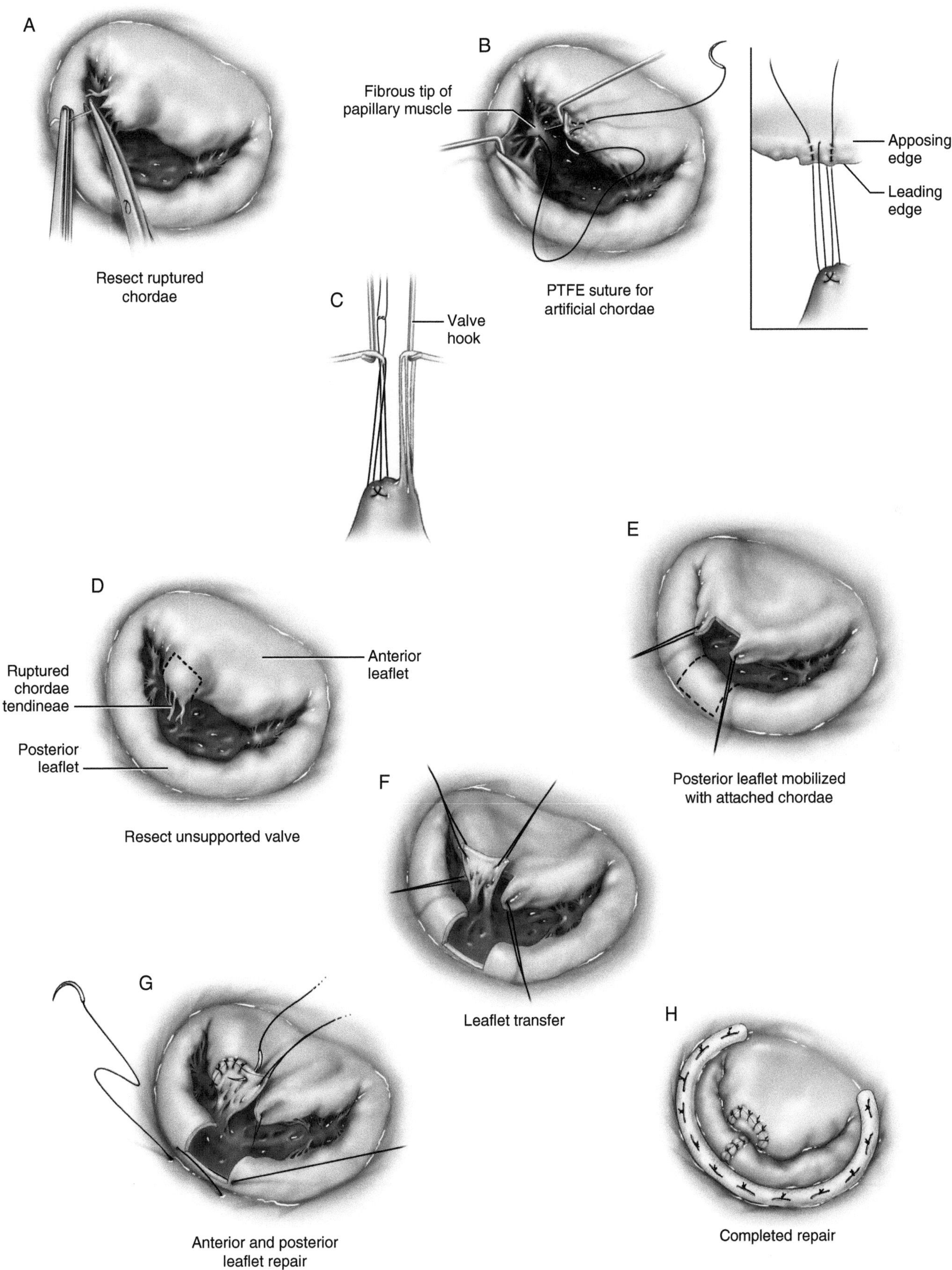
A
Resect ruptured chordae
B
Fibrous tip of papillary muscle
PTFE suture for artificial chordae
Apposing edge
Leading edge
C
Valve hook
D
Ruptured chordae tendineae
Posterior leaflet
Anterior leaflet
Resect unsupported valve
E
Posterior leaflet mobilized with attached chordae
F
Leaflet transfer
G
Anterior and posterior leaflet repair
H
Completed repair

chapter 33 MITRAL VALVE REPLACEMENT

Mitral valve replacement is performed when the mitral leaflet tissues are thickened or calcified to the point that repair is impossible, likely to result in inadequate hemodynamic performance of the valve, or unlikely to be long lasting.

Morphology

Valves that do not qualify for repair and must be replaced have often been damaged by the rheumatic process. This manifests as marked thickening and scarring of leaflet tissue, with reduction of leaflet mobility; thickening and shortening of supporting chordae tendineae, fixing the leaflets to the papillary muscles and further reducing leaflet mobility; and calcification of leaflets. Some extreme cases of myxomatous degenerative disease may result in marked deformity of the valve leaflets and thinning and lengthening of chordae tendineae, making repair unpredictable and even undesirable.

Figure 33-1

A Operative specimen of rheumatic-type mitral valve stenosis and regurgitation. The leaflets are thick, and the commissures are fused. There is inadequate leaflet tissue to close the mitral orifice.

B Operative specimen of rheumatic-type mitral valve stenosis and regurgitation, viewed from the ventricular aspect to demonstrate leaflet supporting structures. Chordae tendineae are markedly thickened and shortened.

C Operative specimen of mitral valve regurgitation due to severe myxomatous degeneration. The specimen shows marked "hooding" of leaflet tissue and inadequate leaflet tissue to close the mitral orifice.

D Operative specimen of mitral valve regurgitation due to severe myxomatous degeneration, viewed from the ventricular aspect to demonstrate leaflet support. Chordae tendineae are thinned and degenerated, with no uniformity. Such chordae would not likely support a valve repair for very long.

E Operative photograph of rheumatic-type mitral valve stenosis and regurgitation. The mitral leaflets are scarred, thickened, and calcified; the commissures are fused. Repair of this type of valve would not restore leaflet flexibility and mobility to provide adequate hemodynamic performance.

A

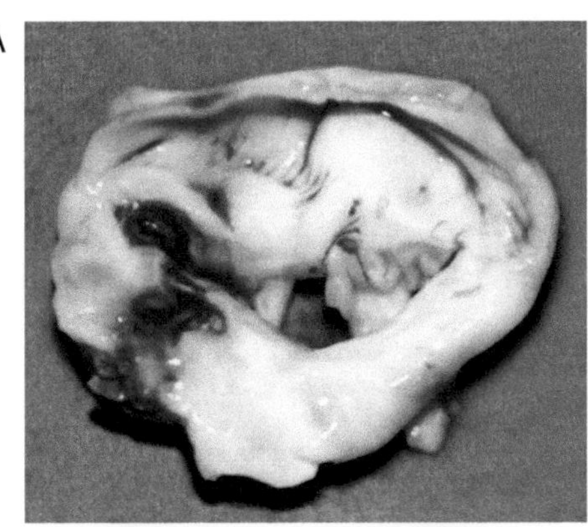

Mitral stenosis and regurgitation, rheumatic type, fused commissures

B

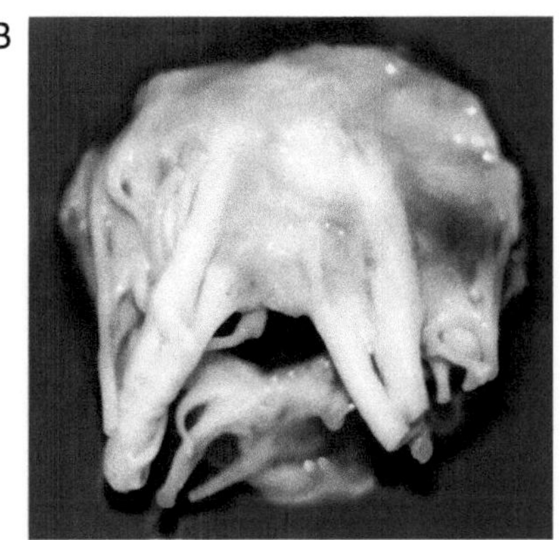

Mitral stenosis and regurgitation, rheumatic type, thick, short chordae tendineae

C

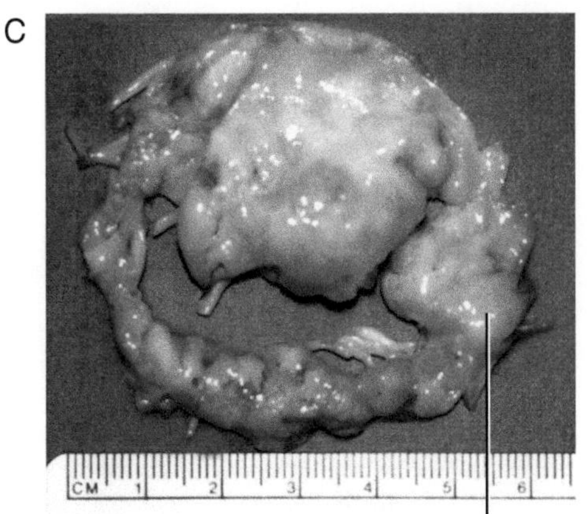

Myxomatous degeneration with "hooding"

D

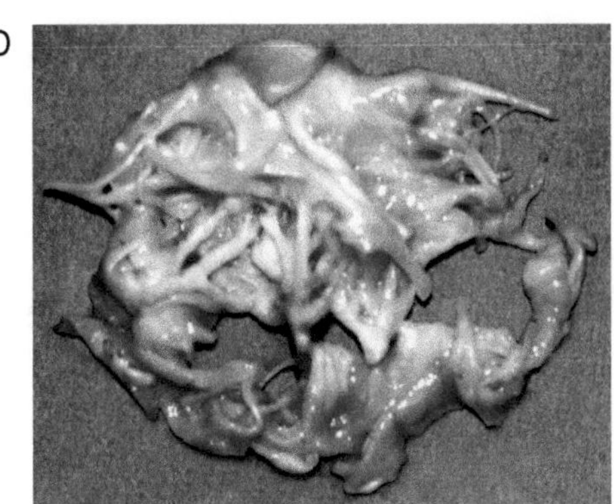

Myxomatous degeneration with thin chordae tendineae

E

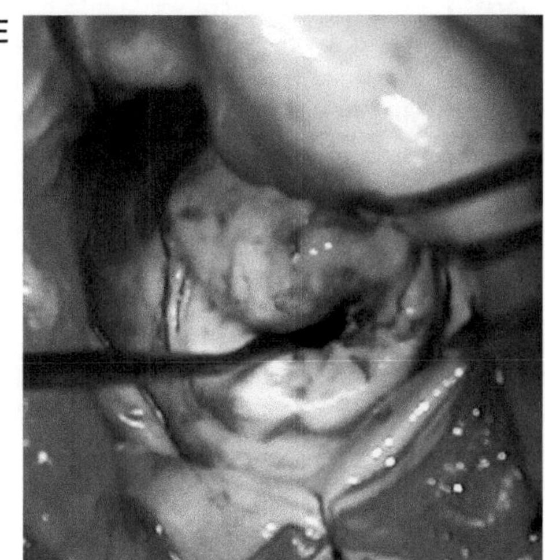

Mitral stenosis and regurgitation with thick, calcified leaflets and fused commissures, reducing valve mobility

Incisions

Mitral valve replacement operations are performed with the patient on cardiopulmonary bypass under cold cardioplegic conditions. Usually a single (two-stage) cannula suffices for venous drainage. When the need for greater exposure is anticipated or when the operation is being performed along with another procedure on the tricuspid valve or other right heart structure, two venous cannulae are employed. The use of suction to remove pulmonary venous blood from the left atrium is also required. A short, pediatric left atrial drainage cannula with multiple holes passed through the right superior pulmonary vein, across the posterior wall of the left atrium, to the left inferior pulmonary vein works well for left atrial drainage. There are three types of incisions in the left atrium to expose the mitral valve: inferior, superior, and transseptal.

Figure 33-2

A **Inferior approach.** This incision is the most common method of exposing the mitral valve and can be considered standard. An incision is made in the left atrium just behind and parallel to the interatrial groove on the right side. The pericardial reflection over the inferior vena cava is opened to allow access to the posterior wall of the left atrium. The incision is extended posteriorly behind the inferior vena cava. This incision provides adequate access to the mitral valve in most situations.

B **Superior approach.** The superior vena cava is mobilized to provide access to the roof of the left atrium. An incision is made in the left atrium just behind the interatrial groove over the pulmonary veins. The incision is extended into the superior aspect of the left atrium, behind the superior vena cava and aorta. The incision may extend to the base of the left atrial appendage with retraction of the superior vena cava and aorta.

Excellent exposure of the mitral valve is achieved with this approach. The incision will not enter the atrioventricular groove if it is directed high on the roof of the left atrium toward the right pulmonary artery. It should be recognized, however, that there is strong evidence that the incidence of supraventricular arrhythmia is higher with this approach than with inferior incisions.

C **Transseptal approach.** Two venous cannulae and vena cava tourniquets are required. An incision is made in the right atrium parallel to the atrioventricular groove. The incision passes medial to the right atrial appendage and extends along the medial aspect of the right atrium to the junction with the left atrium. It should be recognized that this incision is likely to divide the artery that supplies blood to the sinoatrial node. Normal sinus rhythm may not be present after the operation, so this incision is best reserved for patients with atrial fibrillation that is not being treated concomitantly.

D The atrial septum is opened through the foramen ovale. The septal incision is extended superiorly to join the right atrial incision. The incision is then continued over the roof of the left atrium to provide a wide opening. The incision may be carried to the base of the left atrial appendage and should be directed toward the right pulmonary artery to keep it high on the roof of the left atrium and away from the atrioventricular groove.

E A self-retaining retractor is placed in the tricuspid orifice to pull the right ventricle anteriorly. Retraction stitches are placed on the atrial septum rather than using mechanical retraction of the septum; this avoids pressure on the atrioventricular node and the bundle of His. This incision provides the best possible exposure of the mitral valve. It is especially useful in mitral valve reoperations and for procedures combined with tricuspid valve operations.

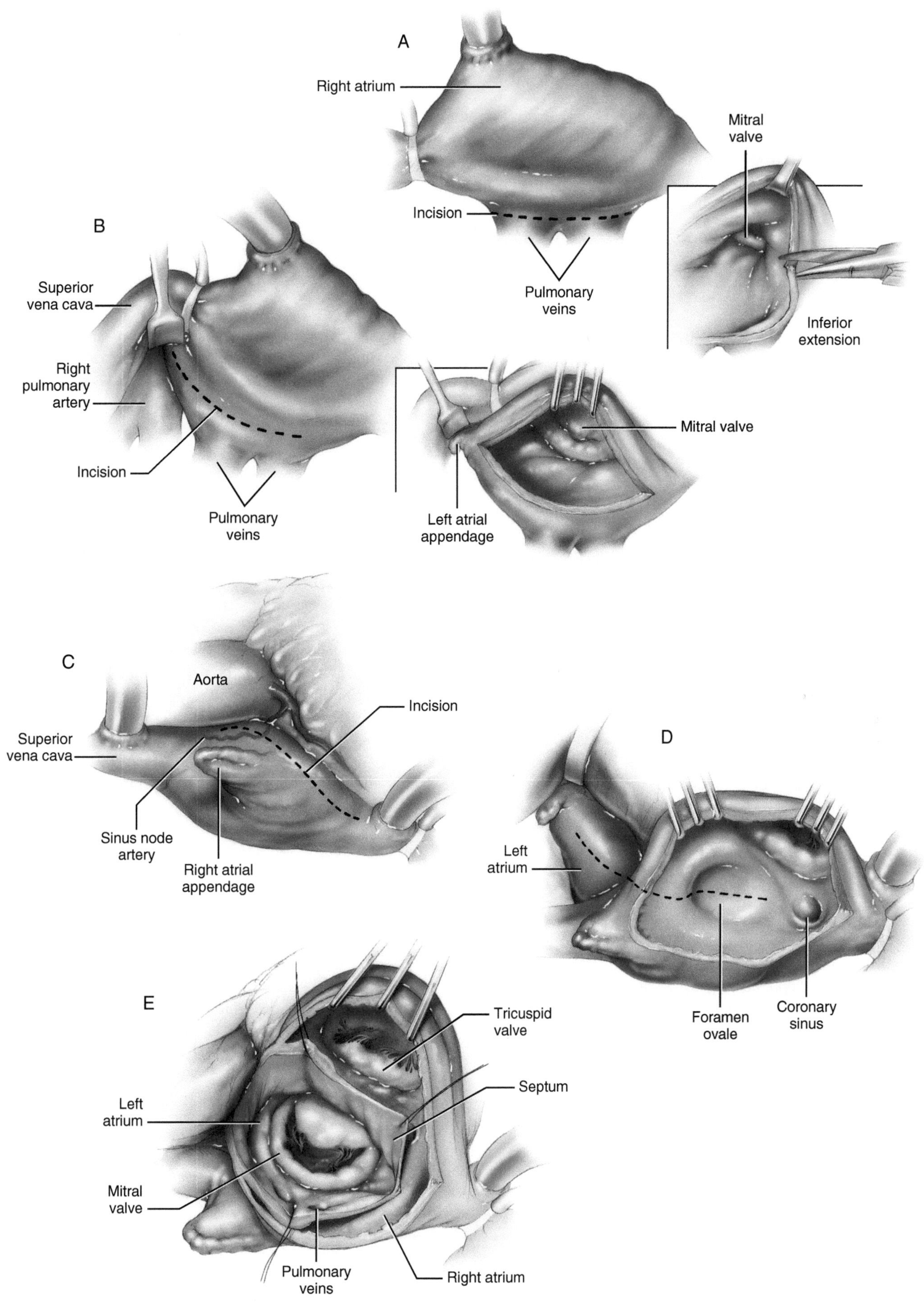

A
Right atrium
Incision
Pulmonary veins
Mitral valve
Inferior extension
B
Superior vena cava
Right pulmonary artery
Incision
Pulmonary veins
Mitral valve
Left atrial appendage
C
Aorta
Incision
Superior vena cava
Sinus node artery
Right atrial appendage
D
Left atrium
Foramen ovale
Coronary sinus
E
Tricuspid valve
Septum
Left atrium
Mitral valve
Pulmonary veins
Right atrium

Preservation of Chordae Tendineae

There is ample evidence that preservation of the attachment of the chordae tendineae and papillary muscles to the mitral valve annulus improves ventricular function after mitral valve replacement in both the short and long term.

Figure 33-3

A Self-retaining retractors are placed anteriorly beneath the atrial septum to expose the mitral valve. A curved hemostat (Shall-Cross) or forceps is placed on the anterior leaflet of the mitral valve, and the valve is retracted posteriorly to expose the annulus. The mitral valve is perforated through the anterior leaflet with a scalpel.

B The mitral valve is separated from the fibrous annulus using a scalpel and scissors, beginning on the anterior leaflet and continuing circumferentially around the posterior leaflet. About 2 mm of the leaflet tissue is left attached to the annulus. Care should be taken during excision at the posteroinferior aspect of the annulus because it is easy to exit the heart and enter the atrioventricular groove. In addition, it is the most difficult area to visualize clearly, especially if chordal attachments are thick and short.

C The anterior leaflet of the mitral valve is divided through its midpoint to facilitate working with the valve and chordae. Normal chordae tendineae are left attached to small remnants of the mitral valve leaflet.

D Only normal length chordae tendineae should be preserved. Thick, short chordae and those that are greatly elongated should be divided at the papillary muscles. In nearly all valves, sufficient normal chordae can be identified to provide secure attachment of the papillary muscles to the mitral annulus.

E The chordae are reattached to the mitral annulus by figure-eight double-loop stitches using 3/0 braided suture. The chordae are attached at appropriate points on the annulus to provide a normal distribution of tension on the papillary muscles. Favored points are the 2, 4, 8, and 10 o'clock positions on the annulus. A large group of normal chordae can be reattached by retaining a larger rim of leaflet tissue that can be sewn to the annulus by continuous stitches of 3/0 or 4/0 polypropylene.

F The entire posterior leaflet may be retained if it is relatively thin and flexible. A continuous stitch of 3/0 or 4/0 polypropylene is used to reef up the posterior leaflet to the annulus.

G Stitches used to attach the prosthetic valve to the mitral annulus should pass around the annulus and penetrate the leaflet remnant retaining the chordae tendineae.

H When the chordae have been hopelessly destroyed by rheumatic processes, the abnormal chordae must be totally divided.

I New chordae tendineae should be created to attach the papillary muscles to the mitral annulus. Polytetrafluoroethylene (PTFE) suture is a good substitute for chordae tendineae. Teflon pledget–reinforced 4/0 or 5/0 PTFE suture is attached to the tips of the papillary muscles and passed through the annulus of the mitral valve. Pledgets are added to prevent the prosthetic chordae from pulling through the papillary muscles. The sutures are tied at an appropriate length to retain support of the mitral valve annulus by the papillary muscles during ventricular systole.

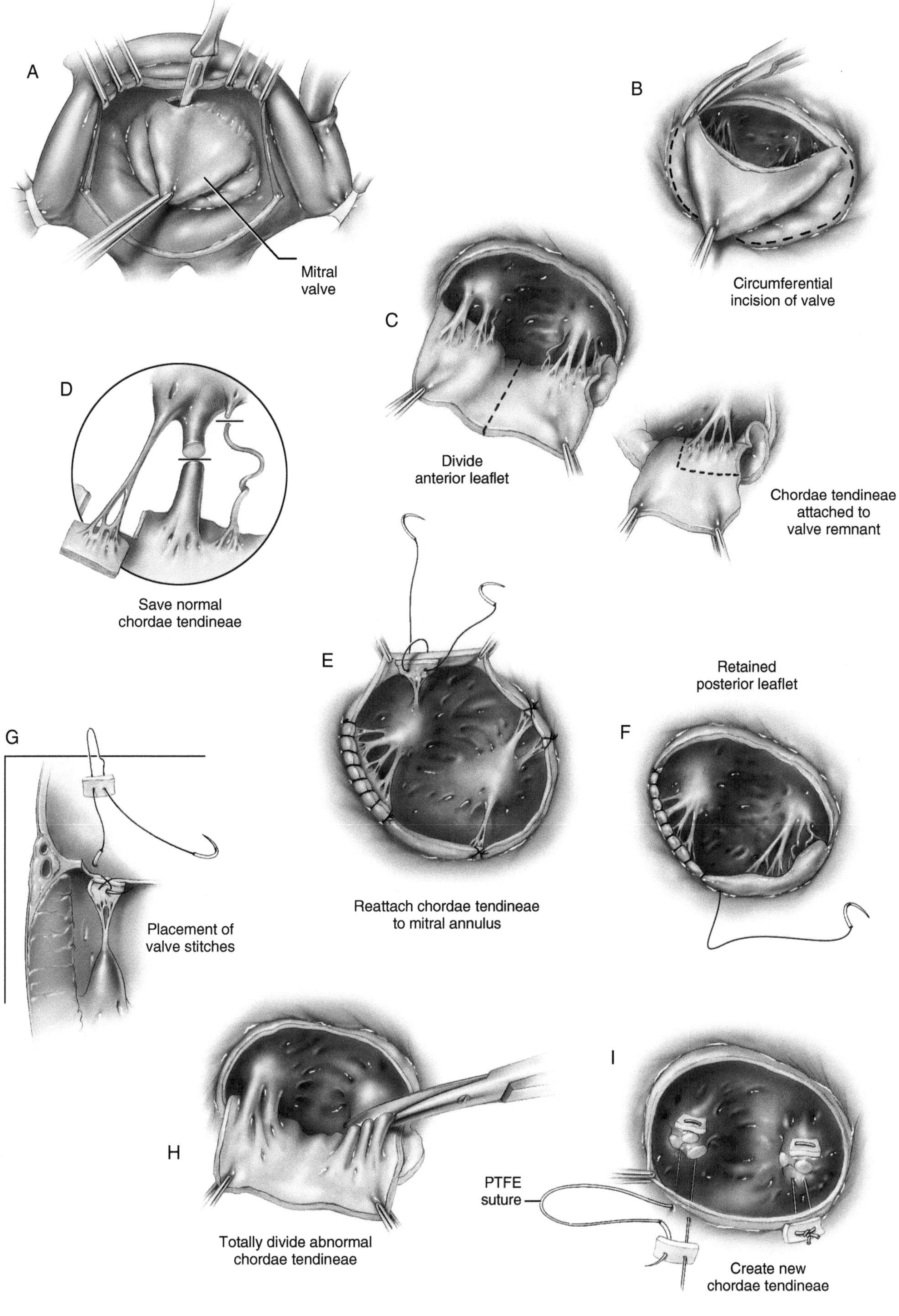
A
Mitral valve
B
Circumferential incision of valve
C
Divide anterior leaflet
Chordae tendineae attached to valve remnant
D
Save normal chordae tendineae
E
Reattach chordae tendineae to mitral annulus
Retained posterior leaflet
F
G
Placement of valve stitches
H
Totally divide abnormal chordae tendineae
I
PTFE suture
Create new chordae tendineae

Interrupted Suture Technique

The most common method of attaching a prosthetic valve to the mitral annulus is the interrupted suture technique. Reinforcement of the sutures with Teflon felt pledgets affords maximal strength and security of the repair.

Figure 33-4

A Traction stitches are placed through the annulus at the superior and inferior aspects to facilitate exposure. A prosthesis holder is used, and all the stitches are placed prior to approximating the prosthesis to the valve annulus. Interrupted mattress stitches of 2/0 braided synthetic material of alternating colors (blue/green, white) are used. Compressed Teflon felt pledgets can be used to strengthen the repair.

In the posterior aspect of the mitral valve annulus, the needles should pass from the ventricular surface below the annulus up into the atrium. The natural curve of the needle guides it away from the circumflex coronary artery and the coronary sinus and prevents inadvertent penetration into the fat of the atrioventricular groove. The stitches can be placed accurately at the ventricle-annulus junction and well back into the floor of the left atrium. The mattress stitches are placed through the sewing ring of the prosthesis and then through the annulus of the mitral valve posteriorly, incorporating the chordae tendineae. The Teflon pledgets are then threaded on separately. The initial stitches are taken superiorly on the annulus, working inferiorly in a counterclockwise fashion. The valve prosthesis is held anterior and to the left of the mitral valve annulus so that the sutures provide traction to expose the annulus.

B Following completion of the posterior half of the mitral annulus, the valve prosthesis is drawn to the right side. Stitches are placed through the anterior portion of the annulus, beginning superiorly and working inferiorly in a clockwise fashion. Here the stitches are taken from the atrial surface through the mitral annulus and then brought through the sewing ring of the prosthesis. Traction on the sutures provides exposure for subsequent stitches. Teflon pledgets are preplaced centrally on double-needle suture.

C When all the stitches have been placed, strong traction is applied to the sutures as the valve prosthesis is slid over them into the annulus of the mitral valve. Sorting of the sutures is facilitated by the alternating colors and helps prevent inadvertent joining of discontinuous sutures as they are tied. Accurate approximation of the sewing ring of the prosthesis to the mitral annulus must be ensured as each suture is tied. Sutures are tied in the same order as they were placed, beginning posteriorly and working in a counterclockwise fashion.

D The anterior sutures are tied in a clockwise fashion to complete the repair.

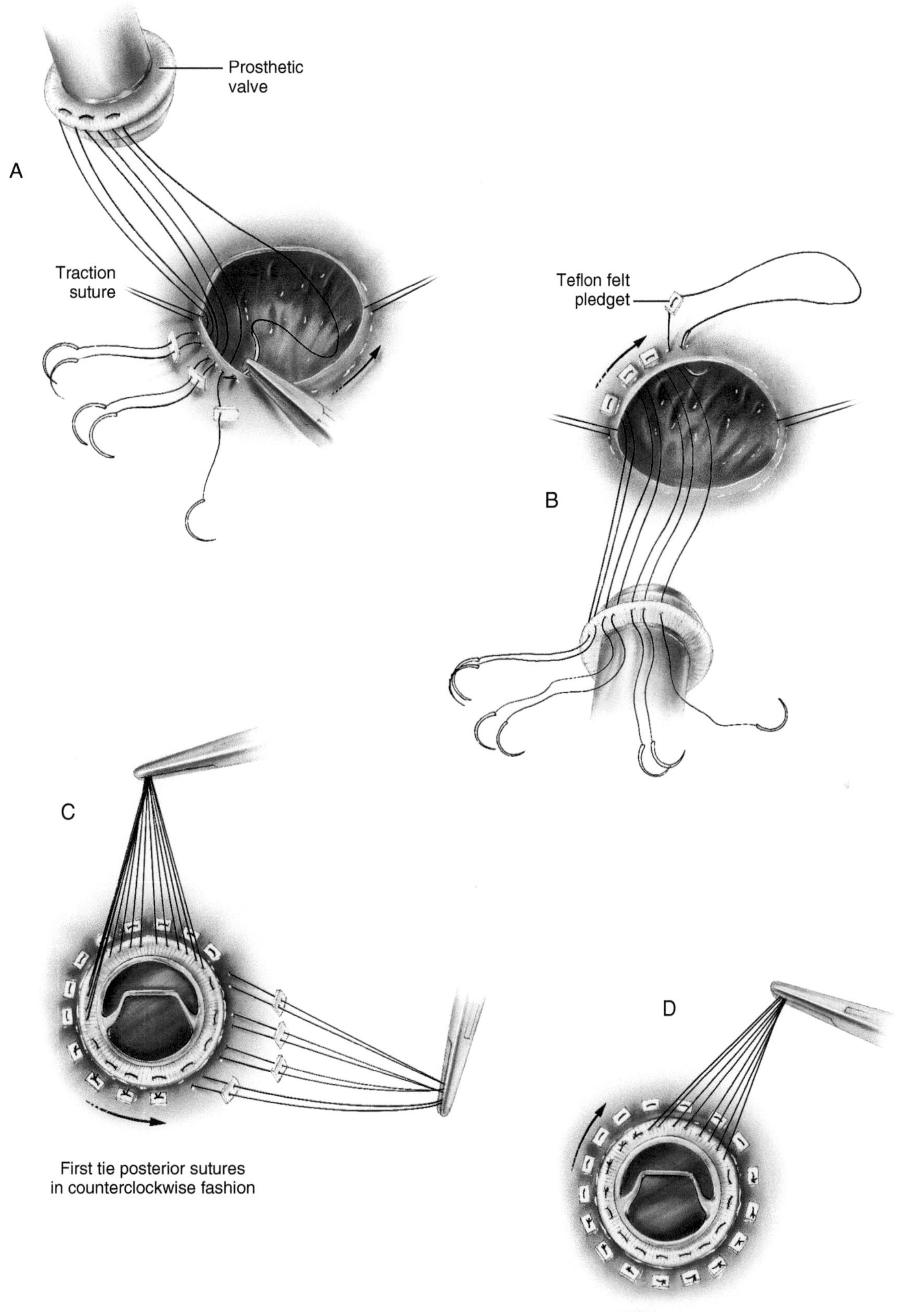
A
Prosthetic valve
Traction suture
B
Teflon felt pledget
C
First tie posterior sutures in counterclockwise fashion
D
Tie anterior sutures in clockwise fashion

Continuous Suture Technique

Continuous suture technique is employed for efficiency and because the stitch loops are always precisely located between the prosthesis and the annulus. Strong annular tissues are a prerequisite for this method of repair.

Figure 33-5

A Continuous stitches of 2/0 polypropylene are used for the repair. A mattress stitch is passed through the sewing ring of the prosthesis and brought up through the annulus of the mitral valve from the ventricular surface to the atrium at the midportion of the posterior leaflet. The suture is passed through a compressed Teflon felt pledget. The valve prosthesis is placed in the left ventricular cavity, below the anterior annulus, and drawn up tight against the posterior region of the mitral annulus. Traction stitches of 2/0 silk are placed through the annulus at the superior and inferior aspects of the mitral valve to facilitate the exposure.

B Continuous sutures are placed from the sewing ring of the prosthesis to the mitral valve annulus. The sutures are placed along the posterior annulus of the mitral valve in a cephalad fashion toward the superior traction suture. Tension on the suture loop is maintained while the needle is placed through the sewing ring of the prosthesis. Tension is released as the needle is passed through the annulus of the mitral valve so that the annulus and ventricle are accurately exposed. The needle must pass just below the annulus and cannot include any ventricular myocardium. The needle may include a good portion (3 to 5 mm) of the left atrial floor. With the opposite needle, the mitral annulus is approximated to the sewing ring of the valve prosthesis; the stitches are placed in a counterclockwise fashion toward the inferior traction suture. Tension on the traction suture aids exposure.

C At the inferior traction stitch on the mitral annulus, the direction of suture placement is reversed. A mattress stitch is placed through a compressed Teflon felt pledget, and the needle is directed from the atrium through the sewing ring of the prosthesis. The application of forceps on the sewing ring forces the prosthesis down over the needle as it emerges from beneath the annulus. The mitral annulus is then approximated to the sewing ring of the prosthesis anteriorly, with the stitches placed in a counterclockwise fashion.

D The final stitches are taken in the area of the aortic valve. The suture loops in the final quadrant are left loose until all have been placed so that the aortic valve annulus can be accurately visualized. After placement of the final stitch, the suture loops are drawn up tight, and the ends of the suture are joined by a knot to complete the repair.

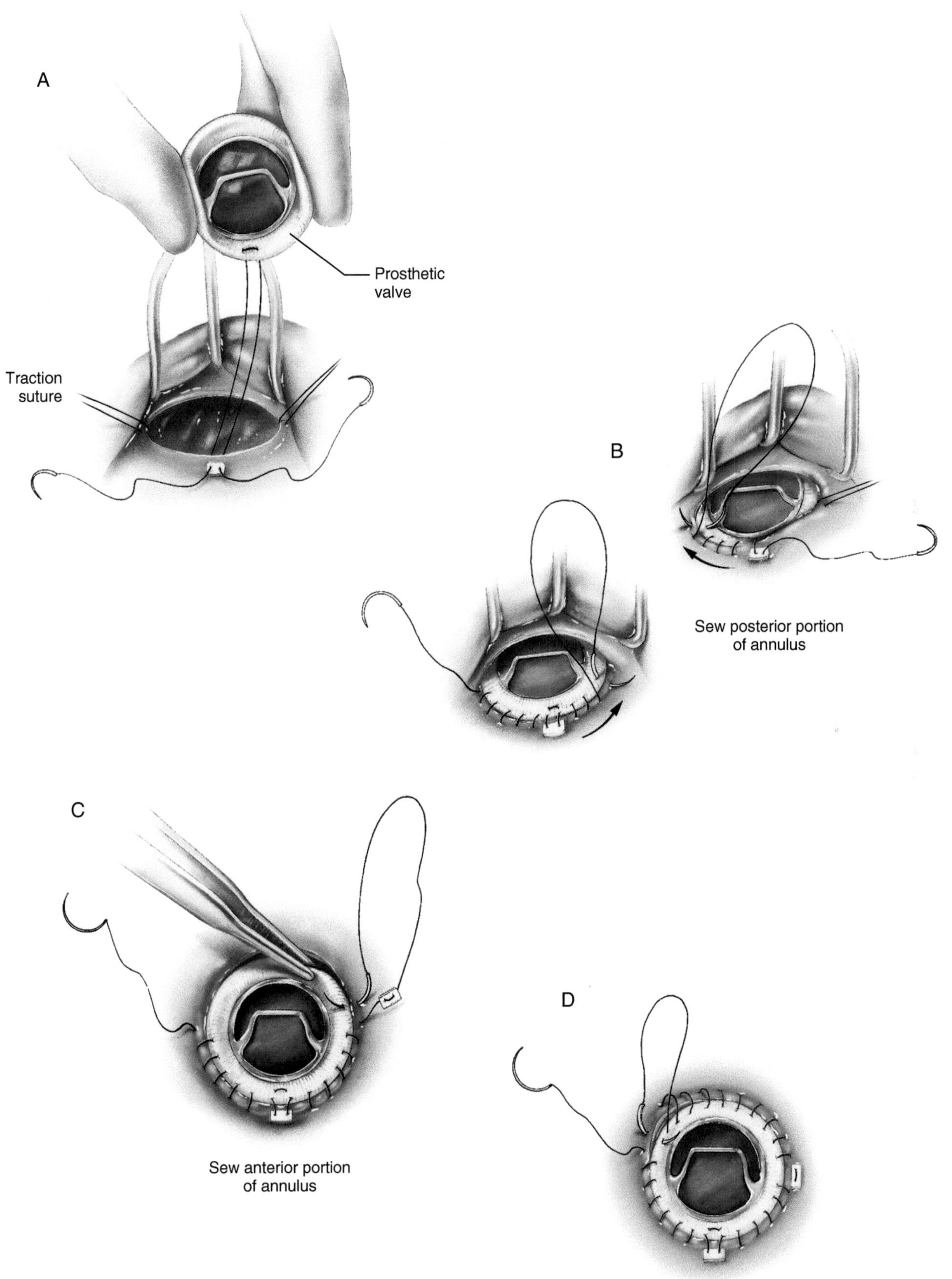
A
Prosthetic valve
Traction suture
B
Sew posterior portion of annulus
C
Sew anterior portion of annulus
D
Completed repair

Mitral Valve Homograft

Mitral valve replacement with homograft is reserved for young patients in whom anticoagulation is undesirable or contraindicated and for prosthetic valve replacement in drug-resistant endocarditis.

Figure 33-6

A The left atrium is opened on the right side through the interatrial groove. A self-retaining retractor is used for optimal exposure. The mitral valve is removed by circumferential incision near the fibrous annulus of the valve. Some of the anterior leaflet is retained, especially in the region near the aortic valve.

B The chordae tendineae are removed from the tips of the papillary muscles. Each papillary muscle must be a single- or double-head muscle. Muscular trabeculations (bands) that attach the papillary muscles to the ventricular wall (inset) are divided, creating space between the papillary muscles and the free wall of the left ventricle in which the graft papillary muscles will be placed.

C The size of the homograft is determined by measuring the diameter of the patient's mitral valve annulus and choosing a graft of nearly the same diameter. While the cryopreserved homograft is thawing, mitral valve annuloplasty in performed by placing horizontal mattress stitches using 2/0 braided polyester around the perimeter of the mitral annulus. These stitches are divided into four groups and placed under secure tension to enhance exposure below the annulus. After the valve is thawed, it is trimmed. The myocardium of the atrium and ventricle is cut away from the annulus of the valve, leaving just enough tissue to allow needle penetration without entering leaflet tissue. The papillary muscles are shortened, leaving 10 mm of muscle below the chordal attachments. The implantation begins with fixation of the papillary muscles. Exposure is enhanced by placing a retractor blade through the mitral valve annulus into the left ventricle anteriorly.

D The posterior papillary muscle is implanted first. Two mattress stitches of 5/0 Cardionyl are placed in the graft papillary muscle and then passed through the patient's papillary muscle. The stitches are placed deep at the base of the papillary muscle so that the homograft papillary muscle is oriented side by side with the patient's papillary muscle, and the tips of the muscles are at the same level when the graft muscle is drawn into place between the papillary muscle and the ventricular wall. Exposure is enhanced by placing a traction stitch through the papillary head that supports the commissure, which is invariably at the apex of the patient's papillary muscles. Traction on the mattress stitches brings the papillary muscles into approximation. The stitches are tied to securely approximate the muscular tissues without weakening or cutting through them.

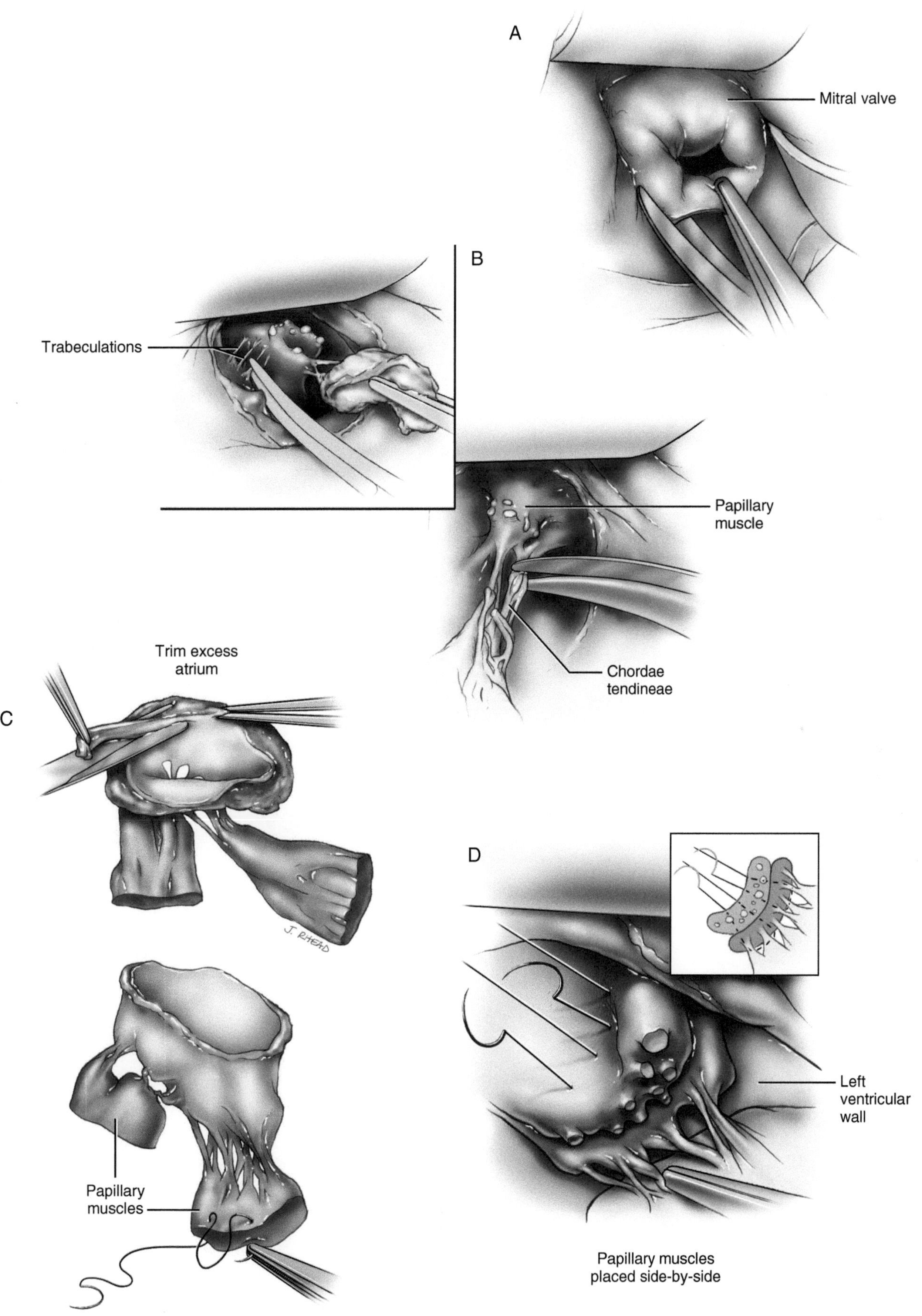
A
Mitral valve
B
Trabeculations
Papillary muscle
Chordae tendineae
Trim excess atrium
C
J. RHEAD
Papillary muscles
D
Left ventricular wall
Papillary muscles placed side-by-side

Figure 33-6 (continued)

E Two interrupted stitches are placed at the anterior margin of the papillary muscles to secure their side-by-side approximation.

F Two interrupted stitches are placed posteriorly on the muscles to finish lining them up. Multiple stitches are then placed to secure the tips of the papillary muscles. Care is taken not to interfere with the chordae tendineae. Vertical mattress sutures may be required. The anterior papillary muscles are approximated in a similar fashion.

G The mitral homograft annulus is attached to the mitral annulus using continuous stitches of 4/0 polypropylene. The fibrous trigones of the graft are lined up with the patient's fibrous trigones. The graft leaflet tissues are distributed uniformly around the annulus. The replaced valve is supported by an annuloplasty ring. The size of the device should match the size of the graft anterior leaflet. The device is attached to the annulus by the previously placed sutures (inset). Competence of the repair is tested by infusing saline under pressure into the left ventricle and by echocardiography after closing the atrium and resuscitating the heart.

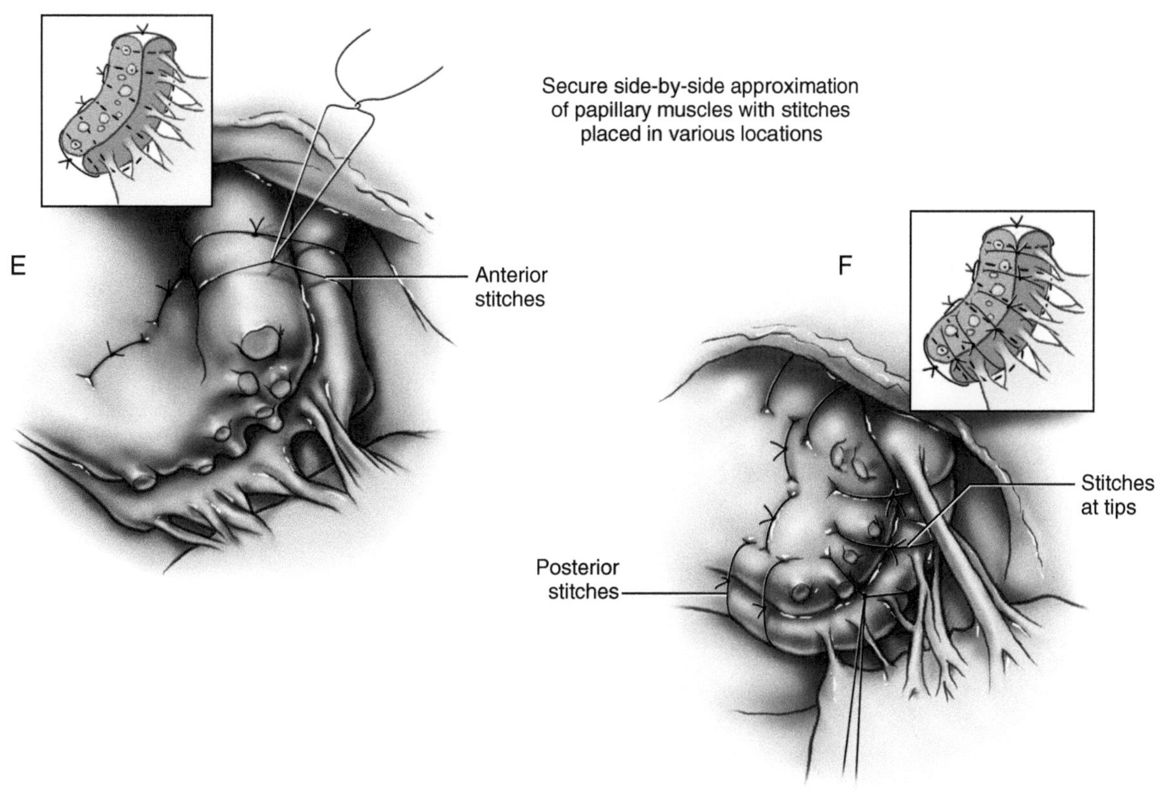
Secure side-by-side approximation of papillary muscles with stitches placed in various locations
E
Anterior stitches
F
Stitches at tips
Posterior stitches

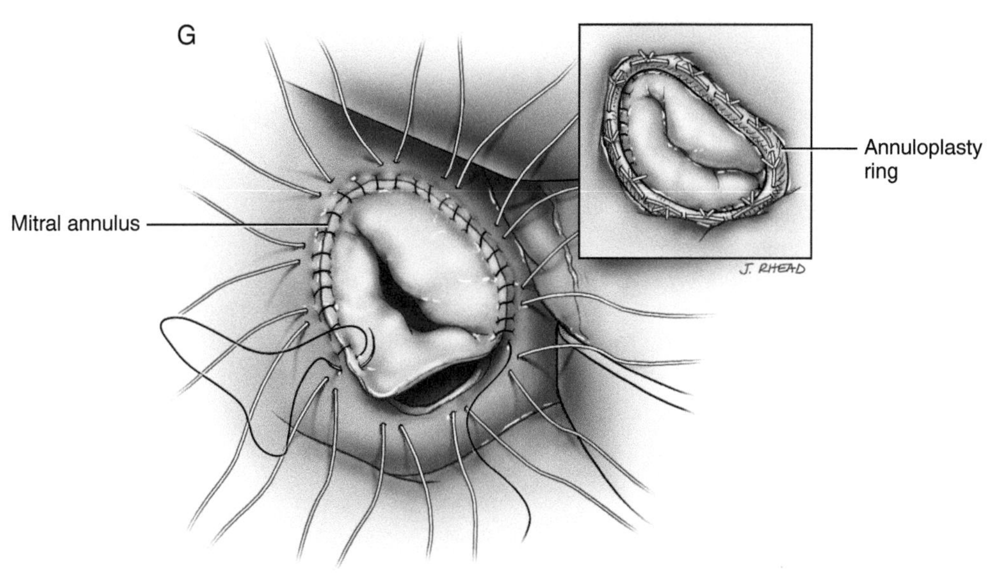
G
Mitral annulus
Annuloplasty ring
J. RHEAD
Annuloplasty stitches placed previously

Calcified Mitral Annulus

Replacement of the mitral valve in the presence of marked annular calcification is a formidable technical challenge. There is substantial risk of atrioventricular groove perforation during decalcification of the annulus by rongeur or forceps. The annulus may be substantially contracted by calcium deposits, and implantation of a prosthetic valve in the atrium above the annulus may not relieve the obstruction. Implantation of a mechanical prosthesis risks impinging on the annular calcium deposits unless the annulus is thoroughly débrided.

Figure 33-7

A Extensive calcareous deposit in the posterior mitral annulus is depicted. The mitral orifice may be significantly narrowed by this process.

B The entire anterior leaflet of the mitral valve is removed. Easily accessible posterior leaflet tissues are removed or débrided. No effort is made to deeply débride the annulus with forceps, rongeurs, or scissors. Normal chordae tendineae are preserved. Usually there are enough normal chordae to the anterior leaflet to allow fixation of the papillary muscles to the annulus.

C An ultrasonic aspirating device is used to completely débride calcareous deposits from the mitral annulus and atrioventricular groove. Ultrasound breaks up the large calcium deposits—turning rocks into sand that can be removed by suction. Soft tissues are spared by the ultrasound, so healthy, viable myocardium and connective tissue are preserved. There is little risk of perforating the atrioventricular groove by this method of débridement. The annular diameter increases as the hard, calcareous deposits are removed and normal soft tissues are exposed.

D This diagram shows extensive calcification of the mitral annulus and atrioventricular groove. The ultrasonic aspirator removes calcareous deposits to the level of the normal soft tissues.

E The débridement is complete when nearly all the calcareous deposits have been removed. Only a few fine bits of calcium are left at the depth of the débridement. The annulus is enlarged by this procedure to accommodate a larger prosthetic valve.

F A pericardial patch is fashioned to cover the area of débridement. This reduces the risk of embolus and strengthens the tissues. The patch is soaked in glutarldehyde solution to strengthen it and make it easier to handle. The patch is attached to ventricular myocardium at the edge of the débrided area by continuous stitches of 4/0 polypropylene. The pericardial patch is left unattached at the annulus to allow accurate suture placement during prosthetic valve implantation.

G Anterior leaflet chordal remnants supporting the papillary muscles are attached to the annulus at appropriate locations by double-loop stitches of 3/0 braided suture. Posterior leaflet chordae are usually fused to the posterior wall of the left ventricle and do not require reattachment. A prosthetic valve (usually mechanical) is attached to the mitral annulus by interrupted pledget-reinforced mattress stitches of 2/0 braided suture. The stitches are placed through the pericardial patch and the posterior mitral annulus.

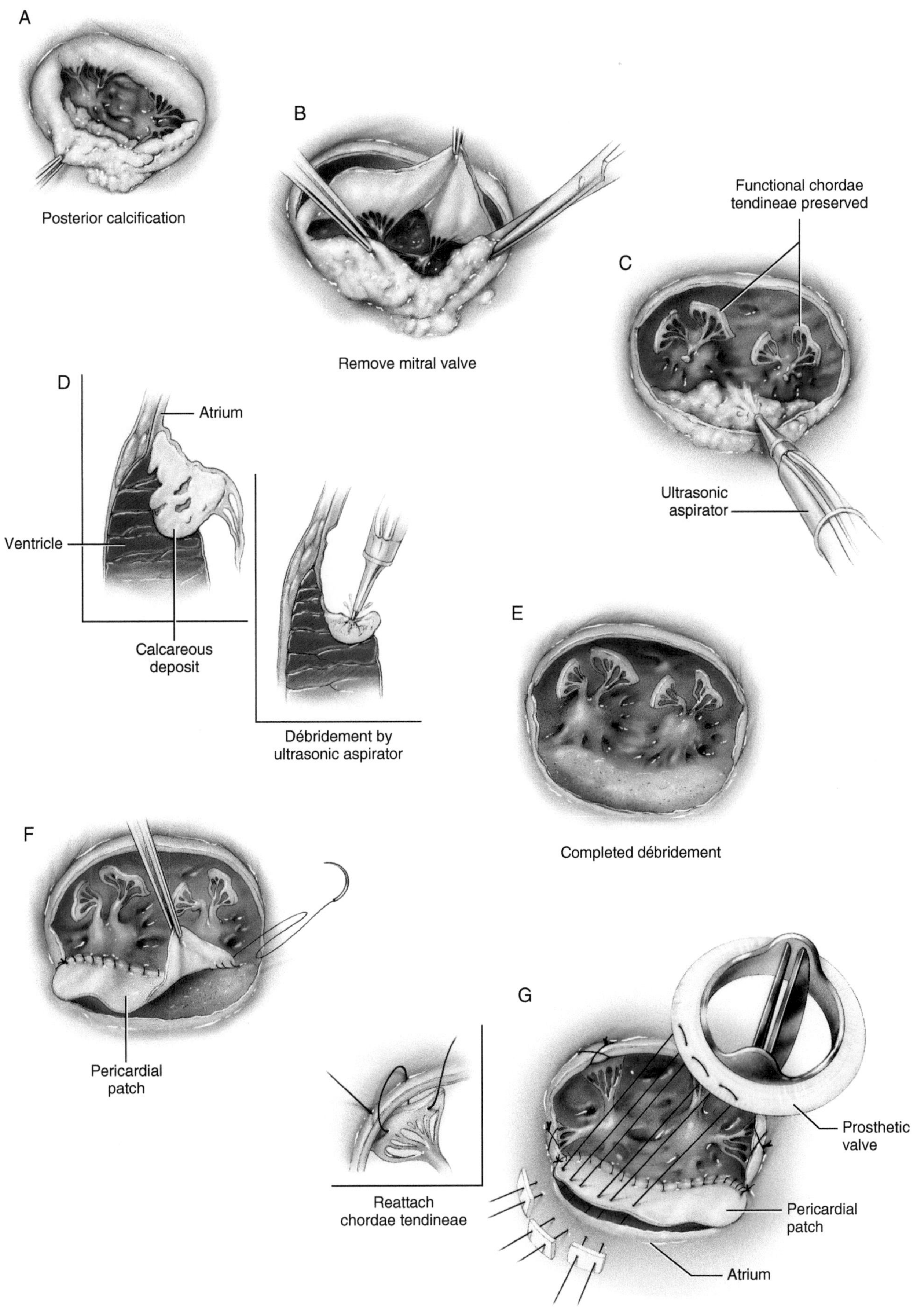
A
Posterior calcification
B
Remove mitral valve
Functional chordae tendineae preserved
C
Ultrasonic aspirator
D
Atrium
Ventricle
Calcareous deposit
Débridement by ultrasonic aspirator
E
Completed débridement
F
Pericardial patch
G
Reattach chordae tendineae
Prosthetic valve
Pericardial patch
Atrium

chapter 34 TRICUSPID VALVE RECONSTRUCTION

Ring Annuloplasty (Carpentier Operation)

The tricuspid valve may be repaired when leaflet tissues and supporting chordae are adequate. The morphology of tricuspid incompetence is often related to simple annular dilation, making reconstruction possible by annuloplasty techniques.

Figure 34-1

A Reconstruction of the tricuspid valve is performed with the patient on cardiopulmonary bypass using two venous cannulae with tourniquets secured around them. The aorta is cross-clamped, and cold cardioplegic solution is perfused into the aortic root. The incision is made in the right atrium parallel to the atrioventricular groove. Exposure is achieved by anterior and posterior retraction stitches placed on the edge of the atriotomy.

B Reference stitches are placed at the commissures between the septal and anterior leaflets and the septal and posterior leaflets of the tricuspid valve. Chordae tendineae of the papillary muscles may be used to guide the placement of reference sutures if commissures are incomplete and poorly defined. The septal portion of the annulus of the tricuspid valve has been shown to remain constant even during gross dilation of the remainder of the annulus. Thus, reduction of the anterior and posterior annular dimensions is required to correct the relationship with the septal portion and achieve an accurate repair. Carpentier tricuspid valve annuloplasty calibrators are used in all cases. Reference grooves in these calibrators are placed against the reference stitches to obtain an accurate estimation of the final desirable dimensions of the tricuspid valve annulus.

C An appropriately sized annuloplasty (Carpentier) ring is selected for symmetric narrowing of the tricuspid valve annulus, based on the measurements obtained from the valve calibrators. Using double-needle 2/0 braided synthetic suture, the surgeon places the stitches through the annulus of the tricuspid valve and through the sewing ring of the annuloplasty ring. A single pass through the annular tissue is converted to a horizontal mattress stitch by passing needles at each end of the suture through the annuloplasty ring. Alternating the color of the suture material will be helpful later on when sorting the sutures and also prevents the inadvertent joining of discontinuous sutures. Stitches are taken in sequential fashion, beginning at the commissure between the septal and anterior leaflets and working in a clockwise fashion to the commissure between the posterior and septal leaflets of the tricuspid valve. Stitches are considerably wider in the annulus of the tricuspid valve than in the annuloplasty ring, especially in the portion of the annulus supporting the posterior leaflet. Reference markings on the prosthetic ring are useful in determining suture width as the various portions of the annulus are repaired.

D The annuloplasty ring is slid over the sutures, which are held under tension, and the sutures are joined tightly to approximate the annuloplasty ring to the floor of the atrium and the tricuspid valve annulus. Tricuspid valve competence is tested by infusing an electrolyte solution into the right ventricle via a catheter across the tricuspid valve. The longer anterior and posterior leaflets should approximate the septal leaflet and keep the valve competent if the annulus diameter has been reduced appropriately. The correctly seated annuloplasty ring should be open over the area occupied by the bundle of His. Competence of the repair is evaluated by transesophageal or surface echocardiography after the heart is filled and beating.

E Operative photograph of a completed tricuspid valve ring annuloplasty (Carpentier operation). The annuloplasty ring has been placed properly, and there is adequate normal-appearing tricuspid leaflet tissue within the ring. A pulmonary artery catheter crosses the tricuspid valve, the repair having been made around it.

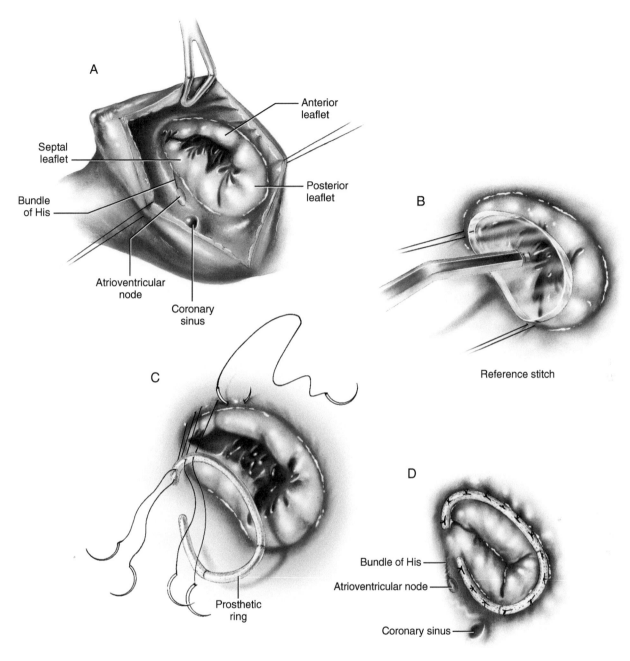

A

Anterior leaflet

Septal leaflet

Posterior leaflet

Bundle of His

Atrioventricular node

Coronary sinus

B

Reference stitch

C

Prosthetic ring

D

Bundle of His

Atrioventricular node

Coronary sinus

Completed ring annuloplasty

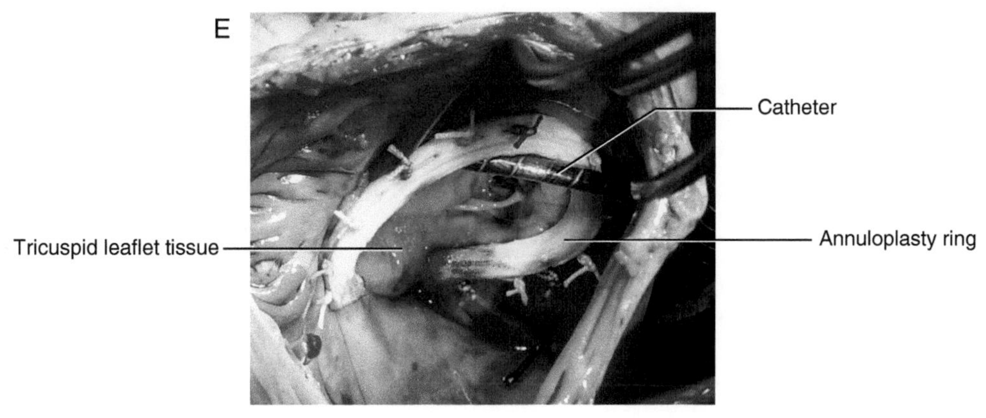

Suture Annuloplasty (DeVega Operation)

The DeVega technique involves narrowing the annulus supporting the anterior and posterior leaflets of the tricuspid valve.

Figure 34-2

DeVega Operation

A A DeVega annuloplasty is formed using 2/0 polypropylene suture material with a pledget placed centrally and needles at each end. The suture is started at the commissure between the septal and anterior leaflets of the tricuspid valve. Sequential stitches are taken through the tricuspid valve annulus, leaving only a small space between each stitch and taking up a segment of annular tissue with each stitch. The suture line is completed at the commissure between the septal and posterior leaflets of the tricuspid valve.

B The opposite end of the suture is then used to make a second suture row in the floor of the atrium just outside the annulus of the tricuspid valve. This stitch is also completed at the commissure between the septal and posterior leaflets. Both suture and needles are passed through a second compressed Teflon pledget.

C Using a Carpentier tricuspid valve annuloplasty calibrator, the annuloplasty suture is tightened to narrow the annulus in a symmetric fashion to the size of the preselected tricuspid valve calibrator. The tricuspid valve is tested for competence by distending the right ventricle with isotonic electrolyte solution infused through a Robinson catheter. Other surgeons use less precise techniques, such as narrowing the valve orifice to two fingerbreadths. Another approach is the beating heart technique, in which the suture is passed to the outside of the atrium, the atriotomy is closed, the heart is filled with blood, and the suture is secured with the heart beating. Then the suture, guided by a finger in the right atrium, is tightened until tricuspid valve competence is achieved. The visual technique guided by valve calibrators seems to be the most reproducible and the least likely to leave residual tricuspid valve incompetence.

Partial Suture Annuloplasty

D Unfortunately, in some cases of annular dilation in the presence of pulmonary hypertension, the tension on the DeVega annuloplasty suture exceeds the strength of the annular tissues. The annuloplasty suture may pull through the tissues, releasing the repair and leaving the suture stretched tightly across the tricuspid orifice. To overcome this deficiency in the repair, surgeons have performed suture annuloplasty of only the posterior leaflet or have included only a portion of the anterior leaflet. A pledget-reinforced 2/0 polypropylene suture is placed in the tricuspid valve annulus, beginning slightly anterior to the commissure that separates the anterior and posterior leaflets of the tricuspid valve. The stitches are continued to the commissure separating the posterior and septal leaflets of the tricuspid valve. Two suture rows are placed.

E The repair is completed by tightening the suture and tying over the reinforcing pledget. The size of the tricuspid annulus is determined by annuloplasty ring sizers, as described previously. The resultant suture line, which is straighter than the more circumferential suture line of the classic DeVega operation, is probably less prone to dehiscence.

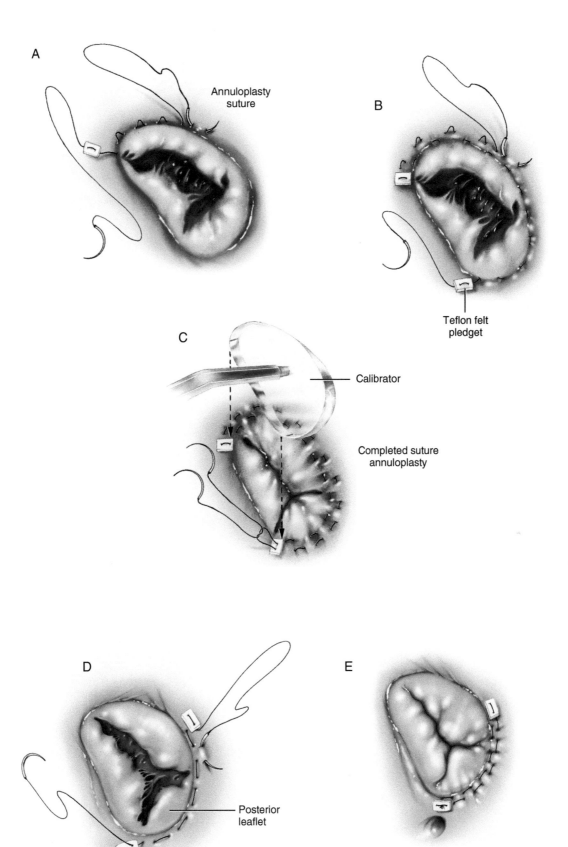

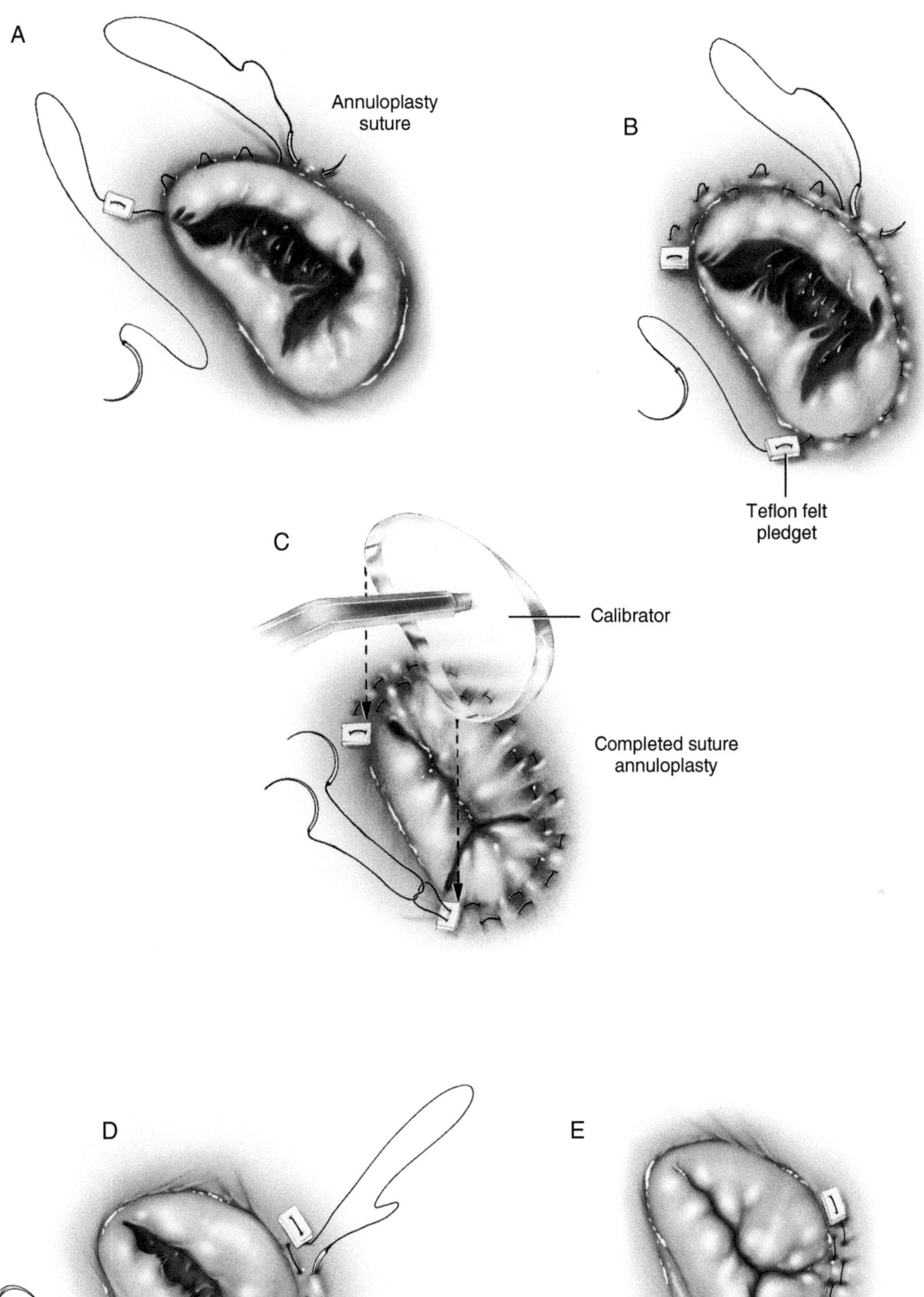
A
Annuloplasty suture
B
Teflon felt pledget
C
Calibrator
Completed suture annuloplasty
D
Posterior leaflet
E
Completed partial annuloplasty

chapter 35 TRICUSPID VALVE REPLACEMENT

Replacement of the tricuspid valve is indicated when leaflet tissue has been so altered by pathologic processes that the valve is judged to be unrepairable.

Morphology

Pathologic processes resulting in tricuspid valve commissural fusion or scarring and contraction or destruction of the leaflet tissue typically disqualify valve repair.

Figure 35-1

Tricuspid valve regurgitation, operative photograph. This image demonstrates near-complete destruction of tricuspid valve leaflet tissue and chordae tendineae by repeated right heart biopsy after cardiac transplantation.

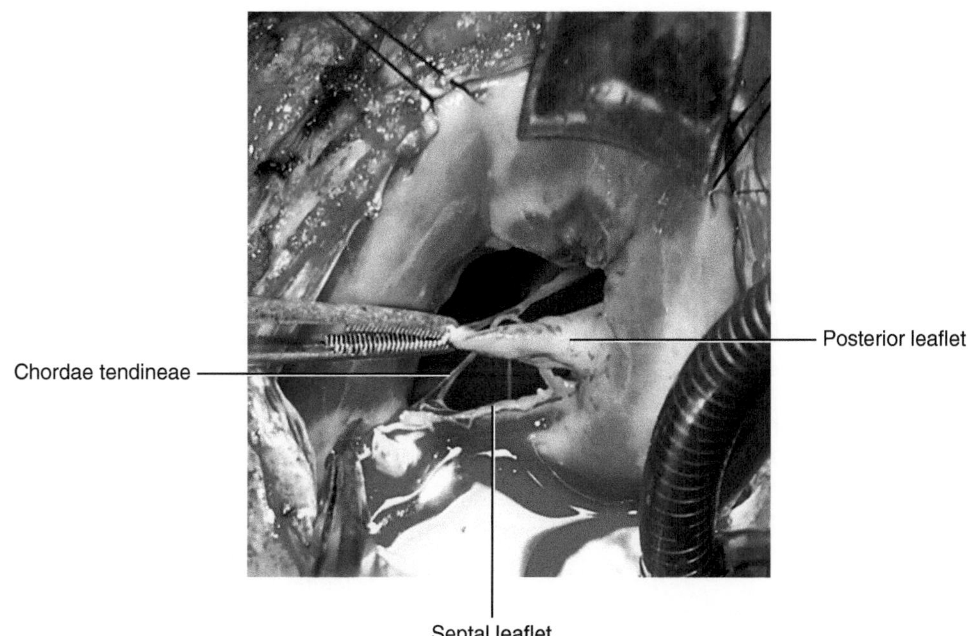
Posterior leaflet
Chordae tendineae
Septal leaflet
remnant

Figure 35-2

A The tricuspid valve is excised beginning with the anterior leaflet, continuing around the posterior leaflet, and ending with partial excision of the septal leaflet. Nearly all of the septal leaflet of the tricuspid valve, or at least a considerable rim of it, should be preserved for attachment of the valve prosthesis. Selection of an appropriately sized valve prosthesis is based on measurements using valve annulus calibrators.

B The valve prosthesis is usually sutured into the annulus of the tricuspid valve by continuous suture technique with 2/0 polypropylene, provided the annular tissue seems to be sufficiently strong. A mattress stitch is placed through the sewing ring of the prosthesis, brought through the septal leaflet of the tricuspid valve, and secured by a pledget at the midportion of the septal leaflet. The prosthesis is placed in the right ventricle, and the suture is tightened to approximate the sewing ring of the prosthesis to the valve annulus.

C Stitches are placed by passing the needle from the sewing ring of the prosthesis through the septal leaflet of the tricuspid valve, working in a clockwise fashion. To facilitate exposure of the junction of the ventricular myocardium and the annulus, tension is maintained on the suture as it is passed through the sewing ring of the prosthesis, and tension is released as it is passed through the septal leaflet of the tricuspid valve. To prevent injury to the bundle of His of the conduction system, the stitches must be entirely in leaflet tissue and cannot be allowed to penetrate the fiber of the annulus or the septal myocardium. About one fourth of the annular repair is completed to a point corresponding to the 9 o'clock position.

D The remainder of the repair is performed using the needle at the opposite end of the suture, working in a counterclockwise fashion. The needle is passed from the sewing ring of the prosthesis through the septal leaflet of the tricuspid valve. The needle direction is reversed at the midportion of the posterior leaflet (3 o'clock position) by passing the stitch twice through a compressed Teflon pledget to create a horizontal mattress stitch. The anterior aspect of the tricuspid valve annulus is then approximated to the sewing ring of the prosthesis, passing the needle from the atrium through the annulus and then through the sewing ring of the prosthesis.

E The suture line is continued in a counterclockwise fashion for the remainder of the annulus and completed by joining it to the opposite end of the suture with a knot.

F An alternative technique is to use interrupted pledget-reinforced mattress stitches. This technique is useful when the tricuspid leaflet tissue and annulus are delicate and are not likely to hold securely with continuous suture technique. The pledget-reinforced sutures buttress and strengthen the tissue repair. For the initial step of the repair, the mattress stitches are taken through the septal leaflet of the tricuspid valve, preserving the function of the electrical conduction system of the heart. The septal portion of the annulus is repaired by pledget-reinforced sutures, followed by repair of the rest of the annulus by continuous suture technique.

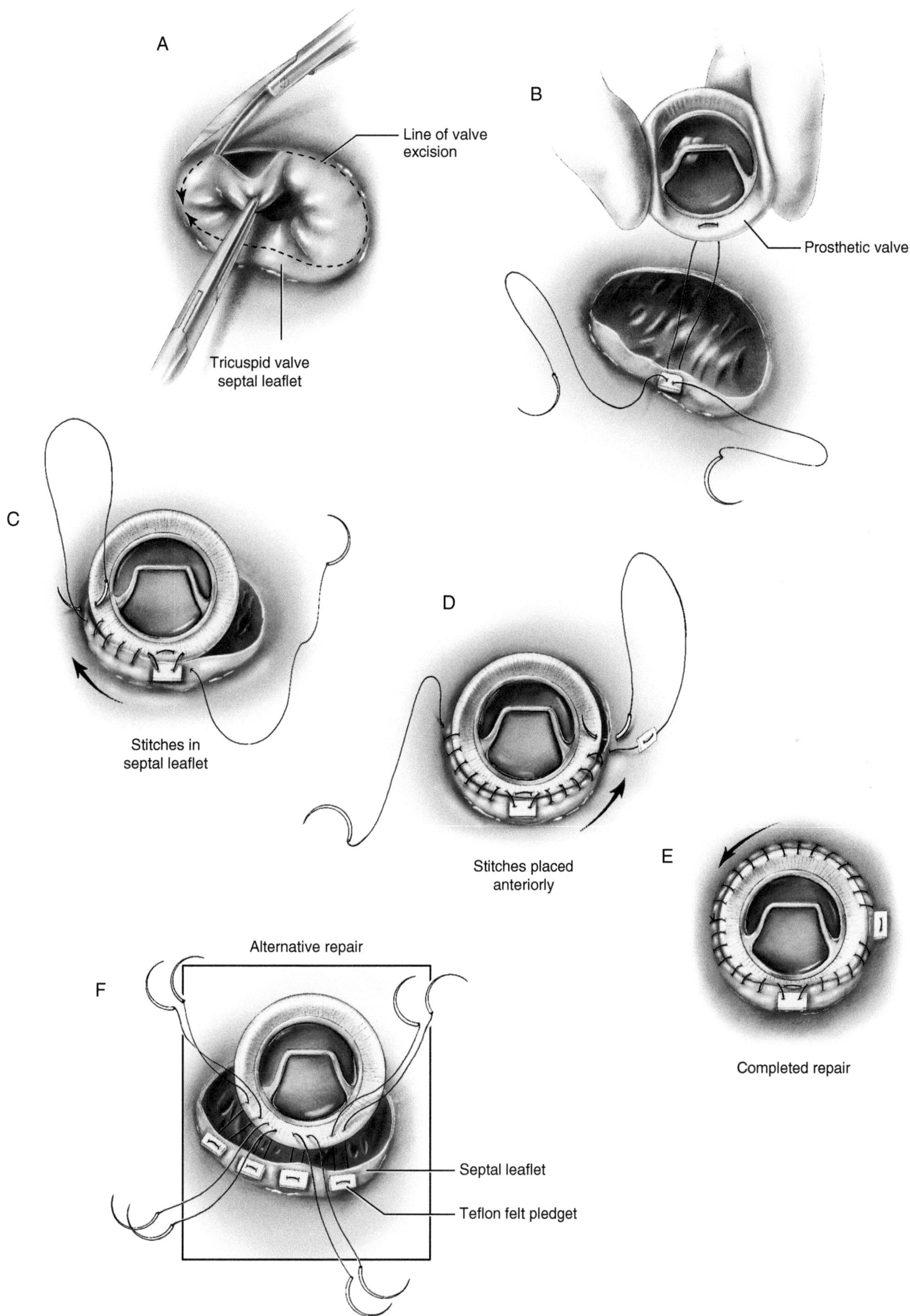
A
Line of valve excision
Tricuspid valve septal leaflet
B
Prosthetic valve
C
Stitches in septal leaflet
D
Stitches placed anteriorly
E
Completed repair
Alternative repair
F
Septal leaflet
Teflon felt pledget

Tricuspid Valve Replacement with Stented Bioprosthesis

The quality of bioprosthetic valves has improved in terms of both durability and hemodynamic performance. These prosthetic valves are usually chosen when tricuspid valve morphology dictates replacement rather than repair.

Figure 35-3

A The operation is performed via a midline sternotomy (complete or lower half) or via an anterior thoracotomy on the right side. Venous uptake cannulae are placed in the superior and inferior venae cavae. Tourniquets are secured around the cannulae to isolate the right atrium. The aorta is occluded, and the heart is arrested and preserved by the infusion of cold cardioplegic solution through a catheter in the coronary sinus. The tricuspid valve is excised beginning with the anterior leaflet and continuing around the posterior leaflet. All or nearly all of the septal leaflet is preserved.

B After selection of an appropriately sized bioprosthesis, pledget-reinforced mattress stitches using braided suture are placed to strengthen the attachment of the bioprosthesis to the septal leaflet. Only leaflet tissue is included in each stitch to protect the bundle of His from injury.

C The bioprosthesis is attached to the rest of the tricuspid annulus by continuous stitches. A pledget-reinforced 2/0 polypropylene mattress stitch is placed around the annulus anteriorly and brought through the sewing ring of the bioprosthesis. The bioprosthesis is approximated to the annulus, and the stent is placed in the right ventricle by tightening the septal mattress stitches and the anteriorly placed mattress stitch. Working clockwise, continuous stitches are placed around the annulus and passed directly through the adjacent sewing ring of the bioprosthesis. Tension is maintained on the suture as stitching proceeds, releasing tension slightly to provide exposure of the junction of the annulus and the sewing ring of the bioprosthesis as the stitch is passed through the sewing ring.

D Stitches are continued posteriorly on the annulus to the previously placed mattress stitches at the junction of the septum and the free wall of the right ventricle. Picking up the opposite needle anteriorly, stitching proceeds in a counterclockwise fashion to the junction of the anterior and septal leaflets.

E The repair is completed by tying the sutures securely.

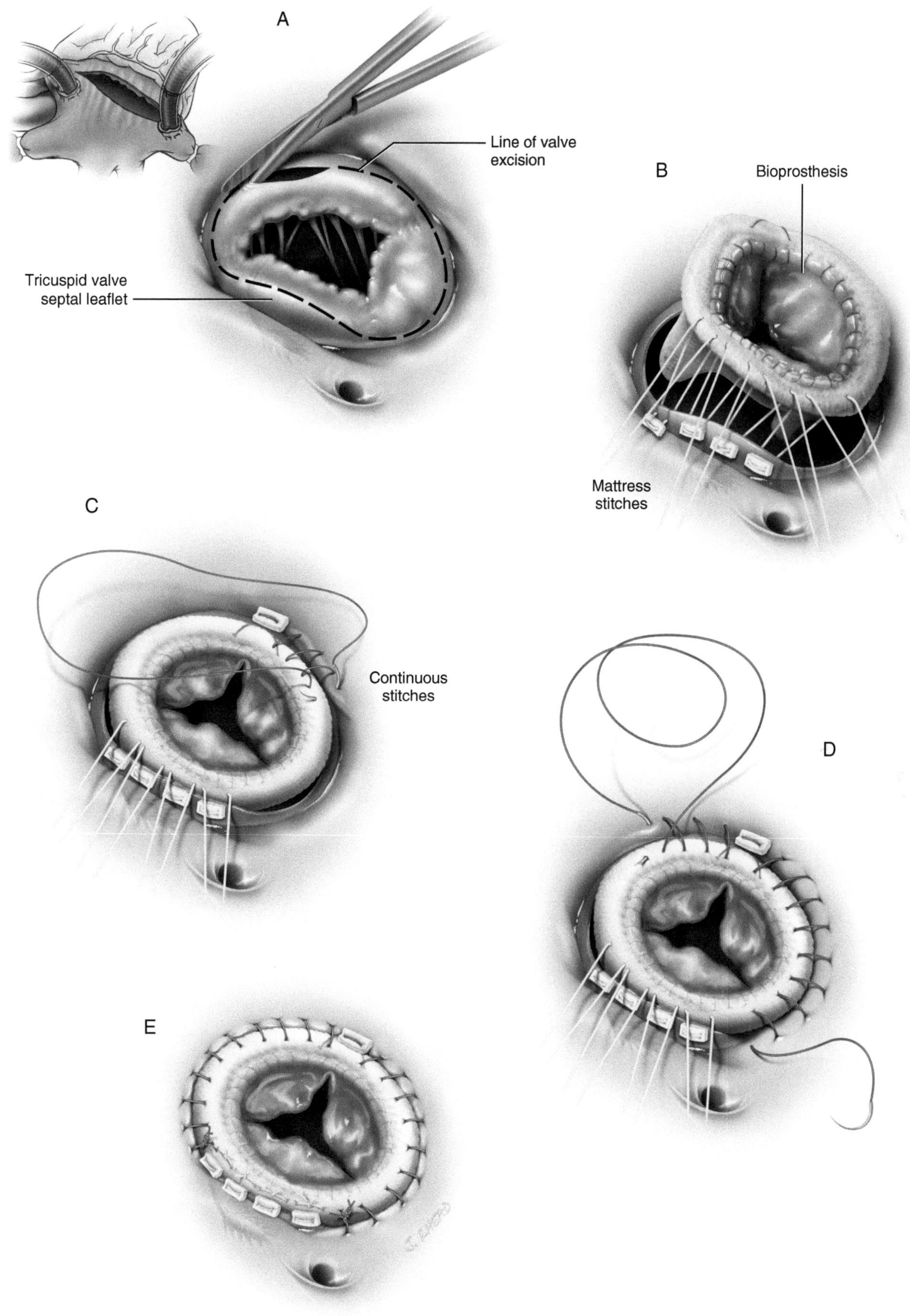
A
Line of valve excision
Tricuspid valve septal leaflet
B
Bioprosthesis
Mattress stitches
C
Continuous stitches
D
E
Completed repair

Tricuspid Valve Replacement with Mitral Homograft

Some cases of mitral valve endocarditis are treated with a mitral valve homograft. This method might be used for recurrent endocarditis in intravenous drug abusers, reinfection of a prosthetic or bioprosthetic tricuspid replacement device, or endocarditis due to antibiotic-resistant organisms.

Figure 35-4

A The entire tricuspid valve is removed, and all evidence of infection is débrided. The tricuspid annulus is measured, and a cryopreserved mitral valve homograft of the same size is selected. The homograft cannot be trimmed until thawing is complete and the tissue is softened; this takes approximately 20 minutes. Myocardium of the atrium and ventricle is then cut away from the annulus of the valve, leaving just enough tissue to allow needle penetration without entering leaflet tissue. The papillary muscles are shortened, leaving 10 mm of muscle below the chordal attachments.

B While the homograft is thawing, horizontal mattress stitches of 2/0 braided polyester are placed through the annulus of the tricuspid valve, except for the area occupied by the septal leaflet. These stitches will be used for annuloplasty. Placing these stitches as the initial step of the operation enhances exposure as the stitches are attached securely to the drapes under some tension. The anterior papillary muscle of the tricuspid valve is the only one suitable for attachment of the graft papillary muscle. The anterior papillary muscle supports the entire anterior leaflet and part of the posterior leaflet of the tricuspid valve and is continuous with the moderator band, which lends additional support.

C The mitral homograft is oriented with the anterior (septal) leaflet to the ventricular septum (septal leaflet of the tricuspid valve). Orientation is maintained by placing 4/0 propylene sutures through the fibrous trigones of the mitral homograft and passing each stitch through the tricuspid annulus at each end of the septal leaflet. The anterior papillary muscle of the mitral homograft is attached side-by-side to the anterior papillary muscle of the tricuspid valve. Multiple simple stitches of 5/0 Cardionyl are used to provide secure attachment and protect the native papillary muscle from necrosis.

D A channel is made through the anterior wall of the right ventricle at an appropriate location to accommodate the posterior papillary muscle of the graft. The papillary muscle of the homograft is pulled through the channel, and it is secured to the epicardial surface of the right ventricle with multiple stitches of 5/0 Cardionyl. The graft papillary muscle is also secured to the endocardial surface of the right ventricle with multiple stitches.

E The annulus of the homograft is attached to the annulus of the tricuspid valve by continuous stitches of 4/0 polypropylene, using the stitches previously placed through the fibrous trigones of the graft.

F An annuloplasty band (prosthetic or autogenous pericardium) is used to support the tricuspid annulus anteriorly and posteriorly. The septal leaflet portion is not supported. The annuloplasty band is attached to the tricuspid annulus by the previously placed mattress sutures. Tying the sutures securely completes the valve replacement.

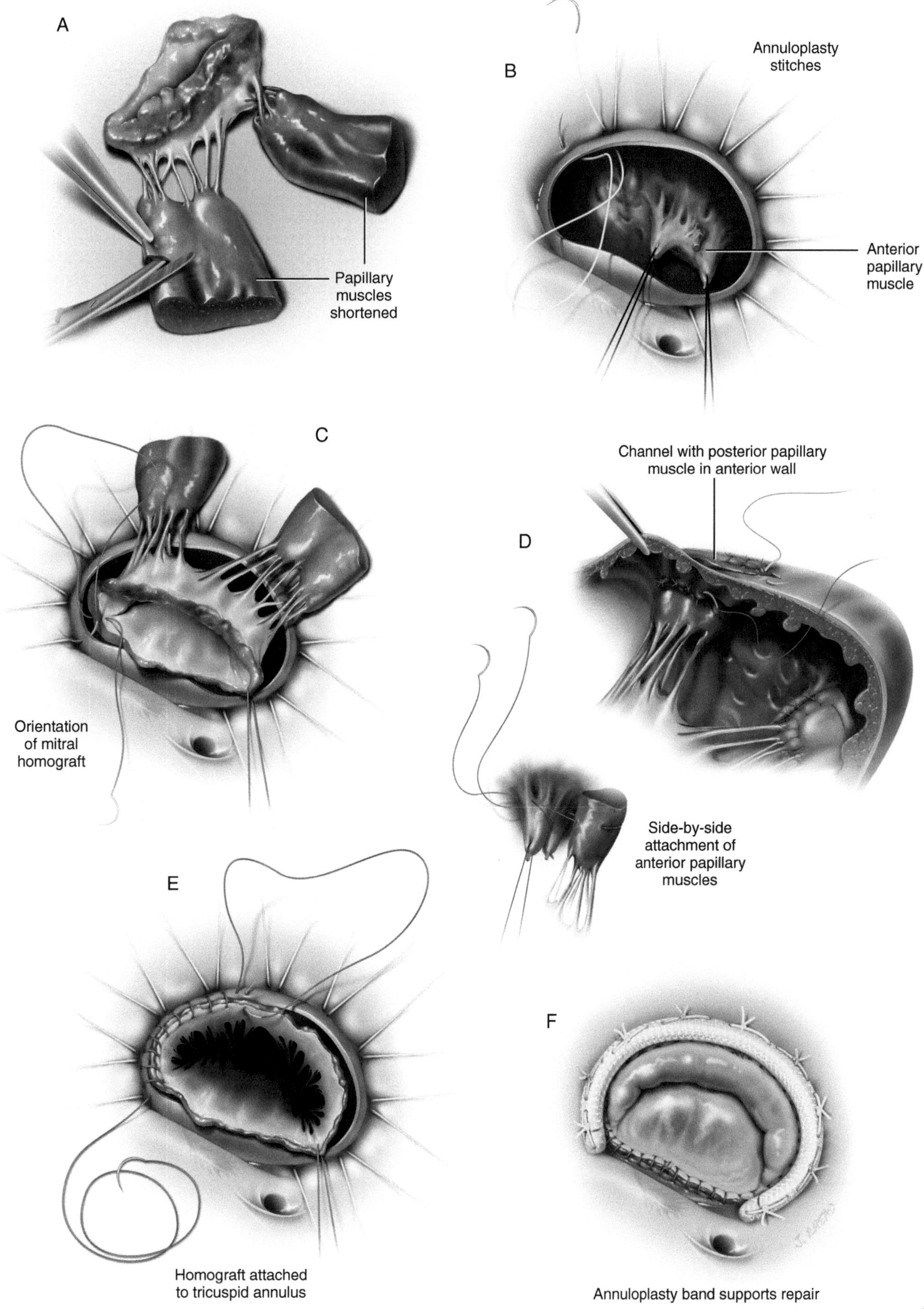
A
Papillary muscles shortened
B
Annuloplasty stitches
Anterior papillary muscle
C
Orientation of mitral homograft
D
Channel with posterior papillary muscle in anterior wall
Side-by-side attachment of anterior papillary muscles
E
Homograft attached to tricuspid annulus
F
Annuloplasty band supports repair

part X

Ischemic Heart Disease

chapter 36 CORONARY ARTERY BYPASS GRAFT

Coronary artery bypass graft operations are effective in the treatment of ischemic heart disease. Although these operations have become quite standard, there seems to be an infinite variety of presentations of atherosclerotic disease and combinations of operations to revascularize the ischemic myocardium.

Figure 36-1

Combinations for Saphenous Vein Bypass Grafts

A Sequential grafts conserve the amount of saphenous vein required for complete revascularization. A number of combinations and sequences can be used. One common sequence is that used in the left anterior descending coronary artery system. The graft is anastomosed side-to-side to the diagonal branch and end-to-side to the left anterior descending coronary artery.

B Another common sequence is anastomosis to the marginal branches of the circumflex coronary artery. The vein graft is anastomosed to the proximal marginal branches in a side-to-side fashion and to the most distal marginal branch in an end-to-side fashion.

C Posterior sequential grafts to the circumflex marginal branches can be continued to include branches of the right coronary artery, such as its posterior lateral or posterior descending branch.

D The right posterior descending coronary artery and a left ventricular branch of the distal right coronary artery can be used in sequence.

E Posterior sequential grafts that include both the right coronary artery and branches of the circumflex coronary artery eliminate the requirement for one proximal anastomosis. The direction is chosen based on the premise that placing the largest coronary artery branch at the end of the sequence will provide runoff that is greatest to the end of the graft.

Combinations for Internal Mammary Artery Bypass Grafts

F The left internal mammary artery is commonly used for bypass to the left anterior descending artery. Sequential graft techniques may include the diagonal branch of the left anterior descending artery. The right internal mammary artery can be used for bypass to the right coronary artery.

G The left internal mammary artery can be anastomosed to the obtuse marginal branch of the circumflex coronary artery. The right internal mammary artery can be brought across the midline to the left anterior descending coronary artery; however, most surgeons avoid this configuration because the right internal mammary artery is placed in proximity to the sternotomy increasing the hazard of re-entry.

H When extensive revascularization of the posterior surface of the heart is required, a posterior sequential vein graft in combination with a left internal mammary artery graft to the left anterior descending coronary artery is usually performed.

I The radial artery can be used to sequentially bypass arteries on the posterior surface of the heart. The radial artery is anastomosed to the left internal mammary artery, which is used to revascularize the anterior circulation.

J Visceral arteries, such as the right gastroepiploic artery or the splenic artery, can be used for posterior revascularization. Combined with a left internal mammary artery bypass graft for anterior revascularization, this achieves total artery revascularization.

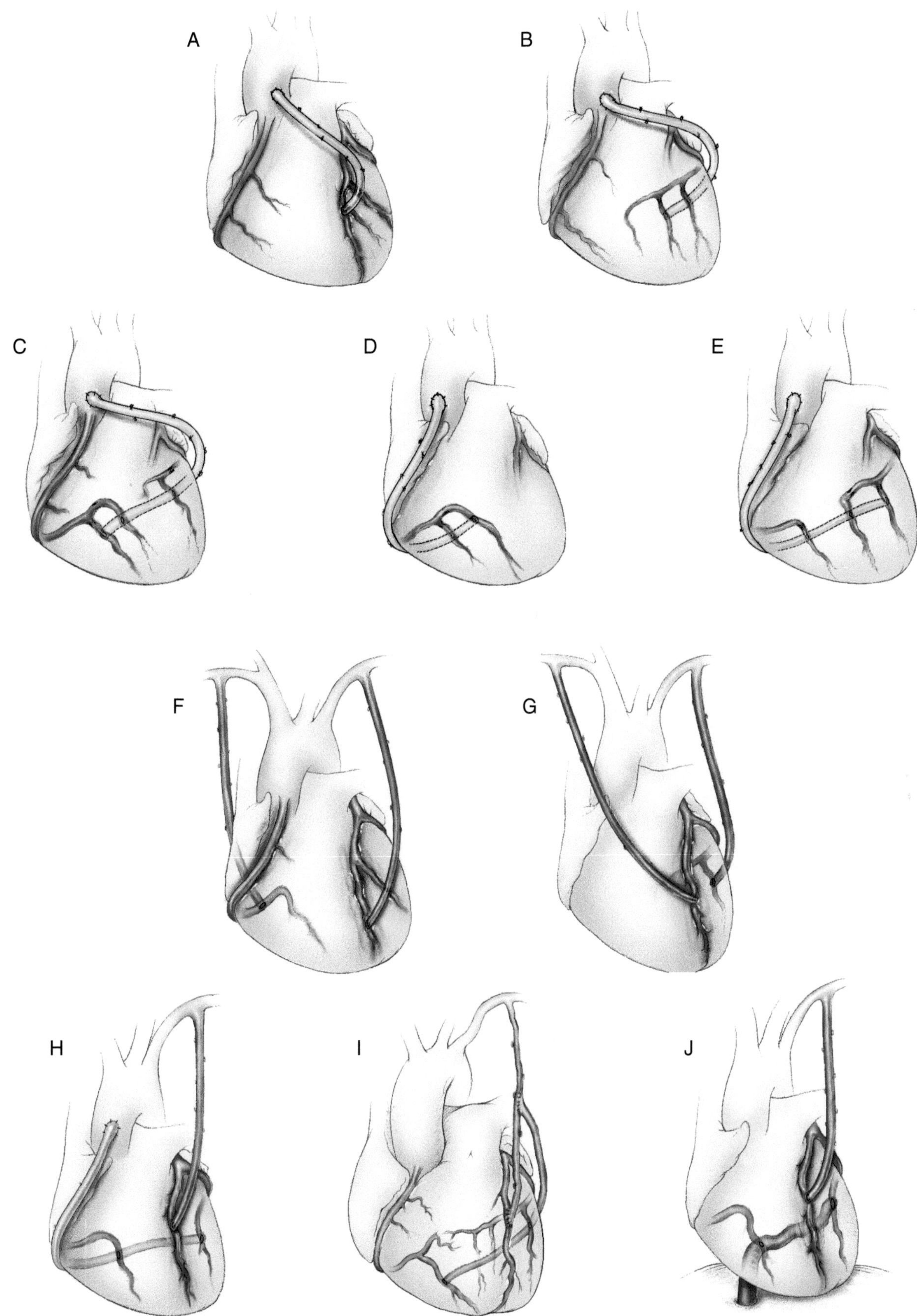
A
B
C
D
E
F
G
H
I
J

Preparation of Saphenous Vein Graft

Figure 36-2

A While the midsternal incision is made and preparations for cardiopulmonary bypass are under way, a simultaneous incision is made in the left leg over the course of the greater saphenous vein. The leg is abducted and rotated laterally by placing a roll under the knee. The foot is draped so that the ankle is exposed. With the leg in the dependent position, the vein becomes distended, allowing its course to be easily marked on the skin with a fine needle or marking pen before making the incision. The skin is opened sharply down to the level of the saphenous vein. Beginning at the ankle—to ensure a constant location anterior to the medial malleolus and easy identification of the vein—the connective tissue overlying the vein is removed. Curved Mayo scissors are ideal for this dissection. These scissors can be placed easily and safely into the plane between the connective tissue and adventitia of the saphenous vein, allowing the plane to be opened without injuring the vein. The scissors are opened perpendicular to the vein to lift the connective tissue from the top of the vein. Lateral blunt dissection should be avoided to prevent tearing of the side branches. The dissection must be limited to tissues directly over the vein. The scissors are then used to divide the connective tissue and expose the vein. Most of the side branches of the vein come into view without any lateral dissection. The entire length of the vein should be exposed before attempting to remove any of it. For a single segment of vein graft, the incision extends from the ankle to the midportion of the leg below the knee. For two grafts, the vein from the ankle to just below the knee is sufficient; for three or more grafts, the vein should be exposed to the midportion of the leg above the knee.

B The saphenous vein is ligated at the ankle over the medial malleolus. The vein is divided, and an angled peripheral vascular clamp is applied to the end to serve as a handle for retraction. For ease of dissection, firm upward retraction is applied to expose the posterior connective tissue and the side branches of the vein as they are encountered. Connective tissue must be cleanly removed from each branch's junction with the main vein so that the branch can be accurately ligated. A ligature of 4/0 silk is passed on a curved hemostat around the branch. The branch is tied precisely on the side of the saphenous vein. A small hemoclip is applied to the branch at the tissue level, and the vein branch is divided. Ligatures placed too close to the saphenous vein or that include any connective tissue not completely removed from the junction will distort and narrow the saphenous vein as its adventitia is drawn into the ligature. If the ligatures are placed away from the side of the vein, thereby leaving a length of branch between the vein and the ligatures, there is the potential for thrombus formation where stasis occurs. These errors in technique should be avoided.

C The desired length of saphenous vein is removed and prepared for bypass grafting by gentle distension using heparinized isotonic electrolyte solution. Some surgeons prefer to use the patient's blood to distend the vein. The addition of papaverine to the solution is optional. A Dietrich vascular clamp is placed on the distal end of the saphenous vein as a matter of routine to ensure proper orientation of the valves. As the vein is distended, side branches that have not been ligated are identified. A small hemostat can be applied, and the branch can simply be ligated with 4/0 silk suture or a hemoclip.

D When the branch consists of a hole in the vein, the site is closed by a double-loop stitch of 7/0 polypropylene. This technique provides the most accurate and secure closure of the vein perforation and results in the least chance of vein distortion by the pulling in of adventitial connective tissue. The right coronary system, anterior descending coronary system, and circumflex coronary system can be bypassed using individual grafts for each system. When more than one anastomosis is required in any of the three systems, sequential graft techniques are used. Alternatively, various combinations of graft sequences can be employed to conserve the length of vein required to accomplish complete revascularization of the coronary arteries.

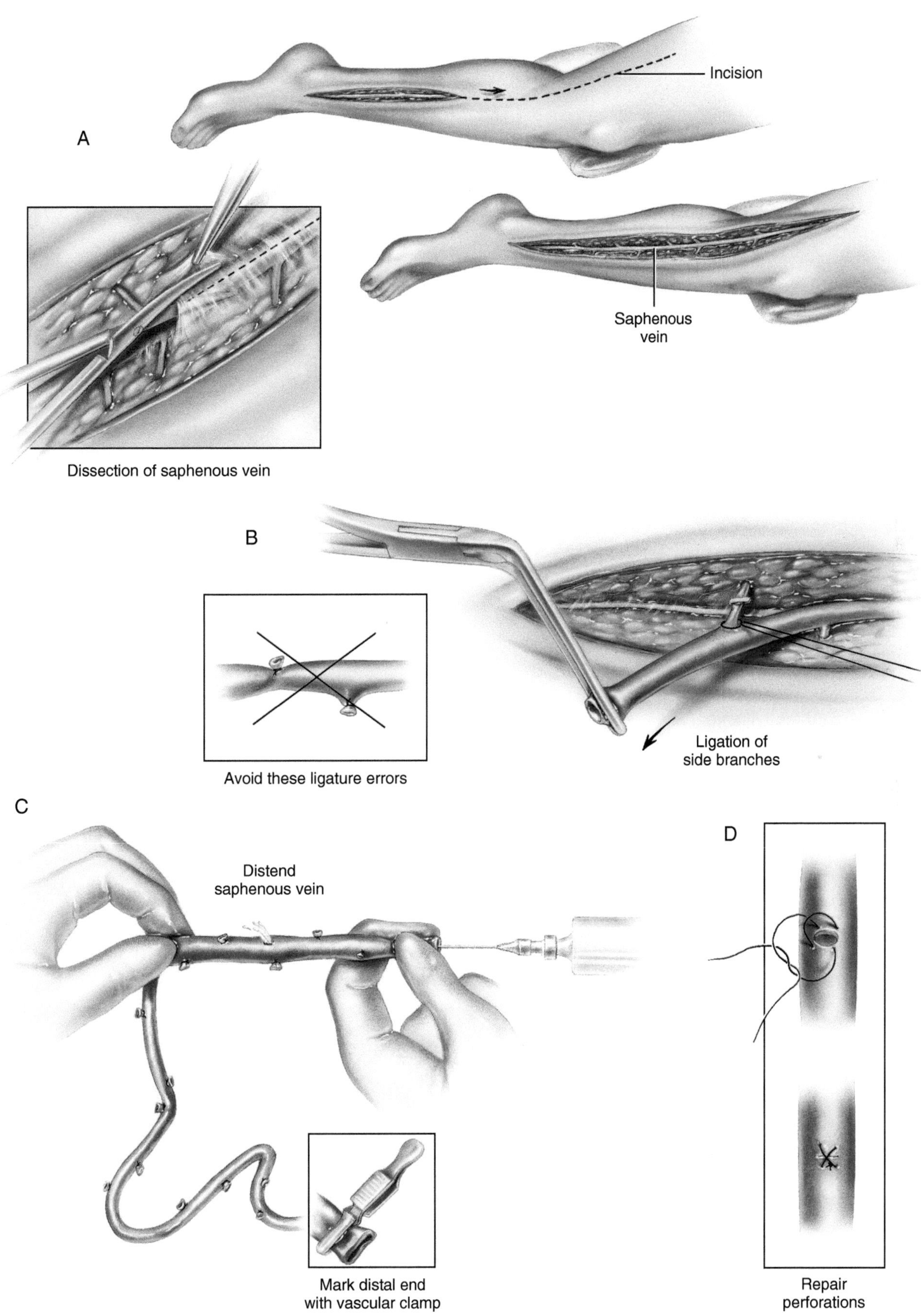
A
Incision
Saphenous
vein
Dissection of saphenous vein
B
Avoid these ligature errors
Ligation of
side branches
C
Distend
saphenous vein
Mark distal end
with vascular clamp
D
Repair
perforations

Endoscopic Saphenous Vein Harvest

Endoscopic dissection and excision of the saphenous vein have the advantages of requiring smaller skin incisions, which heal better; produce less postoperative pain and patient discomfort; and reduce the incidence of infection of the leg incision. Minimally invasive harvest of the greater saphenous vein also improves cosmesis. Nearly the entire saphenous vein can be removed with this technique, using just a few small incisions.

Figure 36-3

A A small incision is made on the medial aspect of the knee. Direct or endoscopic visualization is used to locate the greater saphenous vein, which can be encircled with a vascular snare if necessary. Prior to inserting the endoscopic system, intravenous heparin is administered to prevent intraluminal clot.

B The endoscopic port is inserted into the incision. The balloon on the port is inflated to maintain the seal if necessary. Continuous carbon dioxide insufflation is used to expand the tunnel and subcutaneous tissues for better visualization.

C A tunnel is created along the course of the saphenous vein in the thigh by gradually advancing the cone of the dissector under videoscopic guidance. The vein and side branches are freed from the subcutaneous tissue anteriorly, posteriorly, and bilaterally. The side branches are then cauterized and divided to free the vein within the tunnel in the thigh.

D A similar tunnel is created along the course of the saphenous vein in the calf by reversing the direction of the endoscopic system within the primary incision. The vein and side branches are freed from the subcutaneous tissue, and the side branches are divided to free the vein within the tunnel in the lower leg.

E Using videoscopic guidance, a small stab wound is made through the skin and into the tunnel above the vein at both the proximal and distal ends of the tunnel. The vein is gently retrieved through the stab incision and divided under direct vision. Alternatively, an endoloop can be used to ligate the proximal and distal ends; the vein is then divided with electrocautery.

F The entire saphenous vein is removed through the knee incision. The remnants of the side branches are reinforced with fine silk ligatures. A pressure dressing is applied to the leg.

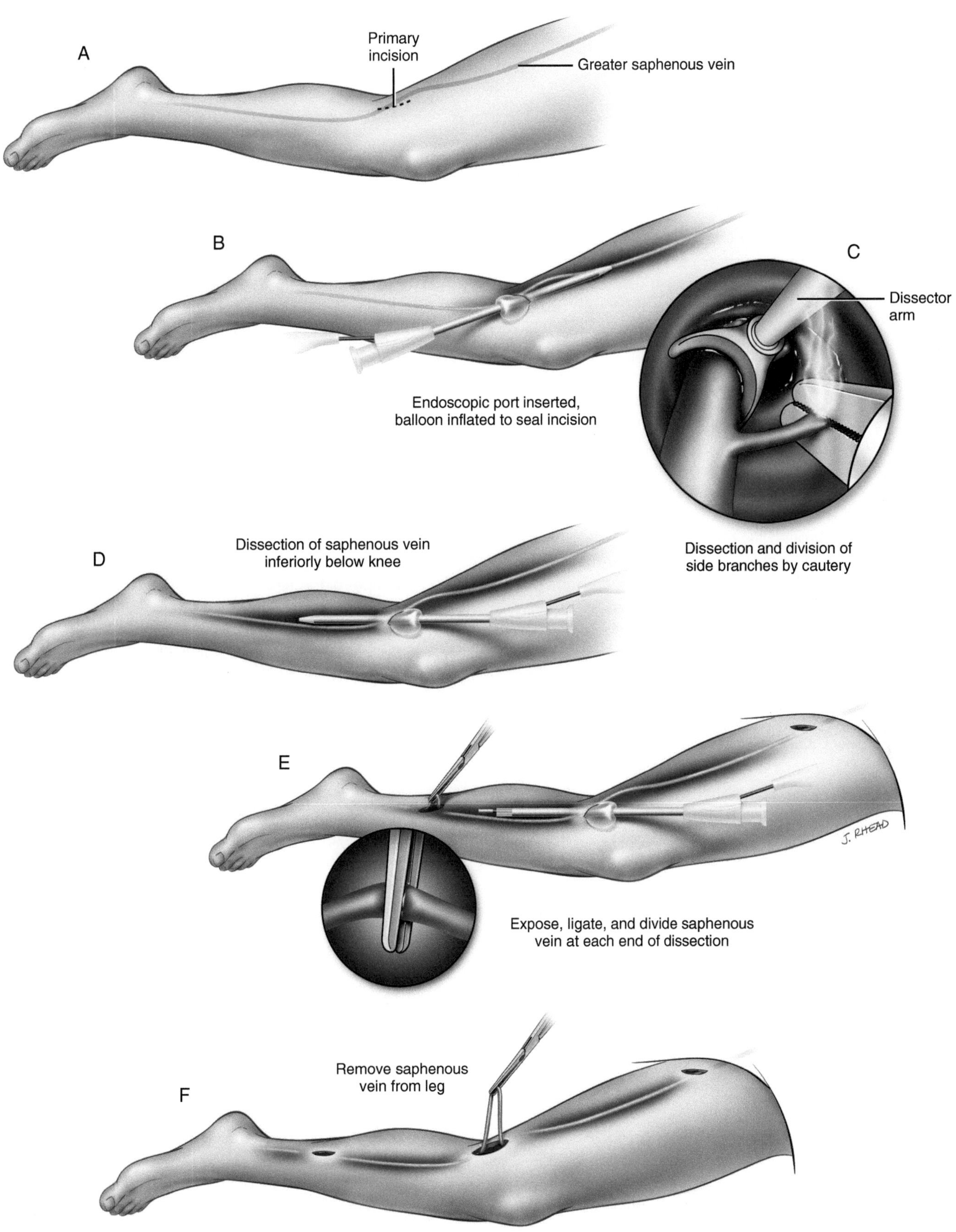
A
Primary incision
Greater saphenous vein
B
C
Dissector arm
Endoscopic port inserted, balloon inflated to seal incision
Dissection and division of side branches by cautery
D
Dissection of saphenous vein inferiorly below knee
E
J. RHEAD
Expose, ligate, and divide saphenous vein at each end of dissection
F
Remove saphenous vein from leg

Saphenous Vein–Coronary Artery (Distal) Anastomosis
Figure 36-4

A Cardiopulmonary bypass is established using a single cannula (two stage) for venous drainage, with oxygenated blood returned to the ascending aorta through a cannula placed just below the pericardial reflection. The left ventricle is decompressed by a right-angled vent catheter or a pediatric vent catheter passed via the right superior pulmonary vein to the left atrium and left ventricle. The aorta is occluded by a vascular clamp high on the ascending aorta. Revascularization is accomplished during a single aortic occlusion period. Cold cardioplegic solution (blood-based) is injected into the ascending aorta, retrograde through the coronary sinus; alternatively, a combination of antegrade and retrograde perfusion can be used. The myocardium is perfused intermittently during the procedure. Exposure of the coronary arteries for the distal anastomosis of the saphenous vein to the coronary arteries can be accomplished by a number of techniques. The common practice of having an assistant retract the heart under a gauze sponge or with a cotton glove may cause unwanted cardiac trauma. The quality of the exposure depends on the attention of the assistant. Static exposure of the distal right coronary artery and its posterior descending branch can be obtained by placing three or four traction stitches on the acute margin of the heart. One of the stitches should be near the atrioventricular groove. These stitches are held with a hemostat, which is retracted cephalad either by an assistant or by attaching it to a rubber band secured to the drapes.

B Exposure of the left coronary branches is accomplished by a net device tied to umbilical tape. The ends of the tape are drawn through the transverse sinus and through an opening below the right inferior pulmonary vein behind the inferior vena cava. The net is placed behind the heart and drawn tight to the atrioventricular groove by right lateral retraction and by securing the tape to hemostats on the right anterior chest wall. Elevating the net and securing the end of it to the left anterior chest wall expose the left anterior descending coronary artery.

C By retracting the net to the right and securing it to the right anterior chest wall, the cardiac apex is tipped up, exposing the posterior surface of the left ventricle and providing access to the left circumflex coronary artery. Sections of the net can be removed for improved access to the surface coronary arteries.

Incision of the Coronary Artery

D The coronary artery is exposed and incised directly through the epicardium, without mobilization. Lateral traction with forceps fixes the coronary artery in place. A No. 15 scalpel is gently stroked on the coronary artery until the lumen is entered. The part of the scalpel blade near the tip is used so that neither the scoring nor the subsequent arteriotomy is too long. Entry of the coronary artery is confirmed by observing cardioplegic solution exiting the artery. Optical magnification (2.5 to 3.5×) is essential for precise and accurate visualization of the coronary artery.

E The arteriotomy is extended at each apex using Dietrich coronary artery scissors. The 20- or 45-degree scissors are used to open the artery at the proximal end. The scissors should be placed carefully into the lumen of the artery so that the tips do not damage the intima. The tips of the scissors should never be used to probe the lumen of the coronary artery. The cut should be to the tips of the scissors so that the length of the incision is precisely controlled. Should there be any question about the identification of the actual coronary artery lumen, calibrated coronary probes should be employed judiciously.

F The distal end of the arteriotomy is completed in a similar fashion using 130-degree Dietrich scissors. The length of the coronary artery incision should approximate the diameter of the saphenous vein, measuring about 4 to 5 mm. Care should be taken to ensure that the completed arteriotomy extends for the full length of the scoring to avoid potential weakness at the ends of the arteriotomy.

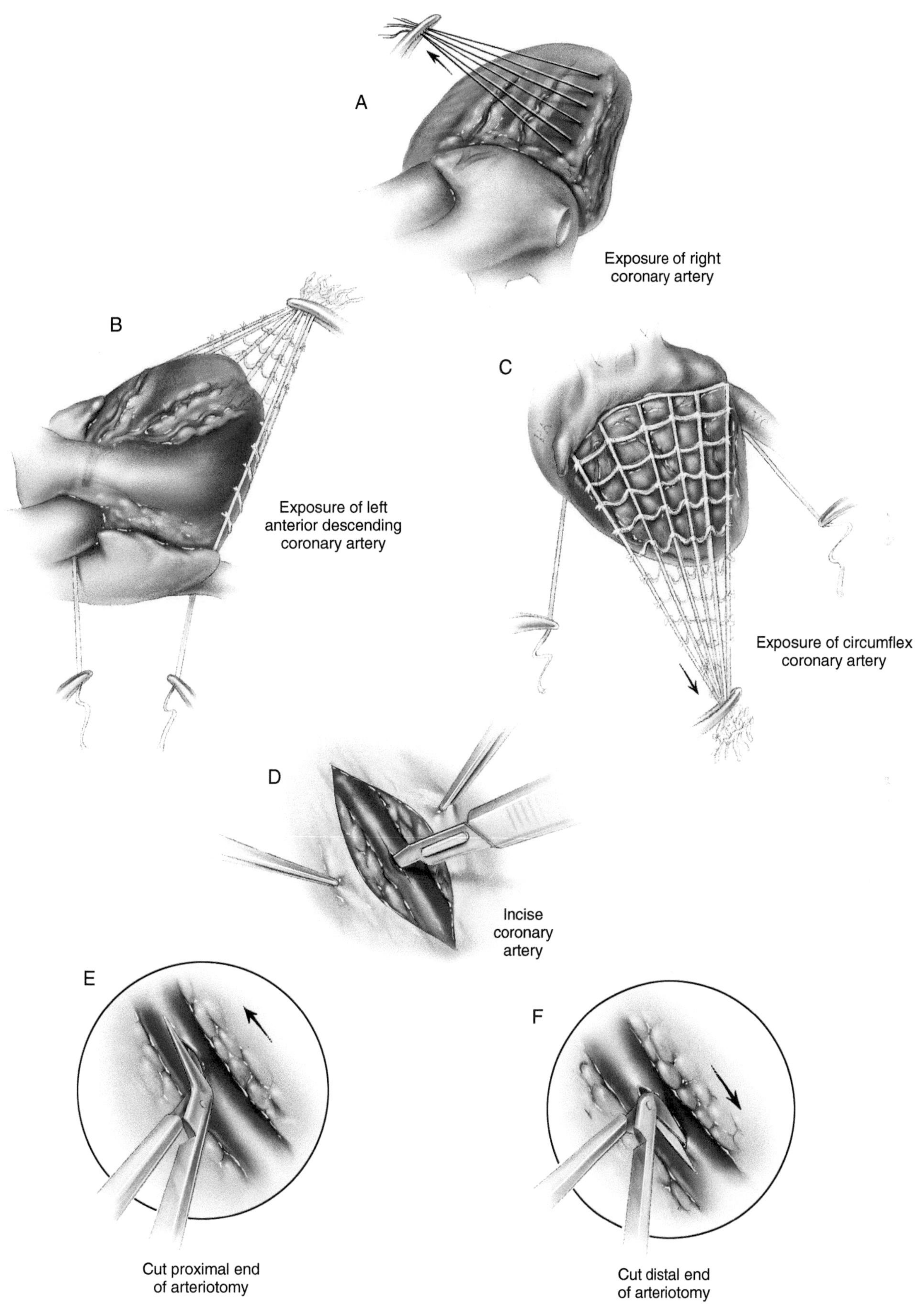
A
Exposure of right
coronary artery
B
Exposure of left
anterior descending
coronary artery
C
Exposure of circumflex
coronary artery
D
Incise
coronary
artery
E
Cut proximal end
of arteriotomy
F
Cut distal end
of arteriotomy

Figure 36-4 (continued)

End-to-Side Anastomosis: Left-Side Grafts

G The distal end of the saphenous vein segment is beveled at a 30- to 45-degree angle, and an adequate length is ensured for its course over the surface of the heart. A 10-stitch anastomosis is constructed using 7/0 polypropylene. Performing the anastomosis in precisely the same fashion in every case ensures a standardized technique and reproducible patency results. Five stitches are taken around the "heel" of the graft: two stitches to the side of the apex of the vein graft and coronary artery, one stitch through the apex, and two stitches on the opposite side of the apex. The graft is held apart from the coronary artery while these stitches are taken. Tension on the suture and retraction of the vein graft to the side provide exposure of the subsequent stitch. The vein graft is held by fine forceps at the side so that the intima at the tip is not injured. Suturing for left-side grafts is performed clockwise on the vein and counterclockwise on the artery.

H The suture loops are drawn up, and the suture is pulled straight through to prevent a purse-string effect. The ends of the suture provide lateral traction on the coronary artery for exposure of the distal apex of the coronary arteriotomy.

I Five stitches are taken around the "toe" of the graft, with the third stitch placed precisely at the apex of the coronary arteriotomy. Loops of the five sutures are left lax for exposure of the distal portion of the anastomosis. For the proper wagon-wheel effect, the needle direction is changed after the apex stitch is placed. Retraction of the vein graft and opposing traction on the epicardium expose the intima of the coronary artery. The ends of the sutures are tied precisely with tension to approximate the tissue without causing a purse-string effect.

End-to-Side Anastomosis: Right-Side Grafts

J The arteriotomy in the right coronary artery is generally made in the distal portion near the takeoff of the posterior descending coronary artery or in the posterior descending coronary artery itself as it courses along the posterior aspect of the ventricular septum. With right coronary artery grafts, it is usually easier to place the initial five stitches around the toe of the graft. Careful orientation of the graft prevents confusion. Stitches are placed around the toe of the graft in a counterclockwise fashion and around the distal end of the coronary arteriotomy in a clockwise fashion. The graft is held by fine forceps at the side. Retraction of the graft and suture tension help achieve exposure of the apex of the coronary arteriotomy. Suture loops are drawn up to approximate the graft to the artery and to provide lateral traction on the coronary arteriotomy.

K The vein graft is retracted inferiorly with forceps to expose the proximal end of the coronary arteriotomy. Five stitches are placed at the heel in a clockwise fashion to complete the anastomosis. As the apex of the arteriotomy is passed with a suture placed directly in line with the coronary artery, the suture is passed beneath the vein graft.

L The final two stitches are placed accurately by retracting the graft laterally and applying opposing traction on the epicardium medially. The suture ends are joined to complete the anastomosis.

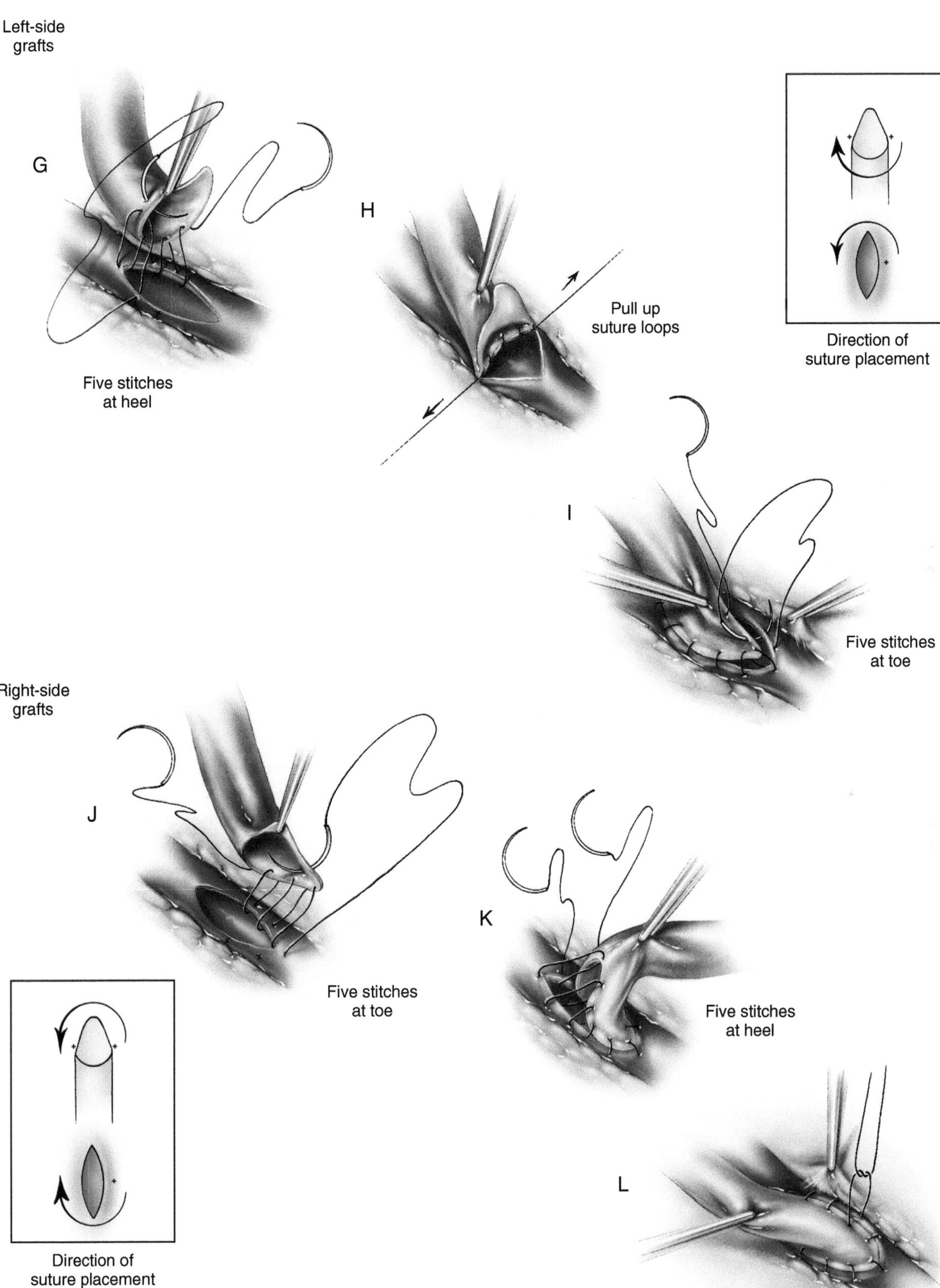
Left-side
grafts
G
Five stitches
at heel
H
Pull up
suture loops
Direction of
suture placement
I
Five stitches
at toe
Right-side
grafts
J
Five stitches
at toe
K
Five stitches
at heel
Direction of
suture placement
L
Completed anastomosis

Figure 36-4 (continued)

Sequential Grafts

M When more than one graft is required in a coronary artery system, sequential graft techniques are used by creating proximal side-to-side anastomoses and completing the graft as an end-to-side anastomosis. A No. 11 scalpel is used to incise the vein in an appropriate orientation. In most cases a transverse incision is necessary; however, diagonal and longitudinal incisions may be more suitable, depending on the orientation of the graft relative to the coronary artery. As the pointed scalpel perforates the wall of the saphenous vein, the incision through the wall should not exceed one third of the circumference of the vein.

N The five stitches placed around the heel of the graft and the coronary arteriotomy are used to provide lateral traction while the five stitches around the toe are placed. It is easiest to work in a counterclockwise fashion around the coronary arteriotomy for the most proximal of the sequential anastomoses. The more distal anastomoses are performed in a clockwise fashion to prevent unnecessary traction on the more proximal anastomoses. This technique of reversing the direction of the continuous suture anastomosis allows the graft to be retracted toward the more proximal anastomoses, providing exposure without exerting any tension on the completed anastomoses. Only four stitches are placed around the proximal end of the arteriotomy because once the suturing has passed the apex, it is no longer possible to retract the vein graft for exposure without pulling on the proximal anastomoses. The vein graft and the arteriotomy are nicely approximated at this point, and the walls of graft and the artery are easily sutured together.

O The last anastomosis in a sequential graft is an end-to-side connection of the graft to the coronary artery. This arteriotomy is, of necessity, somewhat larger than those for the side-to-side anastomoses. Suturing proceeds clockwise around the arteriotomy, allowing use of the suture and retraction of the vein graft to provide exposure without distorting the completed proximal anastomoses. Again, it is of no advantage to place more than four stitches around the apex of the arteriotomy before approximating the vein graft and the artery. Determining the length of graft to use between the coronary artery sequences is a simple matter because the distensibility of the vein graft is approximately the same as the expansion of the heart when it is filled. Simply place the graft on the surface of the heart and make the anastomoses where the graft seems to fit. This results in a graft that lies without stretch or excess length when blood distends the graft and the heart.

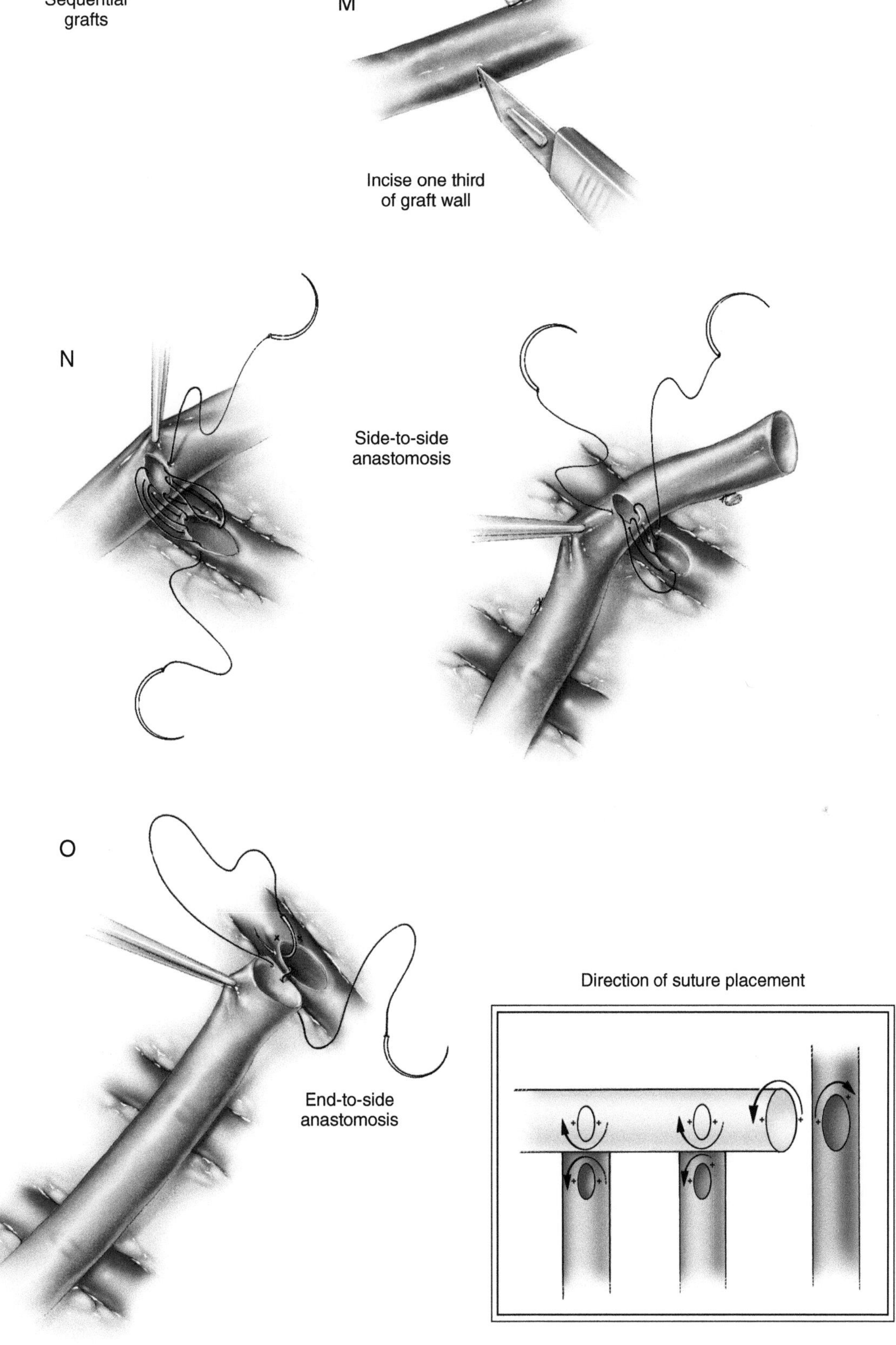
Sequential
grafts
M
Incise one third
of graft wall
N
Side-to-side
anastomosis
O
End-to-side
anastomosis
Direction of suture placement

Aorta–Saphenous Vein (Proximal) Anastomosis
Figure 36-5

A Anastomosis of the saphenous vein to the aorta is usually performed after construction of the distal anastomosis to the coronary artery. We favor this technique and use a single period of aortic occlusion and intermittent retrograde perfusion of the myocardium via the coronary sinus for both distal and proximal anastomoses. Alternatively, some surgeons prefer to perform the proximal anastomosis as the initial step to ensure aortic input to the graft and to allow antegrade perfusion of cardioplegia solution through the graft via the aorta as the revascularization proceeds.

The pericardial layer covering the aorta is removed over its anterior wall. Small openings (4 to 5 mm in diameter) are made into the ascending aorta using an aortic punch. The opening for the right coronary artery graft is directly anterior to or to the right lateral side of the aorta, whereas openings for left-side grafts are made on the left lateral side. The end of the saphenous vein is cut back longitudinally for a distance of approximately 1 cm. A Cooley infant vascular clamp is placed across the tip of the saphenous vein to flatten it for exposure of the vein's shorter, beveled end. Five suture loops of 5/0 polypropylene are then placed around the heel of the graft and passed through the aortic wall. Two stitches are placed to the side of the apex, the third stitch is placed precisely through the apex of the incision in the saphenous vein, and the final two stitches are placed on the opposite side of the apex. Traction on both the suture and the vein graft helps expose the edge of the aortic opening for accurate needle placement. Stitches include about 3 to 5 mm of the aortic wall to ensure adequate strength of the anastomosis.

B The suture loops are pulled up to approximate the vein graft to the aorta. The anastomosis is completed by placing stitches in a wagon-wheel fashion around the opening in the aorta. The placement of each stitch should be accurately visualized by observing the edge of the vein graft and the intima of the aorta. Retraction of the vein graft with forceps and slight relaxation of suture tension as the needle passes from the graft to the aorta provide exposure. Wide stitches are taken along the lateral edge of the saphenous vein as it is approximated with narrow stitches to the aorta to ensure that the maximal length of saphenous vein is positioned laterally. The completed anastomosis should bulge anteriorly above the aortic wall, achieving a "cobra head" appearance.

C Left-side grafts are oriented so that the shorter, beveled end of the saphenous vein graft (the heel) directly faces the left side. The stitches are placed in a clockwise fashion around the heel of the graft and in a counterclockwise fashion around the aortic opening. The right coronary graft is placed so that the heel is oriented caudally; the stitches are placed in a counterclockwise fashion around the heel of the graft and in a clockwise fashion around the aorta.

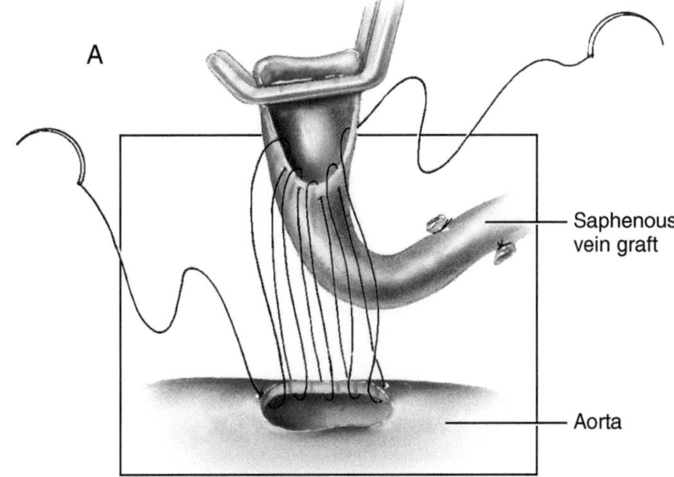

Five stitches around heel

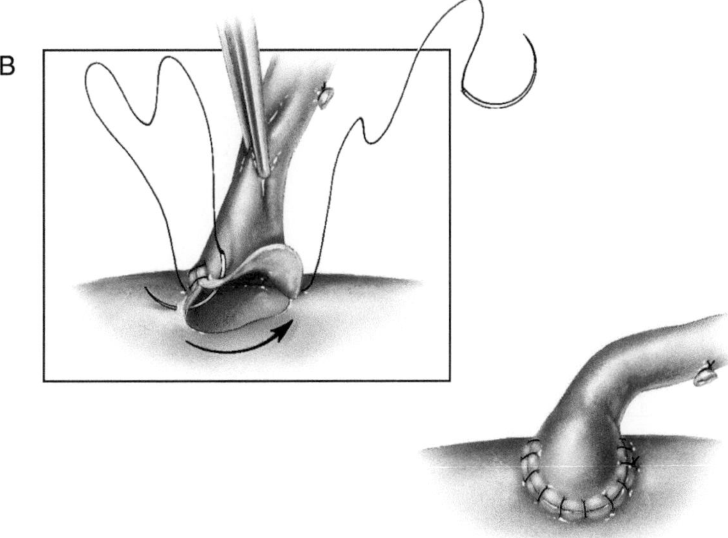

Completed anastomosis

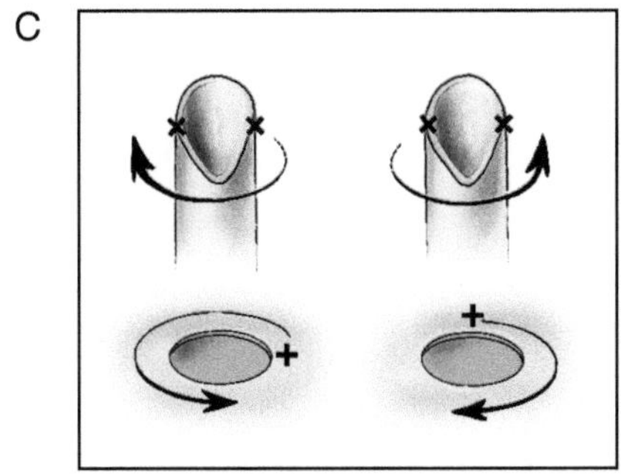

Direction of suture placement

Preparation of the Internal Mammary Artery Pedicle

Coronary artery bypass using the internal mammary artery for the bypass conduit has become established practice. Long-term outcome data show favorable results and excellent patency.

Figure 36-6

A A midsternal incision is made, and the pleura is swept back from the sternal edge with a gauze sponge. The posterior surface of the sternum and ribs are exposed using specially modified self-retaining rake retractors to elevate the anterior chest wall. The internal mammary artery is dissected from the anterior chest wall by electrocautery. An incision is made at the edge of the sternum for its entire length using electrocautery. The dissection of the artery is started inferiorly, just above the diaphragm. The artery is mobilized from the ribs by blunt dissection where there are no arterial branches.

B Strong tension is exerted posteriorly on the vascular pedicle to expose the branches located in the rib interspaces. The blade of the electrocautery is angled so that the tissue can be cut deep in the interspace, allowing a considerable length of arterial branch to be retained with the internal mammary artery when it is divided. The internal mammary artery, along with the venae comitantes and the chest wall fat, muscle, and fascia, is mobilized as a pedicle.

C The internal mammary artery is mobilized for its entire length. The dissection should be continued until the artery is completely freed from the parasternal tissues to the level of the diaphragm. Electrocautery is used to complete the pedicle dissection by incising the chest wall tissues and pleura for the length of the dissection.

D Heparin is administered for systemic anticoagulation, and cardiopulmonary bypass is established. The internal mammary artery pedicle is divided, and the distal end of the pedicle is ligated. Division of the internal mammary artery should result in forceful blood flow from the proximal end, but on cardiopulmonary bypass, the flow may be minimal. A Dietrich vascular clamp is applied to the pedicle to control blood flow. The pedicle is soaked with 5% dextrose containing sodium nitroprusside to obtain vasodilation of the internal mammary artery.

E The aorta is occluded, and the heart is arrested by administering cold cardioplegic solution in the aortic root. The coronary artery is incised as described for a saphenous vein bypass graft, with special care taken to make a short, controlled arteriotomy. An appropriate length of the internal mammary artery is dissected free of the pedicle to approximate the coronary arteriotomy. Dissecting scissors are used to separate the veins and other tissues from the artery. The pedicle is cut just short of the proposed location of the anastomosis.

F Venae comitantes and arterial branches are ligated with small hemoclips. During the dissection and subsequent anastomosis, the internal mammary artery is handled only at the tip, which will be discarded later.

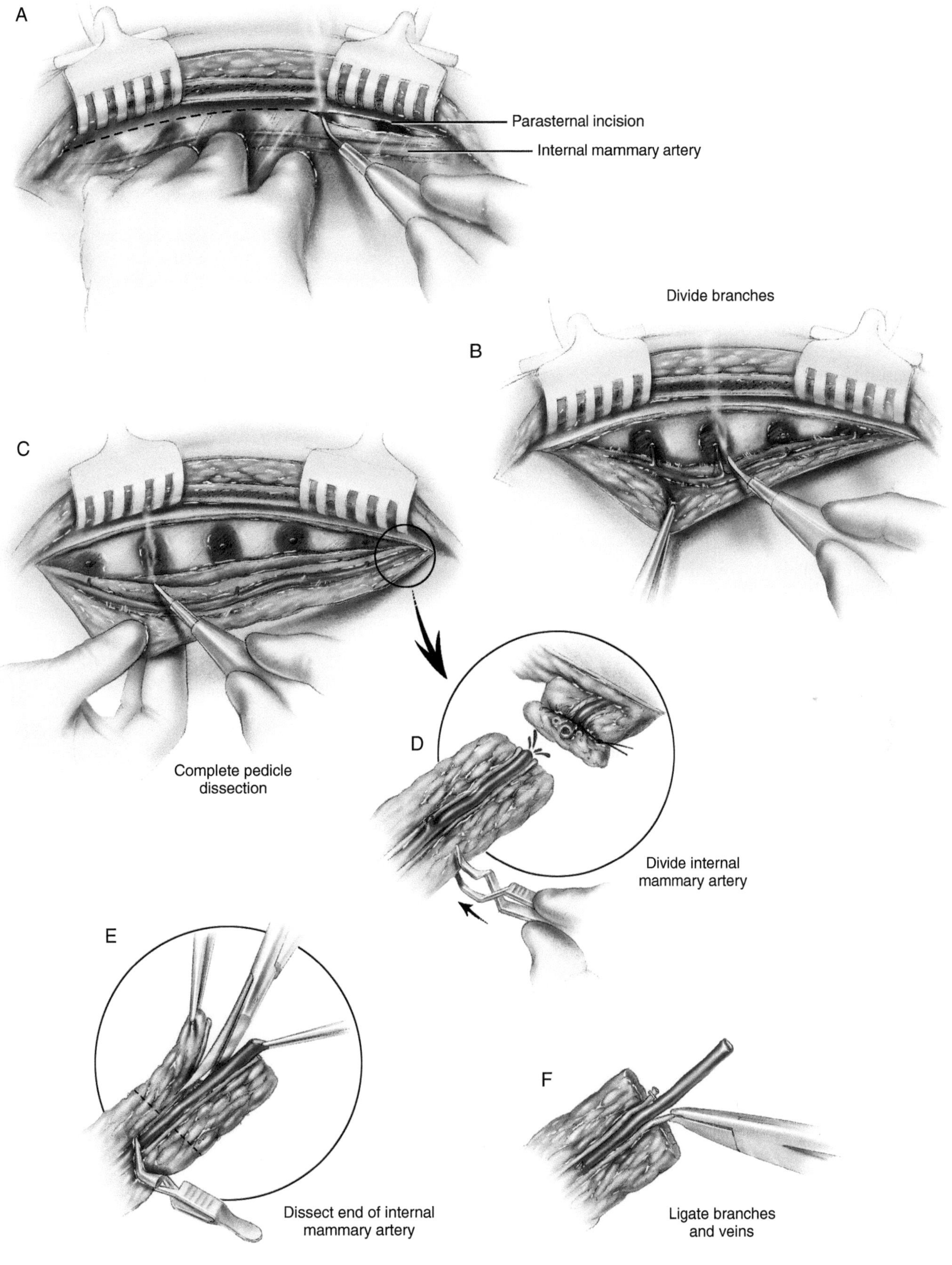
A
Parasternal incision
Internal mammary artery
Divide branches
B
C
Complete pedicle dissection
D
Divide internal mammary artery
E
Dissect end of internal mammary artery
F
Ligate branches and veins

Internal Mammary Artery–Coronary Artery Anastomosis
Figure 36-7

A The internal mammary artery is pulled back to expose its posterior surface. A longitudinal incision is made to cut back the artery to the appropriate length for anastomosis. The artery can be manipulated by firm traction on the tip if that portion will be excised later. During incision of the artery, care must be taken to avoid injuring the intimal surface when the tips of the scissors are inserted into the artery.

B A 10-stitch anastomosis is constructed by continuous suture technique using 7/0 polypropylene. At an appropriate distance from the apex of the incision in the mammary artery to approximate half the length of the coronary arteriotomy, five stitches are placed through the heel of the mammary artery and the coronary arteriotomy. The initial stitch is placed at the midpoint on the arteriotomy; the second stitch is placed halfway between the initial stitch and the apex of the arteriotomy; the third stitch is placed precisely at the apex, in line with the coronary artery lumen; and the fourth and fifth stitches are placed in similar positions on the arteriotomy opposite the first two stitches. The internal mammary artery is held away from the coronary artery until all five stitches are placed.

C The suture loops are pulled up to approximate the mammary artery to the coronary artery. The suture is pulled straight through to eliminate the chance of a purse-string effect. Lateral tension on the suture ends separates the edges of the coronary arteriotomy to accurately expose the apex of the arteriotomy.

D The internal mammary artery is held at the tip with forceps in the correct orientation so that scissors can be used to shorten it to the correct length to cover the remainder of the coronary arteriotomy. The mammary artery is folded edge-to-edge so that an angle is created at the tip during incision with the scissors.

E The 10-stitch anastomosis is completed by placing five stitches around the toe of the graft in exactly the same manner as the heel was approximated. Two stitches are placed at the side of the apex; the third stitch is placed precisely at the apex, in line with the coronary artery lumen; and the fourth and fifth stitches are placed on the opposite side of the apex to complete the anastomosis. The suture ends are joined by a knot at the midpoint of the side of the coronary arteriotomy.

F The pedicle is sutured to the epicardium just behind and to the side of the anastomosis with 5/0 polypropylene. This attachment stabilizes the anastomosis and prevents tension from being placed on it.

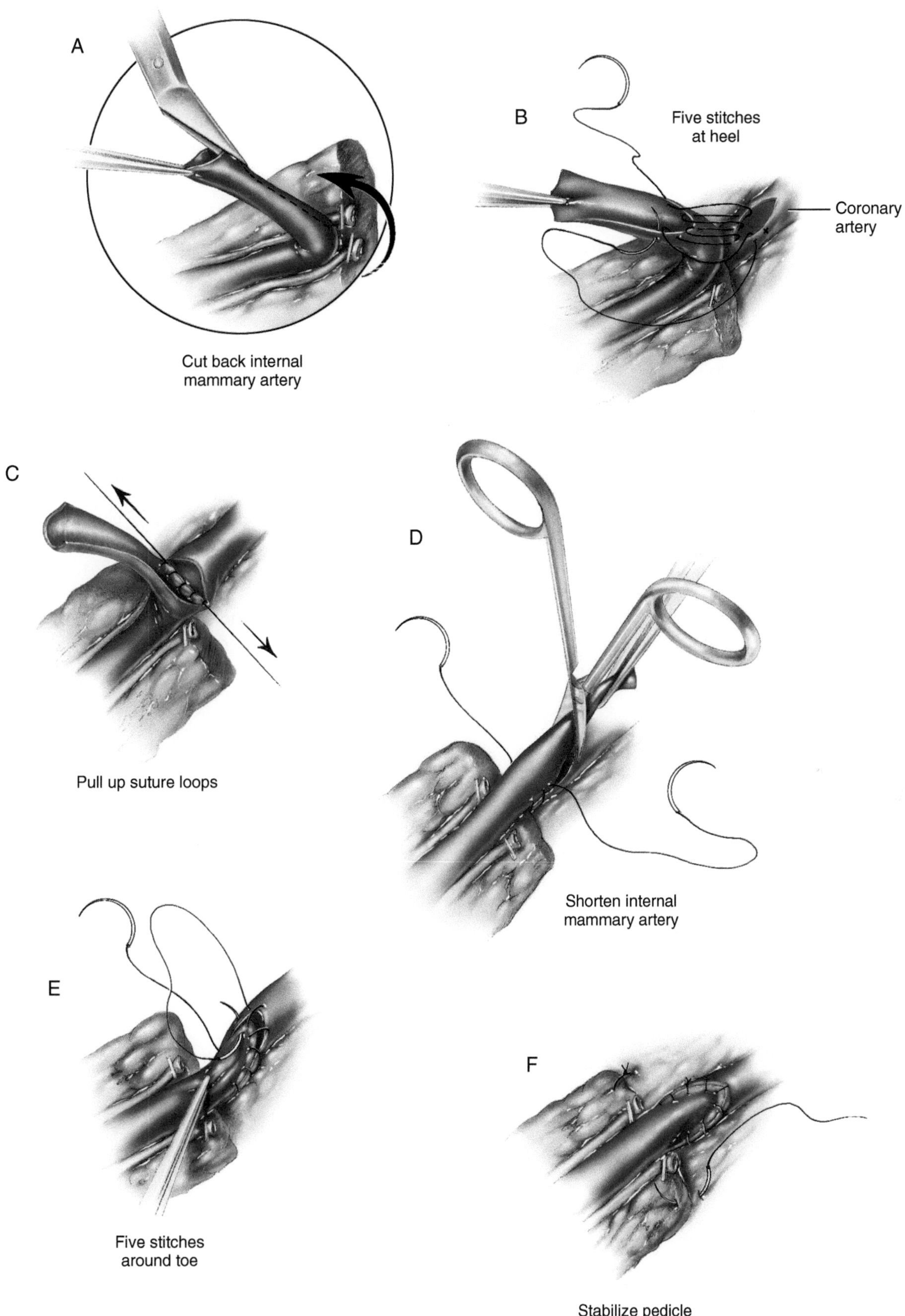
A
Cut back internal mammary artery
B
Five stitches at heel
Coronary artery
C
Pull up suture loops
D
Shorten internal mammary artery
E
Five stitches around toe
F
Stabilize pedicle

Figure 36-7 (continued)

G Sequential anastomoses of the internal mammary artery to the coronary arteries can extend the use of this conduit. This bypass design requires a side-to-side anastomosis technique. The sequence most frequently used and the one that best conforms to the course of the left internal mammary artery is side-to-side anastomosis to the diagonal branches of the left anterior descending coronary artery, with termination in an end-to-side anastomosis to the left anterior descending coronary artery. The internal mammary artery may naturally course across the anterior surface of the left ventricle and conform to longitudinal side-to-side anastomoses without much distortion. A separate incision in the pericardium anterior to the phrenic nerve on the left side allows entry to the pericardial sac from the opened left hemithorax adjacent to the diagonal branches of the left anterior descending coronary artery.

H An incision is made into the pedicle through the endothoracic fascia and muscle directly over the internal mammary artery. Distal occlusion of the mammary artery distends it, and the lumen is entered by making a longitudinal stroking incision with a No. 15 scalpel.

I With the vessels held apart, five stitches are placed between the apex of the internal mammary arteriotomy at the heel and the apex of the coronary artery incision, also at the heel. The suture loops are drawn up to approximate the vessels.

J Suturing proceeds along the side closest to the surgeon to the opposite apex (the toe) of the arteries. Continuous stitches of 7/0 polypropylene are used.

K The pedicle is rotated to the right to allow the suturing to be completed on the side opposite the surgeon. About 8 to 10 stitches are used for the entire anastomosis.

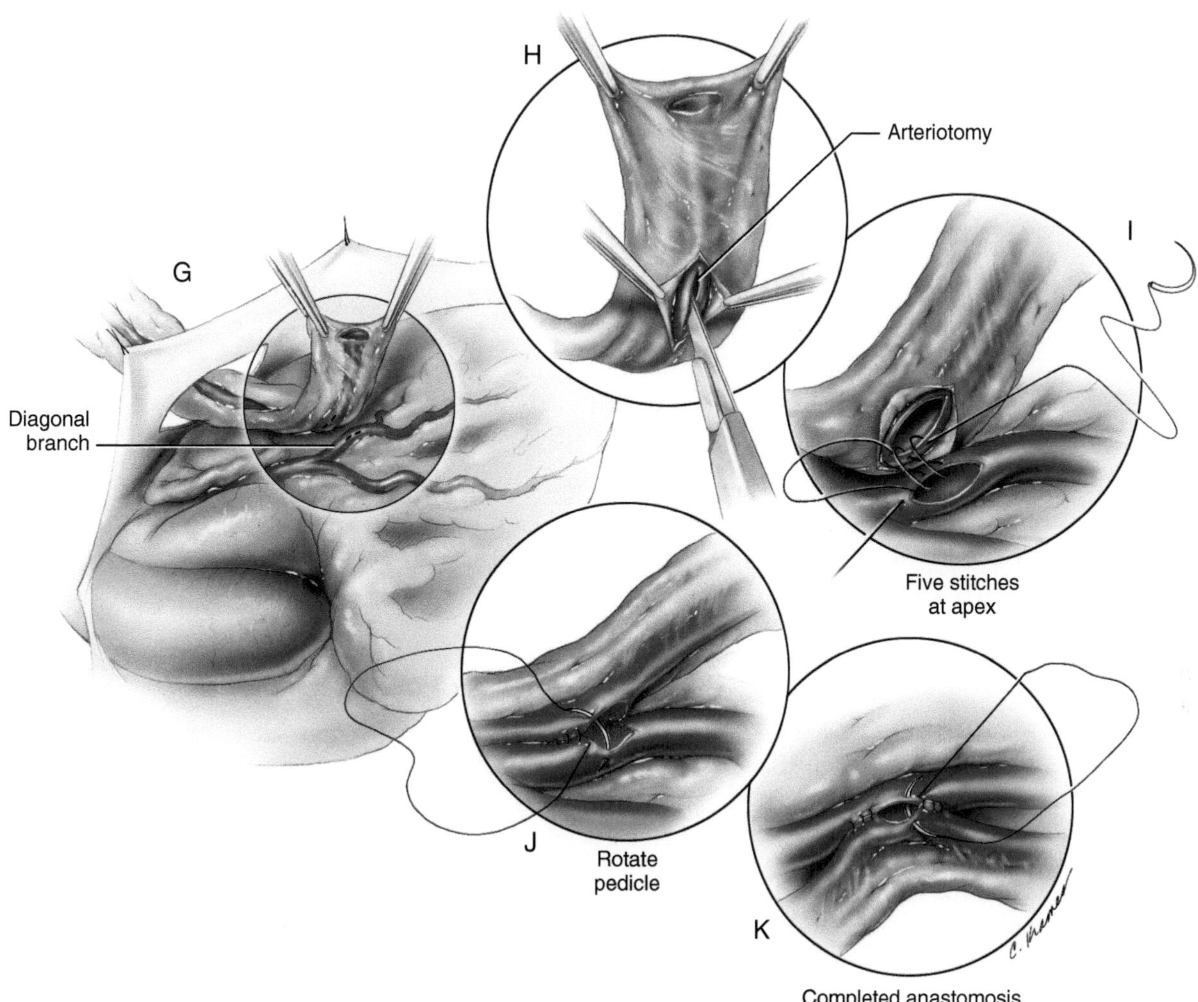
H
Arteriotomy
I
G
Diagonal
branch
Five stitches
at apex
J
Rotate
pedicle
K
Completed anastomosis

Right Internal Mammary Artery–Circumflex Coronary Artery Bypass

The left internal mammary artery is best utilized to bypass the left anterior descending coronary artery and its diagonal branches. The right internal mammary artery can be used to bypass selected vessels more posteriorly, such as the distal right coronary artery. It can also be used to bypass selected marginal branches of the left circumflex artery. Marginal branches high on the obtuse margin can be reached by the right internal mammary artery passed through the transverse sinus. More distal marginal branches can be reached by taking the graft through the oblique sinus.

Figure 36-8

A The pericardium is reflected posteriorly over the left atrium at its superior margin. Dividing the two leaves of the reflection that are near each other opens up a space between the right and left pulmonary veins behind the left atrium. This is called the oblique sinus of Haller. The free pericardial space behind the left atrium extends almost to the superoposterior aspect of the atrium. This passageway is the shortest bypass graft route from the right side to the posterior surface of the left ventricle.

B The opening into the oblique sinus should be large enough to easily accommodate the right internal mammary pedicle. Anteriorly, the pericardium is cut back to the superior vena cava.

C The heart is retracted superiorly and to the right to expose the marginal branches of the circumflex coronary artery. The bypass graft can be seen emerging from the posterior surface of the left atrium. There is usually sufficient pedicle length to reach reasonable positions on the marginal arteries.

D Care should be taken to maintain the proper graft orientation. As the graft is brought around the atrium and up onto the surface of the left ventricle, the side of the graft with the endothoracic fascia is on top of the pedicle. Thus, the anastomosis is made on the side of the internal mammary artery opposite that used for anterior anastomoses. The longitudinal incision of the end of the artery is made on its anterior aspect. With the vessels held apart, five stitches are taken to join the heel end of the internal mammary artery and the marginal branch of the circumflex coronary artery. The suture loops are drawn up to approximate the arteries. A continuous suture technique with 7/0 polypropylene is used.

E The toe end of the anastomosis is completed, and the pedicle is secured to the epicardium with two stitches.

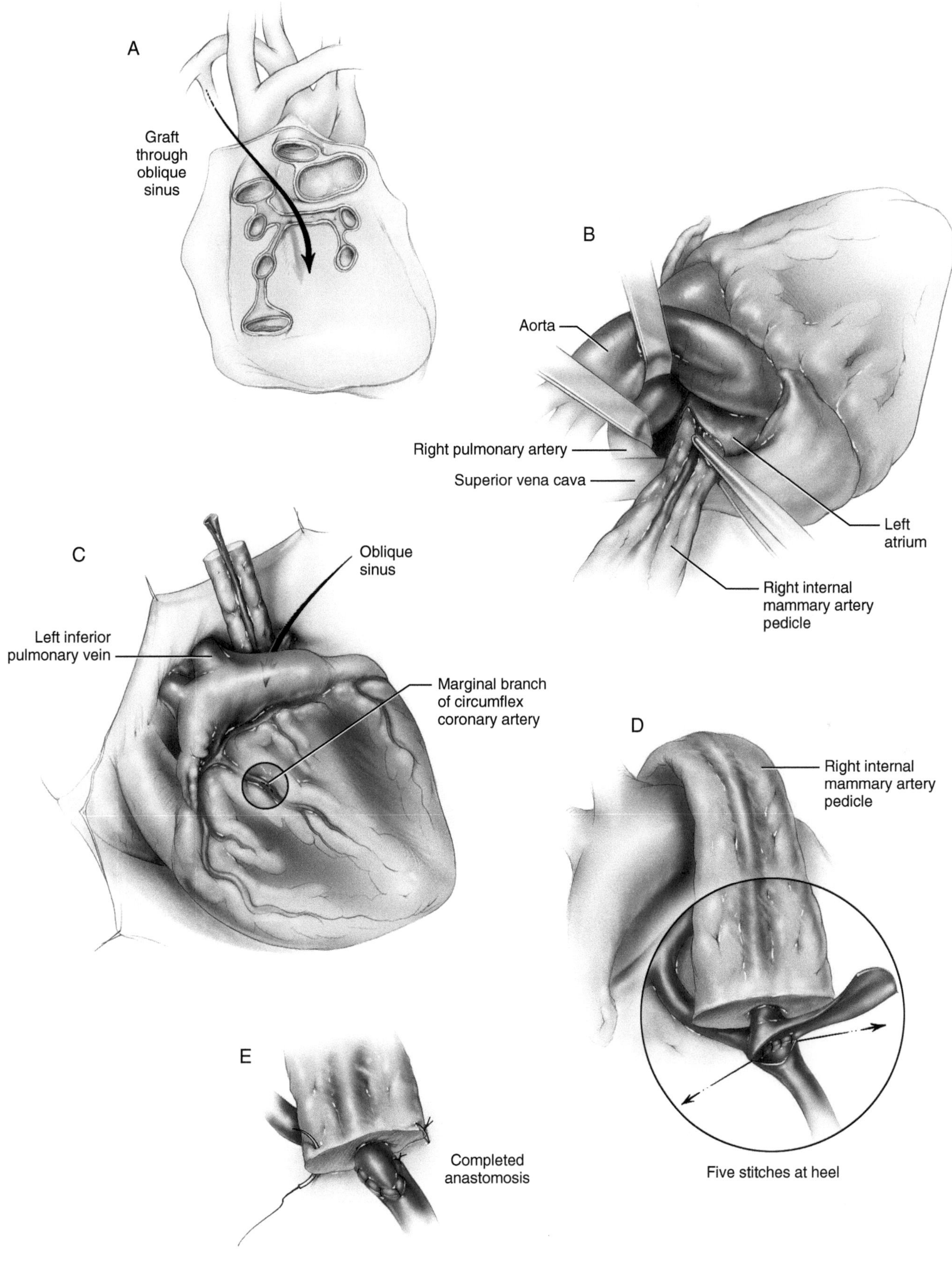
A
Graft through oblique sinus
B
Aorta
Right pulmonary artery
Superior vena cava
Left atrium
Right internal mammary artery pedicle
C
Oblique sinus
Left inferior pulmonary vein
Marginal branch of circumflex coronary artery
D
Right internal mammary artery pedicle
Five stitches at heel
E
Completed anastomosis

Radial Artery Bypass Grafts

The radial artery can be used in combination with the left internal mammary artery to achieve complete revascularization of the heart with an all-arterial conduit. Using the artery as a pedicle with its venae comitantes and employing calcium channel blockers for vasodilation have proved to be very satisfactory, with late patency rates approaching those of internal mammary artery grafts.

Open Radial Artery Harvest
Figure 36-9

A An Allen test is performed on the nondominant hand (usually the left). The radial and ulnar arteries are compressed while the hand is opened and closed vigorously to produce blanching of the skin on the palm. The ulnar artery is released while maintaining compression over the radial artery. The skin on the palm of the hand should immediately become red as blood flow is restored through the ulnar artery to the palmar arch. This hyperemic response is taken as evidence that the radial artery can be removed without risk to the blood supply to the hand.

The arm is positioned on an arm board at the patient's side. As a practical matter, the left radial artery is used so that it can be removed simultaneously as a median sternotomy is performed and the left internal mammary artery is mobilized. An incision is made in the forearm. The incision takes a gentle curve, following the brachioradialis muscle belly. The lateral antebrachial cutaneous nerve is lateral to the incision and is carried laterally as the incision is deepened. Some surgeons recommend continuous intravenous infusion of diltiazem to prevent vasoconstriction in the radial artery, but we have not found this to be particularly helpful.

B The deep fascia of the forearm is opened, exposing the radial vascular pedicle. The lateral antebrachial cutaneous nerve is now far lateral to the dissection; the superficial radial nerve is also lateral to the vascular pedicle. As dissection proceeds along the anterior surface of the vascular pedicle and the incision is deepened, the muscles of the forearm are displayed. This is a deep forearm dissection, not to be equated with the superficial dissection required for removal of the saphenous vein. The anatomy of the forearm should be clearly understood, and the dissection plane should be limited to the vascular pedicle to avoid injury to deep forearm structures.

C The radial vascular pedicle is mobilized at its midpoint, which is the easiest location for gaining control of the pedicle. A Silastic vessel loop is used to retract the pedicle. The dissection proceeds proximally to the recurrent radial artery branch. Further dissection to the brachial artery bifurcation is possible, but this adds considerable difficulty and is seldom required to obtain sufficient length of radial vascular pedicle for posterior heart surface revascularization. The dissection proceeds distally to the fascia enclosing the tendons at the wrist. Again, greater length can be acquired by crossing the wrist, but this is usually not necessary. The side branches of the radial artery are controlled with hemoclips. There are many side branches, so hemoclips are used liberally. The surface of the radial artery is marked with ink or dye to ensure its later correct orientation against the surface of the heart; the side with all the branches is exposed after the artery is attached to the heart as a bypass graft. The arterial graft is gently dilated with blood via an olive-tip needle. The external surface of the graft is irrigated thoroughly with nitroprusside in dextrose and water over a gauze sponge in which the graft is stored.

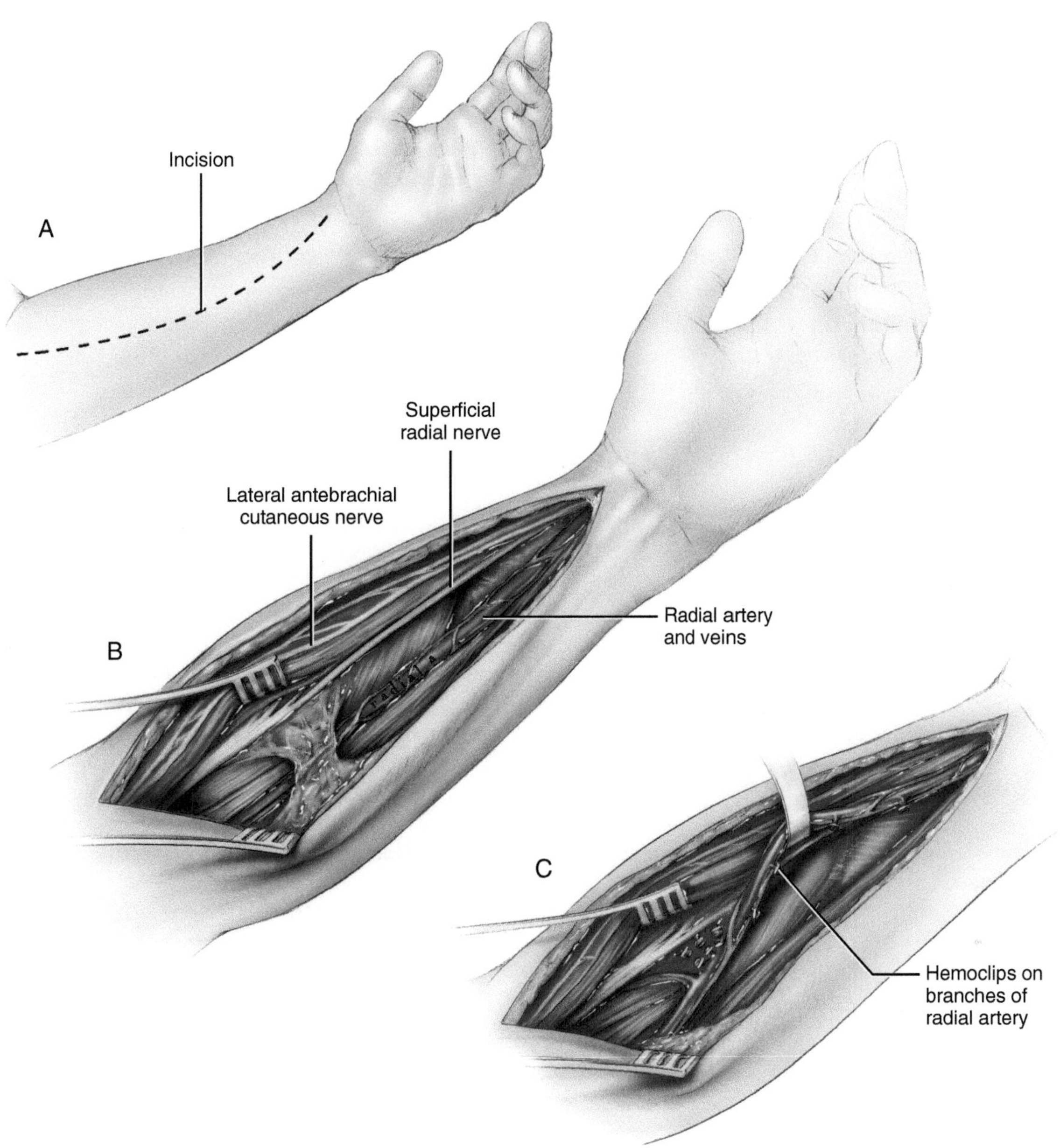
A
Incision
B
Superficial
radial nerve
Lateral antebrachial
cutaneous nerve
Radial artery
and veins
C
Hemoclips on
branches of
radial artery

Endoscopic Radial Artery Harvest

Minimally invasive harvest of the radial artery reduces patient discomfort and improves the appearance of the arm after operation. The artery can be removed through a single incision at the wrist. Adequate perfusion of the hand through the ulnar artery must be verified with an Allen test and ultrasound evaluation before removing the radial artery.

Figure 36-9 (continued)

D A small vertical incision is made directly over the distal aspect of the radial artery proximal to the wrist crease. Direct vision is used to locate the artery and encircle it with a vascular snare. The forearm is exsanguinated via circumferential compression and inflation of a tourniquet placed above the antecubital fossa. This provides a bloodless field for endoscopic harvesting.

E The endoscopic port is inserted into the incision. Continuous carbon dioxide is insufflated to expand the subcutaneous tissue as careful blunt dissection along the anterior and posterior radial artery progresses.

F A tunnel is created proximally along the course of the radial artery by gradually advancing the cone of the dissector anterior and posterior to the artery. The fascia is cut superiorly along the tunnel to provide visualization and to enlarge the tunnel. The arterial side branches are cauterized and divided using bipolar cautery.

G After the entire length of the radial artery is free within the tunnel, an endoloop of 2/0 polypropylene suture is placed around the distal radial artery pedicle. The endoloop is then advanced through the tunnel to the proximal aspect, below the origin of the ulnar artery. The dissector arm of the endoscopic system is used for guidance and countertraction as the knot is gently tightened to occlude the artery. Bipolar cautery is used to divide the artery distal to the knot.

H The tourniquet is released, and the radial artery stump is carefully inspected for hemostasis. The artery is divided distally at the wrist and removed through the incision. The wound is closed with absorbable suture, and a gentle pressure dressing is applied around the entire forearm.

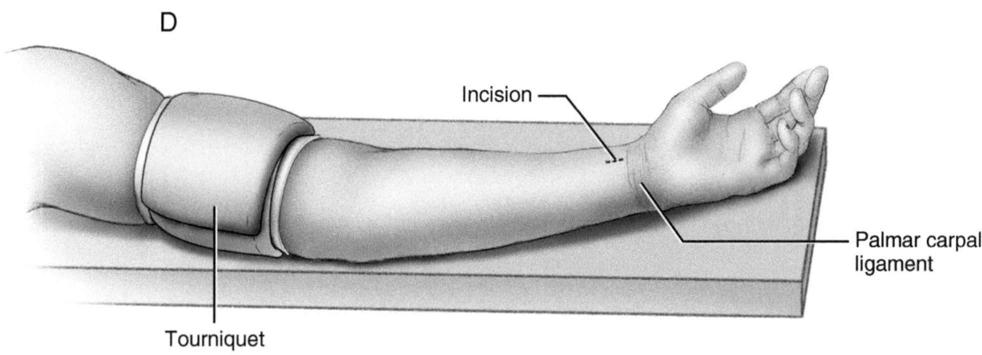
D
Incision
Palmar carpal ligament
Tourniquet

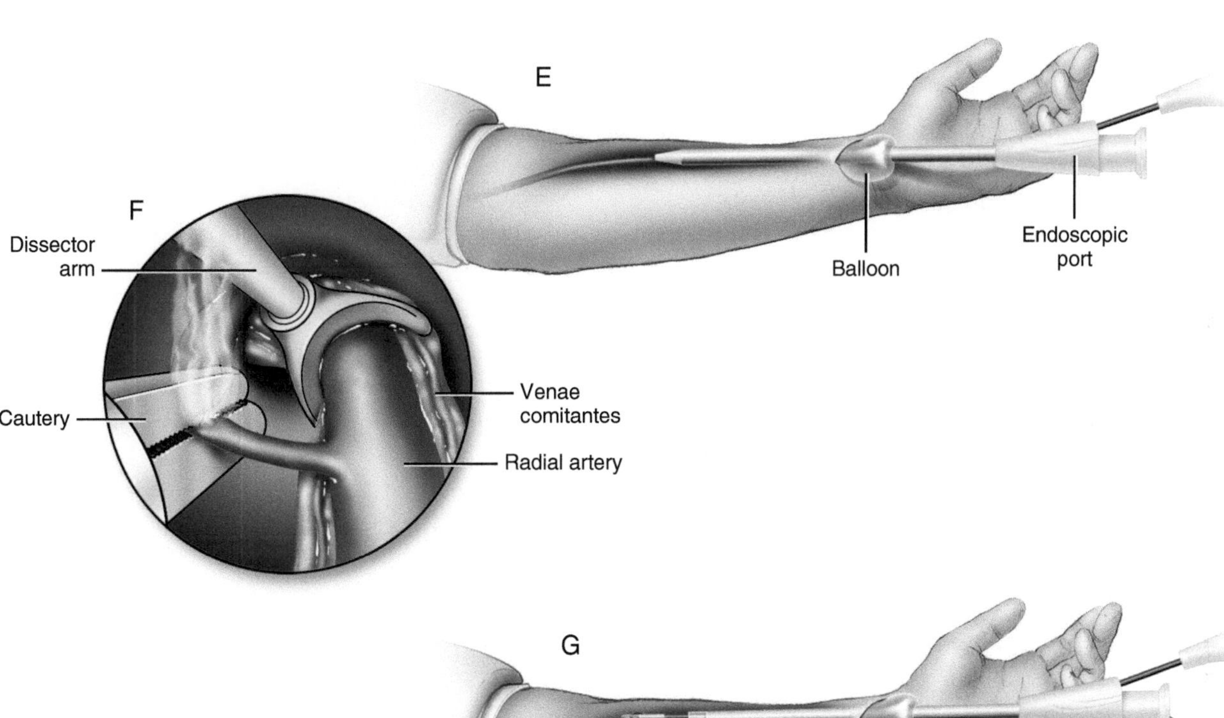
E
F
Dissector arm
Cautery
Venae comitantes
Radial artery
Balloon
Endoscopic port
G
Endoloop

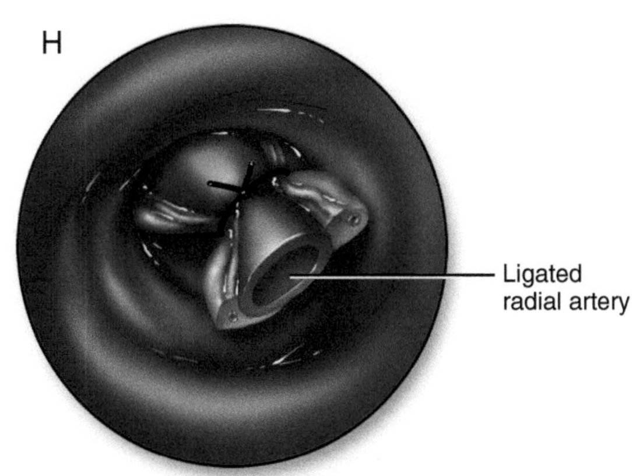
H
Ligated radial artery

All-Arterial Revascularization
Figure 36-9 (continued)

I The left internal mammary artery is used in conjunction with the radial artery to achieve an all-arterial revascularization of the myocardium. The left internal mammary artery is mobilized as a pedicle in the usual fashion. It is used to revascularize the anterior surface of the heart, whereas the radial artery is used to revascularize the posterior surface. The left internal mammary artery is used as the sole conduit for input to the bypass grafts. The radial artery input is based on the left internal mammary artery. Alternatively, the radial artery can be based on the aorta, but it will not reach the distal marginal branches of the circumflex coronary artery or the posterior descending coronary artery. The mammary artery must be thoroughly mobilized to that it can drop posteriorly to enter the pericardial sac through an incision in the pericardium near the left atrial appendage. This is the point at which the radial artery will be anastomosed to the left internal mammary artery.

J A longitudinal incision is made through the pleura and endothoracic fascia into the left internal mammary artery. The incision is extended appropriately to match the diameter of the radial artery.

K An end-to-side anastomosis of the radial artery to the mammary artery is performed. Attention must be paid to the proper orientation of the grafts. The anastomosis to the mammary artery is usually made on the pleural surface, so it may be necessary to rotate the artery to achieve the correct exposure. The toe end of the radial artery is directed toward the proximal end of the arteriotomy in the left internal mammary artery. This orientation allows the anastomosis to direct the radial artery posteriorly and inferiorly toward the atrioventricular groove near the left atrial appendage. The anastomosis is constructed using continuous stitches of 7/0 polypropylene. The wall of the radial artery is thick and may be tough and therefore finer suture material and delicate needles are not useful.

L The anastomosis is completed as the suture line is carried around the heel of the radial artery to the opposite side of the arteriotomy.

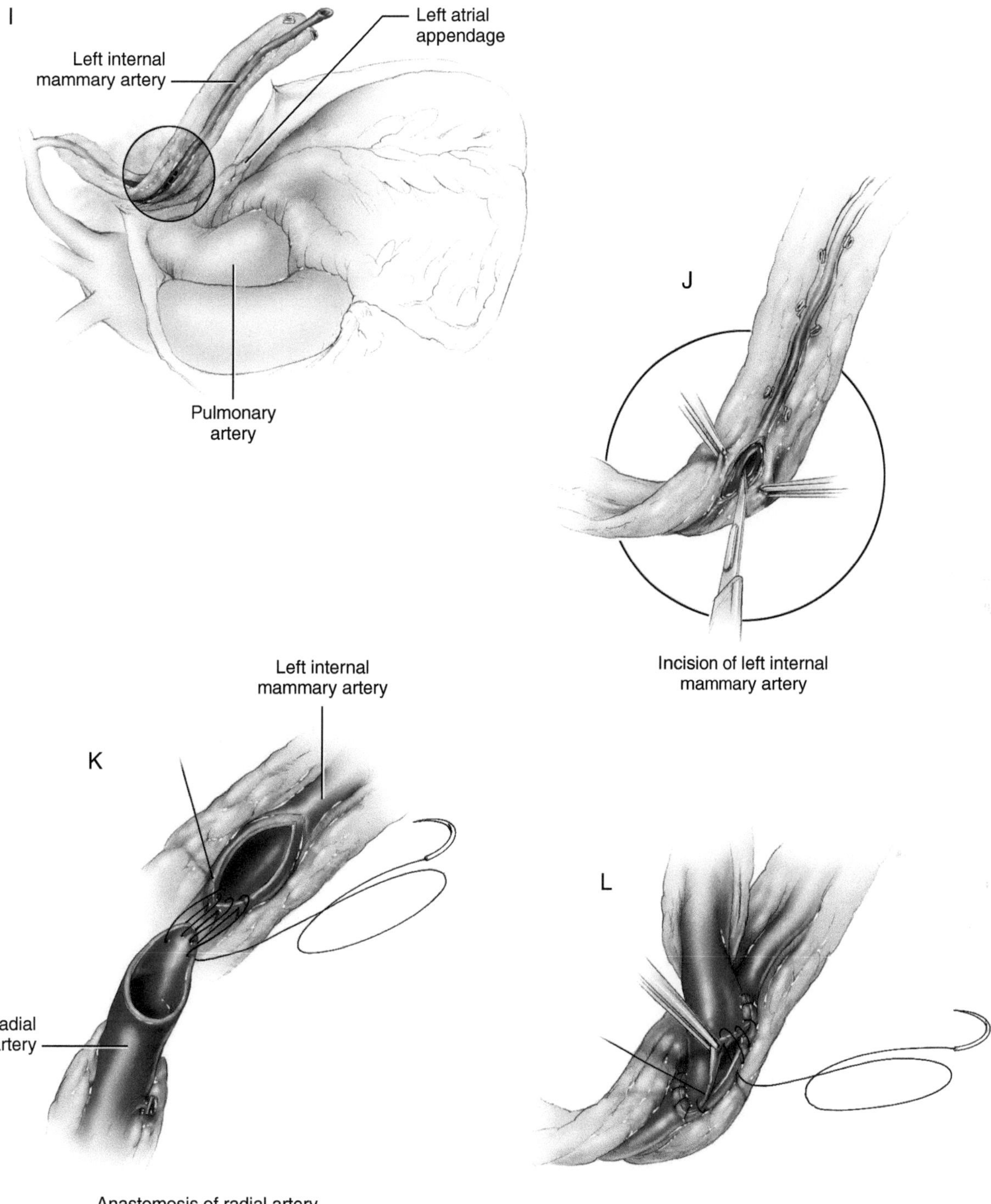

Incision of left internal mammary artery

Anastomosis of radial artery to left internal mammary artery

Completed anastomosis

Figure 36-9 (continued)

M The radial artery pedicle is used to revascularize the posterior circulation. There is sufficient length to reach the posterior descending coronary artery. The radial artery is brought onto the posterior surface of the heart by passing it over the pulmonary artery (PA) near the left atrial appendage (LA).

N Marginal branches of the left circumflex coronary artery are anastomosed to the radial artery in a side-to-side fashion. It is preferable to make each anastomosis in line with both arteries rather than in a crossing fashion. This construction requires a gentle curving of the radial pedicle on the surface of the heart to prevent kinking. If the radial artery is large, crossing or diamond-shaped anastomoses may be used.

O The sequential radial artery bypass graft is completed by constructing an end-to-side anastomosis to the posterior descending coronary artery in the usual fashion. Continuous stitches of 7/0 polypropylene are used for all anastomoses.

P The left internal mammary artery is used to revascularize the anterior surface of the heart. An end-to-side anastomosis of the left internal mammary artery to the left anterior descending coronary artery is constructed in the usual fashion using continuous stitches of 7/0 polypropylene. Side-to-side anastomoses to the diagonal branches can be employed for complete revascularization.

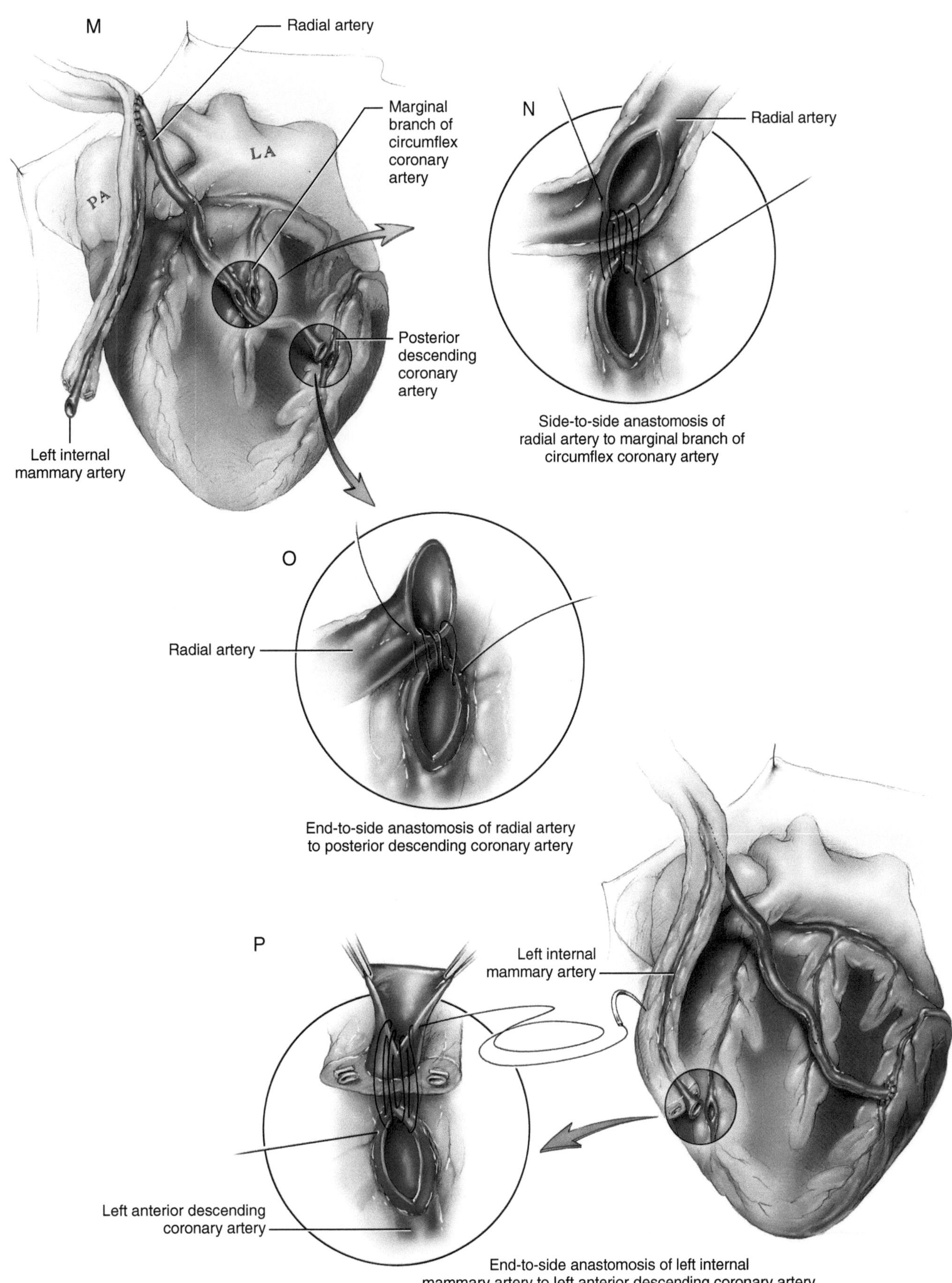

Side-to-side anastomosis of radial artery to marginal branch of circumflex coronary artery

End-to-side anastomosis of radial artery to posterior descending coronary artery

End-to-side anastomosis of left internal mammary artery to left anterior descending coronary artery

Visceral Artery Bypass Grafts

There are some dispensable arteries in the visceral circulation that can be used for bypass grafts. The right gastroepiploic artery can be used because the stomach has an alternative arterial blood supply. The splenic artery can also be used as a bypass conduit.

Figure 36-10

A The right gastroepiploic artery is accessed by extending the midline sternal incision through the midline fascia of the abdomen halfway to the level of the umbilicus. Excellent exposure of the upper abdomen is obtained with the sternum divided. The triangular ligament attaching the left lobe of the liver to the diaphragm is divided. The liver is retracted superiorly and to the right. The right gastroepiploic artery originates from the gastroduodenal branch of the celiac artery. It passes posterior to the stomach and extends to the greater curvature of the stomach just above the pylorus. Arterial branches from the right gastroepiploic artery to the stomach and to the omentum are ligated in continuity and divided. A substantial pedicle is created alongside the gastroepiploic artery to support it. The dissection proceeds from the pylorus along the greater curvature of the stomach until the right gastroepiploic artery terminates with a final branch into the stomach. The artery becomes smaller near its termination. A long pedicle can be created.

B The right gastroepiploic artery pedicle can be taken superiorly either anterior or posterior to the stomach, depending on the patient's anatomy. In thin patients with a vertical orientation of the viscera, a course anterior to stomach is best, whereas in stocky patients with a horizontal orientation of the viscera, a posterior route may be preferable. An opening is made in the diaphragm just medial to the inferior vena cava. The arterial pedicle is passed through this opening into the pericardial sac.

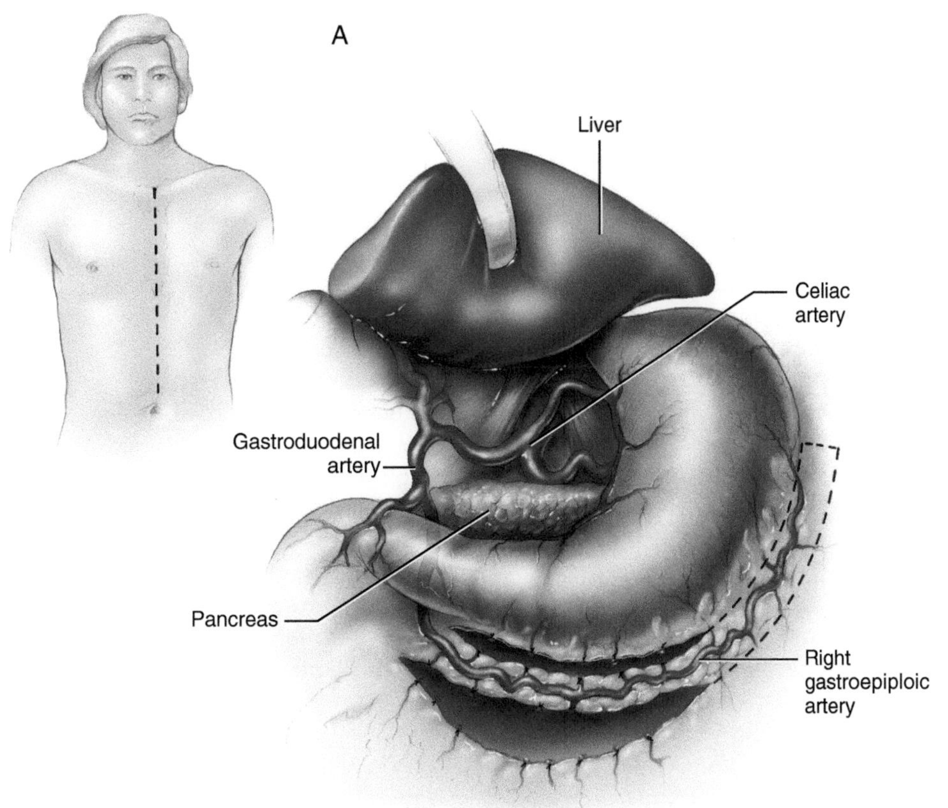
A
Liver
Celiac artery
Gastroduodenal artery
Pancreas
Right gastroepiploic artery

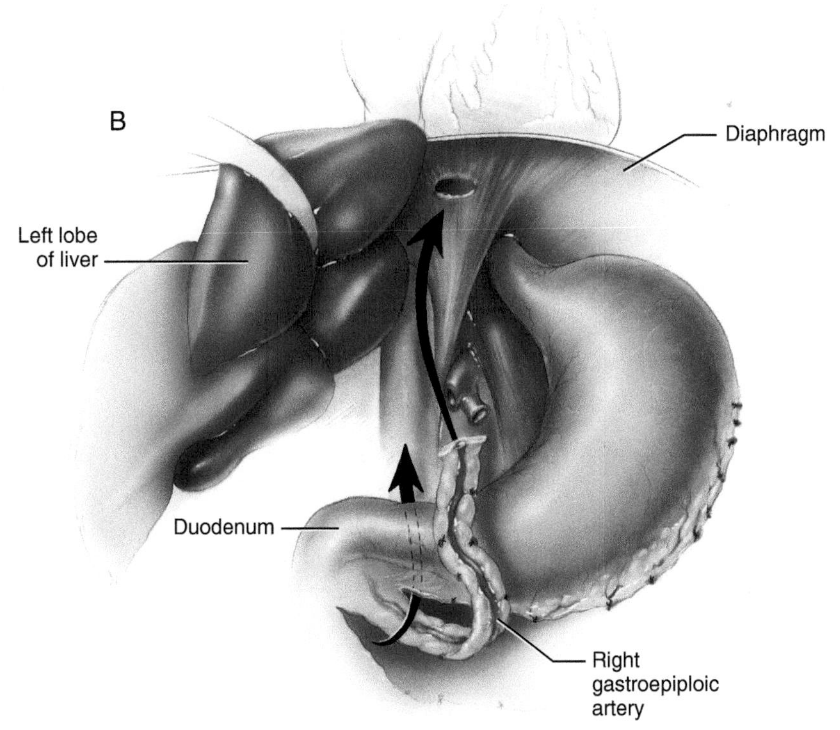
B
Diaphragm
Left lobe of liver
Duodenum
Right gastroepiploic artery

Figure 36-10 (continued)

C The right gastroepiploic artery can be used to revascularize nearly any artery on the surface of the heart. It is most commonly anastomosed to the distal right coronary artery or the posterior descending branch. These coronary arteries are close to largest part of the right gastroepiploic artery, making it possible to construct a large anastomosis. The right gastroepiploic artery can be brought anteriorly across the acute margin of the heart to approximate the left anterior descending coronary artery. There has been considerable experience with this revascularization operation, and the results appear to be acceptable. The right gastroepiploic artery pedicle can also follow a course along the atrioventricular groove posteriorly and be used to revascularize marginal branches of the circumflex coronary artery. The pedicle reaches high onto the obtuse margin of the heart; however, in this bypass construct, the diameter of the gastroepiploic artery is quite small at the anastomosis site.

D The anastomosis of the right gastroepiploic artery to the coronary artery is performed with a standard end-to-side technique. A side-to-side technique can also be used for sequential anastomoses, but this is difficult because of the small size of the right gastroepiploic artery.

E In unusual circumstances the splenic artery can be used as a bypass conduit. The artery is large and tortuous, and atherosclerosis often affects the artery at points of tortuosity. It is rarely stenosed, however, because of its large diameter. The splenic artery is a branch of the celiac artery. It is exposed through a midline abdominal extension of a midsternal incision. The lesser peritoneal sac is opened to gain access to the artery, which courses along the superior margin of the pancreas. Branches of the artery to the pancreas are ligated and divided. The artery is mobilized into the hilum of the spleen, where it is ligated and divided. It is not necessary to remove the spleen because it has a dual blood supply. Although it is supplied mainly from the splenic artery, it also receives blood from the short gastric branches of the left gastric artery. The splenic artery is passed into the pericardial sac through a hole created in the diaphragm medial to the inferior vena cava. The artery is usually used to revascularize posterior coronary arteries. As a bypass conduit, the splenic artery works best when anastomosed to the distal right coronary artery, but it is long enough to reach marginal branches of the circumflex coronary artery.

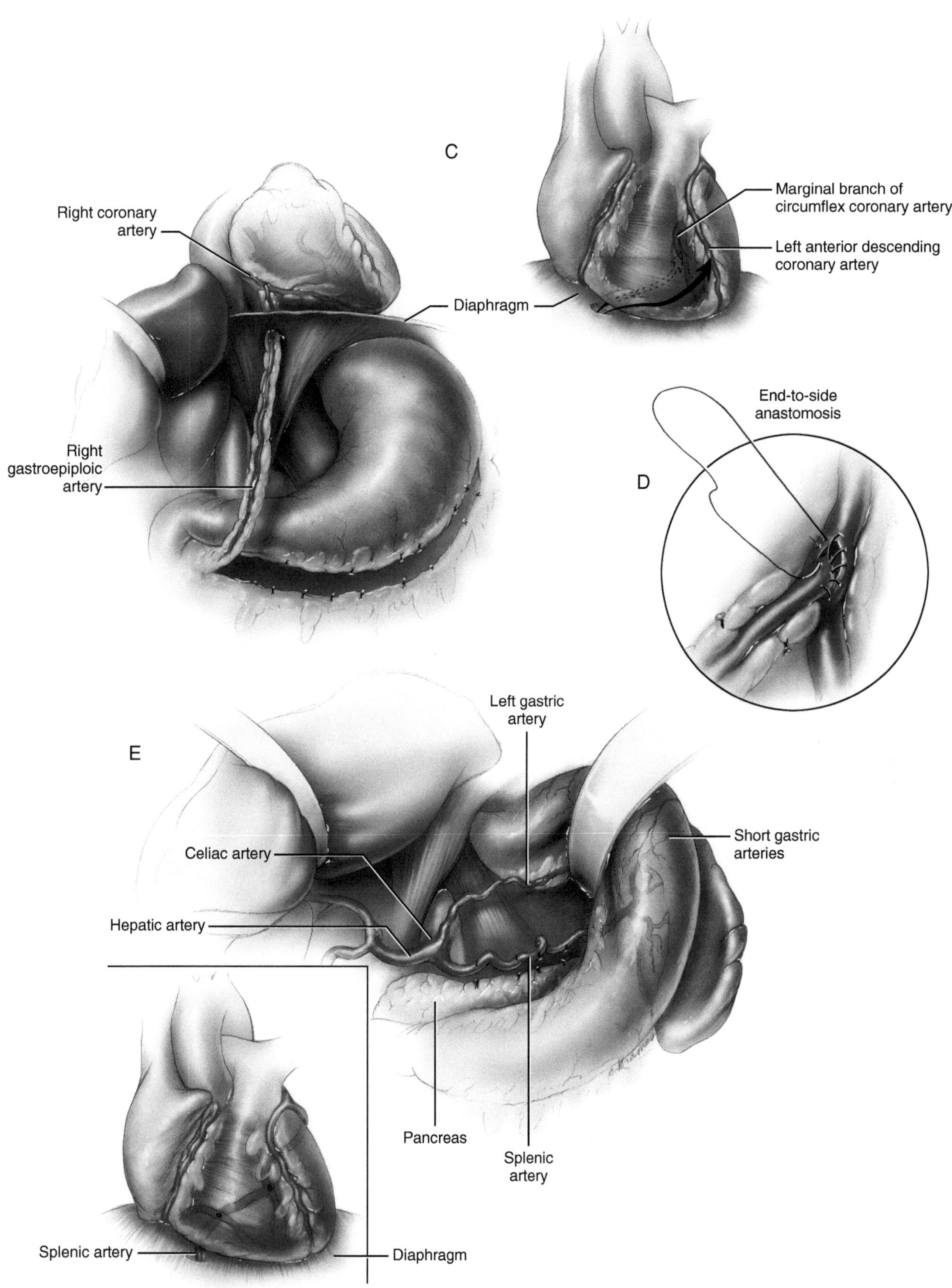
C
Right coronary artery
Diaphragm
Marginal branch of circumflex coronary artery
Left anterior descending coronary artery
Right gastroepiploic artery
D
End-to-side anastomosis
E
Left gastric artery
Celiac artery
Short gastric arteries
Hepatic artery
Pancreas
Splenic artery
Splenic artery
Diaphragm

Coronary Thromboendarterectomy

Coronary obstructive disease may be treated by coronary thromboendarterectomy in certain circumstances, such as occlusion of a dominant right coronary artery in which there are small but significant distal branches to the posterior wall of the left ventricle that cannot be treated effectively using bypass grafts. Thromboendarterectomy involves an increased risk of intraoperative myocardial infarction compared with bypass graft operations. Removal of the thrombotic core also removes the arterial intima, which has likely been irreversibly injured by the atherosclerotic process. Thromboendarterectomy is best performed in the right coronary artery and should be used sparingly in the left coronary artery.

Figure 36-11

A A longitudinal arteriotomy is made in the distal right coronary artery close to the origin of the posterior descending artery. The arteriotomy should be kept short because it will lengthen during removal of the atherosclerotic core.

B Dissection of the core starts in the plane between the adventitia and media of the artery. An ophthalmologic spatula (Wheeler cyclodialysis spatula) is the most versatile instrument to use because of its shape, blade length, and malleability. The core is carefully separated from the ends of the arteriotomy to minimize stretching of the incision during manipulation.

C A small clamp is passed around the core, which is then divided.

D The distal portion of the atherosclerotic core is dissected with the endarterectomy spatula by gently passing the instrument into the plane between the core and the adventitia and advancing it past all points of resistance while gently retracting the core with vascular forceps. The spatula should be used to cut through the core's points of attachment at branches rather than pulling on the core, which could break it off prematurely.

E Once all points of attachment have been severed, the atherosclerotic core can be removed from the coronary artery with ease. The spatula naturally finds its way into the coronary artery lumen and tapers the end of the core once it extends beyond the plaque. The inclination to forcefully pull out the plaque must be avoided, lest it break off and leave a flap of residual disease or intima. Should this happen inadvertently, a Jacobsen forceps can be used to grasp the remaining plaque and complete the dissection. Alternatively, a second arteriotomy may be required if the entire plaque cannot be extracted to a tapered end point. The end points should always be carefully checked to ensure that the plaque has been fully removed and tapered. It is easier to divide the plaque and remove the posterior descending artery plaque separately from the distal right coronary artery plaque.

F An eversion endarterectomy is performed to remove the atherosclerotic core proximal to the arteriotomy. The core is grasped firmly with forceps, and the proximal right coronary artery is pushed back from the core with a second pair of forceps. The core usually breaks off spontaneously at the location of the worst proximal disease, or it can simply be cut off once enough has been extracted to free it from the proximal end of the arteriotomy.

G The arteriotomy is closed by placing a saphenous vein bypass graft into it. The lumen of the coronary artery is irrigated, and any residual debris is removed. The tissue of the right coronary artery is remarkably strong after thromboendarterectomy, so no special suture techniques are required. In fact, because the lumen is usually very large at the arteriotomy site, substantial bites of the arterial wall can be taken as the vein bypass graft is being attached.

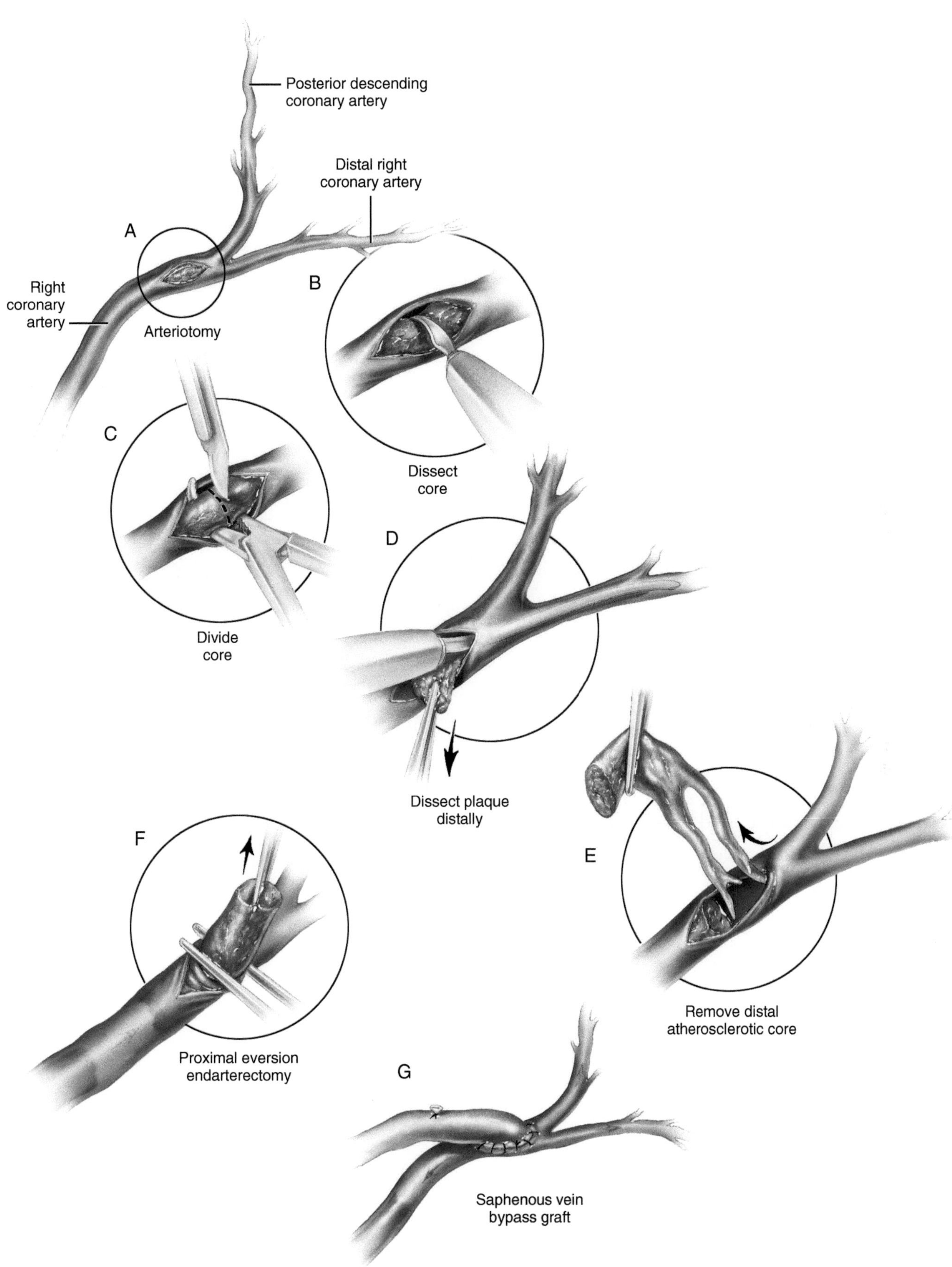
Posterior descending
coronary artery
Distal right
coronary artery
A
Right
coronary
artery
Arteriotomy
B
Dissect
core
C
Divide
core
D
Dissect plaque
distally
E
Remove distal
atherosclerotic core
F
Proximal eversion
endarterectomy
G
Saphenous vein
bypass graft

Minimally Invasive Direct Coronary Artery Bypass (MIDCAB)

Isolated bypass of the left anterior descending artery can be performed through a minimally invasive approach using the left internal mammary artery as the bypass graft. Sternotomy is not required, and cardiopulmonary bypass is not employed.

Figure 36-12

A A small anterior thoracotomy is made in the left fourth intercostal space. The left internal mammary artery is identified at the medial aspect of this incision.

B The left internal mammary artery is dissected off the chest wall in a pedicle fashion. A retractor is used to elevate the fourth rib for improved visualization. It is important to mobilize the artery as high as possible superiorly to ensure an adequate length to reach the anterior wall of the heart without tension and to conform to its contour. The internal mammary artery pedicle is divided, and the proximal end is occluded with a small vascular clamp.

C The pericardium is opened over the anterior wall of the heart and suspended on the chest wall. A stabilizing device is positioned to expose the left anterior descending artery. Soft Silastic snares are placed proximally and distally around the left anterior descending coronary artery to isolate the intended site for vascular anastomosis.

D The internal mammary artery is prepared for grafting by making an angled cut to create a tip and making a short cut back at the heel. A longitudinal incision is made in the coronary artery. Excessive bleeding is controlled with combined carbon dioxide and saline mist irrigation or by placement of an intracoronary shunt (inset). Continuous stitches of 7/0 polypropylene are used to construct an end-to-side anastomosis of the left internal mammary artery to the left anterior descending coronary artery.

E The coronary artery snares are released, and the temporary occlusion clamp is removed from the internal mammary artery. The internal mammary artery pedicle is tacked to the epicardium, and the wound is drained and closed in standard fashion.

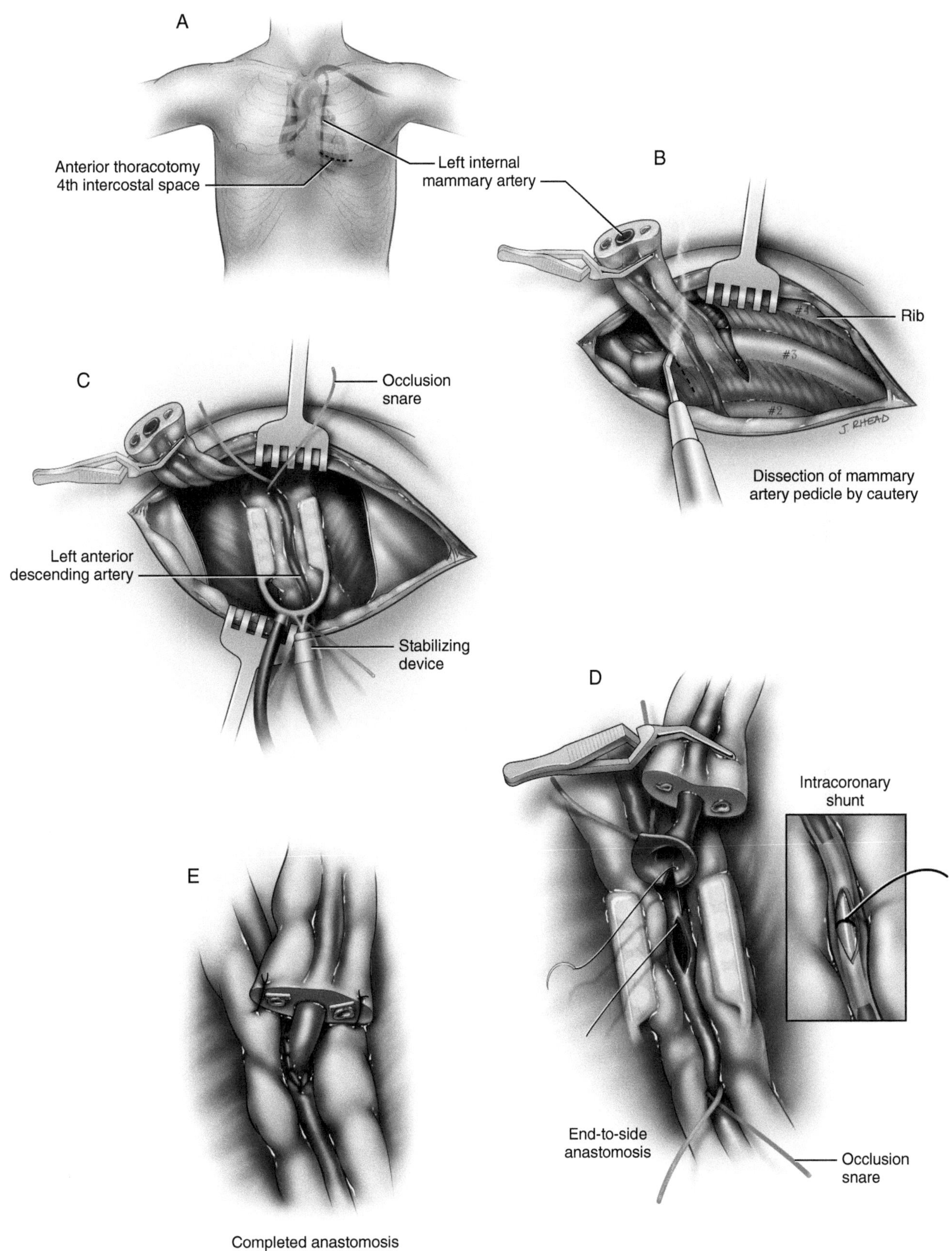
A
Anterior thoracotomy
4th intercostal space
Left internal
mammary artery
B
Rib
#4
#3
#2
J. RHEAD
Dissection of mammary
artery pedicle by cautery
C
Occlusion
snare
Left anterior
descending artery
Stabilizing
device
D
Intracoronary
shunt
End-to-side
anastomosis
Occlusion
snare
E
Completed anastomosis
with tacking stitches

chapter 37 VENTRICULAR ANEURYSM

Anterior Left Ventricular Aneurysm

One of the most common sequelae of severe transmural myocardial infarction is development of an aneurysm of the left ventricle. Acquired ventricular septal defect occurs as a consequence of myocardial infarction with necrosis of the septal myocardium and perforation of the ventricular septum.

Morphology

Acquired left ventricular aneurysm is usually caused by extensive transmural infarction of the anterolateral wall of the left ventricle and the anterior portion of the ventricular septum in the distribution of the blood supply from the left anterior descending coronary artery. Less common but even more complicated is a posterior aneurysm caused by infarction in the distribution of the distal dominant right coronary artery with associated circumflex coronary artery disease.

The usual location of acquired ventricular septal defect is the anterior portion of the ventricular septum near the apex of the heart, in the distribution of the left anterior descending coronary artery. Less common are high and posterior septal perforations, which are the consequence of interruption of myocardial blood flow in the distribution of the posterior descending coronary artery.

Figure 37-1

A Operative photograph of postinfarction ventricular septal defect, anterior type. There is extensive scarring surrounding a defect in the ventricular septum. This appearance of the endocardium is also typical for postinfarction left ventricular aneurysm. The approach to the septum is by incision of the thinned-out (aneurysmal) anterior wall of the left ventricle. Septal scarring and thinning of the left ventricle indicate that this is more than three months after the myocardial infarction and healing is complete.

B Operative photograph of repaired postinfarction ventricular septal defect, anterior type. The ventricular septal defect has been closed with a Dacron patch.

A

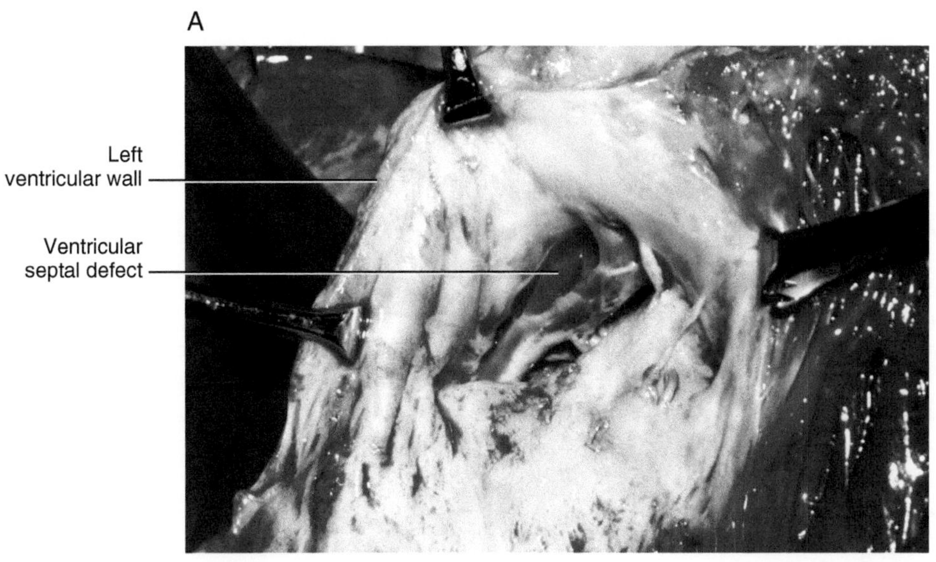
Left
ventricular wall
Ventricular
septal defect

B

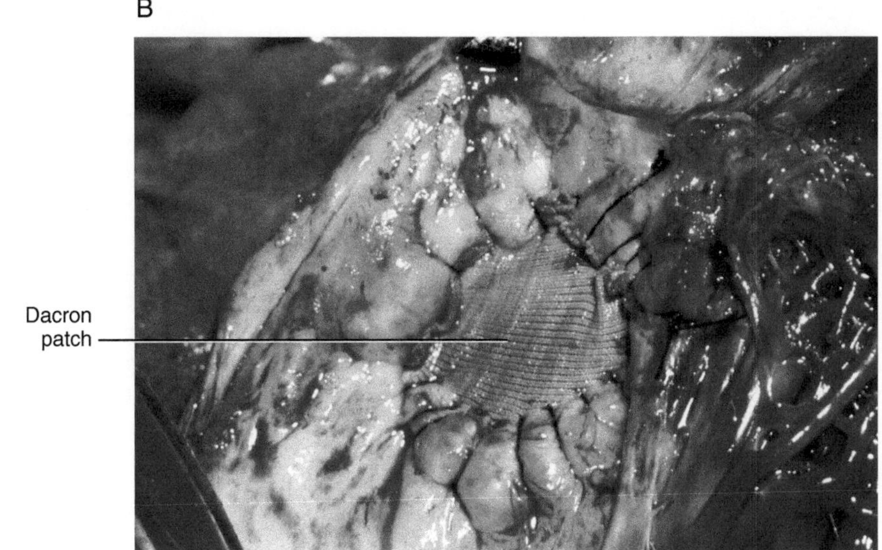
Dacron
patch

Figure 37-2

A It is not possible to resect all scarred and thinned portions of the left ventricle. The septal portion cannot be conveniently excised without entering the right ventricle, and reconstruction of the heart would be unnecessarily complicated. To avoid sacrificing normal contractile myocardium, the line of resection is just inside the confines of the aneurysm on the free wall of the left ventricle anteriorly and laterally, preserving a rim of scar for secure closure of the ventricle. Cardiopulmonary bypass is established prior to manipulating or mobilizing the left ventricle or the aneurysm because there is often mural thrombus in the left ventricle attached to the inside of the aneurysm. To reduce the chance of embolism during manipulation, the aorta should be occluded and the heartbeat arrested with cold cardioplegia before the adhesions between the aneurysm and the pericardium are divided. A vent catheter placed in the left ventricle via the right superior pulmonary vein collapses the thin parts of the ventricle. The aneurysm is opened in its center portion, parallel to the ventricular septum. Allis clamps are placed at each end of the incision into the aneurysm. Mural thrombus is removed from the left ventricle. Removing all the clot from the trabeculations of the left ventricle may be quite tedious. The wall of the aneurysm is excised, retaining about 1 cm of scar at the rim. The medial edge of the excision is near the septum but does not enter the right ventricle. The left ventricle, left atrium, and aortic root are thoroughly irrigated with cold electrolyte solution and carefully inspected for retained debris.

B The illustrated method of repair is still considered standard by many surgeons. The left ventricle is repaired by closure of the large ventriculotomy between strips of Teflon felt to strengthen the suture line and enhance hemostasis. Interrupted mattress stitches of 0 polypropylene are placed through the felt and the rim of the scarred ventricle. The stitches may be placed obliquely in the ventricular septum so that the closure is inverted against the septum, eliminating some of the paradoxical septal motion. The mattress stitches are tied to approximate the edges of the ventriculotomy. To ensure hemostasis, a second layer of closure stitches of 2/0 polypropylene is placed as a continuous row down and back over the ventriculotomy. As these stitches are pulled up, the edges of the ventriculotomy are compressed with the fingers rather than by applying tension on the suture, in order to avoid cutting through the heart.

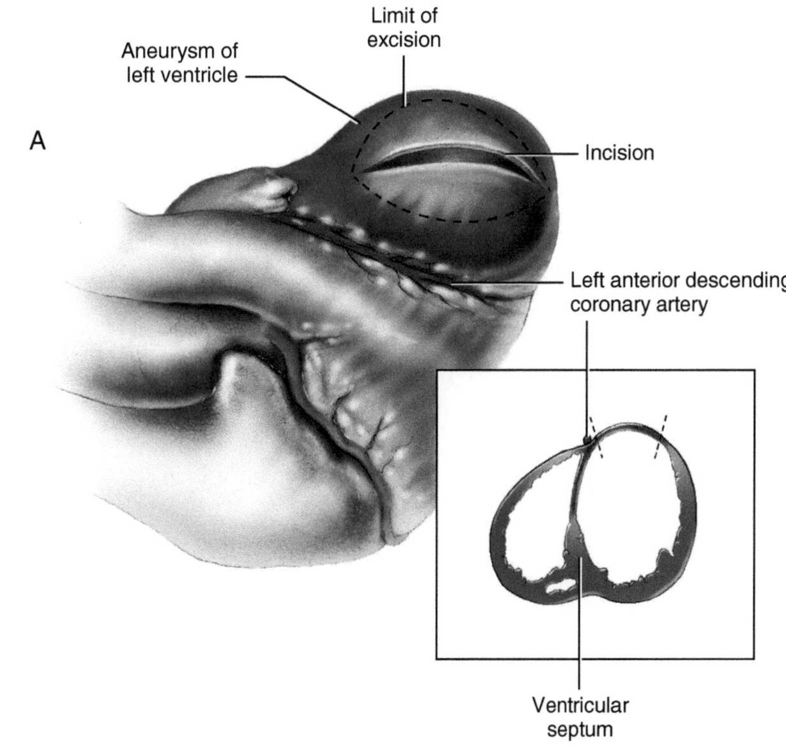
A
Limit of excision
Aneurysm of left ventricle
Incision
Left anterior descending coronary artery
Ventricular septum

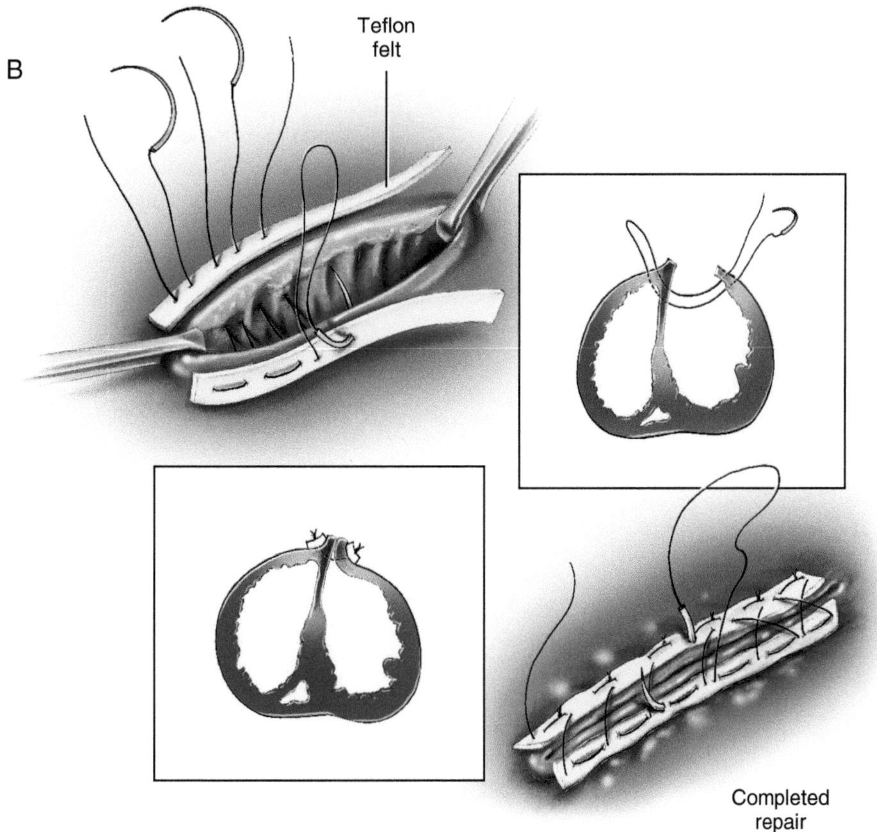
B
Teflon felt
Completed repair

Endoaneurysmorrhaphy Technique

An aneurysm of the left ventricle located on the anterior apical portion of the heart is repaired using the principles described by Daggett, Jatene, and Cooley. A small akinetic area remains on the anterior wall of the left ventricle after this method of repair, but the geometric shape of the ventricle is nearly normal. This is thought to be preferable to methods that attempt to approximate normal myocardium by eversion and leave an abnormal ventricular shape.

Figure 37-3

A The ventricular aneurysm is incised in the usual manner. The ventricular wall is carefully débrided, removing all mural thrombus. The thinned-out scar is retracted to expose its junction with normal myocardium.

B A purse-string stitch of 0 polypropylene is placed circumferentially around the junction of scar and normal myocardium. This junction is easy to identify on the free wall of the ventricle but more difficult to discern on the septum. The stitch is sometimes placed some distance back on the septum, below the anterior wall of the heart. The stitch may come close to the base of the anterior papillary muscle. The stitch is drawn down and tied to narrow the neck of the aneurysm. The opening that remains is usually about the size of a quarter.

C The defect in the heart is closed with a composite patch cut from Teflon felt. The patch should be somewhat larger than the defect. The felt is covered with autogenous pericardium. The felt and pericardium are held together with hemoclips. The patch is attached to the perimeter of the defect using continuous stitches of 2/0 polypropylene. The hemoclips are removed sequentially as the patch is secured to the myocardium.

D The repair is completed by closing the aneurysm scar over the patch closure using 0 or 2/0 polypropylene. A double suture line is constructed using both needles on the suture to achieve a secure closure.

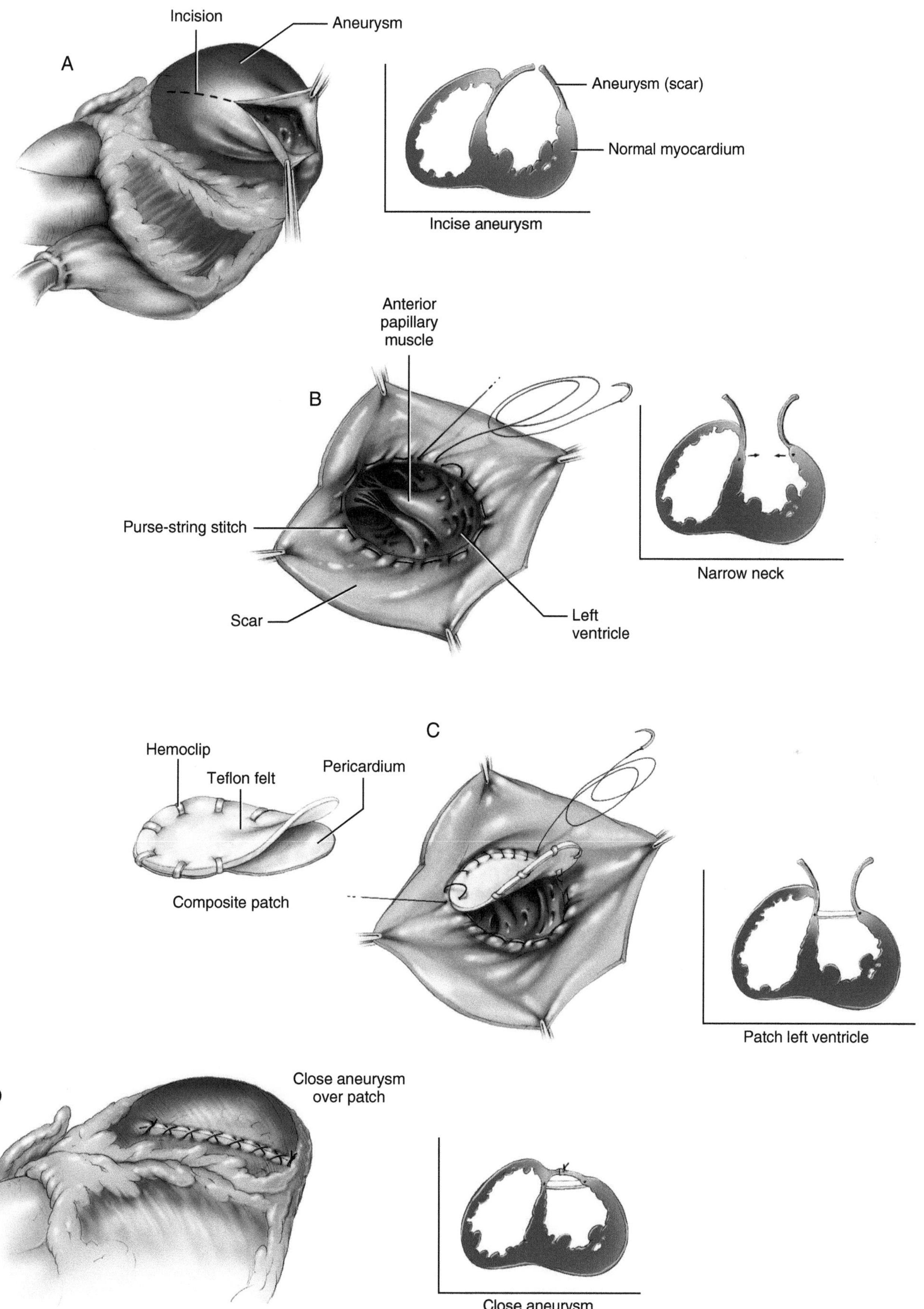
A
Incision
Aneurysm
Aneurysm (scar)
Normal myocardium
Incise aneurysm
Anterior papillary muscle
B
Purse-string stitch
Scar
Left ventricle
Narrow neck
C
Hemoclip
Teflon felt
Pericardium
Composite patch
Patch left ventricle
D
Close aneurysm over patch
Close aneurysm

Ventricular Aneurysm: Mitral Valve Replacement

The mitral valve may become incompetent after myocardial infarction owing to rupture or dysfunction of the papillary muscles, rupture of chordae tendineae, or dilation of the left ventricle and mitral valve annulus. Papillary muscle disorders usually require replacement of the mitral valve, whereas the other pathologic conditions can sometimes be repaired by valvuloplasty techniques. When mitral valve replacement is required in association with operations for left ventricular aneurysm, it is easy to replace the valve working through the left ventriculotomy.

Figure 37-4

A The chordae tendineae are divided at the tips of the destroyed papillary muscles. Functional chordae should be preserved and reattached to the mitral annulus, or prosthetic chordae should be constructed to attach to functional papillary muscles (see Figure 33-3). The mitral valve is excised while carefully observing the location of the annulus.

B Interrupted mattress stitches of 2/0 braided synthetic suture material reinforced with Teflon felt pledgets are placed through the mitral valve annulus from within the left atrium. The stitches are passed through the sewing ring of the mitral valve prosthesis as they are placed in the annulus. Alternating the color of the sutures makes sorting easier. Thought must be given to the proper orientation of the prosthesis, recognizing that this exposure is on the outlet side of the valve.

C Through this exposure it is easy to lower the prosthesis into position in the mitral valve annulus and secure it there by tying the sutures.

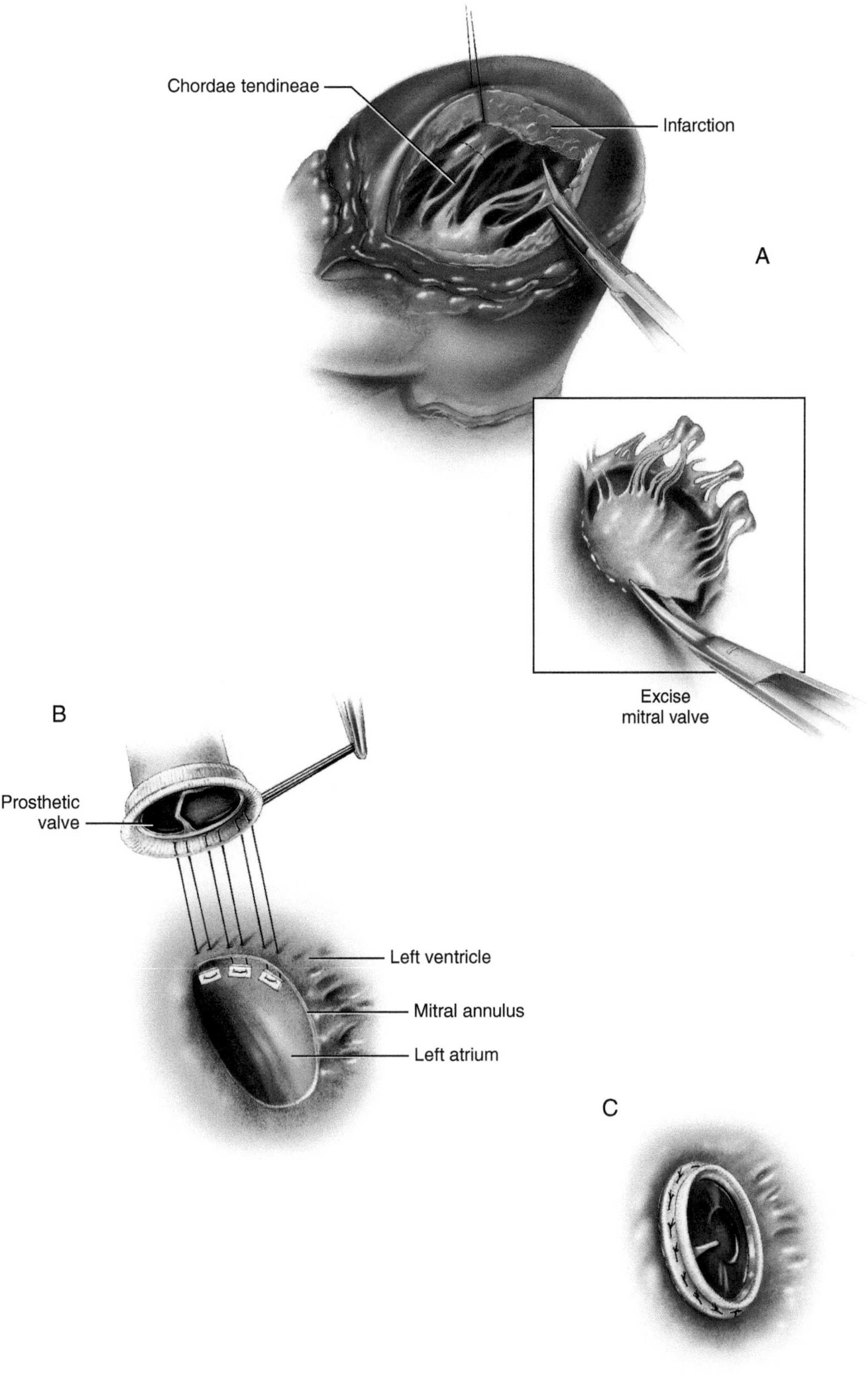
Chordae tendineae
Infarction
A
Excise
mitral valve
B
Prosthetic
valve
Left ventricle
Mitral annulus
Left atrium
C
Prosthesis in place

Anterior Septal Rupture

Patients with these defects are usually seriously ill with recent myocardial infarction and severe congestive cardiac failure. Insertion of an intraaortic balloon catheter and institution of diastolic balloon counterpulsation are useful preoperative interventions and may be continued intraoperatively to provide pulsatile cardiopulmonary bypass flow.

Figure 37-5

A The ventricular septal defect is approached via an incision of the infarcted myocardium. This incision provides access to the left ventricle, where the septal perforation is most easily visualized. Coarse trabeculation makes right ventricular approaches difficult and undesirable.

B After recent infarction, the edges of the septal perforation are usually ragged and poorly defined. If the patient is operated on later in the course of the healing process, the edges of the defect are better defined by scarring.

C A large patch of collagen-sealed, knitted, double-velour Dacron is fashioned for closure of the ventricular septal defect. One edge of the patch is rounded, while sufficient fabric is retained on the opposite side to extend through the ventriculotomy after the patch is in place against the septum. Rather than suturing the patch to the weakened, necrotic myocardium at the edges of the defect, it is sutured to more normal myocardium some distance from the defect. The patch, being on the left side of the septum, is pressed against the septum by pressure in the left ventricle. Interrupted mattress stitches of 2/0 braided suture reinforced with Teflon felt pledgets are placed in the ventricular septum, away from the edge of the septal defect. Substantial bites of the septum are taken for maximal suture security. The suture line surrounds the septal defect and is continued anteriorly on the septum on both sides of the defect until the ventriculotomy on the free wall of the left ventricle is reached.

D The patch used to close the septal defect is brought out through the ventriculotomy. The ventriculotomy is closed over strips of Teflon felt using the closure technique for ventricular aneurysm repair. The only modification is that the septal defect patch is incorporated into the ventriculotomy closure. The 0 polypropylene mattress sutures include the Teflon felt bolster, ventricular myocardium, and Dacron patch, all sandwiched together.

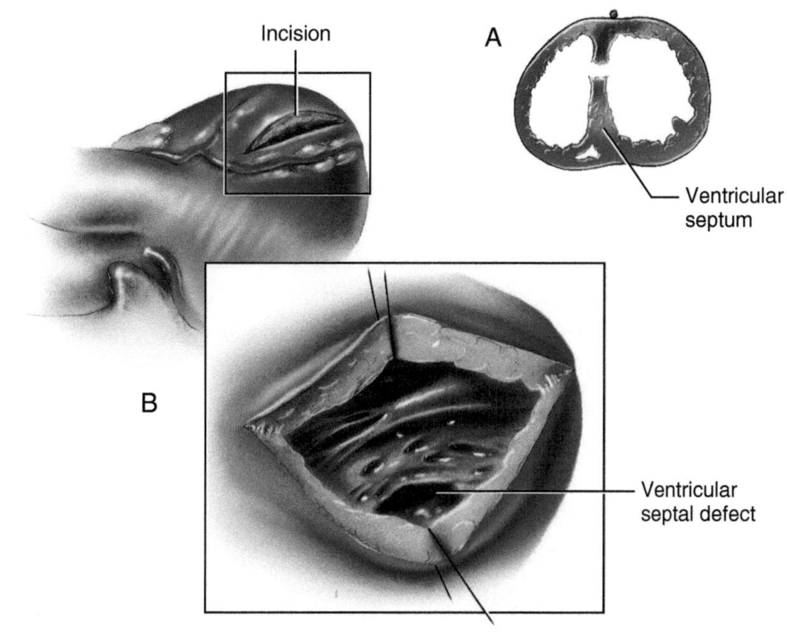
Incision
A
Ventricular
septum
B
Ventricular
septal defect

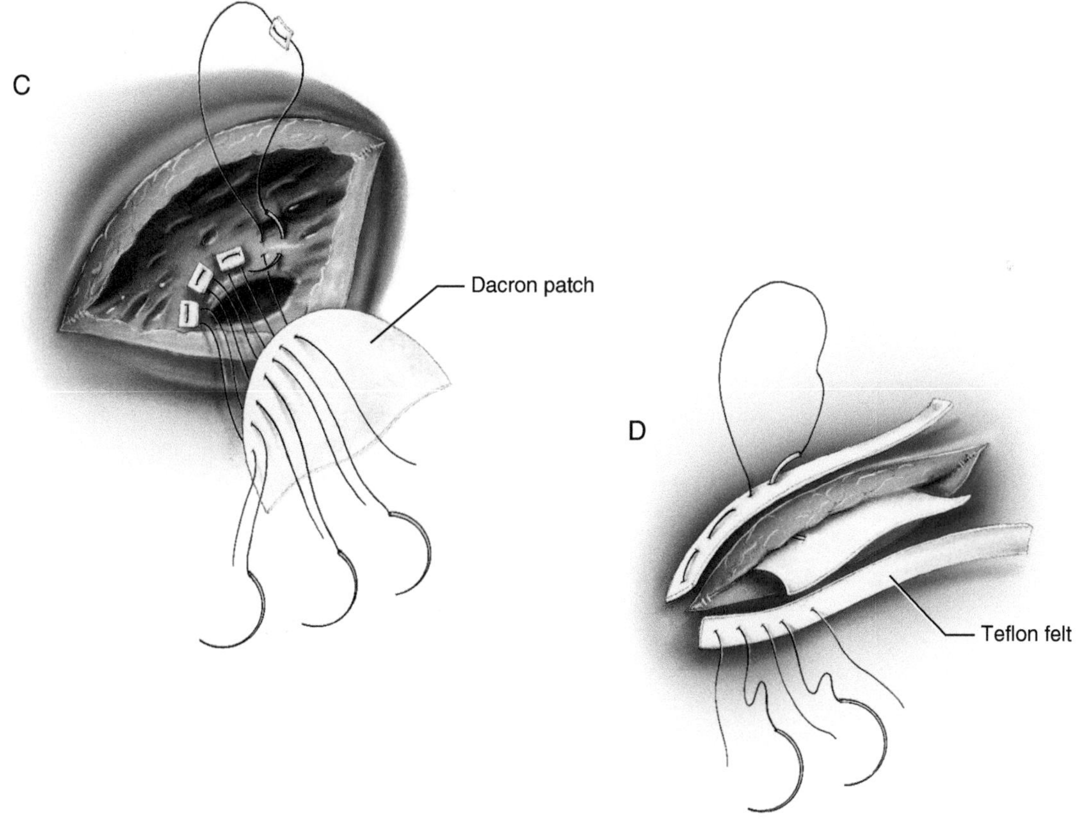
C
Dacron patch
D
Teflon felt

Posterior Septal Rupture

Rupture of the posterior ventricular septum due to myocardial infarction in the distribution of the distal right and posterior descending coronary arteries is more difficult to repair than ruptures in the anterior and apical portions of the septum. Because the defect is on the posterior wall of the left ventricle, on the diaphragmatic surface of the heart, and adjacent to the atrioventricular groove, it is less accessible. The mitral valve annulus is usually close to the infarcted myocardium, so the repair could distort the ventricular geometry in this area, resulting in mitral valve incompetence. There may be substantial loss of myocardium on the posterior wall of the ventricle, so excision of the infarcted tissue often results in a significant free wall defect that must be closed, as well as the defect in the ventricular septum. Repairs in which the tissues of the free wall of the ventricle are bunched or everted have been largely unsuccessful because of residual ventricular septal defect, mitral valve incompetence, and worst of all ventricular rupture with uncontrollable hemorrhage. Daggett's method overcomes many of the problems associated with this technically difficult repair.

Figure 37-6

A The apex of the heart is retracted superiorly and to the left to expose the posterior portion of the left ventricle at the crux. A left ventriculotomy is made through the infarcted myocardium parallel to the posterior descending coronary artery and ventricular septum. The border of the necrotic myocardium can be defined once the inside of the ventricle is visualized.

B The infarcted myocardium is excised. This usually means removing a good-sized piece of the posterior wall of the left ventricle near the atrioventricular groove and possibly some of the right ventricle over the septum.

C Mattress stitches of 2/0 braided synthetic suture bolstered with large Teflon pledgets are placed through the ventricular septum from the right ventricular side into the left ventricle. The stitches should be placed a good distance from the necrotic edge of the septal defect. These stitches are continued until the free wall of the ventricle is reached. Alternating the color of the sutures makes sorting easier.

D In Daggett's original description, Teflon pledgets are placed on both sides of the septum by adding the pledget after the stitch is passed through the septum. It seems reasonable to modify this technique somewhat by simply passing the stitches directly through a prosthetic patch, which acts as its own pledget. The patch material is usually collagen-sealed, velour knitted Dacron. Alternative patch material that might be even more effective includes pericardium-backed Teflon felt or a thick polytetrafluoroethylene (PTFE) graft. For optimal exposure, all the septal defect closure stitches are placed through the graft before the graft is actually placed into the ventricle.

E The patch is approximated to the ventricular septum and secured.

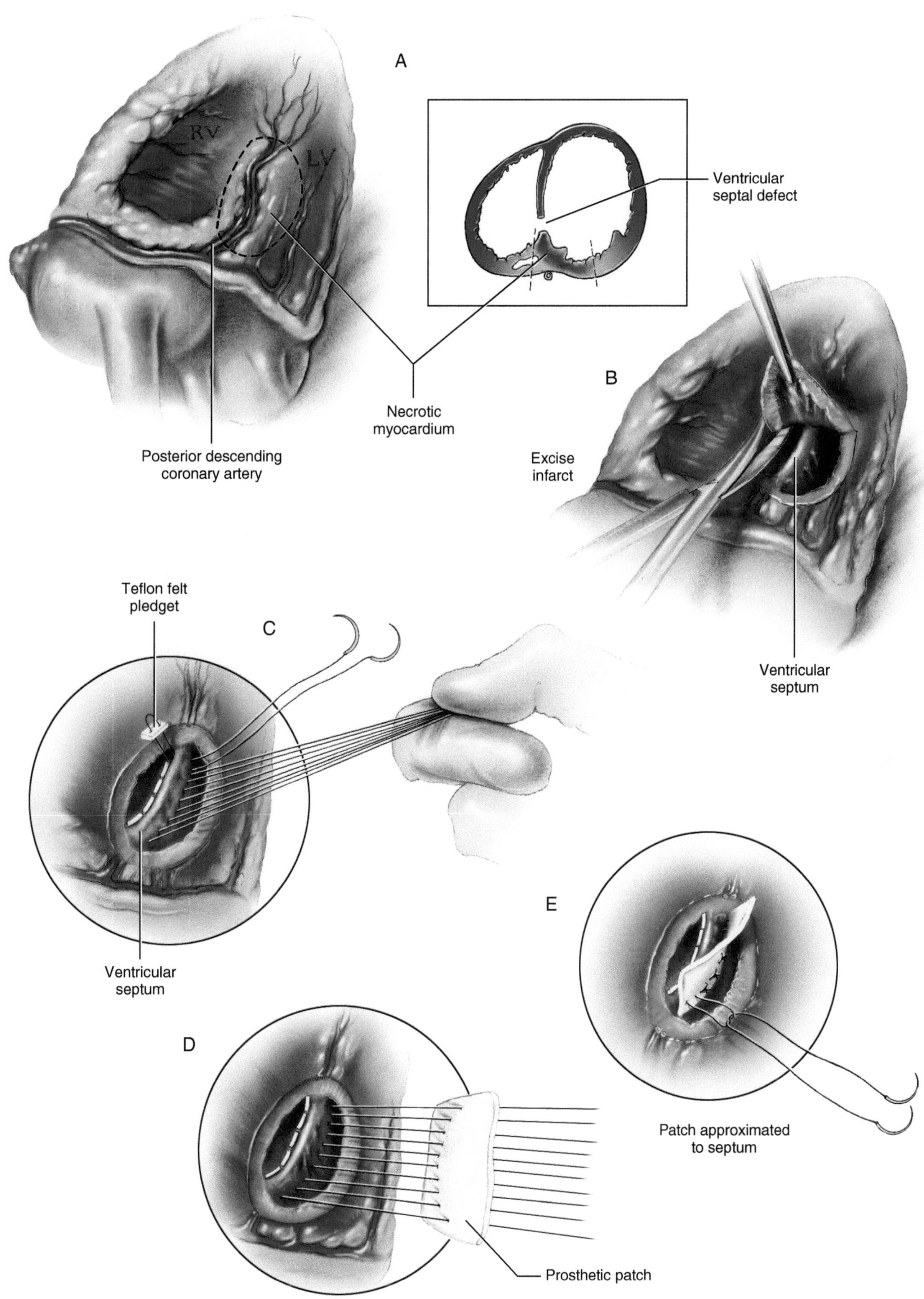
A
RV
LV
Ventricular
septal defect
Necrotic
myocardium
Posterior descending
coronary artery
B
Excise
infarct
Ventricular
septum
Teflon felt
pledget
C
Ventricular
septum
E
Patch approximated
to septum
D
Prosthetic patch

Figure 37-6 (continued)

F A row of mattress sutures is used to approximate the patch to the right ventricular free wall. The mattress stitches are passed through the prosthetic patch and then from the inside of the right ventricle to the free wall. Teflon pledgets are placed on the sutures on the outside of the ventricle. Again, Daggett described pledget material on both sides of the myocardium, but using the prosthetic patch as its own pledget is adequate. All the needles from this step of the repair are retained for later use.

G A second set of pledget-reinforced mattress sutures is passed from within the left ventricle to the outside of the free wall. Daggett described the addition of another pledget on the free wall. When all the sutures are in place, the stitches should circumferentially ring the defect created by excision of the necrotic myocardium of the left ventricular free wall.

H An appropriately sized prosthetic patch is fashioned to cover the ventricular free wall defect. The previously placed stitches are passed through the prosthetic material, and the defect is closed by securing the prosthesis to the heart.

I When viewed in cross section, it can be appreciated that the defect has been repaired in anatomic fashion and adequately reinforced to prevent tearing of the sutures when cardiac contraction resumes. It is recognized that akinetic areas are left in the wall of the left ventricle (LV), but the repair is more secure than methods that attempt to pull the normal myocardium together to eliminate nonfunctional heart tissue. RV, right ventricle.

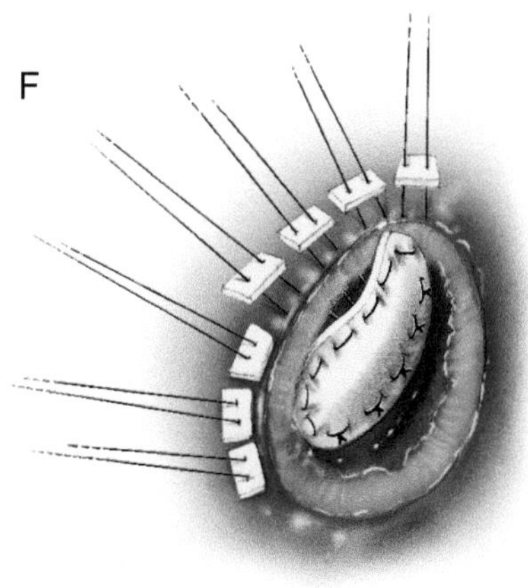

Attach ventricular septal defect patch to right ventricle

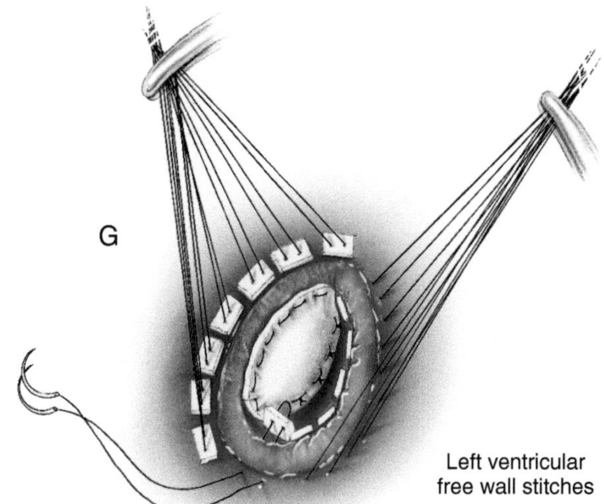

Left ventricular free wall stitches

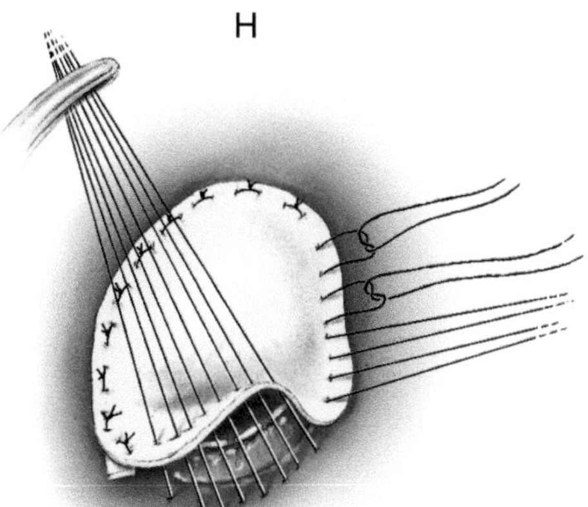

Close free wall defect with prosthetic patch

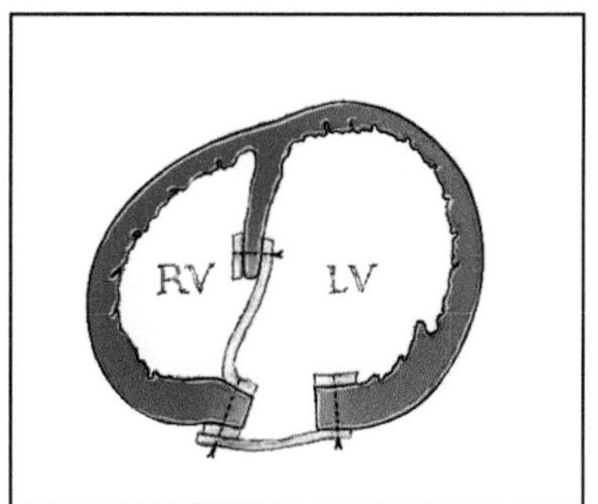

Completed repair

part XI

Thoracic Arteries and Veins (Acquired)

chapter 38 AORTIC ANEURYSM

Aneurysm of the aorta in one of its segments or in its entirety may require replacement of the aorta. The need for operation is determined by the size of the aneurysm and the accompanying risk of rupture, occlusion of the aorta or its branches, thromboemboli originating from the aortic wall, or infection.

Morphology

Figure 38-1

A Operative photograph of aneurysm of the ascending aorta, atherosclerotic type. The aorta is dilated above the sinotubular junction. The aortic dilation extends into the proximal portion of the aortic arch.

B Operative photograph of aneurysm of the ascending aorta, Marfan type. The aortic dilation includes the aortic sinuses. It is often described as onion-shaped.

C Operative photograph of aneurysm of the aorta due to aortic dissection. The blue discoloration is blood within the aortic wall separating the intima and media from the aortic adventitia. The dissection includes the aortic sinuses and continues through the aortic arch.

D Operative photograph of aortic dissection of the ascending aorta. The intima and media have separated from the aortic adventitia.

E Anatomic specimen of aortic dissection of the ascending aorta. There is a tear through the intima and media of the ascending aorta just above the sinuses of Valsalva. Coronary arteries are not involved, and the aortic valve leaflets are normal.

F Operative photograph of aneurysm of the ascending aorta and arch. The aortic dilation continues through the aortic arch.

G Operative photograph of aneurysm of the ascending aorta and arch. This view, from the same patient as in Figure 38-1, *F*, shows the upper portion of the descending aorta, which was previously replaced with a prosthetic graft for aneurysmal disease.

A

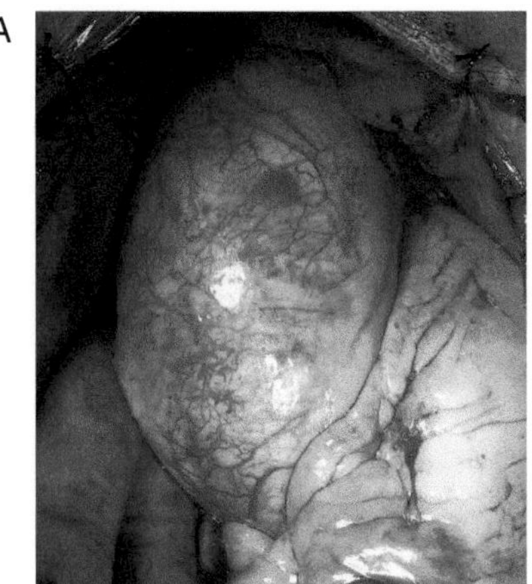

Aneurysm, ascending aorta
atherosclerotic type

B

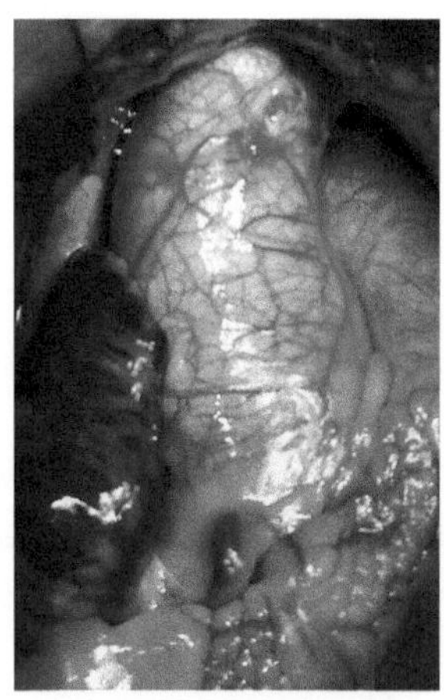

Aneurysm, ascending aorta
Marfan type

C

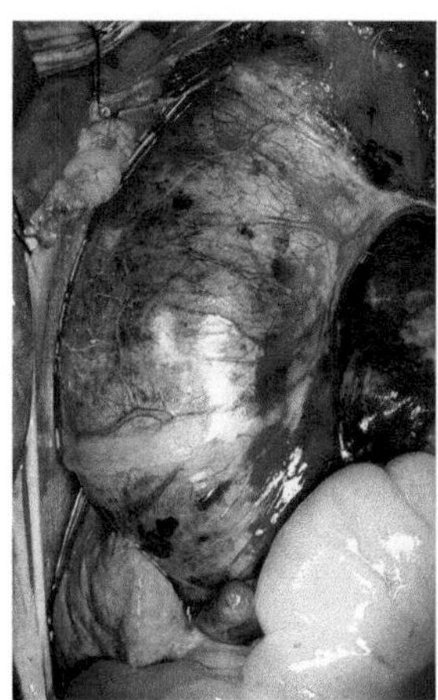

Aneurysm, aorta
due to aortic dissection

D

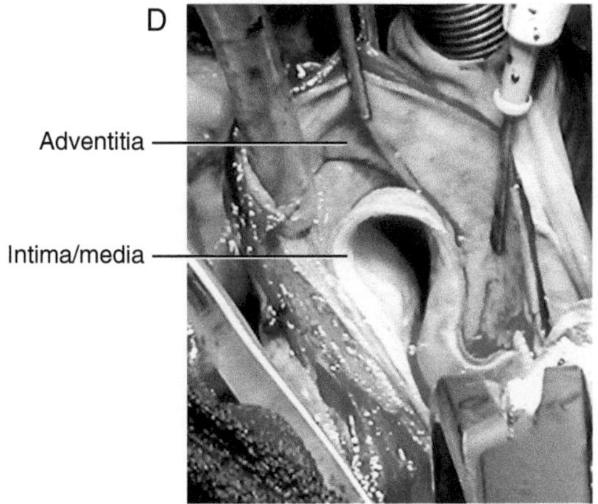

Aortic dissection

E

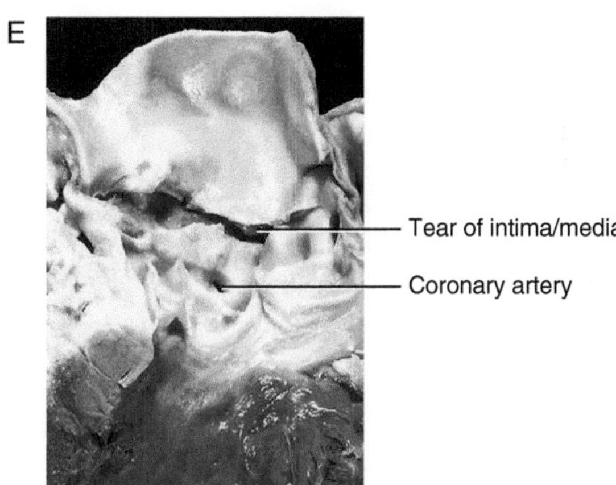

Aortic dissection

F

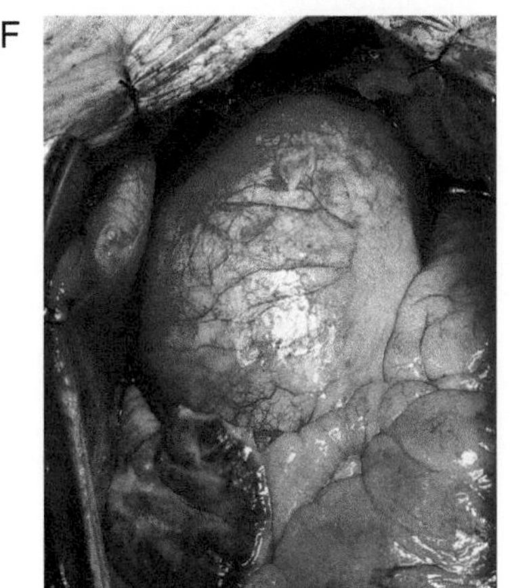

Aneurysm, ascending
aorta and arch

G

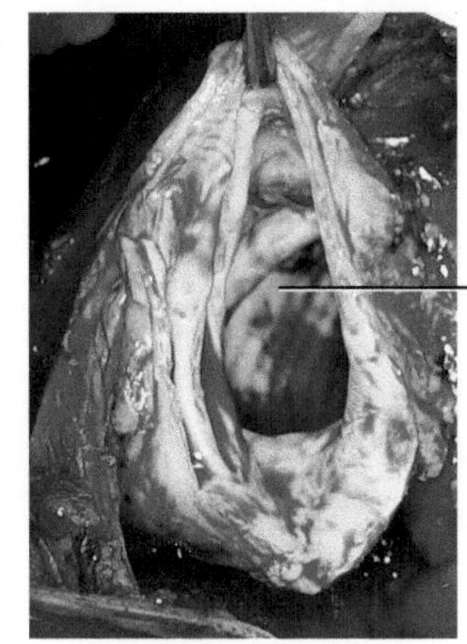

Aneurysm, ascending
aorta and arch

Cannulation Strategies for Aortic Operations

Multiple cannulation techniques are available for cardiopulmonary bypass during aortic operations. Alternative techniques, such as partial cerebral perfusion, can make the operative field more accessible during complex reconstructions.

Figure 38-2

A Femoral-femoral bypass is instituted by placing an arterial cannula in the common femoral artery and a venous return cannula in the common femoral vein. For patients with small or diseased arteries, construction of a "side arm" with a prosthetic graft ensures distal perfusion of the leg. When using this strategy in acute aortic dissection, the surgeon should select the artery with the strongest pulse. High arterial pressure in the return cannula is strongly suggestive of impaired perfusion, and the cannula should be removed and placed in the opposite common femoral artery.

B Antegrade perfusion via the right axillary artery is useful for operations on the aortic arch. It can be used as the sole method for arterial return during cardiopulmonary bypass, or it can be used to provide partial, selective antegrade cerebral perfusion during periods of hypothermic circulatory arrest. An oblique incision is made 1 cm below the right clavicle for exposure of the axillary artery.

C The pectoralis major muscle is separated in the direction of its fibers to enter the subclavicular space. The artery is isolated with vascular loops, taking care to avoid injury to the brachial plexus.

D A longitudinal incision is made in the artery. An 8 mm prosthetic graft is beveled and attached in an end-to-side fashion using continuous stiches of 5/0 polypropylene suture.

E The graft is trimmed to about 20 cm in length, and a 22 F arterial return cannula is inserted into the graft. The cannula is secured with multiple ties around the graft and connected to the cardiopulmonary bypass circuit. Antegrade perfusion is delivered through the axillary graft to the right arm and the aortic arch. During periods of circulatory arrest, the innominate artery is clamped, and selective antegrade perfusion of the brain can be performed through the right common carotid artery.

F When perfusion through a side graft is discontinued, the graft is clamped close to the artery, divided, oversewn with continuous stitches of 4/0 polypropylene, and sealed with BioGlue.

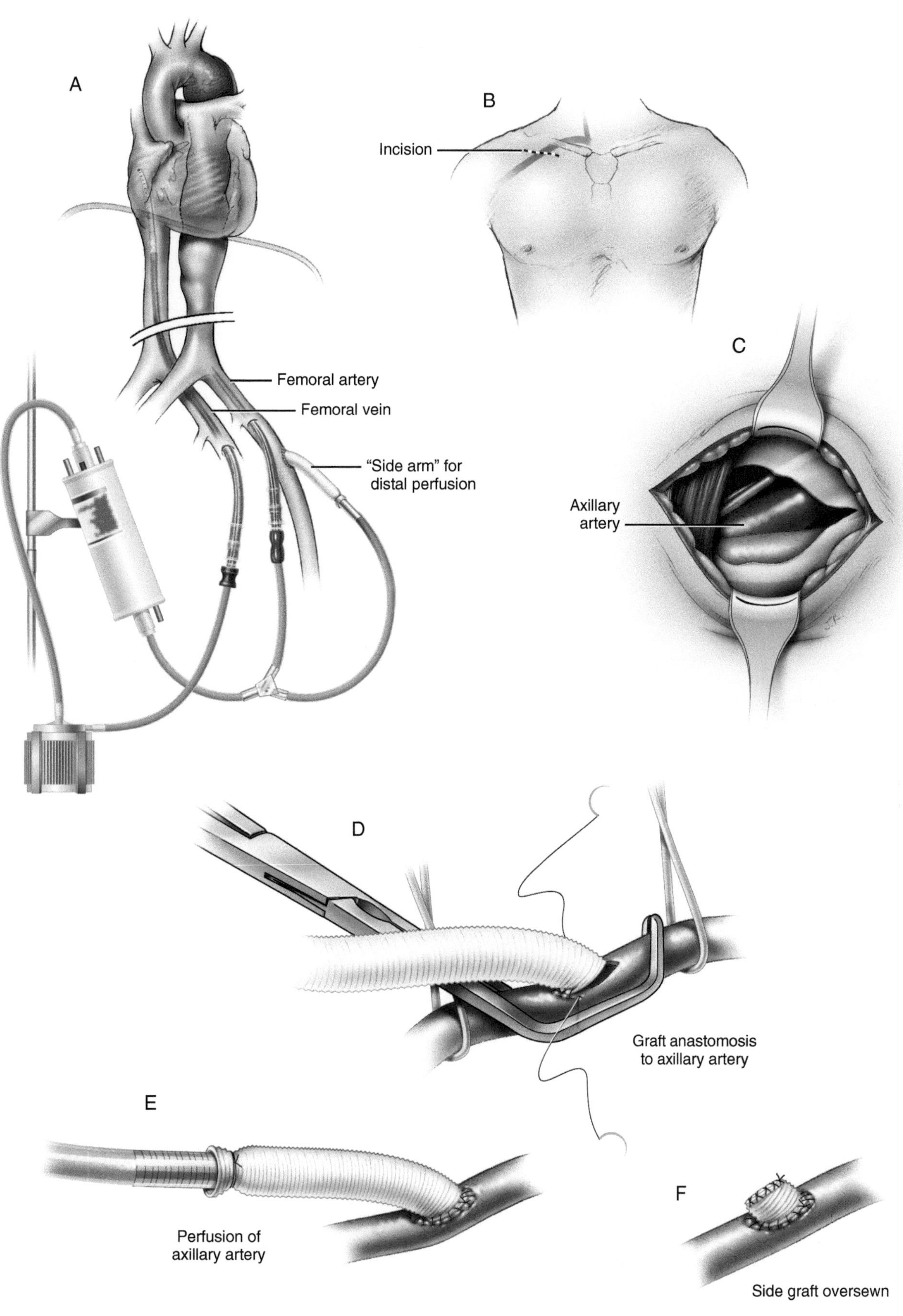
A
Femoral artery
Femoral vein
"Side arm" for distal perfusion
B
Incision
C
Axillary artery
D
Graft anastomosis to axillary artery
E
Perfusion of axillary artery
F
Side graft oversewn

Figure 38-2 (continued)

G In cases of acute aortic dissection, central cannulation can be safely performed using the Seldinger guidewire technique. Under transesophageal echocardiographic guidance, a needle is placed directly into the distal ascending aorta, and the guidewire is advanced into the true lumen.

H Successive dilation is performed over the guidewire, and the arterial cannula is placed through the aortic arch into the descending thoracic aorta. This ensures antegrade perfusion of the true lumen and avoids potential malperfusion and the differential flow patterns that can be associated with femoral artery cannulation.

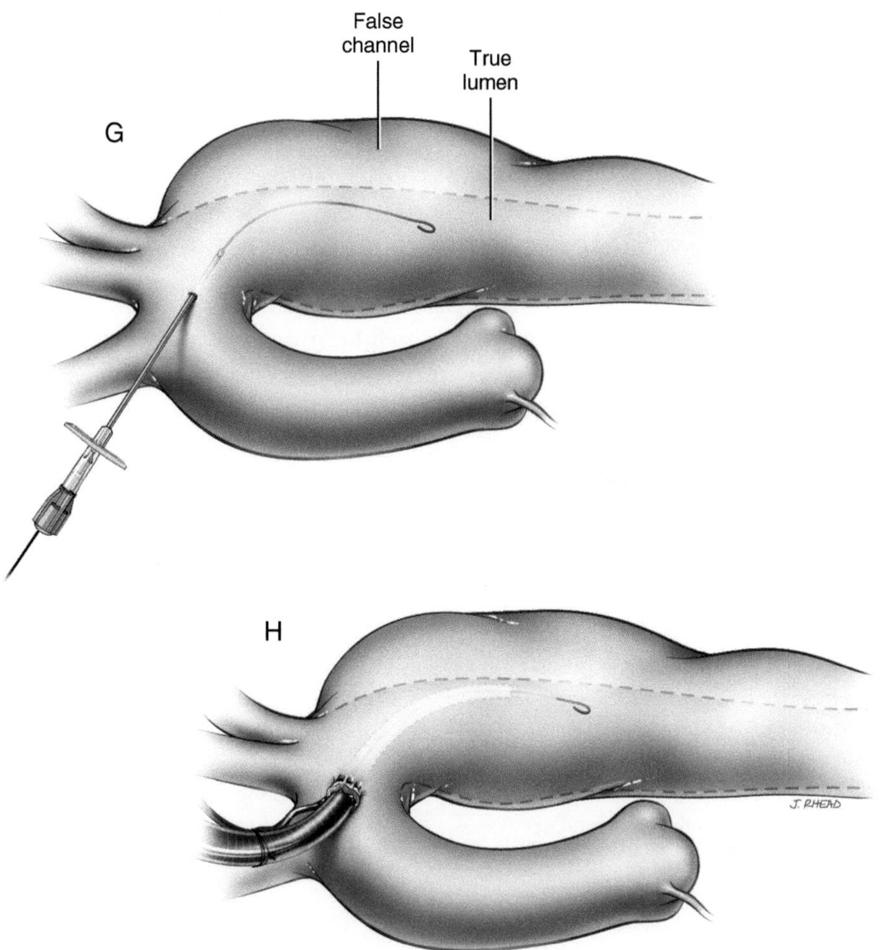

Arterial cannula placed over guidewire

Replacement of Ascending Aorta with Prosthetic Graft

Ascending aortic aneurysm or dissection is repaired by replacing the ascending aorta with a prosthetic graft. Placement of the arterial cannula in the proximal aortic arch facilitates placement of the cross-clamp and construction of the distal aortic anastomosis. If the aneurysm approaches the innominate artery, use of the hemiarch technique may be necessary to extend the repair and effectively resect all aneurysmal tissue. The hemiarch technique is also useful for the repair of acute aortic dissection.

Figure 38-3

A The arterial perfusion cannula is placed in the proximal aortic arch. Cardiopulmonary bypass is established, the aorta occluded, and cardiac arrest achieved with cold cardioplegia given retrograde through the coronary sinus. The aorta is transected 1 cm above the sinotubular junction and 1 cm from the aortic cross-clamp. The entire aneurysmal portion is removed, taking care to avoid injury to the right pulmonary artery, which lies directly behind the ascending aorta.

B A prosthetic graft is attached to the distal aorta in an end-to-end fashion using continuous stitches of 4/0 polypropylene suture. The suture line is first constructed across the back wall of the aorta and then carried up to the front of the anastomosis.

C The prosthetic graft is trimmed appropriately to avoid excess length, which can result in kinking. The graft is attached to the sinotubular junction of the native aortic root using continuous stitches of 4/0 polypropylene suture.

D BioGlue is used to reinforce the suture lines before removing the aortic cross-clamp. This effectively seals the needle holes. More significant areas of bleeding should be reinforced with interrupted pledgetted sutures.

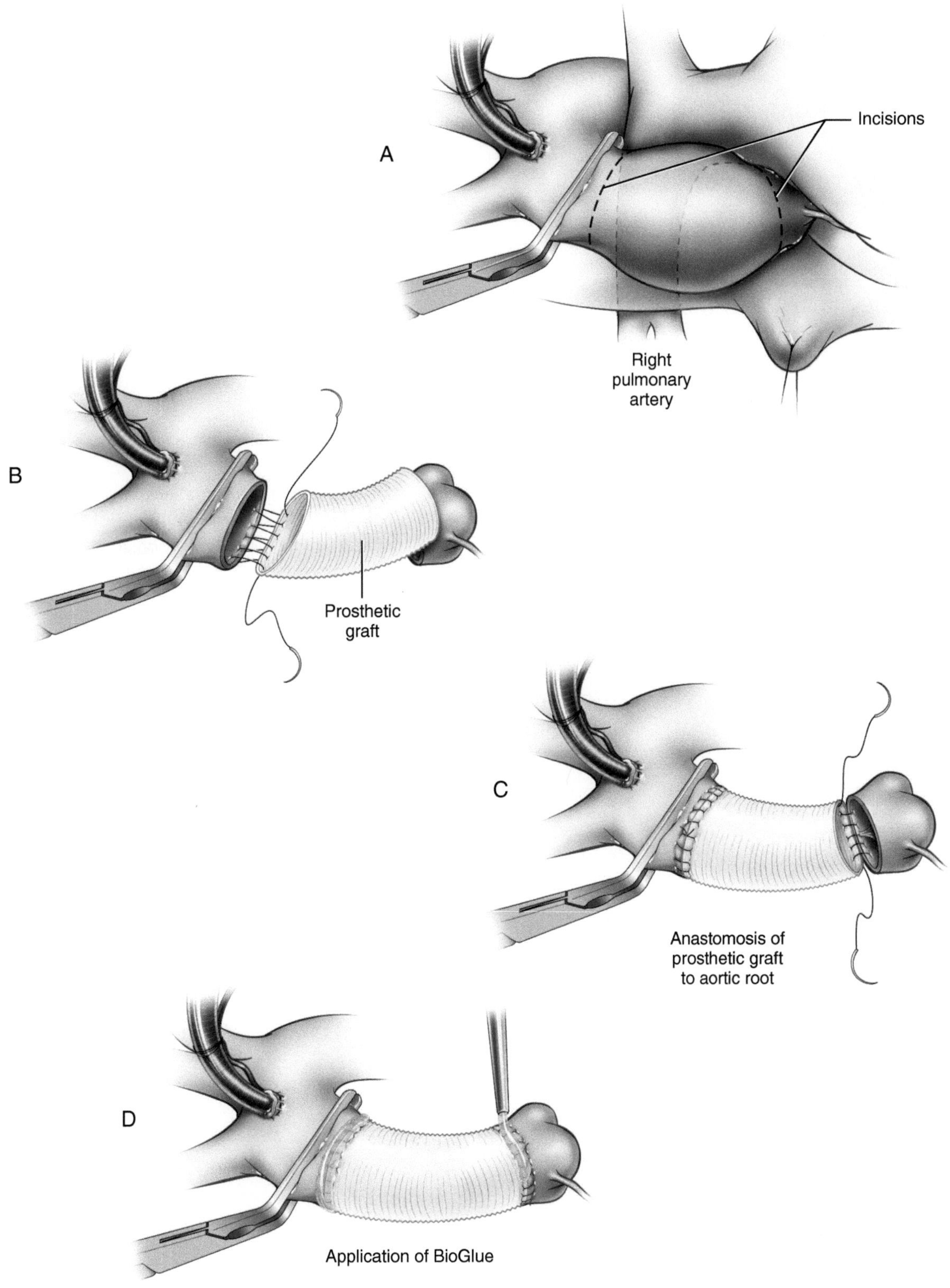
A
Incisions
Right
pulmonary
artery
B
Prosthetic
graft
C
Anastomosis of
prosthetic graft
to aortic root
D
Application of BioGlue

Figure 38-3 (continued)

E If the aneurysm involves the distal ascending aorta or proximal aortic arch, the hemiarch technique should be used to resect all aneurysmal tissue. The arterial perfusion cannula is placed in the distal aortic arch. The cross-clamp is placed at a convenient point on the dilated ascending aorta. The aorta is transected 1 cm above the sinotubular junction and below the cross-clamp.

F A short period of circulatory arrest under deep hypothermia is required to construct the distal aortic anastomosis. The cross-clamp is removed, and the aorta is trimmed to the level of the innominate artery and beveled underneath the aortic arch.

G A prosthetic graft is selected and beveled to match the hemiarch configuration. It is attached in an end-to-end fashion using continuous stitches of 4/0 polypropylene suture. The suture line is first constructed across the back wall of the aorta and then carried up to the front of the anastomosis.

H Cardiopulmonary bypass is reinstituted, and de-airing maneuvers are employed to evacuate air and debris from the arch vessels and the descending thoracic aorta. After appropriate de-airing, the cross-clamp is placed on the distal portion of the prosthetic graft, and full cardiopulmonary bypass flow is reestablished.

I The prosthetic graft is trimmed appropriately and attached to the sinotubular junction of the native aortic root using continuous 4/0 polypropylene suture.

J BioGlue is used to reinforce the suture lines before removing the aortic cross-clamp. This effectively seals the needle holes. More significant areas of bleeding should be reinforced with interrupted pledgetted sutures.

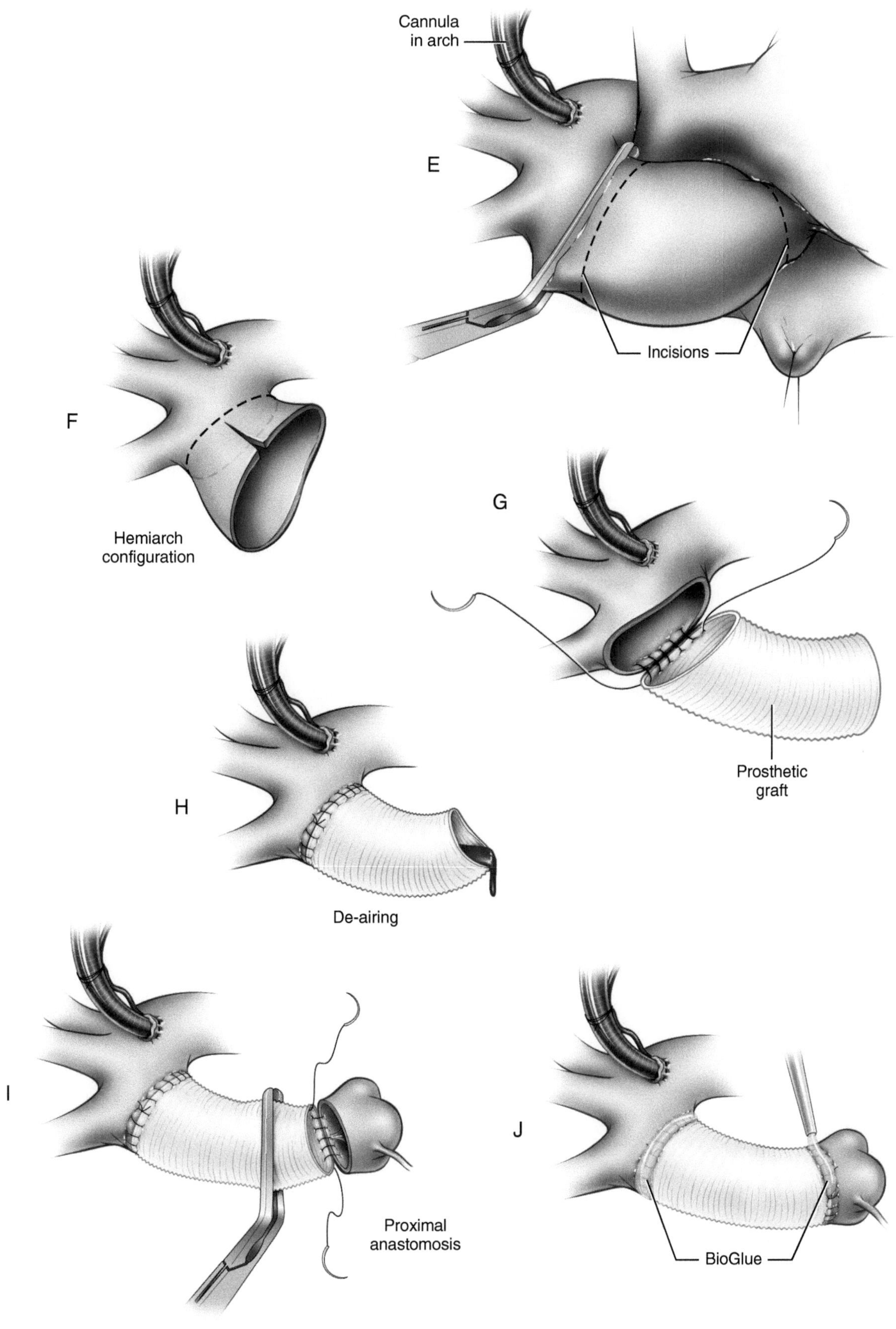
Cannula
in arch
E
Incisions
F
Hemiarch
configuration
G
Prosthetic
graft
H
De-airing
I
Proximal
anastomosis
J
BioGlue

Figure 38-3 (continued)

K In the setting of acute aortic dissection, the arterial cannula is placed in the distal ascending aorta using the Seldinger guidewire technique. Transesophageal echocardiography is used to place the guidewire into the true lumen, and the arterial cannula is advanced over the guidewire out into the descending thoracic aorta.

L The cross-clamp is placed at a convenient point on the ascending aorta. The aorta is transected 1 cm above the sinotubular junction and 1 cm from the cross-clamp.

M The aortic root is inspected, looking for extension of the dissection. If the dissection is limited to the noncoronary sinus or there is minimal extension below the sinotubular junction, BioGlue is used to reapproximate the aortic layers and reinforce the sinotubular junction.

N A short period of circulatory arrest under deep hypothermia is required to construct the distal aortic anastomosis. The cross-clamp and the arterial cannula are removed, and the aorta is trimmed to the level of the innominate artery and beveled underneath the aortic arch. The arch is inspected for evidence of an intimal tear.

O BioGlue is used to reapproximate the aortic layers. A balloon catheter is inflated in the aortic arch while the glue is applied sequentially around the circumference of the aorta. This prevents the glue from flowing down the false lumen into the descending thoracic aorta.

P A prosthetic graft is selected and beveled to match the hemiarch configuration. It is attached in an end-to-end fashion using continuous 4/0 polypropylene suture. The suture line is first constructed across the back wall of the aorta and then carried up to the front of the anastomosis.

Q The arterial cannula is placed back through the prosthetic graft (as shown in Figure 38-3, *R*) and the tip of the cannula positioned in the distal aortic arch under direct vision. Cardiopulmonary bypass is reinstituted, and de-airing maneuvers are employed to evacuate air and debris from the arch vessels and the descending thoracic aorta. After appropriate de-airing, the cross-clamp is placed on the distal portion of the prosthetic graft, and full bypass flow is reestablished.

R The prosthetic graft is trimmed appropriately and attached to the reinforced sinotubular junction of the native aortic root using continuous stitches of 4/0 polypropylene suture.

S BioGlue is used to reinforce the suture lines before removing the aortic cross-clamp. This effectively seals the needle holes. More significant areas of bleeding should be reinforced with interrupted pledgetted sutures. The completed repair is shown with BioGlue sealing the suture lines and arrows demonstrating proper blood flow to the true aortic lumen.

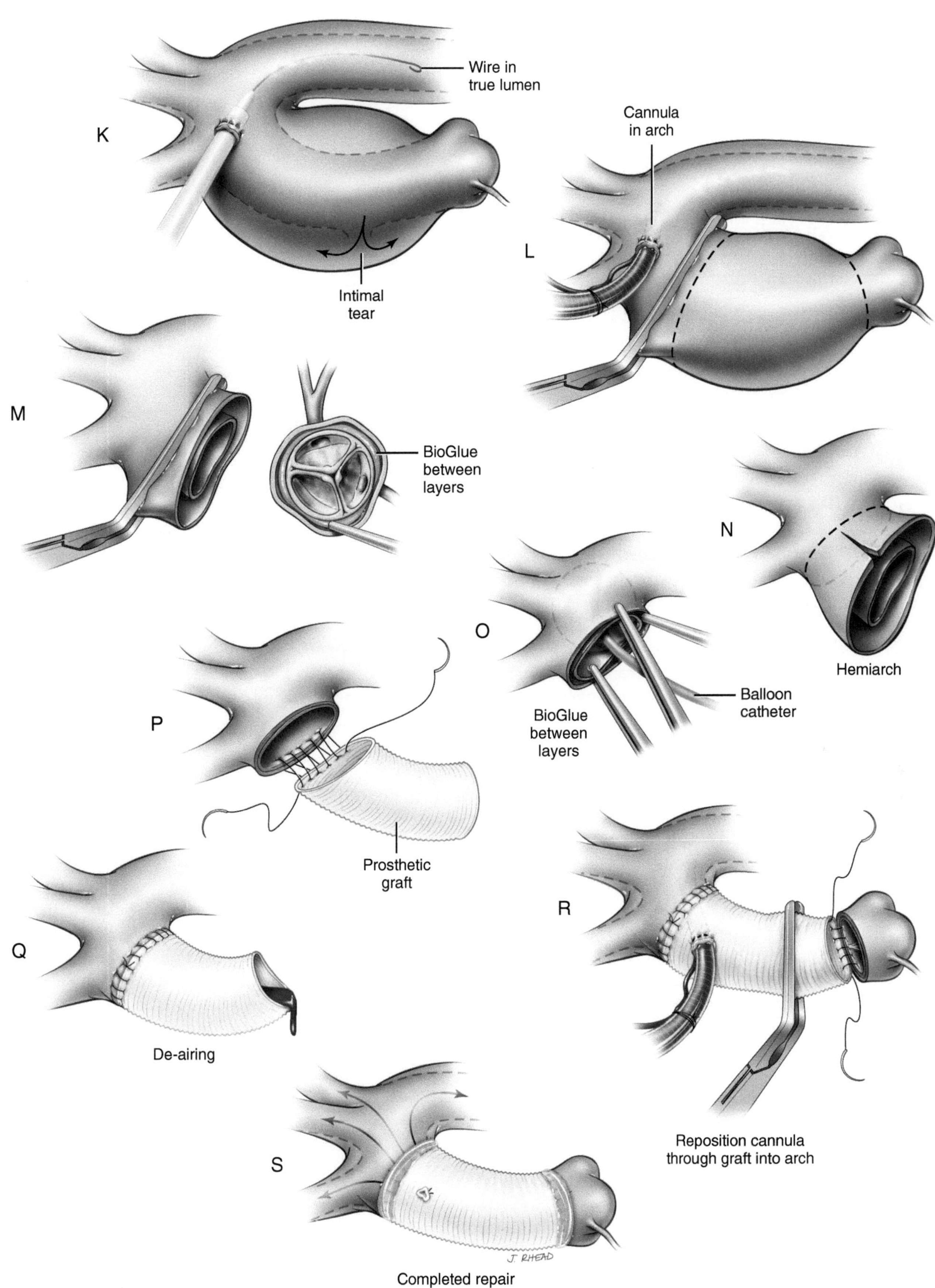
K
Wire in true lumen
Intimal tear
Cannula in arch
L
M
BioGlue between layers
N
Hemiarch
O
BioGlue between layers
Balloon catheter
P
Prosthetic graft
Q
De-airing
R
Reposition cannula through graft into arch
S
J. RHEAD
Completed repair

Replacement of Ascending Aorta and Aortic Root

Concomitant replacement of the ascending aorta and the aortic root is necessary when there is combined disease. Aortic dissection that extends deep into the aortic root, rendering the aortic valve unrepairable, is an indication for replacement of both the ascending aorta and the aortic root. Another common indication is aortic valve incompetence due to root dilation from aneurysmal disease, such as that associated with Marfan syndrome. An additional indication is a bicuspid aortic valve with associated dilation of the ascending aorta. Durable repair is achieved with the use of either a composite mechanical valved conduit or a tissue aortic root bioprosthesis and a prosthetic graft.

Figure 38-4

A The arterial perfusion cannula is placed in the distal ascending aorta or proximal aortic arch, depending on the extent of the ascending aortic aneurysm. The cross-clamp is placed in the ascending aorta distal to the aneurysm, and retrograde cardioplegia is used to arrest the heart. The aorta is transected 1 cm above the sinotubular junction and 1 cm from the aortic cross-clamp. The aneurysmal aorta is resected.

B The aortic valve is excised, and the aortic root exposure is enhanced by placing traction sutures at the top of each commissure. The aortic tissue is removed from each sinus, leaving a 5 to 6 mm rim of aortic tissue along the aortic annulus. The left and right coronary arteries are mobilized on generous buttons of aortic sinus tissue.

C The diameter of the aortic annulus is measured, and a mechanical valved composite graft is selected for the repair. A porcine aortic root prosthesis can also be used. Interrupted mattress stitches of 2/0 braided suture are placed down through the aortic annulus and brought up through the sewing ring of the prosthesis. Suture placement is started in the right coronary sinus and proceeds in a clockwise fashion, similar to standard aortic valve replacement. Repair of the left coronary sinus follows in a counterclockwise fashion, and the repair is completed in a clockwise fashion through the noncoronary sinus.

D The valved composite prosthesis is lowered down on the aortic annulus, ensuring that the valve is seated properly without impinging on the leaflets or valve occlusion mechanism. The sutures are tied down first in the noncoronary sinus in a counterclockwise fashion. The second group of sutures in the left coronary sinus is tied in a counterclockwise fashion, and the repair is completed in the right coronary sinus in a clockwise fashion. A running suture technique is also acceptable, provided the annulus is strong enough to support this type of repair.

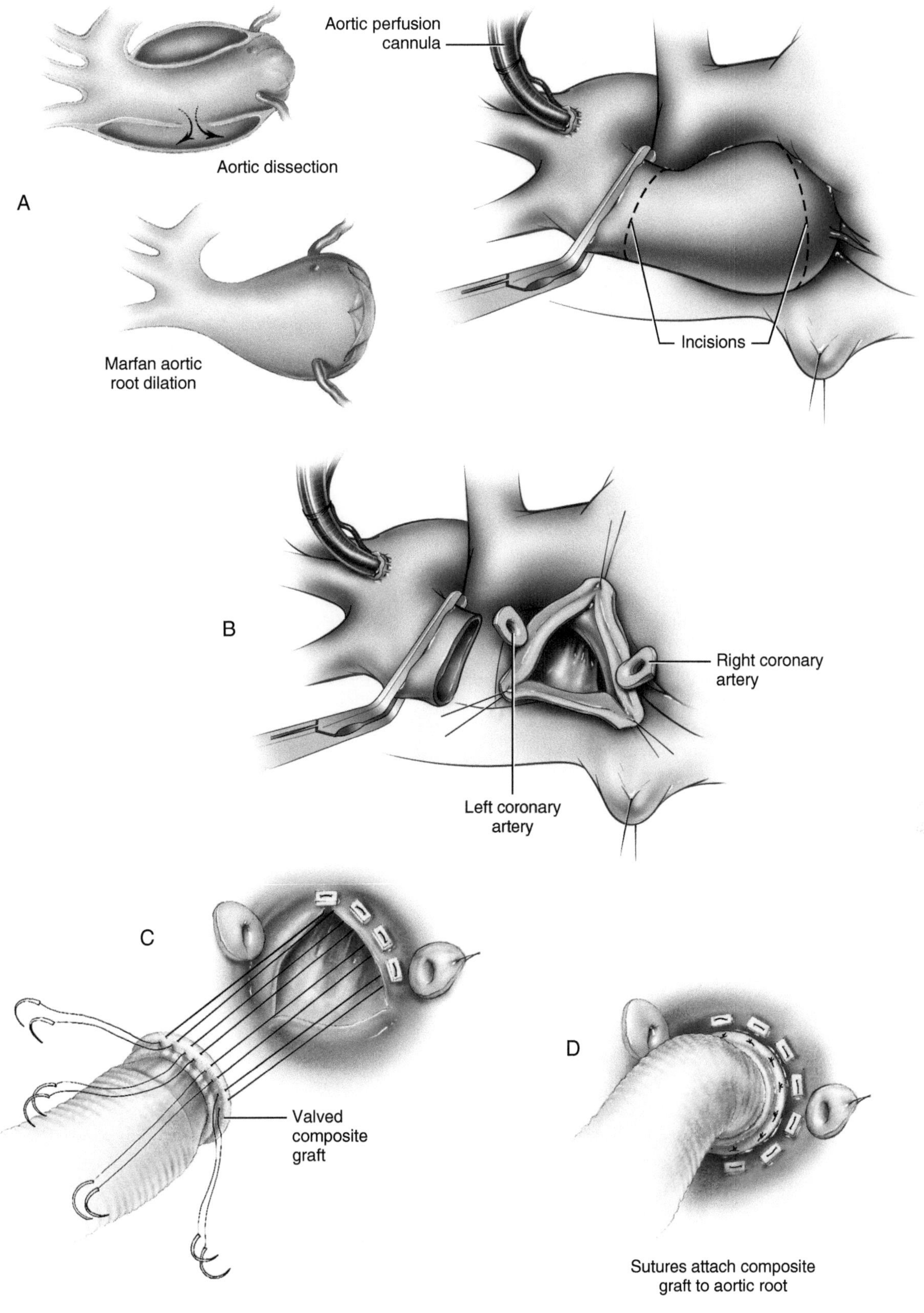
Aortic perfusion cannula
Aortic dissection
A
Marfan aortic root dilation
Incisions
B
Right coronary artery
Left coronary artery
C
Valved composite graft
D
Sutures attach composite graft to aortic root

Figure 38-4 (continued)

E Openings are made into the sides of the Dacron graft exactly opposite the coronary artery ostia using a battery-operated ophthalmic cautery unit. Large openings make the technical aspects of the repair easier and avoid narrowing the anastomosis. An adequate amount of graft should be left between the bottom of these openings and the sewing ring of the prosthesis. The left coronary ostium is attached first using continuous stitches of 5/0 polypropylene. All the suture loops are placed around the inferior rim of the coronary ostium before they are tightened in order to accurately approximate the ostium to the graft opening.

F Both coronary ostia are approximated to the graft in a similar fashion. The right coronary artery anastomosis can be completed either before or after the distal aortic anastomosis if there is concern about the proper orientation of the right coronary artery.

G Secure, accurate stitches must be placed in the coronary artery button wall for secure approximation to the side of the graft. The stitches are placed in a "wagon wheel" fashion, taking wide bites of the surrounding Dacron graft or bioprosthetic aortic sinus tissues. This is particularly important in the case of aortic dissection, because the aortic tissue can be fragile. Use of BioGlue or Teflon felt "washers" is advised to support these critical coronary reimplantations.

H When there has been extensive dissection into the coronary arteries, the main coronary arteries must be trimmed to some degree. Small, short interposition PTFE grafts can then be used to compensate for the loss of coronary artery length. The interposition grafts are attached in an end-to-end fashion to each main coronary artery using continuous stitches of 6/0 polypropylene sutures; then the grafts are attached to the openings in the composite graft using continuous stitches of 5/0 polypropylene suture. Careful attention must be paid to the length of each interposition graft to avoid kinking and improper orientation. BioGlue is applied to reinforce these suture lines.

An alternative method is to use a single interposition graft for the reimplantation. The left main coronary artery (LCA) is trimmed back to healthy tissue, and a small prosthetic graft is attached in an end-to-end fashion using continuous stitches of 6/0 polypropylene. This prosthetic graft is then routed behind the main composite graft and attached to the front of it using continuous stitches of 4/0 polypropylene. The right coronary artery (RCA) is also trimmed back to healthy tissue, and a small opening is made in the side of the small prosthetic graft. The right coronary artery is attached to the side of the graft using continuous stitches of 6/0 polypropylene. In cases of Marfan type aortic aneurysm, the coronary ostia may be widely separated by the size of the aneurysm of the aortic root. An interposition graft may be anastomosed directly to the aorta around the coronary ostia without resection of part of the root aneurysm. The interposition graft may be anastomosed to the posterior aspect of the aortic graft, or interiorly as seems best.

I The distal end of the graft is trimmed to an appropriate length and attached in an end-to-end fashion using continuous stitches of 4/0 polypropylene sutures. The suture line is first constructed across the back wall of the aorta and then carried up to the front of the anastomosis.

J A short "collar" of graft material is used to support the distal anastomosis. The collar must be cut and placed around the graft prior to construction of the anastomosis. The collar is pulled up to cover the anastomosis and BioGlue is inserted beneath the collar to reinforce the suture line.

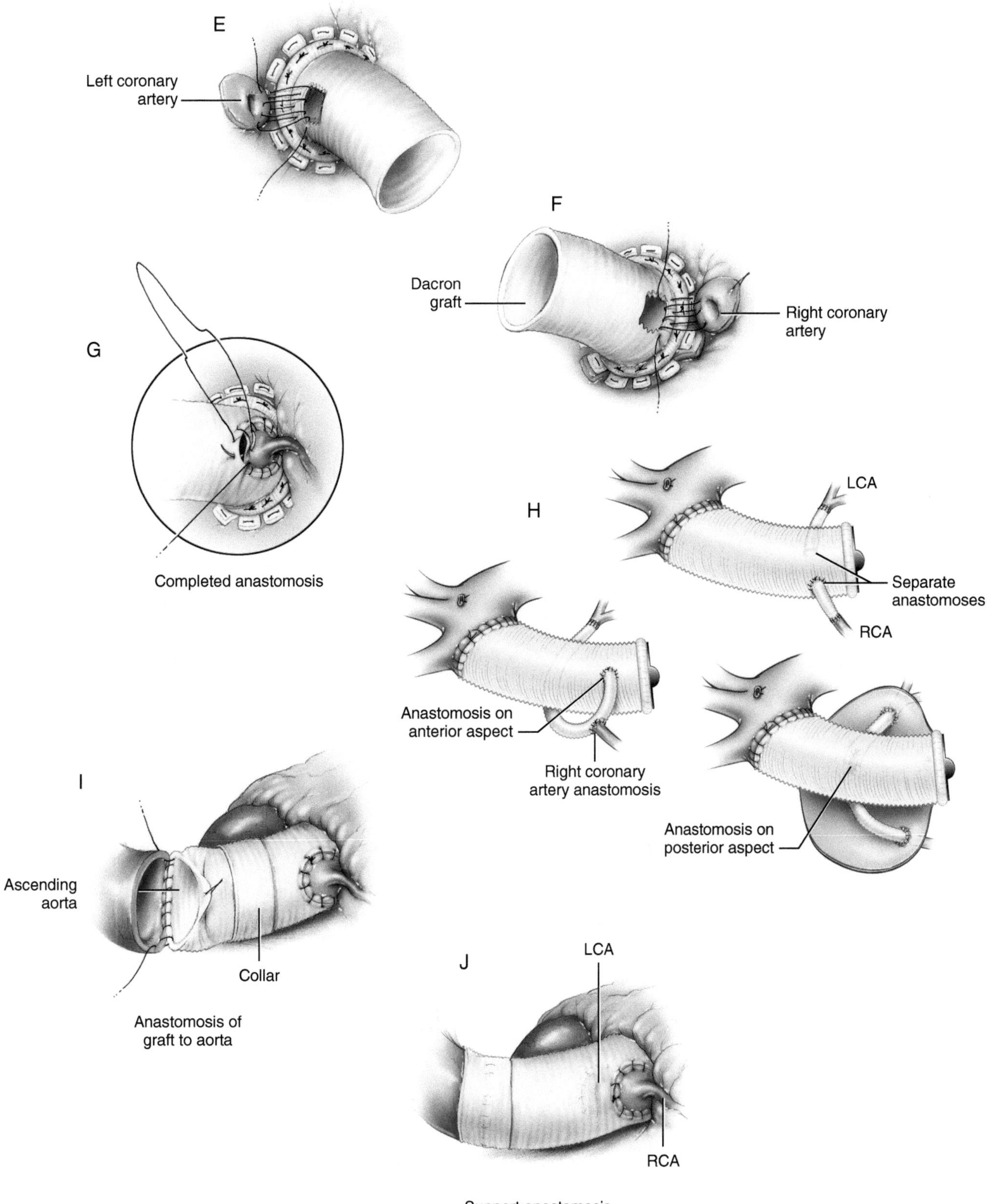
E
Left coronary artery
F
Dacron graft
Right coronary artery
G
Completed anastomosis
H
LCA
Separate anastomoses
RCA
Anastomosis on anterior aspect
Right coronary artery anastomosis
Anastomosis on posterior aspect
I
Ascending aorta
Collar
Anastomosis of graft to aorta
J
LCA
RCA
Support anastomosis with graft collar

Figure 38-4 (continued)

K In patients in whom it is desirable to avoid anticoagulation, concomitant replacement of the aortic root with a Freestyle tissue bioprosthesis provides an excellent alternative to a composite mechanical valved conduit. The initial part of the operation is identical to that for aneurysmal disease of the ascending aorta and aortic root. The arterial return cannula is inserted into the distal aortic arch, and the ascending aorta is resected.

L The aortic root is prepared after placing traction sutures at the top of each commissure. All diseased aortic sinus tissue is removed, and the coronary arteries are mobilized on generous buttons of aortic tissue. The aortic annulus diameter is measured, and an appropriate Freestyle porcine aortic root bioprosthesis is selected. The diameter top of the Freestyle graft is measured, and a prosthetic graft of similar diameter is selected for the ascending aortic repair.

M A short period of circulatory arrest under deep hypothermia is required to construct the distal aortic anastomosis. After trimming the distal aorta in a hemiarch manner, a prosthetic graft is beveled and attached in an end-to-end fashion using continuous stitches of 4/0 polypropylene. The Freestyle sizer is inserted inside the graft to distend the suture line, and BioGlue is applied to reinforce the anastomosis. Cardiopulmonary bypass is reinstituted at low flow. After air and debris are removed from the aortic arch, the graft is clamped, and full cardiopulmonary bypass is reinstituted.

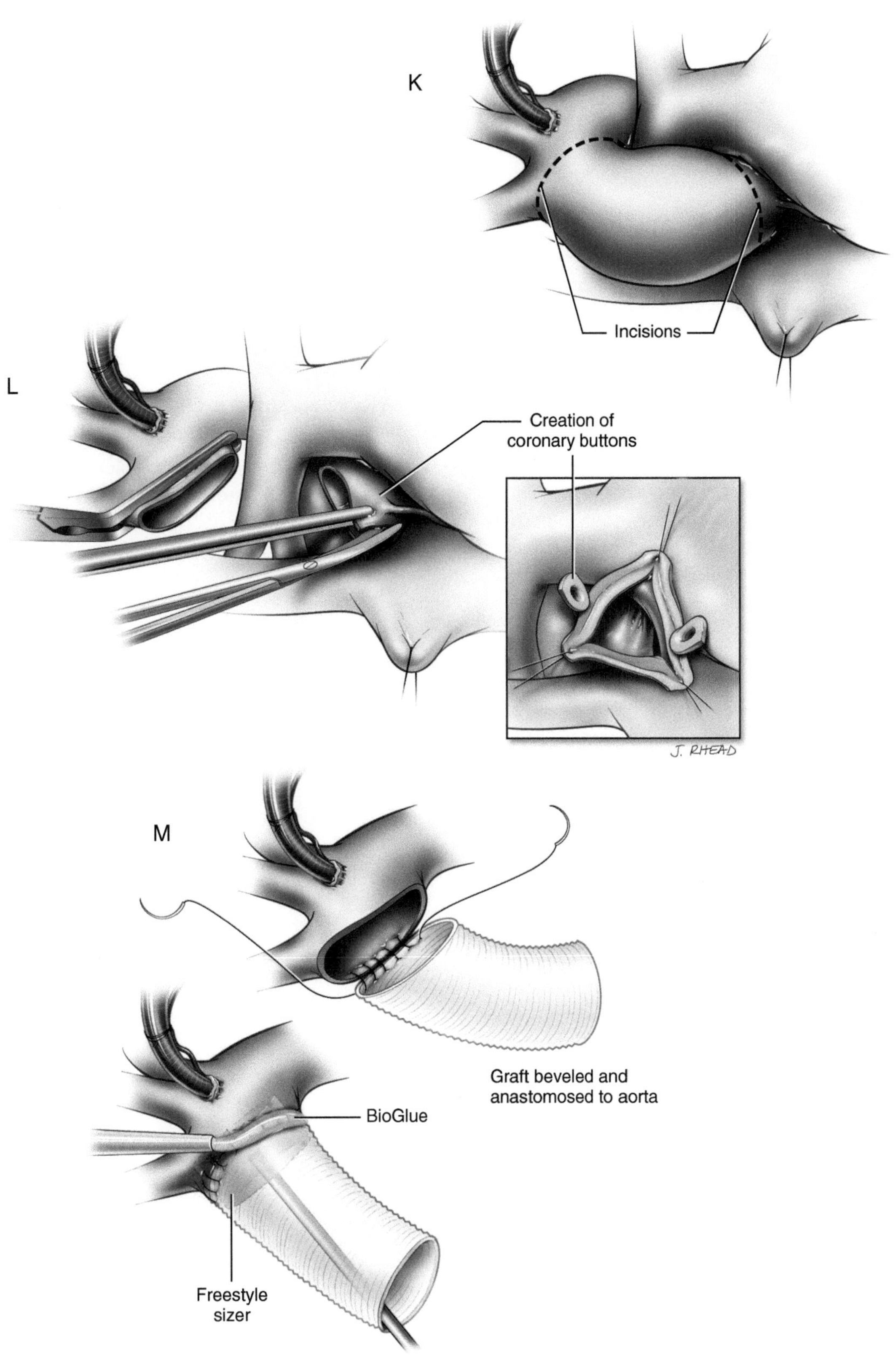
K
Incisions
L
Creation of
coronary buttons
J. RHEAD
M
Graft beveled and
anastomosed to aorta
BioGlue
Freestyle
sizer

Figure 38-4 (continued)

N The Freestyle porcine aortic root bioprosthesis is attached to the left ventricular outflow tract using continuous 3/0 polypropylene sutures. The bioprosthesis is aligned in an anatomic fashion, with the stumps of the porcine left and right coronary arteries facing the native coronary buttons. The suture line is begun at the commissure between the left and right sinuses. The suture is brought in a clockwise fashion along the right coronary sinus to the halfway point of the noncoronary sinus, taking generous bites of the aortic annulus and bringing the needle up through the collar of the Freestyle tissue bioprosthesis just below the dashed marker line. The other end of the suture is brought in a counterclockwise fashion along the left coronary sinus to the halfway point of the noncoronary sinus, meeting the previous suture. Silk sutures are looped around every third stitch, acting as "pulleys" that are gently tightened as the bioprosthesis is lowered into position. This ensures even, symmetric tightening of the anastomosis without breaking the suture. BioGlue is used to reinforce the suture line.

O The left coronary stump of the Freestyle porcine aortic root bioprosthesis is removed to create an opening in the porcine root. The left coronary ostium is attached using continuous 5/0 polypropylene sutures. Several suture loops are placed along the inferior rim of the left coronary ostium before tightening the suture line; this ensures precise placement of the stitches. The right coronary stump of the Freestyle bioprosthesis usually does not align exactly opposite the patient's right coronary artery. A second opening is made in the right coronary sinus of the bioprosthesis at the approximate location, and the right coronary ostium is attached in a similar fashion. Both coronary artery anastomoses are reinforced with BioGlue.

P The bioprosthetic graft is trimmed to appropriate length and beveled to match the bevel of the aorta. Beveling re-creates the natural contour of the ascending aorta, forming a small curvature on the central or leftward part of the graft.

Q The Freestyle tissue bioprosthesis is attached to a prosthetic graft using continuous stitches of 4/0 polypropylene. A short "collar" of graft is used to support the anastomosis. The collar is cut from the unused portion of the graft and must be placed over the graft prior to performing the anastomosis. The collar is pulled over the completed anastomosis and BioGlue is inserted beneath the collar to reinforce the suture line.

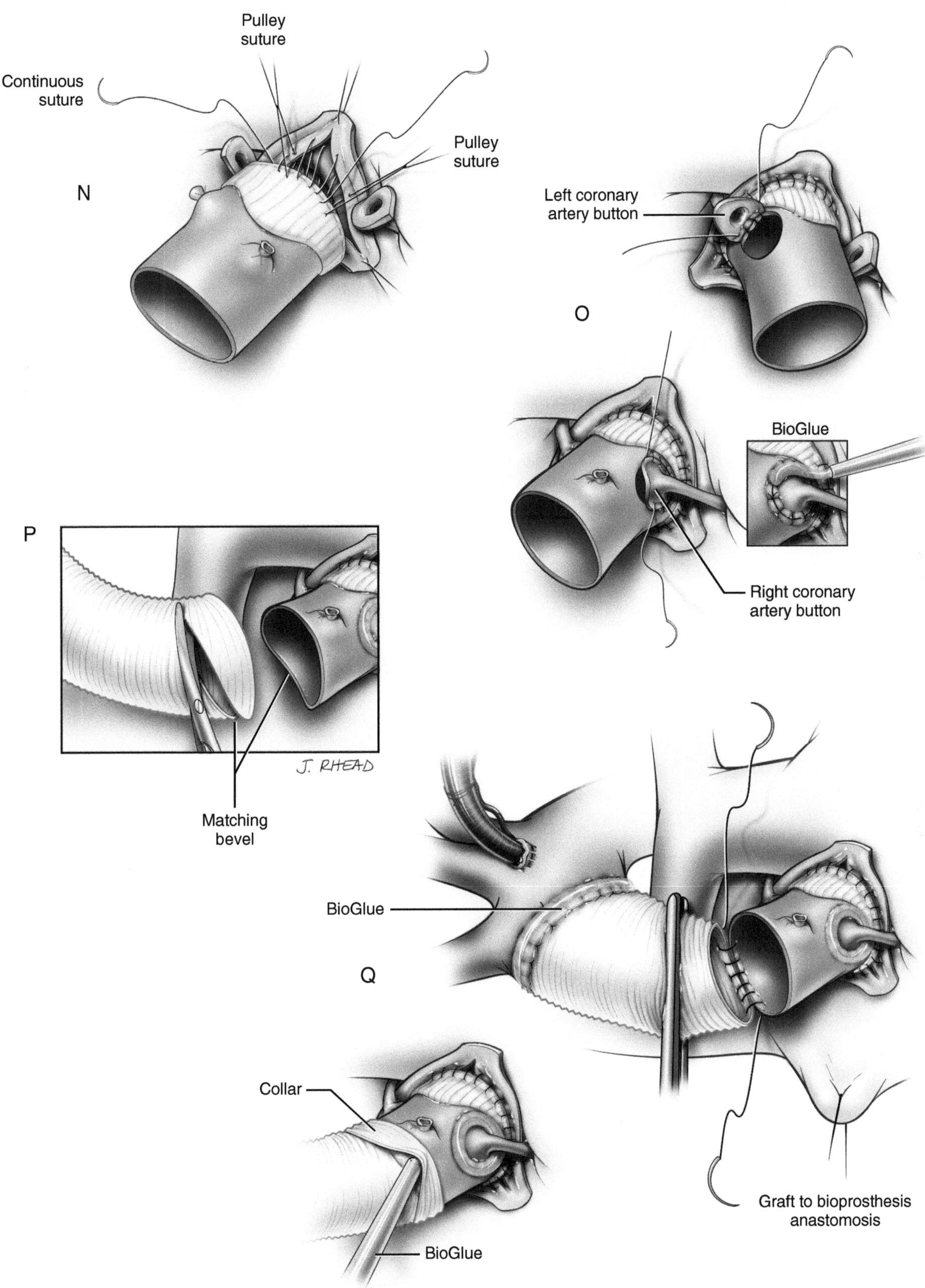
Pulley
suture
Continuous
suture
Pulley
suture
N
Left coronary
artery button
O
BioGlue
Right coronary
artery button
P
J. RHEAD
Matching
bevel
BioGlue
Q
Collar
BioGlue
Graft to bioprosthesis
anastomosis

Aortic Arch

Reconstruction of the aortic arch may be necessary for atherosclerotic aneurysm or dissection of the aorta that extends into the arch, making repair impossible or inadvisable proximal to the innominate artery. This region was once accessible only with great difficulty and risk using continuous-flow cardiopulmonary bypass techniques. The application of circulatory arrest with the patient under deep body hypothermia has made the aortic arch much more accessible.

Ascending Aorta and Hemiarch Replacement with Arch Thromboendarterectomy

Atherosclerotic disease with aneurysm of the ascending aorta may extend into the aortic arch. There may be ulcerated atherosclerotic plaques in the aorta, placing the patient at risk for intraoperative stroke due to atheroemboli. Addressing this risk factor during ascending aorta and partial arch (hemiarch) replacement should improve survival and reduce neurologic comorbidity.

Figure 38-5

A An aortic perfusion cannula is placed in the distal part of the aortic arch, with the tip in the upper portion of the descending thoracic aorta beyond the origin of the left subclavian artery. A two-stage venous uptake cannula is placed in the right atrium. The patient is perfused with blood cooled to 12°C until the body temperature (nasopharyngeal) reaches 16 to 18°C. An induction dose of thiopental sodium (Pentathol), corticosteroids, and mannitol are useful pharmacologic adjuncts. Circulatory arrest under these conditions should be well tolerated for 60 minutes. This period can be extended by interval hypothermic perfusion of the brain. Some surgeons favor retrograde cerebral perfusion via the superior vena cava as a means of cerebral protection, but data on the efficacy of this method are not conclusive. An occlusion clamp is placed on the ascending aorta when ventricular fibrillation occurs. The occlusion clamp must be placed on a disease-free area; this can be determined by gentle palpation of the aorta. The best spot is often just above the sinotubular junction. A vent catheter is placed in the left superior pulmonary vein and passed into the left ventricle. Retrograde perfusion of the coronary sinus is begun, and the heart is cooled to 4°C.

When the target body temperature is reached, cardiopulmonary bypass is discontinued. The occlusion clamp is removed from the aorta. The aorta is divided above the sinotubular junction. It is divided distally just proximal to the origin of the brachiocephalic artery in an oblique manner across to the inferior aspect of the aortic arch, including part of the arch.

B A dissection plane is opened between the aortic intima-media and the adventitia, working through the open end of the aorta.

C Endarterectomy of the portions of the arch affected by atherosclerotic disease is performed. Removal of all the arch intima and media may be required, extending the dissection into the arch branches. A smooth transition to the arterial intima, with firm attachment, must be present at the end points of the endarterectomy. Extending the endarterectomy into the branch vessels beyond visualization (blind endarterectomy) may be required, but this adds risk to the procedure.

D A tubular Dacron vascular graft is tailored obliquely when part of the arch has been removed. The short angle of the graft is placed medially on the aortic arch to avoid kinking as the graft is brought down to the aortic root. An end-to-end anastomosis of the graft to the aortic arch is constructed using continuous stitches of 4/0 polypropylene.

E The anastomosis is sealed with BioGlue. Cardiopulmonary bypass is resumed, with the patient in a head-down position. Air and debris are removed from the arch and its branches by gentle agitation and floated out the open proximal end of the graft. An occlusion clamp is placed on the graft. The proximal anastomosis of the graft to the proximal aorta is completed during the rewarming process.

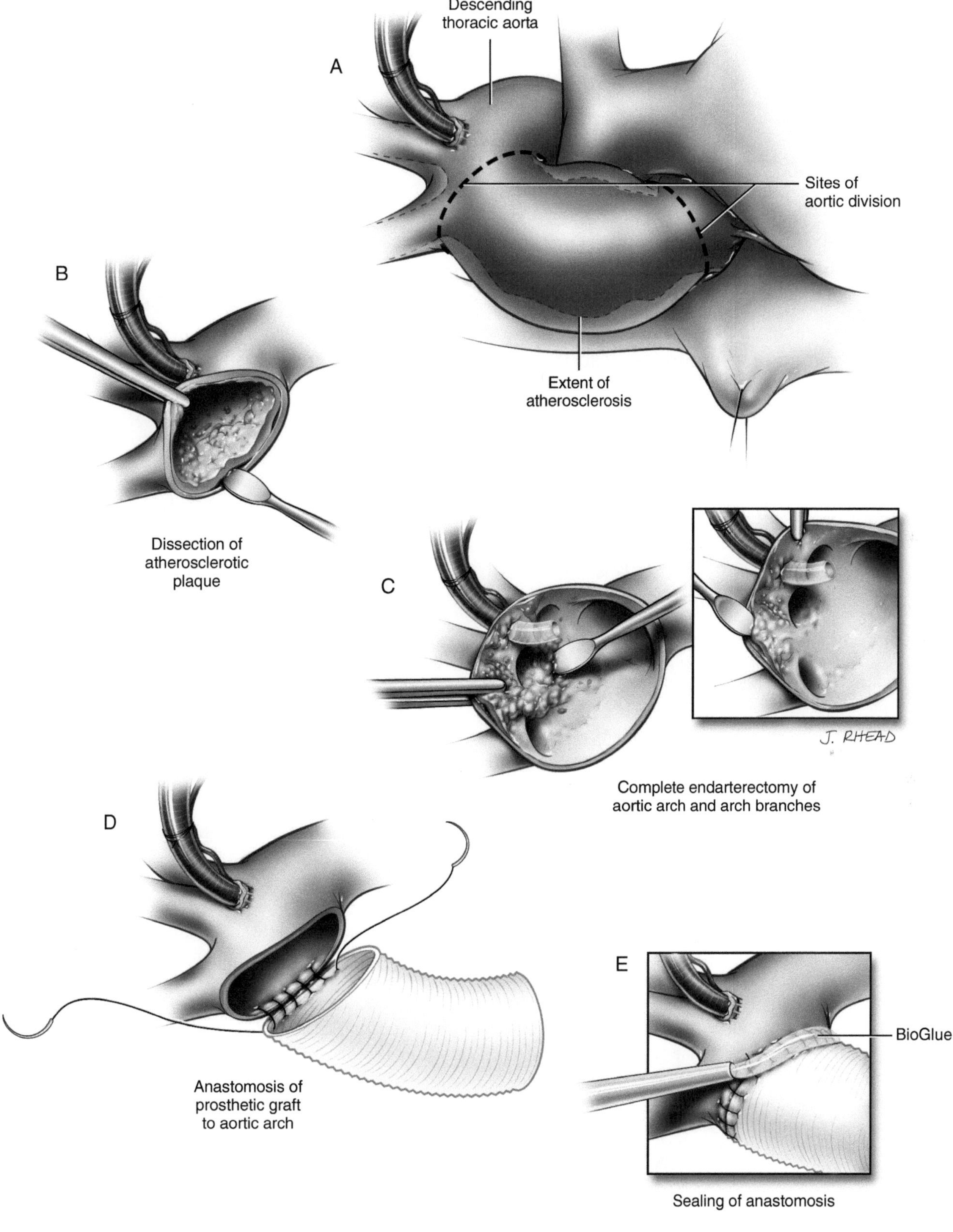
A
Descending
thoracic aorta
Sites of
aortic division
Extent of
atherosclerosis
B
Dissection of
atherosclerotic
plaque
C
J. RHEAD
Complete endarterectomy of
aortic arch and arch branches
D
Anastomosis of
prosthetic graft
to aortic arch
E
BioGlue
Sealing of anastomosis

Valve-Sparing Aortic Root Replacement-Reimplantation Technique (Yacoub/David II Operation)

Occasionally, aneurysmal disease of the ascending aorta is associated with normal aortic valve cusps and no dilation of the aortic valve annulus. It may be possible to preserve aortic valve function in this situation. The principles of repair are based on techniques described by Yacoub and David and on aortic root dimensions detailed by Kunzelman.

Figure 38-6

A Cardiopulmonary bypass is established as usual. The aorta is occluded and retrograde cold cardioplegia given through the coronary sinus. The aneurysm of the ascending aorta is incised longitudinally. The aorta is divided distally above the aneurysm.

B The aortic valve is inspected to determine the feasibility of repair. If the aneurysmal disease is restricted to the aorta, with dilation of the sinuses of Valsalva, it may be possible to preserve the aortic valve. The aortic valve cusps should be normal. There should be no dilation of the aortic annulus, although there are techniques to narrow the annulus. In the situation depicted here, the aortic valve is determined to be incompetent due to separation of the commissures by aneurysmal dilation of the aorta.

C The sinus aorta is excised, retaining only a 3 to 5 mm rim above the fibrous connecting point of the aortic valve (annulus). A button of sinus aorta is retained around ostia of the left and right coronary arteries.

D Average dimensions of the aortic leaflets are obtained. The length of the free margin of the leaflets is determined, and the height of the leaflets is measured. The sinotubular diameter is calculated using dimensions determined by Kunzelman: if the diameter of the aortic root at the ventriculoaortic junction ("the "annulus") is taken as 1.0, the diameter of the sinotubular junction (which will also be the diameter of the prosthetic graft chosen for the repair) is 0.91 of the annulus diameter. For example, if the diameter of the aortic valve annulus measures 25 mm, a 22 mm diameter tubular prosthesis is chosen ($25 \times 0.9 = 22.5$). A practical method for selecting an appropriately sized prosthetic graft is to simply measure "the annulus," as would be done for an aortic valve replacement, and choose a tubular graft diameter that is about 90% of the diameter of the annulus.

E A graft of the appropriate size is selected. Double-velour knitted Dacron that has been collagen coated for hemostasis is usually chosen. The graft is cut at three symmetric points to accommodate the commissures of the aortic valve. The cuts usually extend six or seven crimp ridges into the graft, depending on the height of the leaflets. The graft material between these cuts will become the reconstructed sinuses of Valsalva.

F The edges of the graft are attached to the sinus aortae remnant at the hinge point of the aortic leaflets. Continuous stitches of 3/0 or 4/0 polypropylene are used for the repair. The commissures of the aortic valve are brought into the apices of the cuts in the graft.

G Openings are cut into the graft, opposite the location of the coronary arteries, using a hot cautery. The coronary arteries are anastomosed to the openings in the graft with continuous stitches of 5/0 polypropylene.

H An end-to-end anastomosis of the graft to the aorta completes the repair. All vascular anastomoses are sealed with BioGlue.

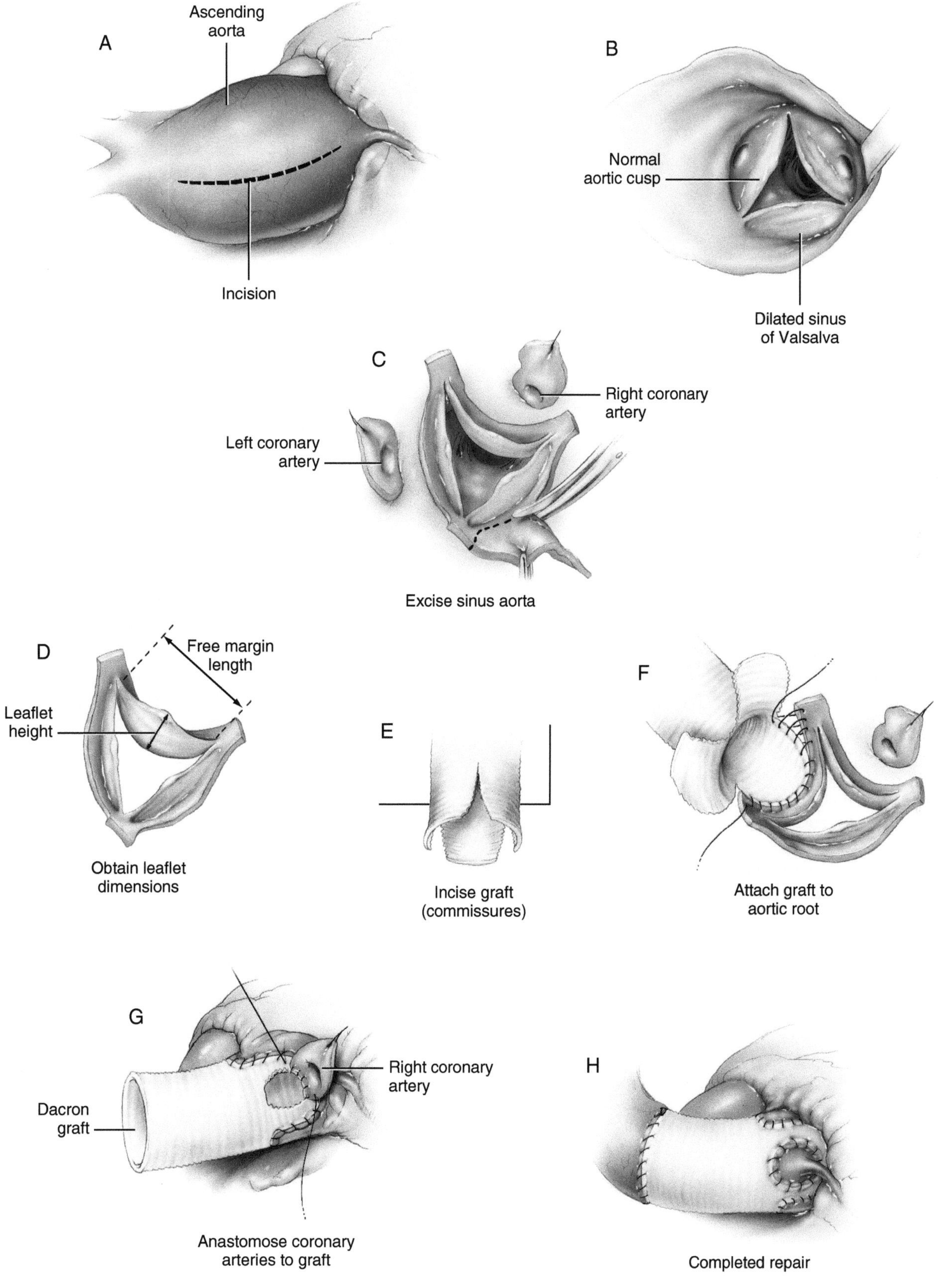
A
Ascending aorta
Incision
B
Normal aortic cusp
Dilated sinus of Valsalva
C
Right coronary artery
Left coronary artery
Excise sinus aorta
D
Free margin length
Leaflet height
Obtain leaflet dimensions
E
Incise graft (commissures)
F
Attach graft to aortic root
G
Right coronary artery
Dacron graft
Anastomose coronary arteries to graft
H
Completed repair

Valve-Sparing Aortic Root Replacement with Valsalva Graft Resuspension Technique (David I Operation)

Preservation of the native aortic valve using the David I reimplantation operation is facilitated by utilizing a prosthetic graft with prefabricated sinuses. The Valsalva graft also has reinforced collars at the annulus and sinotubular junction to provide a more anatomic reconstruction and prevent graft dilation.

Figure 38-7

A The aortic root is dissected well below the aortic annulus. It is particularly important to carry the dissection below the root behind each commissure because the graft will be seated outside the root and below the annulus. The aortic sinus tissue is excised, retaining a 3 to 5 mm rim above the annulus, and buttons of sinus tissue are retained around each coronary ostium. A pledgetted 5/0 polypropylene suture is placed at the top of each commissure, taking care not to impinge on any leaflet tissue.

B Nine 2/0 braided polyester sutures are placed in mattress fashion below the aortic annulus and passed to the outside of the aortic root. Three sutures are placed in each sinus, with one suture at the lowest point of the valve and one suture slightly higher on each side toward the commissure. These sutures should be narrow to avoid crimping and distorting the annulus.

C The diameter of the annulus is measured, and a graft 3- to 4-mm larger than the annulus is selected. The graft is trimmed, leaving two or three rings below the proximal reinforced collar.

D Each of the nine subannular sutures is brought through the lower portion of the graft. Once again, these sutures should be narrow to avoid crimping and distorting the graft.

E The graft is lowered onto the root by gently pulling the three 5/0 polypropylene sutures up through the graft. The braided sutures are also gently tightened to ensure that the graft is seated well down on the root, below the annulus.

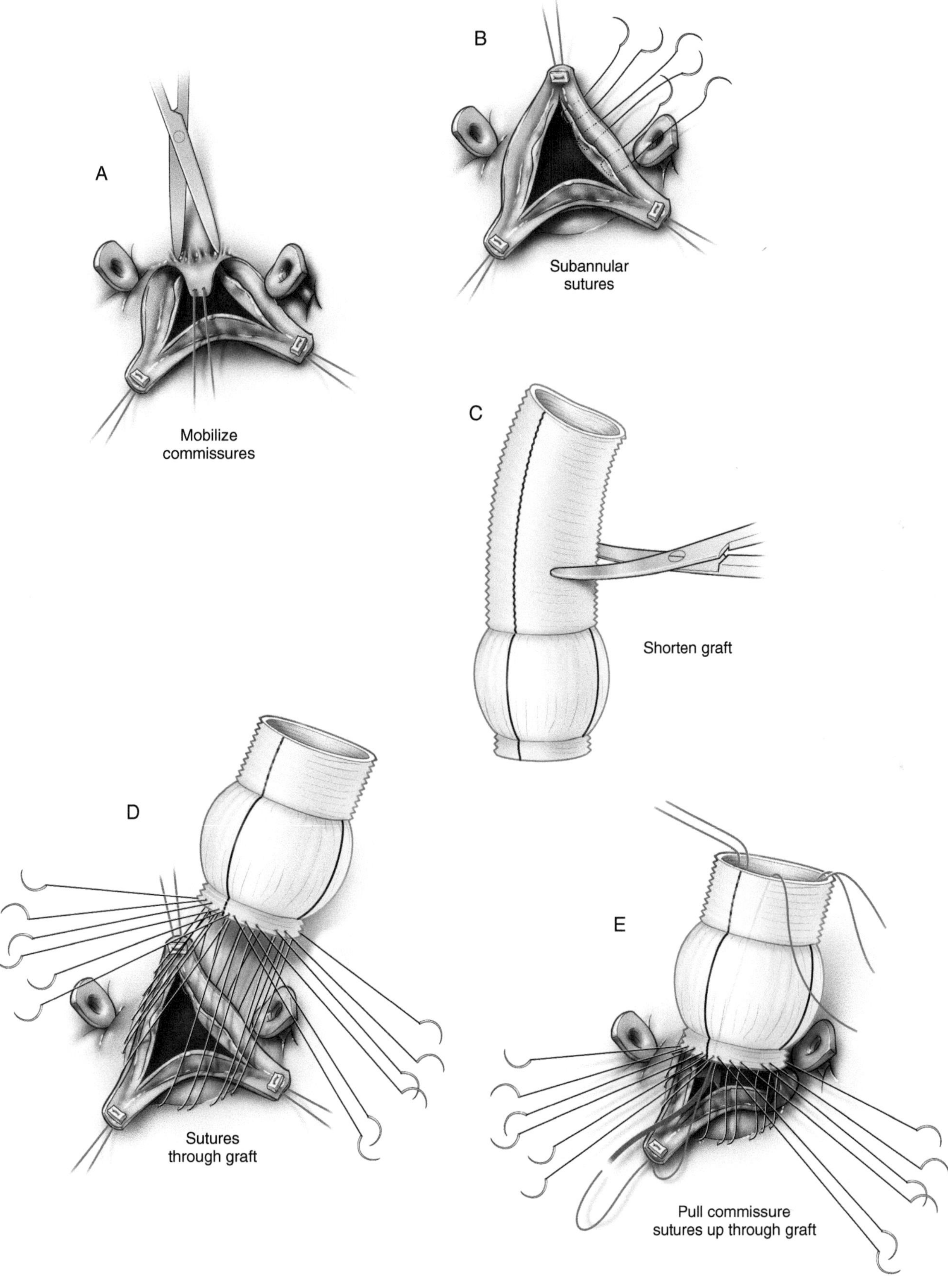
A
Mobilize commissures
B
Subannular sutures
C
Shorten graft
D
Sutures through graft
E
Pull commissure sutures up through graft

Figure 38-7 (continued)

F The braided sutures are tied to secure the graft to the left ventricular outflow tract. The sutures should be tied gently to avoid graft distortion.

G The three 5/0 polypropylene sutures are passed through the graft at the level of the distal reinforced collar. The guidelines on the graft assist in proper location of the stitch. To prevent aortic insufficiency, it is critical to ensure that the commissures are all at the same height. Placing these sutures at the distal reinforced collar maintains the proper elevation and diameter of the valve.

H Three continuous 4/0 polypropylene sutures are used to attach the retained rim of aortic sinus tissue to the graft. The sutures are begun at the lowest point of the sinus and brought up to the top of each commissure. These sutures are then passed outside the graft.

I The 4/0 and 5/0 polypropylene sutures are tied outside the graft to secure the tops of the commissures. The valve is tested for competency.

J The coronary buttons are reimplanted into openings made in the graft in the left and right sinuses of the graft using continuous stitches of 5/0 polypropylene.

K The distal end of the graft is trimmed to the appropriate length and attached in an end-to-end fashion to the aorta using continuous stitches of 4/0 polypropylene. BioGlue is used to reinforce all suture lines.

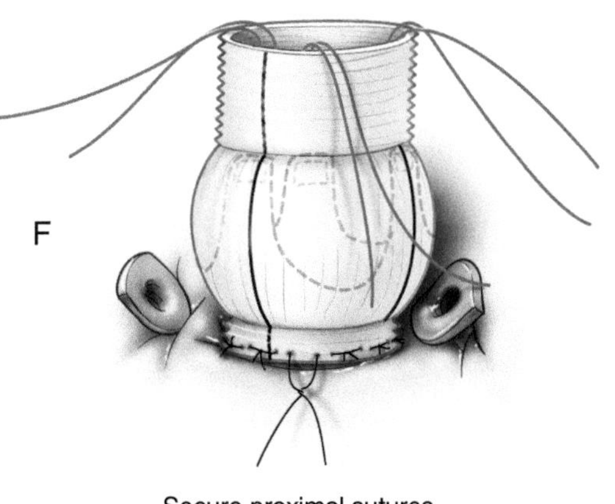

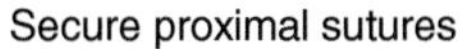

Secure proximal sutures

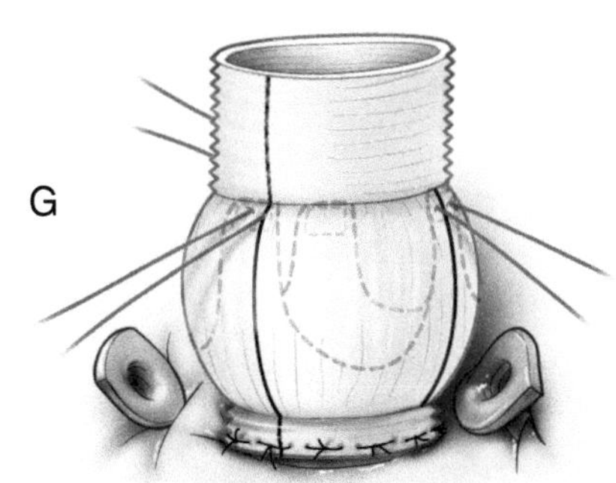

Place commissure sutures through graft

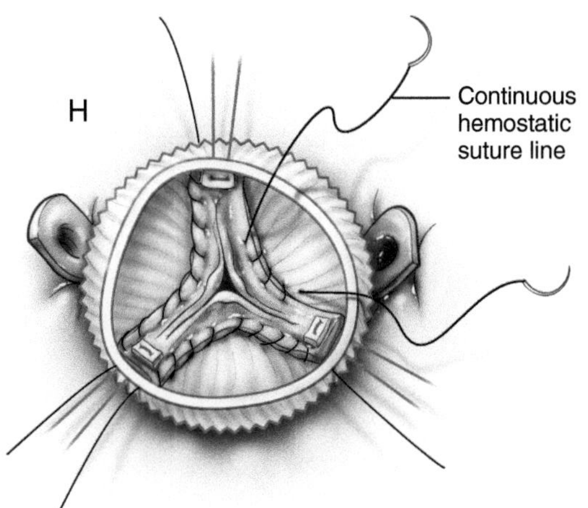

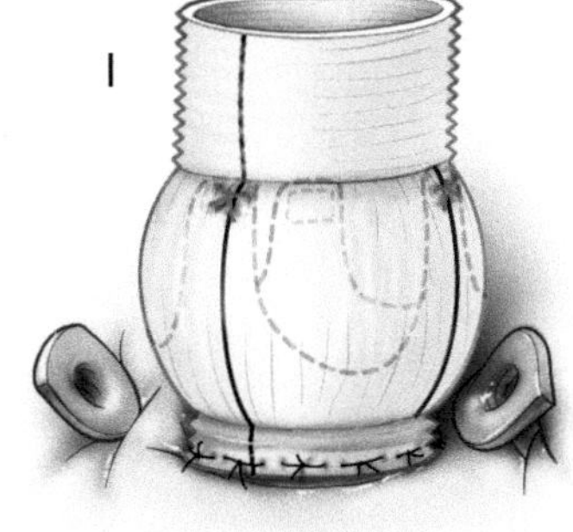

Secure commissure sutures

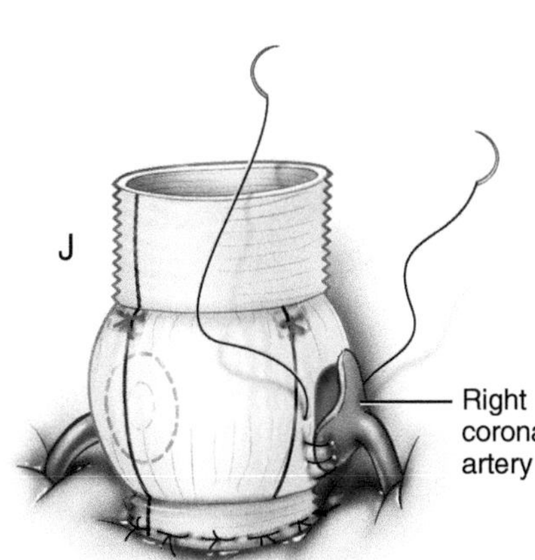

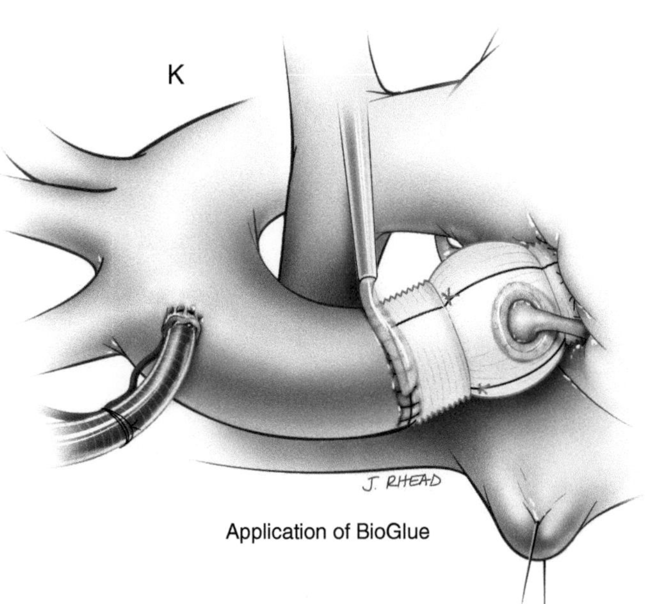

Application of BioGlue

Aortic Arch Replacement: Arch Vessel Island Technique

Total arch replacement requires reimplantation of the arch vessels under hypothermic circulatory arrest. Creation of an "island" of aortic arch tissue that contains the origins of all three arch vessels minimizes the duration of circulatory arrest.

Figure 38-8

A Axillary cannulation with a prosthetic side graft is used to facilitate both full perfusion and low-flow antegrade cerebral perfusion during hypothermic circulatory arrest. The arterial return cannula is inserted into the side graft, allowing the arch to be perfused without compromising flow to the right arm.

B Hypothermic circulatory arrest is initiated, and the arch is resected. An "island" of aortic tissue along the superior aspect of the arch is created that incorporates all three arch vessels. The proximal descending thoracic aorta is trimmed. The aortic root remains intact.

C An appropriate size prosthetic graft is selected and attached in an end-to-end fashion to the descending thoracic aorta, using continuous stitches of 4/0 polypropylene. Particular care is taken to ensure a secure anastomosis because this portion of the repair is difficult to access after the operation is completed.

D An oval-shaped portion is removed along the superior aspect of the prosthetic graft to match the arch vessel island. The island is attached to the prosthetic graft using continuous stitches of 4/0 polypropylene. De-airing maneuvers are used, as cardiopulmonary bypass is reinstituted.

E The graft is occluded proximal to the arch vessel island anastomosis. The proximal end of the graft is trimmed to an appropriate length and attached in an end-to-end fashion to the ascending aorta using continuous stitches of 4/0 polypropylene. Care is taken to bevel the graft and avoid excessive length, which can result in kinking.

F To complete the operation, BioGlue is used to reinforce all suture lines.

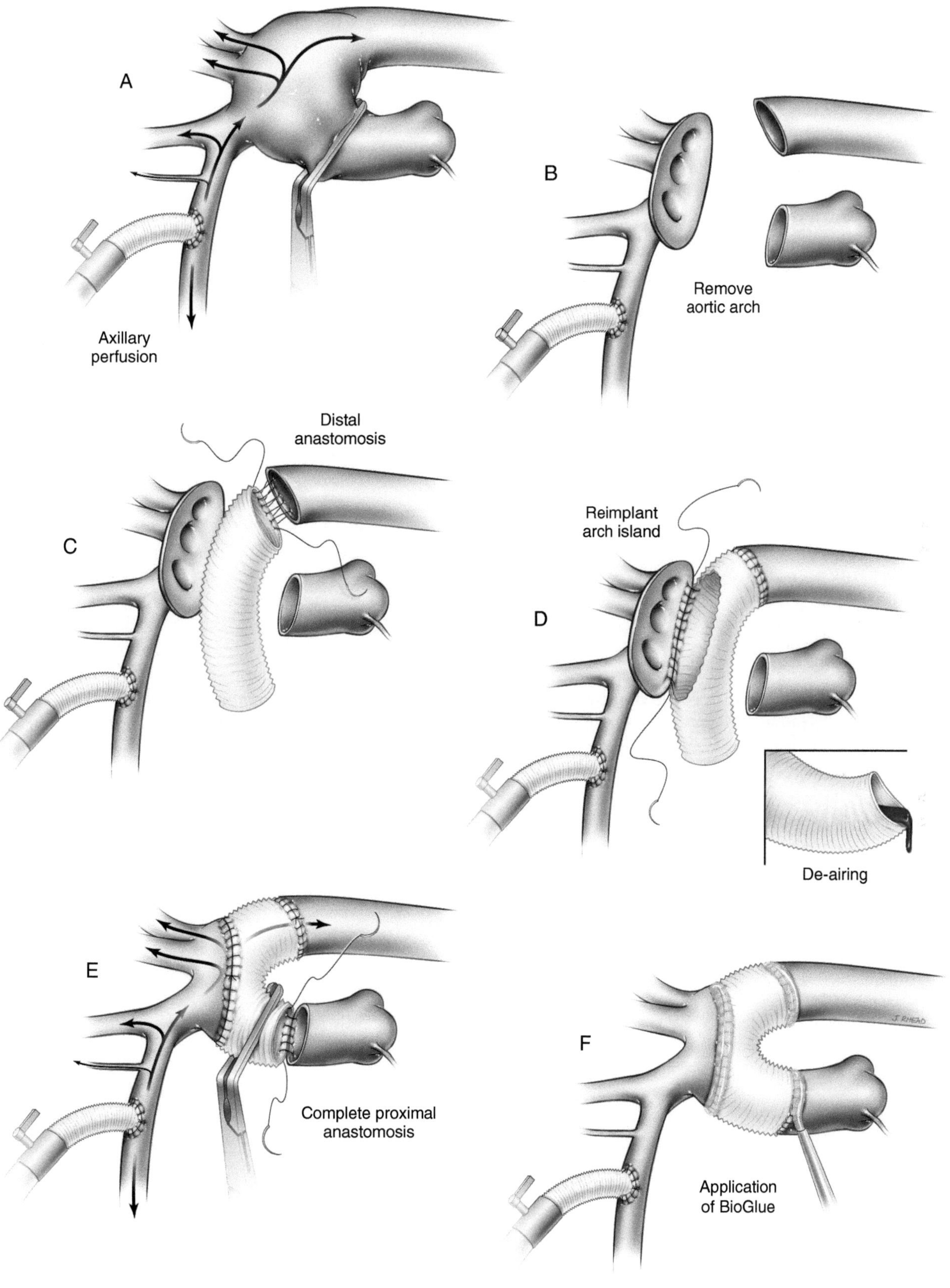
A
Axillary perfusion
B
Remove aortic arch
Distal anastomosis
C
Reimplant arch island
D
De-airing
E
Complete proximal anastomosis
F
Application of BioGlue
J. RHEAD

Aortic Arch Replacement: Prefabricated Triple-Branched Graft with Side Perfusion Branch

Total arch replacement is facilitated by using a prosthetic graft with prefabricated side grafts. The graft has three segments along the exterior curve for reimplantation of the arch vessels, as well as a fourth segment on the opposite side for a perfusion cannula.

Figure 38-9

A This set of illustrations is presented in standard anterior anatomic perspective. Arrows demonstrate direction of blood flow as the procedure progresses. Axillary cannulation is used to facilitate low-flow antegrade cerebral perfusion during hypothermic circulatory arrest. Use of a prosthetic side graft allows uncompromised flow to both the arch and the right arm.

B A short period of circulatory arrest under deep hypothermia is employed to open the aortic arch and transect the aorta above the aortic root and beyond the arch. The arch vessels are transected near their origins from the aortic arch. Each vessel should be trimmed back to relatively healthy tissue.

C The ascending aorta and arch are removed ("ghost" illustration). The innominate artery is occluded and low-flow antegrade perfusion is initiated at low flow to provide additional cerebral protection and to evacuate air and debris from the arch vessels.

D The arch vessels are occluded and prepared for anastomosis. The prosthetic graft is attached in an end-to-end fashion to the proximal descending thoracic aorta using continuous stitches of 4/0 polypropylene suture. The left subclavian artery is then attached to the most distal of the three segments on the exterior curve of the graft using continuous stitches of 4/0 polypropylene.

E A perfusion cannula is placed in the side graft located on the inferior curve of the main graft. A clamp is placed across the main graft just proximal to the left subclavian anastomosis, directing flow through the side graft into the left subclavian artery and down the descending thoracic aorta. The left common carotid artery is attached to the middle segment on the superior curve of the graft using continuous stitches of 4/0 polypropylene.

F The clamp on the main graft is moved proximally to allow perfusion to both the left subclavian artery and the left common carotid artery. The innominate artery is attached to the most proximal of the three segments using continuous stitches of 4/0 polypropylene.

G The clamp is moved proximally again to the main graft to allow perfusion to all the arch vessels and the descending thoracic aorta. The main graft is trimmed to an appropriate length and attached in end-to-end fashion to the ascending aorta using continuous stitches of 4/0 polypropylene.

H BioGlue is used to reinforce all suture lines. Cardiopulmonary bypass is discontinued. The side branch perfusion graft is trimmed nearly flush with the main graft, oversewn with 4/0 polypropylene and imbricated to provide a smooth surface, which will be in direct contact with the pulmonary artery. The side graft on the right axillary artery is also trimmed and oversewn with continuous stitches of 4/0 polypropylene.

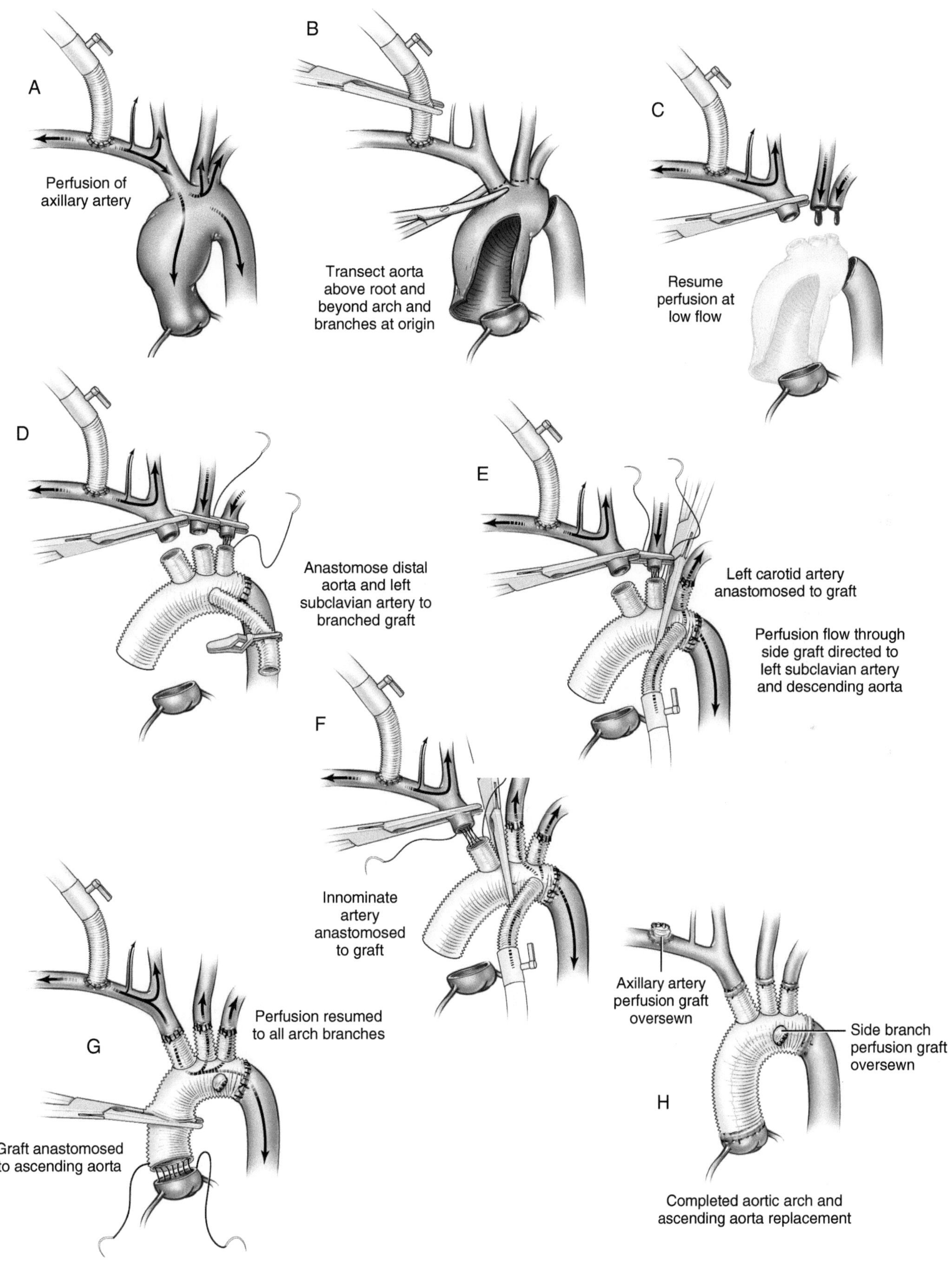
A
Perfusion of axillary artery
B
Transect aorta above root and beyond arch and branches at origin
C
Resume perfusion at low flow
D
Anastomose distal aorta and left subclavian artery to branched graft
E
Left carotid artery anastomosed to graft
Perfusion flow through side graft directed to left subclavian artery and descending aorta
F
Innominate artery anastomosed to graft
G
Perfusion resumed to all arch branches
Graft anastomosed to ascending aorta
Axillary artery perfusion graft oversewn
Side branch perfusion graft oversewn
H
Completed aortic arch and ascending aorta replacement

Aortic Arch Replacement: "Elephant Trunk" Procedure

Figure 38-10

A Perfusion is accomplished by a single venous uptake cannula; oxygenated blood is returned to the femoral artery. The patient is perfused with blood cooled to 12°C until the body temperature (nasopharyngeal) reaches 16 to 18°C. Dissection of the aortic arch is minimal. No occlusion clamps are used. The aortic aneurysm is opened throughout its length, extending through the aortic arch but not dividing the vagus nerve, which lies on the surface of the distal aortic arch.

B The aortic arch vessels are left open and will generally remain covered with blood if the head is lowered. Dissection extending through the aortic arch is illustrated. All the loose intima and media are excised from the ascending aorta and arch. The excision is extended into the descending aorta as far as possible through the arch aortotomy. This provides a large reentry of the dissection in the descending thoracic aorta.

C The arch repair is accomplished by an elephant trunk technique for later reconstruction of the descending aorta by direct graft anastomosis. An appropriately sized collagen-sealed, knitted velour Dacron graft is selected. The graft is invaginated, leaving a folded-back portion approximately 5 cm long. A pull string of 2/0 silk is attached to the proximal end of the invaginated end of the graft and brought back through the lumen. The graft is pushed down into the descending aorta. The folded edge of the graft is anastomosed to the aorta beyond the left subclavian artery. Because all the intima and media have been excised, the anastomosis is made to the inside of the intact adventitia of the aorta with 3/0 polypropylene. Suture loops are placed deep into the adventitial layer to ensure tight approximation of graft to aorta.

D The pull string is used to retrieve the graft from the distal aorta. The graft is pulled back into the arch, leaving 5 cm of graft extending, unattached, beyond the anastomosis. The elephant trunk technique is often performed with a much longer extension of unattached graft, creating the possibility of thrombosis of the space between the graft and the wall of the aorta. A short segment of graft beyond the anastomosis, as illustrated here, should reduce the risk of this complication. Perhaps this repair should be referred to as a "pig snout" rather than an "elephant trunk" technique. The branches of the aortic arch are anastomosed to the graft as a unit. An ellipse of the graft is excised to accommodate the arch branches. A side-to-side anastomosis is constructed by continuous stitches of 3/0 polypropylene.

E After the arch vessels are anastomosed to the graft, circulation can be restored to the head vessels and the rest of the body by retrograde perfusion through the femoral artery at low flow. The head is lowered, and blood is allowed to flow slowly into the carotid arteries to fill them without trapping air. The head vessels are probed gently with a hemostat to dislodge air and debris through the graft and out the open proximal end. The graft is occluded proximal to the arch vessel anastomosis. Full-flow perfusion is established with rewarming of the body. The ascending aorta is reconstructed by anastomosis of the proximal end of the graft to the aorta in end-to-end fashion, working from within the aorta.

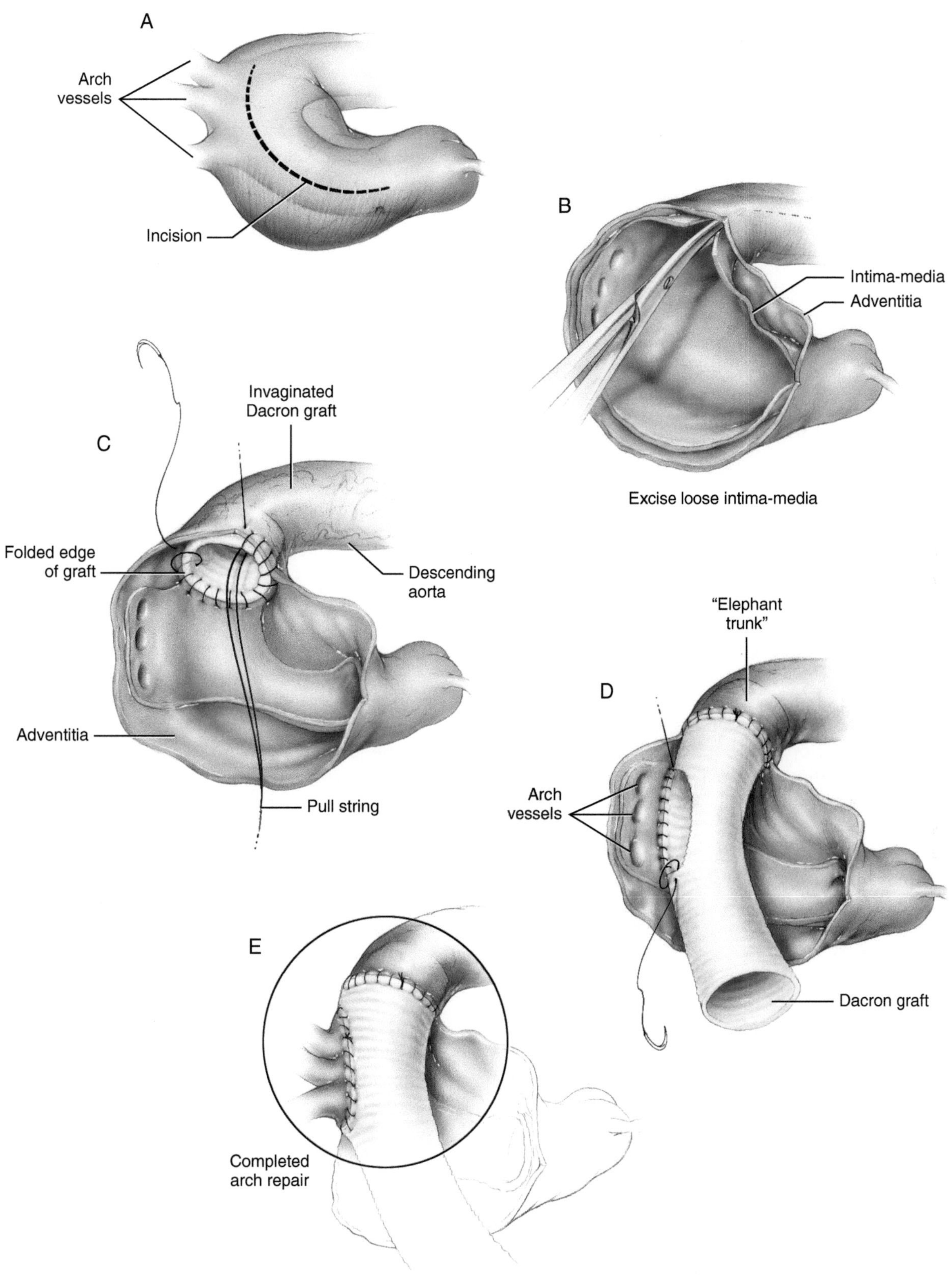
A
Arch vessels
Incision
B
Intima-media
Adventitia
Excise loose intima-media
C
Invaginated Dacron graft
Folded edge of graft
Descending aorta
Adventitia
Pull string
D
"Elephant trunk"
Arch vessels
Dacron graft
E
Completed arch repair

Arch Replacement: Arch First Technique

A staged procedure for replacement of the aortic arch may not be possible in some situations. In cases of marked aneurysmal enlargement—that is, when the diameter of the thoracic aorta exceeds 4.5 cm—safe attachment of an elephant trunk graft just distal to the origin of the left subclavian artery may not be possible. It may be necessary to make an anastomosis to the midportion of the descending thoracic aorta or even farther distally. Some cases of chronic type A aortic dissection that require a second-stage operation for replacement of the aortic arch after replacement of the ascending aorta may benefit from this approach because the upper portion of the descending thoracic aorta may be significantly enlarged, requiring aortic replacement to a more distal point in the thoracic aorta. Kouchoukos described this technique and is credited with developing a safe method of treating such cases, which are associated with a significant risk of hemorrhage or cerebral ischemic injury.

Figure 38-11

A General anesthesia is induced with the patient in the supine position. A double-lumen endotracheal tube is used to allow collapse of the left lung. If arterial perfusion via the left common femoral artery is selected, the catheter is inserted with the patient in the supine position. If the axillary artery is to be used, the arterial catheter is inserted after the thorax is entered. The patient is rotated 20 to 30 degrees to the right, and the left arm is abducted and secured. A bilateral submammary incision is made (inset) in the fourth intercostal spaces, both internal mammary arteries are ligated and divided, and the sternum is divided transversely. The left lung is collapsed. The pericardium is opened minimally over the aorta and right atrium to allow placement of venous uptake cannulae in the superior and inferior vena cavae (with tourniquet tapes around the cavae), a perfusion cannula through the right atrium into the coronary sinus, and a small vent catheter through the right superior pulmonary vein to the left atrium and left ventricle.

B Cardiopulmonary bypass is established, and the body cooled to 16 to 18°C. The left phrenic and left vagus nerves are mobilized on a pleural pedicle. The left inferior pulmonary ligament is divided. The ascending aorta is clamped when ventricular fibrillation occurs or at any point when cardiac distension is observed. If the aortic valve is competent, cold blood cardioplegia can be administered into the aortic root. When the aortic valve is not competent, the aorta is opened, and cold cardioplegic solution is given retrograde through the coronary sinus. The aorta is divided proximal to the occlusion clamp. Aortic valve or aortic root replacement or distal coronary bypass anastomoses can be done during the cooling procedure, if indicated. When the target body temperature is reached, cardiopulmonary bypass is discontinued. The patient's head is surrounded with ice packs, and the head is lowered. The tourniquet around the superior vena cava is tightened around the cannula. About one-quarter of the calculated blood volume is drained from the inferior vena cava cannula to the reservoir of the oxygenator. A clamp is placed on the descending thoracic aorta below the proposed site of distal aortic graft anastomosis. The aortic arch branch arteries are removed from the arch as an island, surrounded by a small aortic arch cuff. The aorta is divided distal to the origin of the left subclavian artery. The descending thoracic aorta is incised longitudinally, beginning distal to the neural pedicle and extending to a point where the aorta approaches near-normal diameter above the occlusion clamp.

C A tubular, crimped, collagen-sealed polyester graft with a 10 mm diameter side graft attached is selected. The graft diameter should match that of the divided ascending aorta and the descending aorta. An elliptical opening the size of the vascular island is made in the graft opposite the side graft. The distal end of the graft is pulled beneath the neural pedicle into the descending thoracic aorta. The vascular arch island is anastomosed to the prosthetic graft with continuous stitches of 3/0 or 4/0 polypropylene. The anastomosis is sealed with BioGlue. The descending thoracic aorta is divided in a beveled fashion.

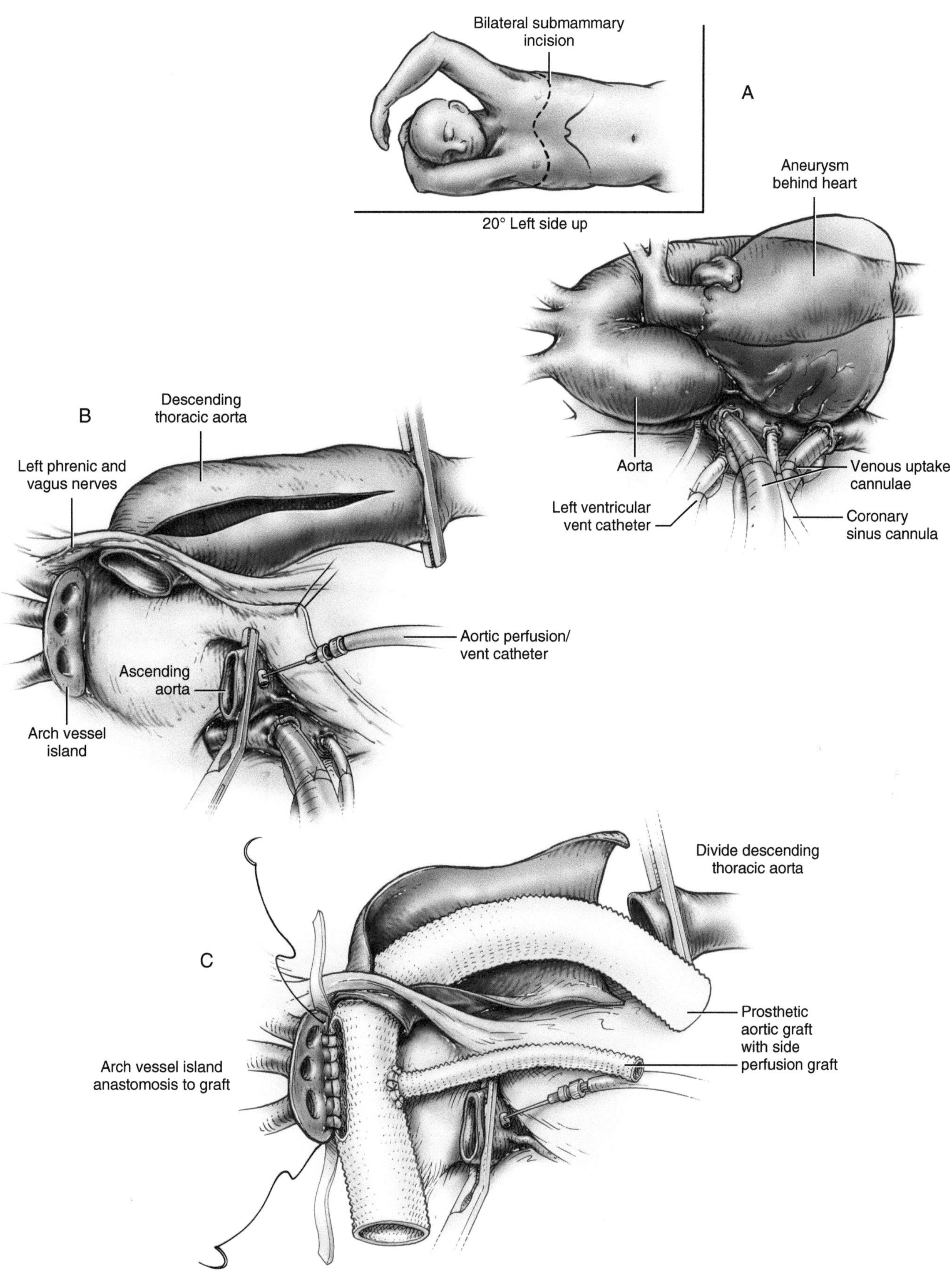
Bilateral submammary incision
A
20° Left side up
Aneurysm behind heart
Aorta
Venous uptake cannulae
Left ventricular vent catheter
Coronary sinus cannula
B
Descending thoracic aorta
Left phrenic and vagus nerves
Aortic perfusion/ vent catheter
Ascending aorta
Arch vessel island
C
Divide descending thoracic aorta
Prosthetic aortic graft with side perfusion graft
Arch vessel island anastomosis to graft

Figure 38-11 (continued)

D Cold (18°C to 20°C), oxygenated blood is infused into the cannula in the superior vena cava to raise venous pressure in the upper compartment sufficiently to force blood to flow retrograde from the brachiocephalic arteries into the arch graft, removing air and debris. A vascular clamp is placed on the arch graft just distal to the arch island anastomosis so that retrograde flow fills the proximal end of the graft. A second arterial perfusion line from the pump oxygenator is attached to the side graft, and flow is established to clear any remaining air and debris from the arch graft. Retrograde perfusion of the superior vena cava is discontinued, the aortic graft is occluded proximal to the arch anastomosis, and antegrade perfusion of the arch vessels with cold (20°C) blood is initiated at a flow rate of about 1,000 mL per minute. The occlusion clamp is removed from the descending aorta, the aorta is beveled appropriately to preserve intercostal arteries below the sixth intercostal space, and the graft is divided and beveled to match the aorta. If there is aortic dissection at the point of anastomosis, a large segment of the intima and media separating the true lumen and false lumen, is removed to ensure perfusion of both aortic channels. An end-to-end anastomosis of the graft to the aorta is constructed with continuous stitches of 3/0 or 4/0 polypropylene. The anastomosis may be reinforced by a Teflon felt strip or a beveled Dacron collar cut from the discarded graft.

E Before final completion of the distal aortic anastomosis, the distal aorta is temporarily occluded to allow a dry field as the anastomosis is sealed with BioGlue. The graft is punctured a few times with an 18 gauge needle to allow air to evacuate as the clamp is removed from the aortic graft proximally, and blood is allowed to enter the graft down to the distal clamp. When air has ceased coming from the puncture holes, the distal clamp is removed, and flow is restored to the lower body. The perfusion flow rate is restored, and rewarming of the body is commenced. Patent intercostal arteries and bronchial arteries in the upper descending aorta are closed by suture ligature. The proximal end of the graft is shortened and anastomosed to the ascending aorta or the aortic root replacement device. A Teflon felt strip or beveled Dacron collar reinforces the anastomosis. The aortic anastomosis is sealed with BioGlue. A needle vent is placed in the graft to evacuate air.

F The last remaining clamp is removed from the aortic graft to allow coronary artery reperfusion. When the heart is beating vigorously and the body temperature has been restored to normal, cardiopulmonary bypass is discontinued. Cannulae are removed, stab sites are closed, and the side graft is removed and oversewn.

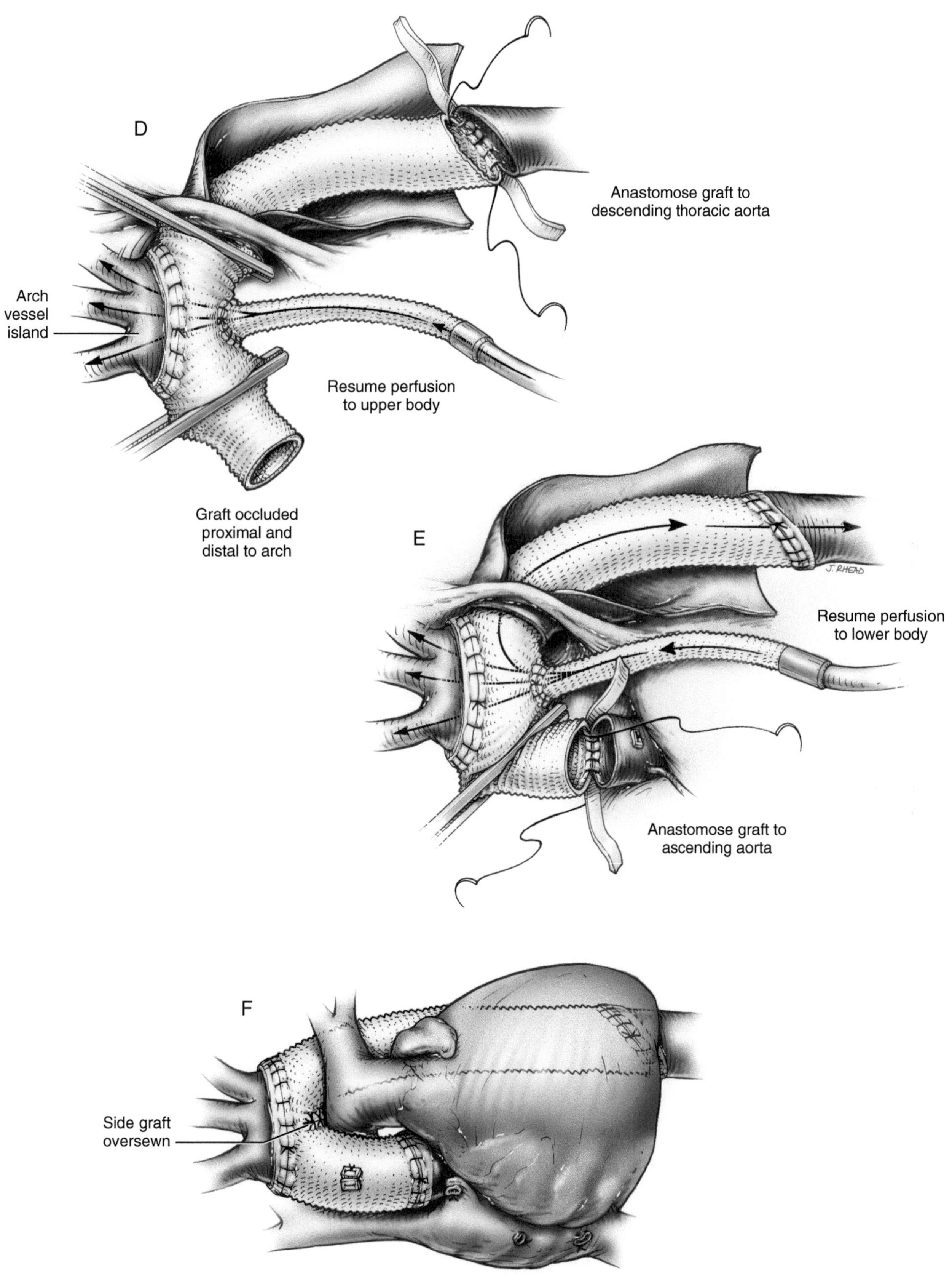
D
Anastomose graft to descending thoracic aorta
Arch vessel island
Resume perfusion to upper body
Graft occluded proximal and distal to arch
E
J. RHEAD
Resume perfusion to lower body
Anastomose graft to ascending aorta
F
Side graft oversewn
Completed repair

Aortic Root, Ascending Aorta, and Hemiarch Replacement, with Bypass of the Descending Thoracic Aorta

Coarctation of the aorta is frequently associated with bicuspid aortic valve and abnormal aortic connective tissue. Patients treated for coarctation during infancy or childhood may present later with residual aortic coarctation at the site of repair. The bicuspid aortic valve frequently degenerates and must be replaced, and the ascending aorta may acquire aneurysmal dilation. Direct re-repair of thoracic aortic coarctation carries considerable risk of hemorrhage and spinal cord ischemic injury. Bypass of the obstructed thoracic aorta, along with replacement of the aortic root, ascending aorta, and part of the arch, is an acceptable single-stage operation to resolve a difficult problem in adults or those with near-adult body size.

Figure 38-12

A Cardiopulmonary bypass is established, and the body is cooled to 16° to 18°C, as previously described. The aorta is occluded, and the heart is cooled to 4°C and arrested by retrograde perfusion of the coronary sinus. The illustration shows the extent of aortic resection relative to the location of coarctation.

B During the body cooling process, and with the heart arrested, the heart is elevated from the pericardial sac and retracted superiorly. The pericardial sac posterior to the heart is opened over the descending aorta. The aorta is minimally dissected to obtain sufficient exposure to occlude the aorta with a C-shaped vascular clamp or with two 20-degree angled vascular clamps. The aorta is incised longitudinally. An externally supported tubular, polytetrafluoroethylene graft measuring 10 mm in diameter is anastomosed to the aorta in end-to-side fashion using continuous stitches of 4/0 or 5/0 polypropylene. Placing several or all of the suture loops before approximating the graft to the aorta simplifies the anastomosis. BioGlue is used to seal the anastomosis. The aortic clamp is removed, and hemostasis is ensured at this point of the operation because bleeding is difficult to deal with after the heart is filled and contracting.

C The arrow indicates the pathway of the graft from the ascending aorta to the descending aorta. An opening is made in the pericardial reflection posterior to the inferior vena cava. The inset shows the graft passing through the opening behind the inferior vena cava to its course through the pericardial sac along the interatrial groove.

D This illustration shows partial replacement of the aortic arch with a tubular Dacron prosthesis. After this portion of the procedure, which is performed under circulatory arrest, cardiopulmonary bypass is restarted, air and debris are removed from the arch through the open end of the graft, and the graft is occluded. Replacement of the aortic root with porcine xenograft aortic root bioprostheses proceeds during rewarming of the body. The aortic root bioprosthesis is anastomosed to the aortic graft. An opening is made on the right lateral wall of the aortic graft. The bypass graft is anastomosed end-to-side to the aortic graft to complete the procedure. All vascular anastomoses are sealed with BioGlue.

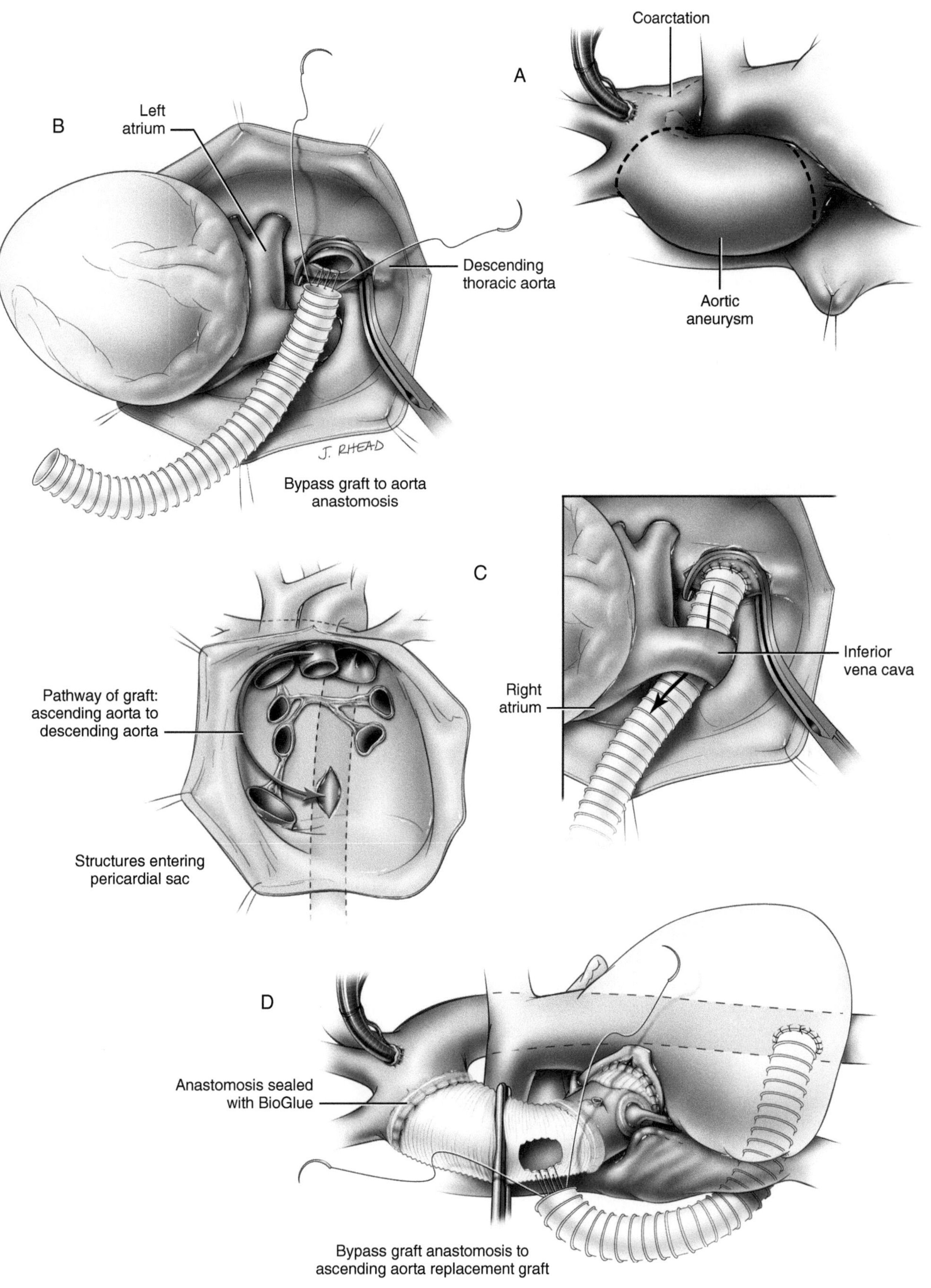
A
Coarctation
Aortic aneurysm
B
Left atrium
Descending thoracic aorta
J. RHEAD
Bypass graft to aorta anastomosis
C
Pathway of graft: ascending aorta to descending aorta
Structures entering pericardial sac
Right atrium
Inferior vena cava
D
Anastomosis sealed with BioGlue
Bypass graft anastomosis to ascending aorta replacement graft

Descending Thoracic Aorta

Repair of an aneurysm of the descending thoracic aorta is accompanied by the risk of paraplegia due to spinal cord ischemia. Although a number of methods of spinal cord protection have been reported, none has proved uniformly successful, and anterior spinal cord ischemia syndrome is a constant hazard of this operation.

Figure 38-13

A Left atrium–to–femoral artery bypass is particularly popular to provide support to the circulation below the aorta, which is isolated to repair the aneurysm. Alternative techniques include femoral vein–to–femoral artery bypass using an oxygenator as shown, ascending aorta–to–descending aorta or ascending aorta–to–femoral artery bypass using a shunt catheter, or simple pharmacologic reduction of afterload without a shunt. The shunt methods offer more control, require heparin, and simplify autotransfusion if a pump is used. The nonshunt methods are simple and direct and may provide better hemostasis because no heparin is used. At present, the most promising method is femoral vein–to–femoral artery bypass using total cardiopulmonary bypass, with an oxygenator and heat exchanger to induce deep systemic hypothermia as a means of protecting the spinal cord. The procedure on the aorta is performed during circulatory arrest. The femoral vessels are exposed and controlled through a skin-line incision in the groin. A 20 F thin-walled percutaneous arterial perfusion cannula is placed in the iliac artery via the common femoral artery. A 28 F thin-walled percutaneous venous uptake cannula is placed in the right atrium via the common femoral vein. It is convenient to perform cannulation with the patient supine as the initial step of the procedure. Then cardiopulmonary bypass can be instituted and systemic cooling started using the heat exchanger. The cannulae and incision are isolated by a stick-on plastic drape to provide sterile access for cannulae removal later.

B An aneurysm of the upper portion of the descending thoracic aorta due to atherosclerosis or aortic dissection is approached through a lateral thoracotomy incision. The patient is placed in the left lateral position with the hips and pelvis turned to maintain exposure of the left groin, where the incision was made to insert the arterial and venous perfusion cannulae. The stick-on plastic drape used to isolate the cannulae and groin incision is included in the skin preparation for the lateral thoracotomy. The thoracic incision is made through the bed of the nonresected fourth rib. For an aneurysm including all or most of the thoracic aorta, a secondary entry to the thorax through the bed of the seventh rib may be necessary.

C Should ventricular fibrillation occur during systemic cooling, a vent catheter is inserted through the left inferior pulmonary vein into the left ventricle. When the body temperature reaches 16°C, extracorporeal circulation is discontinued, and the repair is accomplished during circulatory arrest. Control of the aorta is not required. Vascular occlusion clamps are not used. The aneurysm is incised through its length. Side extensions of the incision define the limits of resection of the aneurysm proximally. The aorta is divided distally beyond the aneurysm. The blood, clot, and debris contained within are removed.

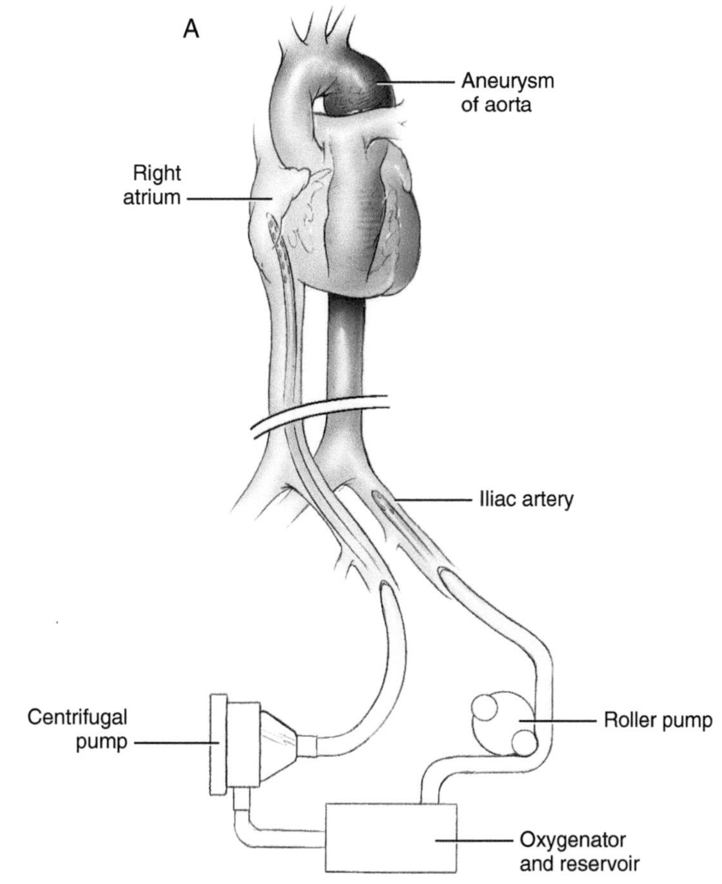
A
Aneurysm
of aorta
Right
atrium
Iliac artery
Centrifugal
pump
Roller pump
Oxygenator
and reservoir

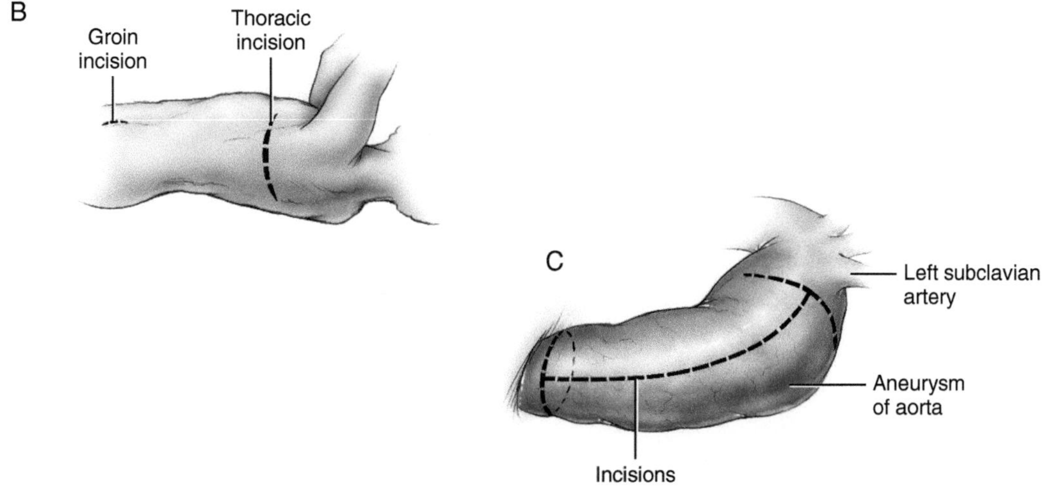
B
Groin
incision
Thoracic
incision
C
Left subclavian
artery
Aneurysm
of aorta
Incisions

Figure 38-13 (continued)

D Intercostal arteries are ligated from within the aneurysm using double-loop stitches of 2/0 silk. If the aneurysm is long and involves several intercostal artery pairs, it may be prudent to preserve one or more large intercostal artery pairs.

E An appropriately sized tubular Dacron graft is chosen for the reconstruction. Double-velour knitted or woven grafts that have been collagen coated are favored. An end-to-end anastomosis of the graft to the proximal aorta is constructed by continuous stitches of 3/0 polypropylene. Several suture loops are placed posteriorly before the sutures are pulled up to approximate the graft to the aorta. Deep bites must be taken so that the full thickness of the aorta is included.

F The anastomosis is completed anteriorly by transition from within the aorta to a full inside-out technique. The needle arc must be controlled so that needle perforations in the tissue do not form slits. An opening can be made in the graft opposite the intercostal artery pair that is to be preserved. The aorta surrounding the intercostal artery pair is anastomosed to the opening in the graft using 3/0 polypropylene suture.

G A collar can be cut from the end of the graft and slipped onto the graft before constructing the distal anastomosis of the graft to the aorta. An end-to-end anastomosis is accomplished by continuous stitches of 3/0 polypropylene.

H The completed distal aortic reconstruction is reinforced by covering the suture line with the Dacron collar. BioGlue is used to seal all vascular anastomoses and is placed under the reinforcing collar. The aneurysm is closed around the graft to isolate it from the lung.

I An alternative technique may be used when additional distal reconstruction of the aorta is anticipated, such as in cases of aortic dissection. An elephant trunk anastomosis can be constructed distally so that the later aortic reconstruction is attached directly to the graft rather than to the aortic wall.

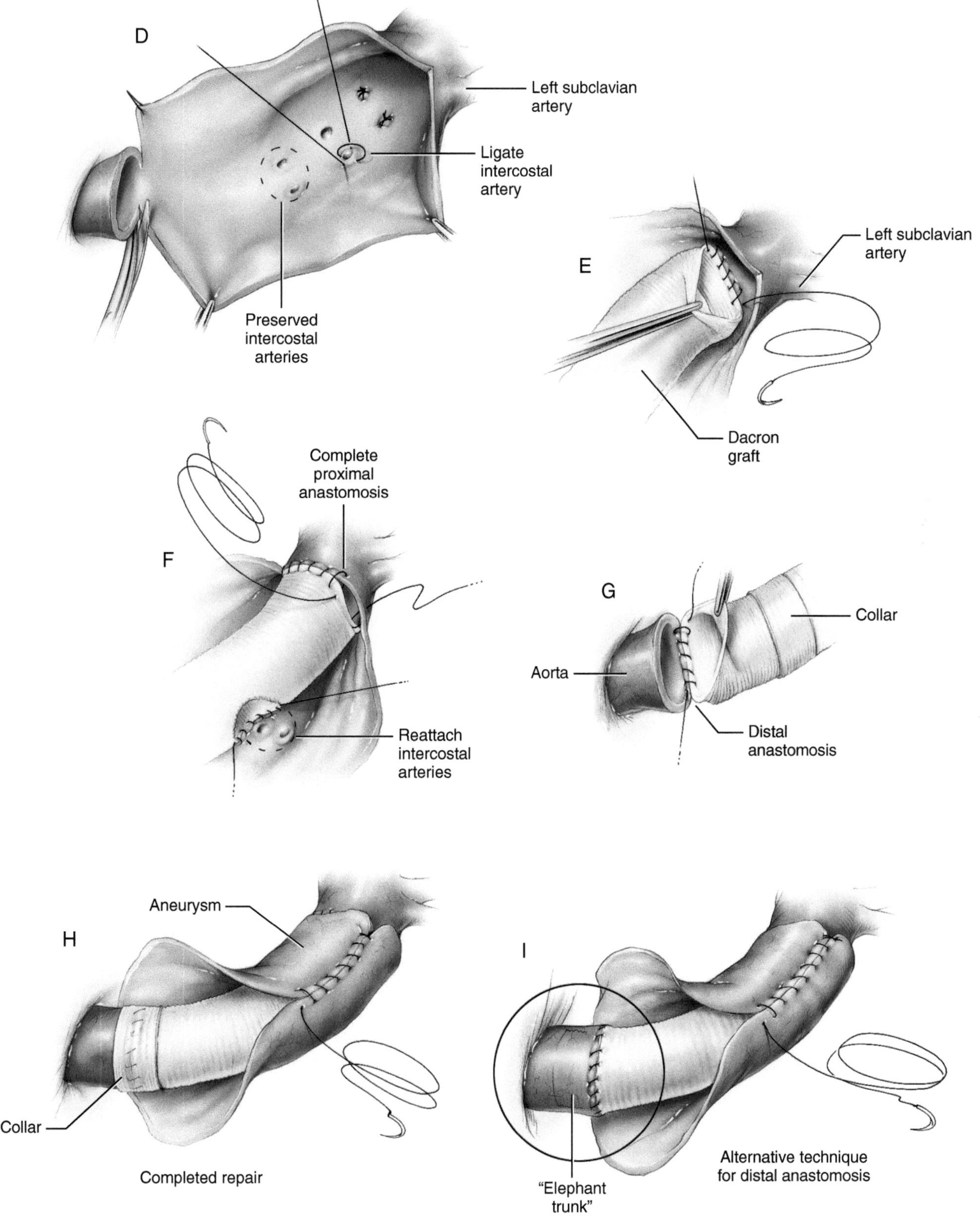
D
Left subclavian artery
Ligate intercostal artery
Preserved intercostal arteries
E
Left subclavian artery
Dacron graft
F
Complete proximal anastomosis
Reattach intercostal arteries
G
Collar
Aorta
Distal anastomosis
H
Aneurysm
Collar
Completed repair
I
"Elephant trunk"
Alternative technique for distal anastomosis

Thoracoabdominal Aorta

An aneurysm extending from the thoracic aorta into the abdominal aorta is amenable to operative treatment. The operation is complex and is associated with significant potential for morbidity because the blood supply to the spinal cord and the kidneys and abdominal viscera is involved, placing these organs at risk for ischemic injury.

Figure 38-14

A The operation is performed with the patient under deep hypothermia for spinal cord protection during circulatory arrest. Arterial and venous perfusion cannulae are introduced by needle catheter technique into the femoral artery and vein, which are exposed through a groin incision with the patient in the supine position. The cannulae are connected to the cardiopulmonary bypass circuit, and perfusion is established (see Figure 38-13, *A*). The cannulae and incision are isolated by stick-on plastic drapes that are reprepared after the patient is repositioned. Alternatively, the arterial perfusion cannula may be placed in the thoracic aorta above the aneurysm after the thorax is opened. The patient is positioned at about a 60-degree angle with the left side up. The operating table can later be rotated to reduce the degree of this angled positioning. A thoracoabdominal incision is used. The thoracic portion of the incision is placed on the chest wall to provide access to the fifth intercostal space. The incision crosses the costal margin to the midline of the upper abdomen and continues in the midline to a point at or below the umbilicus. The periosteum of the fifth rib is elevated from its inferior aspect. The left pleural space is entered through the bed of the nonresected fifth rib. The lung is retracted superiorly to expose the diaphragm. The ribs are separated with a self-retaining retractor. The abdominal portion of the incision is through the linea alba to the preperitoneal space, but it does not enter the peritoneal cavity. Dissection is started in the preperitoneal space to free the peritoneum from the inferior surface of the diaphragm. The diaphragm is perforated in the costophrenic sulcus anteriorly. The costal cartilages are divided without entering the peritoneal cavity. Cardiopulmonary bypass is initiated after the incision is made and continued during the dissection to progressively lower body temperature and allow collapse of the lung.

B The chest retractor is spread more widely. The peritoneum is dissected from the inferior surface of the diaphragm more completely so that the stomach, spleen, and left kidney are mobilized out of the left upper quadrant of the abdomen and retracted medially and anteriorly. The dissection is taken down to the aorta. This prepares the diaphragm for incision without entering the peritoneal cavity. Every effort should be made to leave the peritoneum intact; this keeps the abdominal contents well contained and much easier to control.

C The diaphragm is incised with scissors or a cautery blade in a radial fashion down to and through the aortic hiatus. The retractor is spread more widely, providing complete exposure of the thoracoabdominal aorta. Further dissection and mobilization of the peritoneum from the surface of the aorta inferiorly may be required. The lung is retracted superiorly to gain access to the superior margin of the aneurysm.

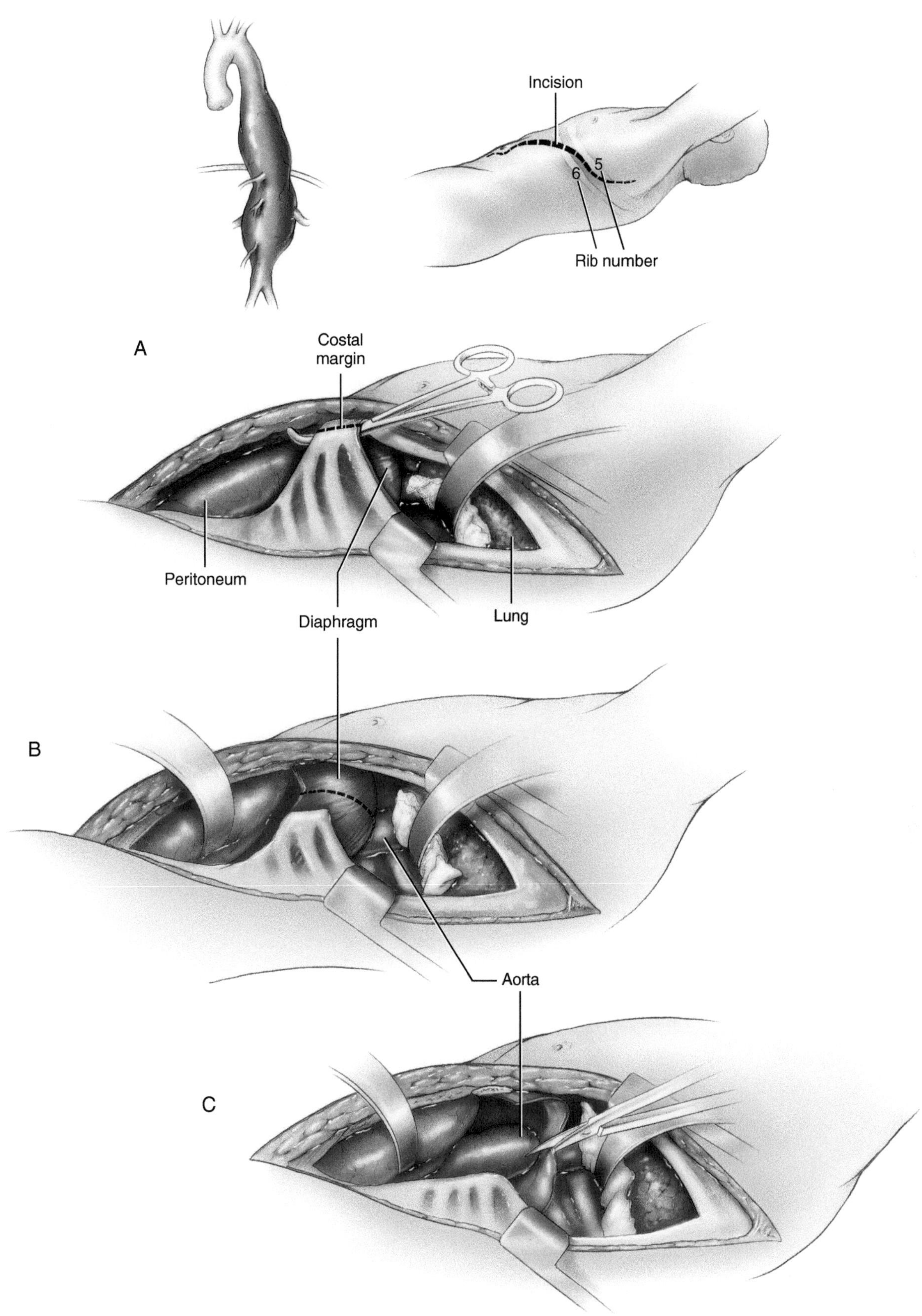
Incision
5
6
Rib number
A
Costal
margin
Peritoneum
Diaphragm
Lung
B
Aorta
C

Figure 38-14 (continued)

D The aorta is exposed for the length of the aneurysm. Only minimal dissection of the vessel is performed to obtain control. The aortic branches are not dissected at all. For clarity, the illustration shows the visceral vessels as if they had been freed from the surrounding tissues; in practice, these vessels are not seen at all. The vessels are buried in the fat and connective tissue anterior to the aorta. Only the lateral wall of the aorta is exposed.

Cardiopulmonary bypass is discontinued when body temperature reaches 16° to 18°C. The aortic branches are not clamped and are simply allowed to backbleed into the aortic lumen. The aorta is opened through the length of the aneurysm. The proximal and distal limits of the aneurysm resection are defined by the extension of the incision.

E Thrombus and other debris within the aneurysm are removed by fingers covered with gauze. The debris should be removed as completely as possible. Retraction stitches are placed on the edges of the aneurysm for exposure.

F The orifices of the visceral arteries are identified from within the aorta. Large intercostal arteries at the level of the diaphragm may be preserved. Lumbar branches are occluded by suture ligature. The aorta is divided proximal to the aneurysm.

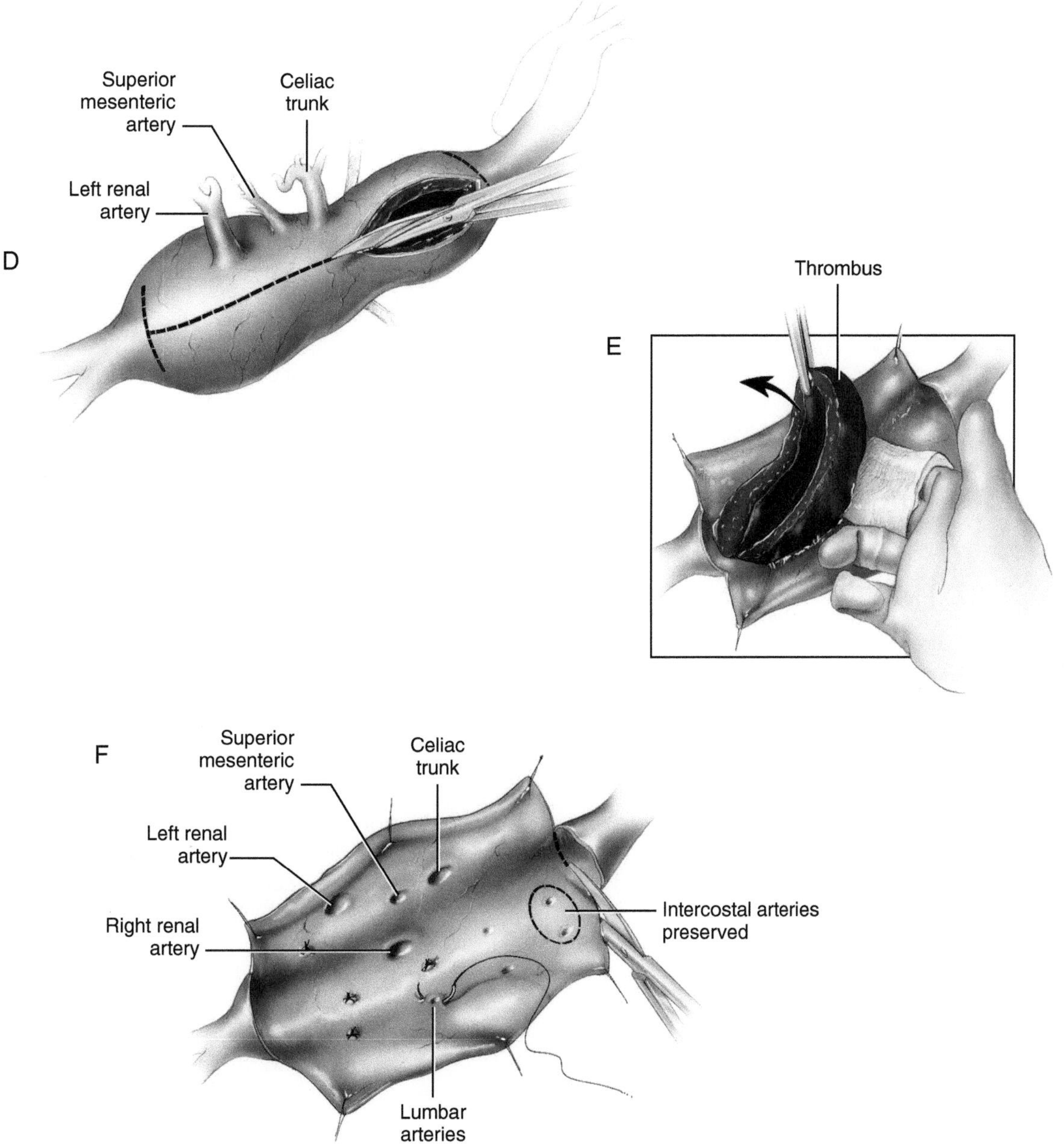
D
Superior mesenteric artery
Celiac trunk
Left renal artery
E
Thrombus
F
Superior mesenteric artery
Celiac trunk
Left renal artery
Right renal artery
Intercostal arteries preserved
Lumbar arteries ligated

Figure 38-14 (continued)

G A collagen-sealed, double-velour knitted Dacron prosthesis is used for the reconstruction. A collar of the graft is fashioned to reinforce the proximal anastomosis. The aorta is divided. An end-to-end anastomosis of the graft to the aorta is constructed using 3/0 polypropylene suture. Suture loops for the entire posterior wall of the anastomosis are placed with the graft held away from the aorta. The suture loops are pulled up to approximate the graft to the aorta. The anterior row of sutures is then placed to complete the anastomosis. Perfusion and rewarming can be reestablished at this point or at any time during the 60-minute safe period. The arterial perfusion cannula is placed into a stab incision in the graft, and the graft is occluded by a soft-jawed clamp below the lowest completed anastomosis.

H The collar is slipped over the anastomosis. If there is a large pair of patent intercostal arteries at about the level of the diaphragm, these can be reimplanted to the graft. A round opening is made into the graft. The graft is simply sewn to the aortic wall around the intercostal artery orifices. Substantial tissue bites are taken for maximal suture line security using continuous stitches of 3/0 polypropylene.

I The visceral arteries are anastomosed to the graft. An opening is made in the graft that is large enough to encompass the origins of the celiac artery, superior mesenteric artery, and right renal artery. Care must be taken to consider the anterior rotation of the visceral artery orifices when planning the graft openings. This usually means making the opening more toward the left side of the graft than might be apparent. The anastomosis is constructed by continuous suture technique using 3/0 polypropylene. Deep tissue bites are taken to ensure security of the suture line.

J The left renal artery is anastomosed to a separate opening in the graft to prevent kinking, using a similar technique. The position of the anastomosis should be planned carefully, taking into account the amount of anterior rotation and displacement of the left renal artery produced by mobilization of the left kidney.

K The distal anastomosis of the graft to the aorta is constructed in end-to-end fashion. The back row of the anastomosis is constructed to the intact wall of the aorta; deep tissue bites must be taken to ensure that the suture engages the aortic adventitia posteriorly. If the aneurysm extends into the common iliac arteries, a bifurcated graft must be used. The limbs of the graft are anastomosed to the iliac arteries in modified end-to-end fashion, keeping the posterior wall of the iliac arteries intact. BioGlue is used to seal all vascular anastomoses. The aneurysm is closed around the graft at the completion of all the anastomoses and after hemostasis of the suture line has been secured.

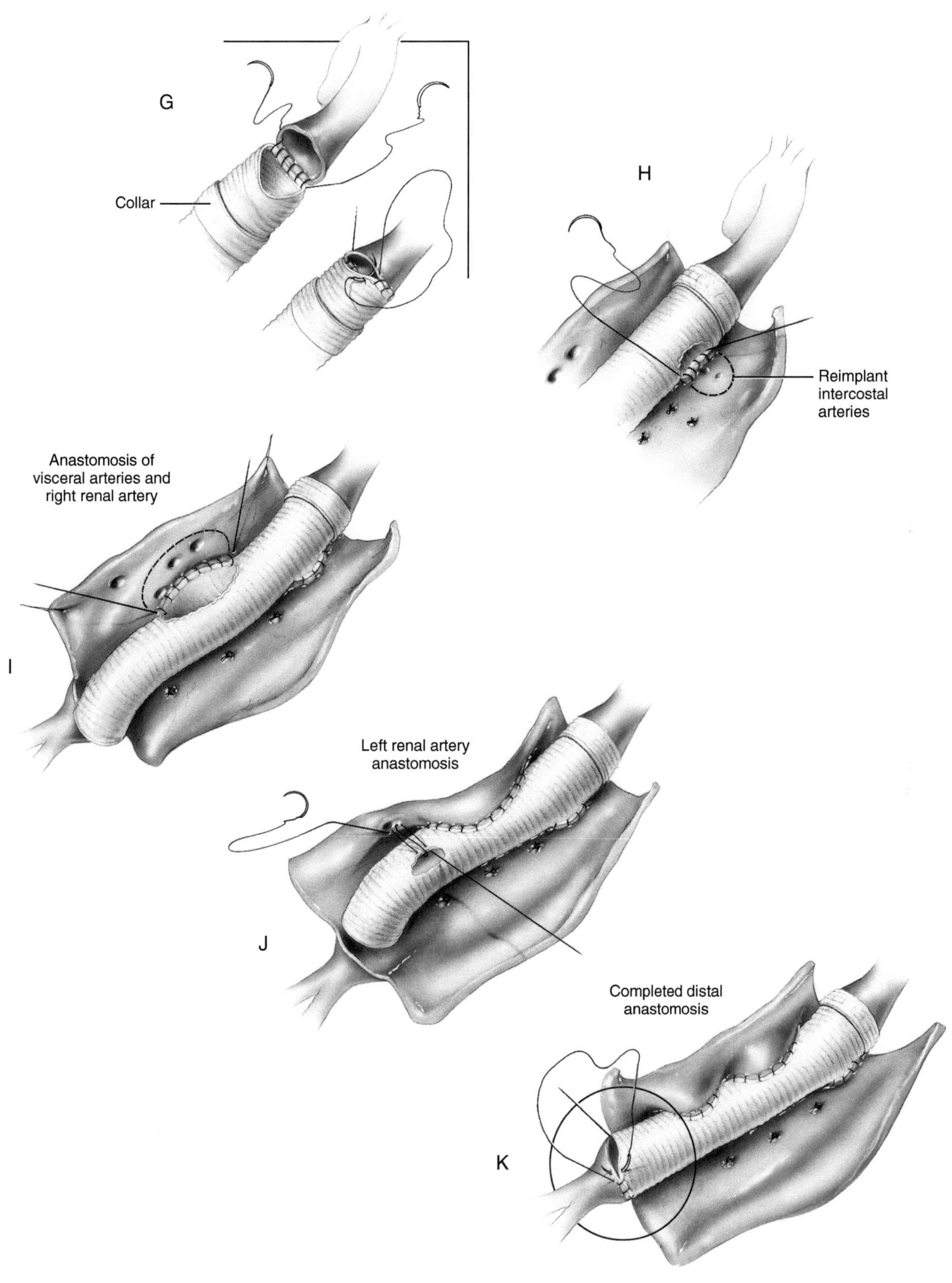
G
Collar
H
Reimplant
intercostal
arteries
Anastomosis of
visceral arteries and
right renal artery
I
Left renal artery
anastomosis
J
Completed distal
anastomosis
K

Figure 38-14 (continued)

L When the aneurysm is very large and the distance from the graft to the orifices of the visceral and renal arteries is long, it may be desirable to use a prefabricated prosthetic graft with side branches for the reconstruction. An aortic arch graft with three arch branch grafts and a side perfusion graft provides the requisite four side branches. The proximal end of the graft is anastomosed to the aorta above the aneurysmal segment. The anastomosis is supported by a collar of the aortic graft. The side branches are anastomosed end-to-end to the aorta surrounding the orifice of the visceral vessels and the renal arteries in sequential fashion, using continuous stitches of 3/0 polypropylene. The reconstruction is completed by anastomosis of the graft to the aortic bifurcation. All anastomoses are sealed with BioGlue.

M Operative photograph of aortic reconstruction with a prefabricated branch graft. The side branches of the graft are anastomosed sequentially to the visceral vessels and the renal arteries without tension. Note that the perfusion side branch is conveniently located (origin out of view) for anastomosis to the left renal artery.

L

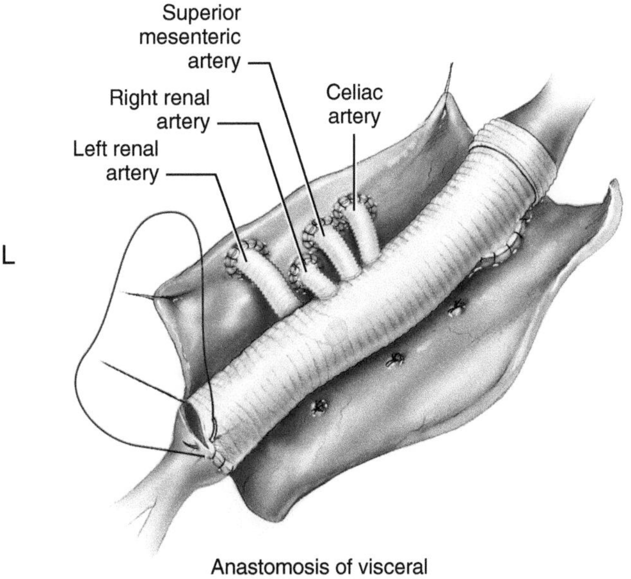

Anastomosis of visceral
and renal arteries

M

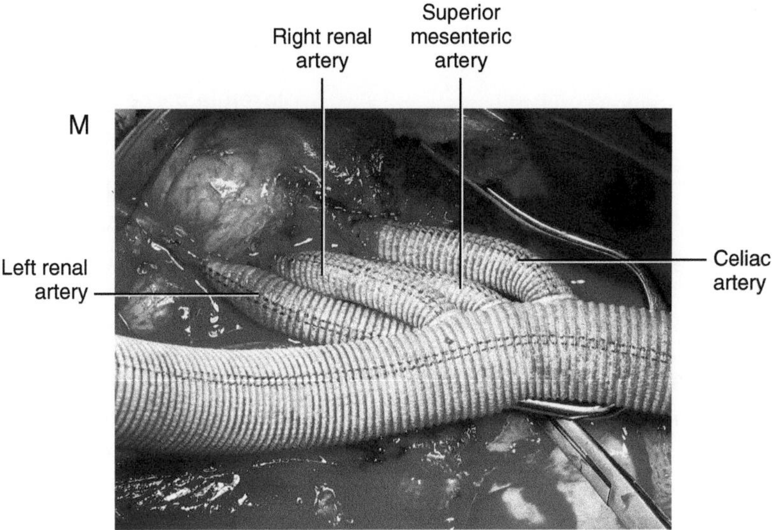

Endovascular Repair of Descending Thoracic Aorta

Thoracic endovascular repair (TEVAR) is indicated for patients with aneurysmal disease isolated to the descending thoracic aorta. This approach is performed under fluoroscopic guidance and avoids thoracotomy and open replacement of the aorta.

Figure 38-15 (The illustrations are presented in anterior anatomic perspective.)

A The thoracic aorta is divided into five zones to describe which of the arch vessels will be covered by the endovascular graft. Zone 0 is the ascending aorta, and the graft will cover all three of the arch vessels. In zone 1, the graft will cover both the left carotid and the subclavian arteries. In zone 2, the graft will cover the left subclavian artery. In zone 3, the graft will encroach on but not cover the left subclavian artery. In zone 4, the graft will be located beyond any of the arch vessels.

B Both common femoral arteries are accessed for the operation. The endovascular graft is inserted through the iliac artery that has the least degree of atherosclerosis and tortuosity. The common femoral artery is exposed on that side, and successive dilation is performed through a small 5/0 polypropylene purse-string suture to allow placement of an access sheath. A stiff wire with a flexible tip is placed into the ascending aorta under fluoroscopic guidance. A pigtail imaging catheter is placed percutaneously through the opposite common femoral artery into the aortic arch.

C An aortogram is performed to localize the aneurysm and evaluate the proximal and distal "landing zones" for the endovascular graft. If there is concern that the graft may encroach on the origin of the left subclavian artery, intravascular ultrasound can be employed for correlation with the aortogram. In general, a graft with a diameter 4 to 5 mm larger than the aorta is selected. The endovascular graft must be long enough to span the aneurysm with additional length on either end to "land" in nonaneurysmal aorta proximally and distally.

D The endovascular device is inserted over the stiff guidewire and positioned in the aortic arch. Care is taken to properly align the graft, which will naturally follow the outer curvature of the aneurysm and arch.

E The graft is partially deployed in the aortic arch and then slowly drawn back into position. It is critical to stabilize the delivery catheter at the groin because the blood pressure in the arch can push the graft beyond the proximal landing zone.

F The graft is fully deployed into the distal landing zone, and the delivery catheter is withdrawn. The pigtail imaging catheter is pulled down below the graft into the distal descending thoracic aorta.

G A balloon catheter is inserted into the graft and is inflated to seal the proximal and distal ends of the graft to the aorta. Care is taken not to overinflate the balloon at the extreme ends of the graft because this may rupture the aorta or dislodge the graft.

H The pigtail catheter is reinserted into the aortic arch, and a completion aortogram is performed. If there is residual endoleak, the balloon catheter can be reintroduced for additional inflations to seal the graft.

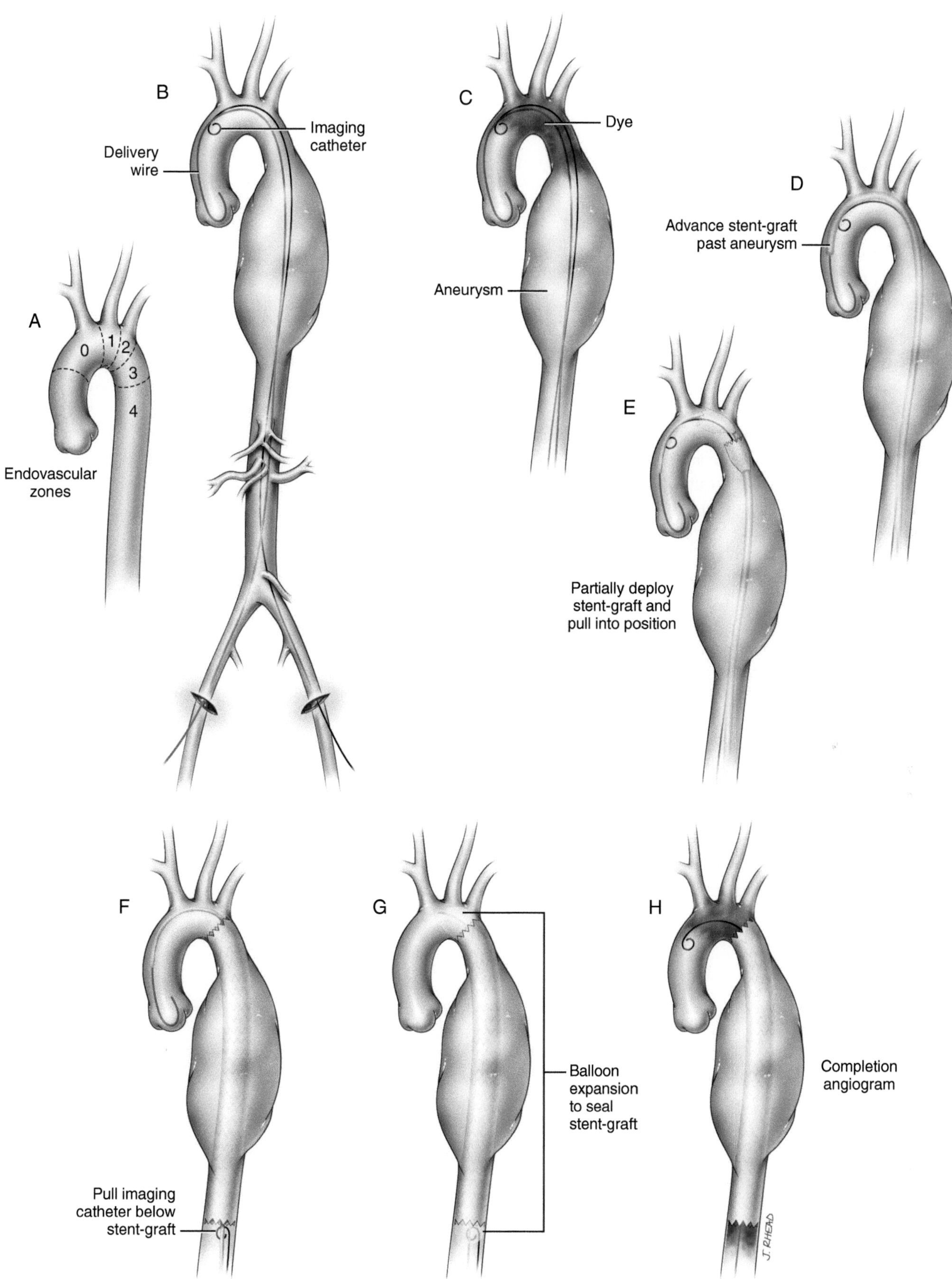
A
0
1
2
3
4
Endovascular
zones
B
Delivery
wire
Imaging
catheter
C
Dye
Aneurysm
D
Advance stent-graft
past aneurysm
E
Partially deploy
stent-graft and
pull into position
F
Pull imaging
catheter below
stent-graft
G
Balloon
expansion
to seal
stent-graft
H
Completion
angiogram
J. RHEAD

Endovascular Repair of Descending Thoracic Aorta—Multiple Endografts

In certain patients with extensive aneurysmal disease of the descending thoracic aorta, endovascular repair necessitates the use of multiple grafts. The endografts are overlapped in a telescoping fashion to adjust for size discrepancies in the proximal and distal aorta.

Figure 38-16

A An aortogram is performed to localize the aneurysm and evaluate the ultimate proximal and distal landing zones for the endovascular grafts. Measurements are taken to ensure the selection of grafts that can be telescoped, with a gradual transition in size between each endograft. This minimizes the potential for endoleak at the points of graft overlap.

B When the proximal landing zone is larger than the distal landing zone, the endovascular repair is constructed in a "top-down" fashion. The largest endograft is placed first in the proximal landing zone. The successive endografts gradually taper in size to the distal landing zone.

C When the distal landing zone is larger than the proximal landing zone, the endovascular repair is constructed in a "bottom-up" fashion. The largest endograft is placed first in the distal landing zone. The successive endografts gradually taper in size to the proximal landing zone.

D A balloon catheter is inserted into the grafts and is inflated to seal the proximal and distal ends of the graft to the aorta. The balloon is also inflated within the grafts to seal the points of graft overlap.

E The pigtail imaging catheter is reinserted into the aortic arch, and a completion aortogram is performed. If there is residual endoleak, the balloon catheter can be reintroduced for additional inflations to seal the grafts or points of overlap.

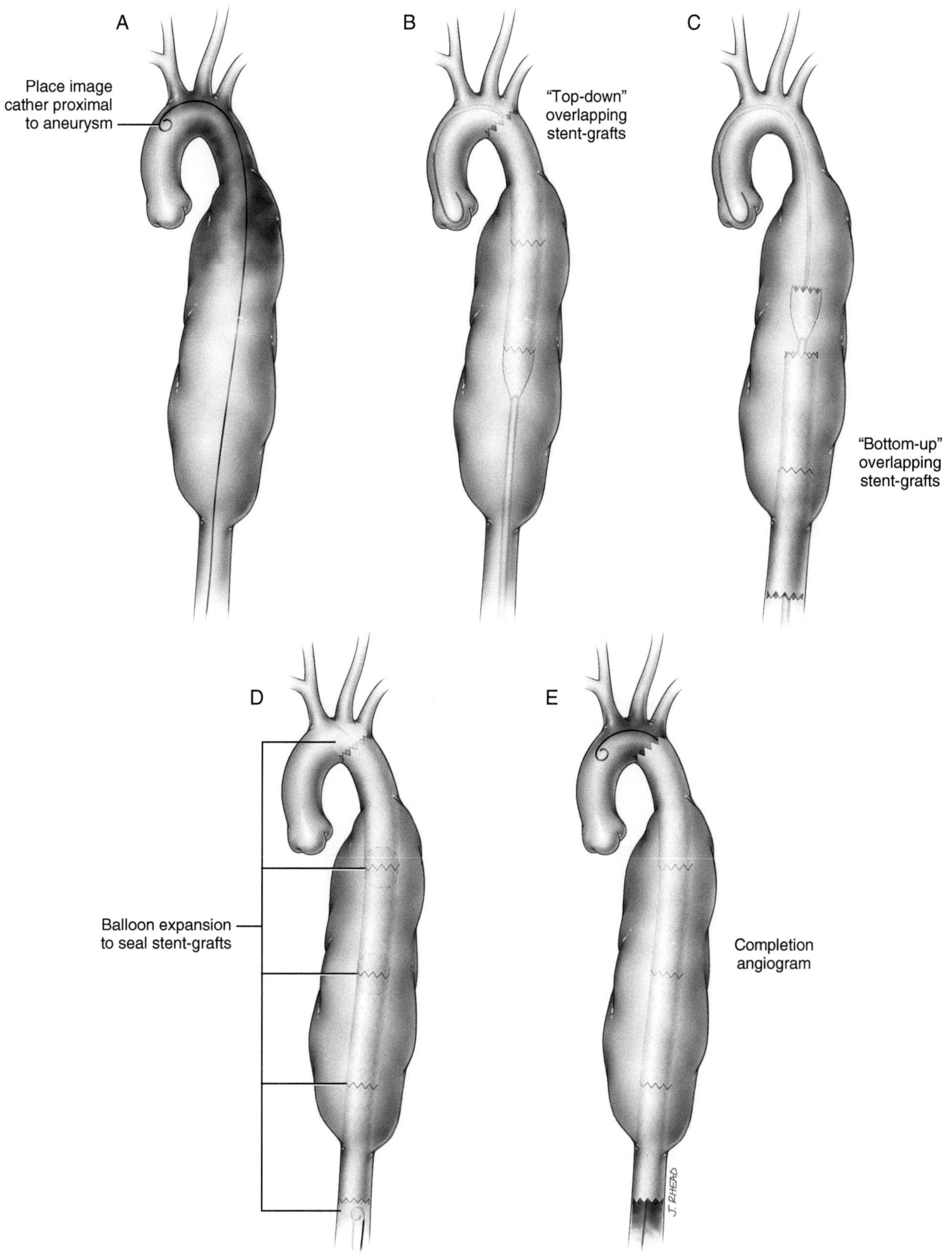
A
Place image
cather proximal
to aneurysm
B
"Top-down"
overlapping
stent-grafts
C
"Bottom-up"
overlapping
stent-grafts
D
Balloon expansion
to seal stent-grafts
E
Completion
angiogram
J. RHEAD

Endovascular Repair of Descending Thoracic Aorta with Occlusion of Left Subclavian Artery

For endovascular repair of an aneurysm that involves the most proximal portion of the descending thoracic aorta, the endograft is placed in zone 2 and covers the origin of the left subclavian artery. In most patients, construction of a concomitant left common carotid–to–left subclavian artery bypass graft is necessary to provide perfusion to the left arm and prevent vertebrobasilar insufficiency (left subclavian steal syndrome). The bypass graft can be constructed either before or after placement of the endograft.

Figure 38-17

A An oblique incision is made above the left clavicle. The lateral head of the sternocleidomastoid muscle is divided to enter the supraclavicular space.

B The left common carotid artery is isolated and mobilized. The proximal portion of the left subclavian artery is isolated proximal to the left vertebral artery. The left subclavian artery is divided as far proximally as is convenient, and the ends are oversewn with 5/0 polypropylene suture.

C A longitudinal arteriotomy is made in the left common carotid artery, and an end-to-side anastomosis is constructed with a ringed prosthetic graft using continuous stitches of 5/0 polypropylene. The graft is then trimmed to length for the left subclavian anastomosis.

D A longitudinal arteriotomy is made in the left subclavian artery, and the graft is attached in an end-to-side fashion using continuous stitches of 5/0 polypropylene. The anastomosis can be placed either proximal or distal to the origin of the left vertebral artery.

E After initial aortography and positioning of the delivery catheter, the endograft is partially deployed in the distal ascending aorta and then slowly drawn back into position in the aortic arch. The proximal end of the graft is placed at the distal margin of the origin of the left common carotid artery.

F The graft is fully deployed into the distal landing zone, and the delivery catheter is withdrawn. The pigtail imaging catheter is pulled down below the graft into the distal descending thoracic aorta.

G The graft is sealed with a balloon catheter, and a completion aortogram is performed. Posterior cerebral circulation is now antegrade through the left carotid–subclavian bypass graft.

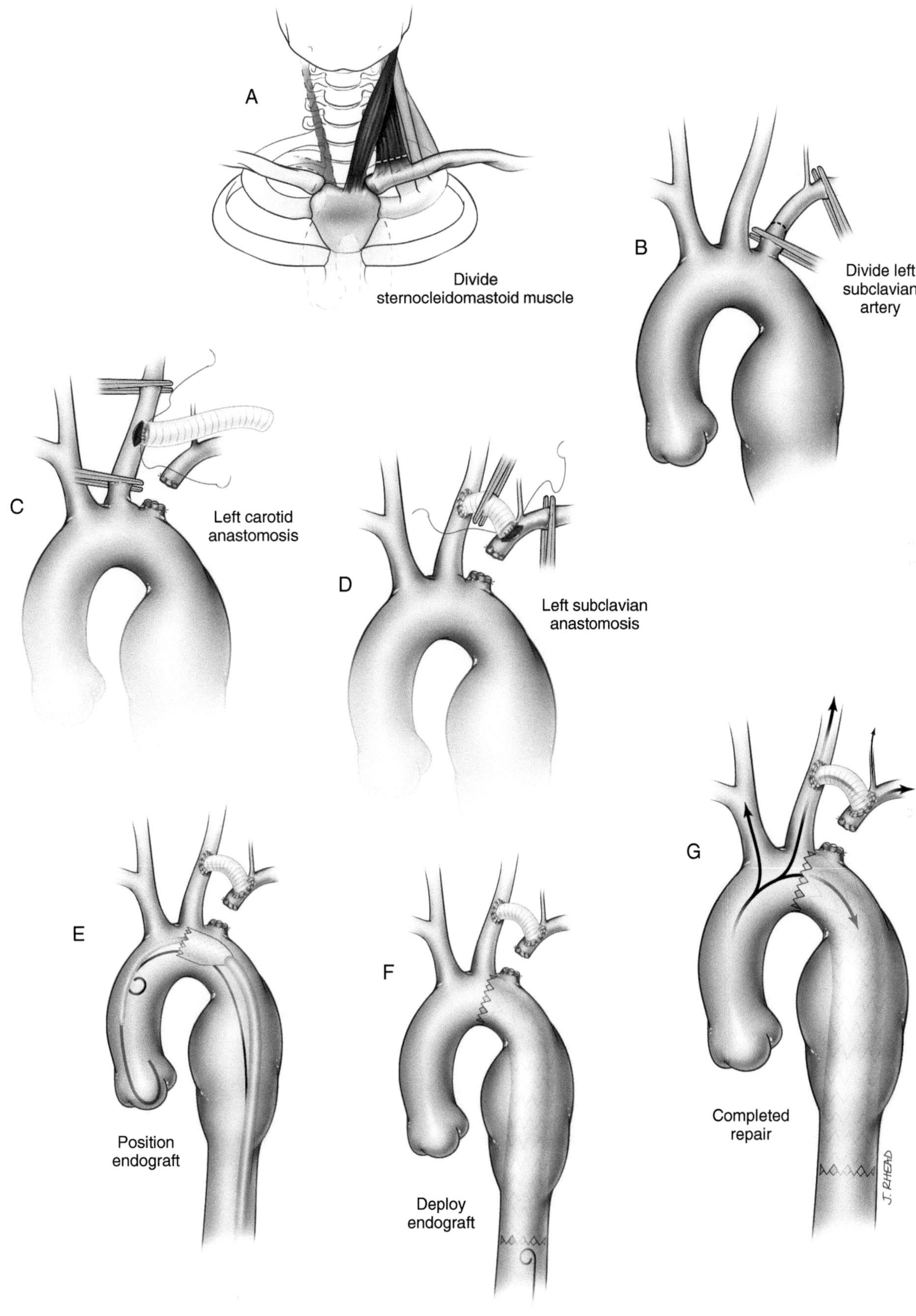
A
Divide
sternocleidomastoid muscle
B
Divide left
subclavian
artery
C
Left carotid
anastomosis
D
Left subclavian
anastomosis
E
Position
endograft
F
Deploy
endograft
G
Completed
repair
J. RHEAD

Total Arch Debranching

Reconstruction of the arterial supply to the arch vessels combined with endovascular repair of the arch is an alternative solution for aneurysmal disease involving the aortic arch. Total arch debranching avoids cardiopulmonary bypass and hypothermic circulatory arrest.

Figure 38-18

A A median sternotomy is performed, and the arch vessels are mobilized. A partial-occlusion vascular clamp is used to facilitate attachment of a branched prosthetic graft to the ascending aorta while maintaining blood flow through the arch branches.

B Beginning with the left subclavian artery, each aortic arch branch is removed sequentially. The proximal end is oversewn with continuous stitches of 4/0 polypropylene. The distal end is anastomosed to the branched prosthetic graft in an end-to-end fashion using continuous stitches of 5/0 polypropylene. The left common carotid is removed from the arch and anastomosed to the branched graft. A similar procedure for the innominate artery follows. Blood flow is restored to each vessel following completion of the anastomosis.

C An endovascular graft is deployed into zone 0, completely covering the entire aortic arch and origins of the arch vessels. Additional endovascular grafts may be deployed, as indicated, to the distal landing zone, thereby covering and isolating the aneurysm.

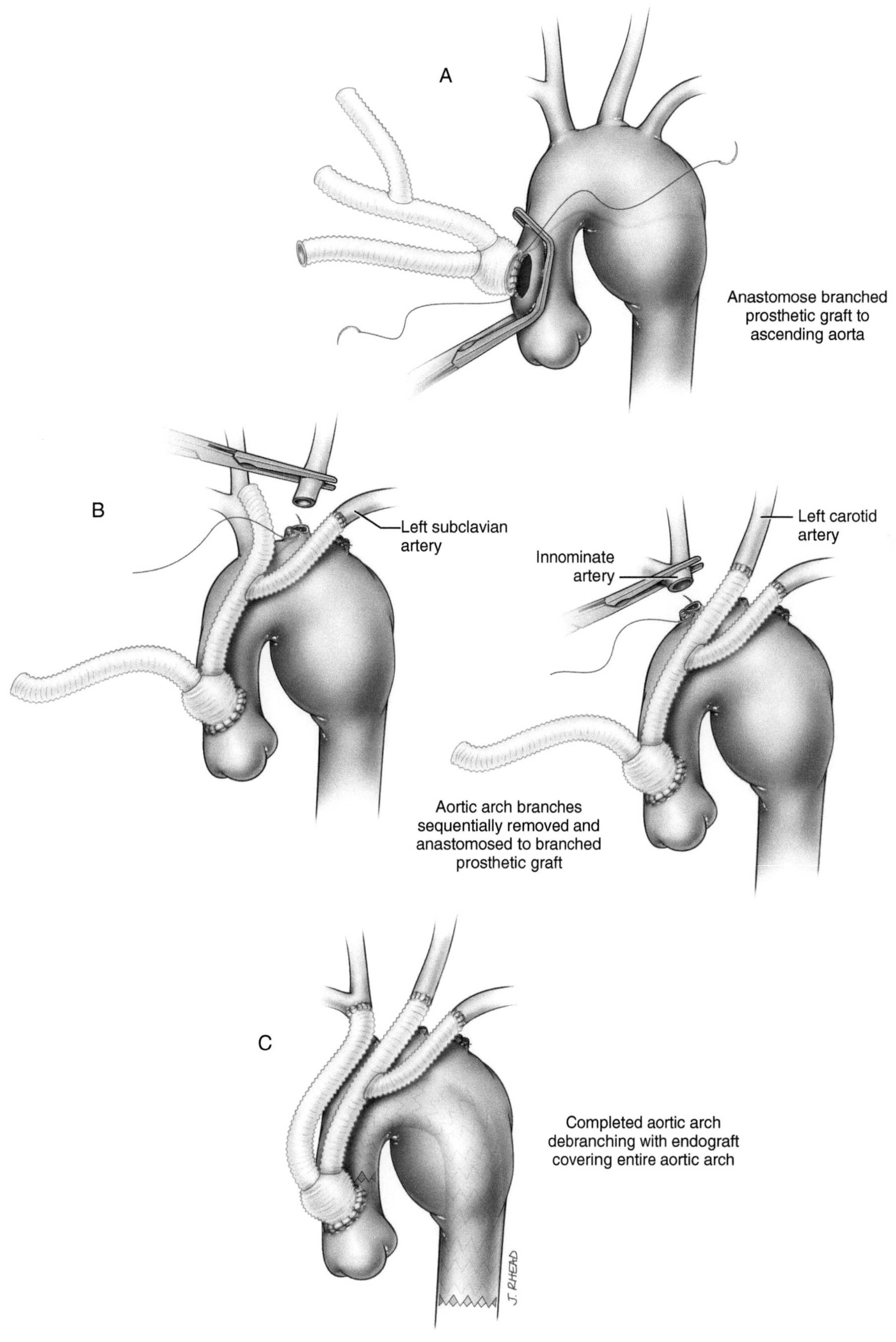
A
Anastomose branched prosthetic graft to ascending aorta
B
Left subclavian artery
Innominate artery
Left carotid artery
Aortic arch branches sequentially removed and anastomosed to branched prosthetic graft
C
Completed aortic arch debranching with endograft covering entire aortic arch
J. R HEAD

Second-Stage Descending Thoracic Aortic Repair after "Elephant Trunk" Arch Repair

In patients with combined disease of the arch and the descending thoracic aorta, complete repair typically requires a staged operative approach. After recovery from arch reconstruction using the elephant trunk technique, the second-stage operation is performed to repair the residual descending thoracic aorta.

Figure 38-19

A A standard posterolateral left thoracotomy is used for operative exposure, and partial left heart bypass is employed. A cannula is placed in the left inferior pulmonary vein for uptake to the partial bypass circuit. A return cannula is placed in either the distal descending thoracic aorta or the left common femoral artery. This allows perfusion of the lower half of the body without the need for cardioplegia or an oxygenator. Alternatively, full cardiopulmonary bypass with hypothermic circulatory arrest can be utilized for additional protection of the spinal cord.

B The descending thoracic aorta is mobilized below the aneurysm. Proximally, the elephant trunk portion of the aorta is identified and mobilized to allow placement of a cross-clamp. Care is taken to avoid injury to the left recurrent laryngeal nerve because this portion of the aorta may be adherent from the previous operation.

C Clamps are placed proximally and distally, and the aorta is opened longitudinally. Back-bleeding intercostals and bronchial arteries are oversewn. One or two sets of larger intercostal arteries are identified as an "island" for later reimplantation.

D The elephant trunk portion of the prosthetic graft is identified and mobilized. A second prosthetic graft is selected and attached in an end-to-end fashion using continuous stitches of 4/0 polypropylene.

E The graft is trimmed to an appropriate length and attached in an end-to-end fashion to the distal descending thoracic aorta using continuous stitches of 4/0 polypropylene. BioGlue is used to reinforce all suture lines.

F If indicated, an opening is made in the graft opposite the intercostal island for reimplantation. A side-to-side anastomosis is constructed using continuous stitches of 4/0 polypropylene.

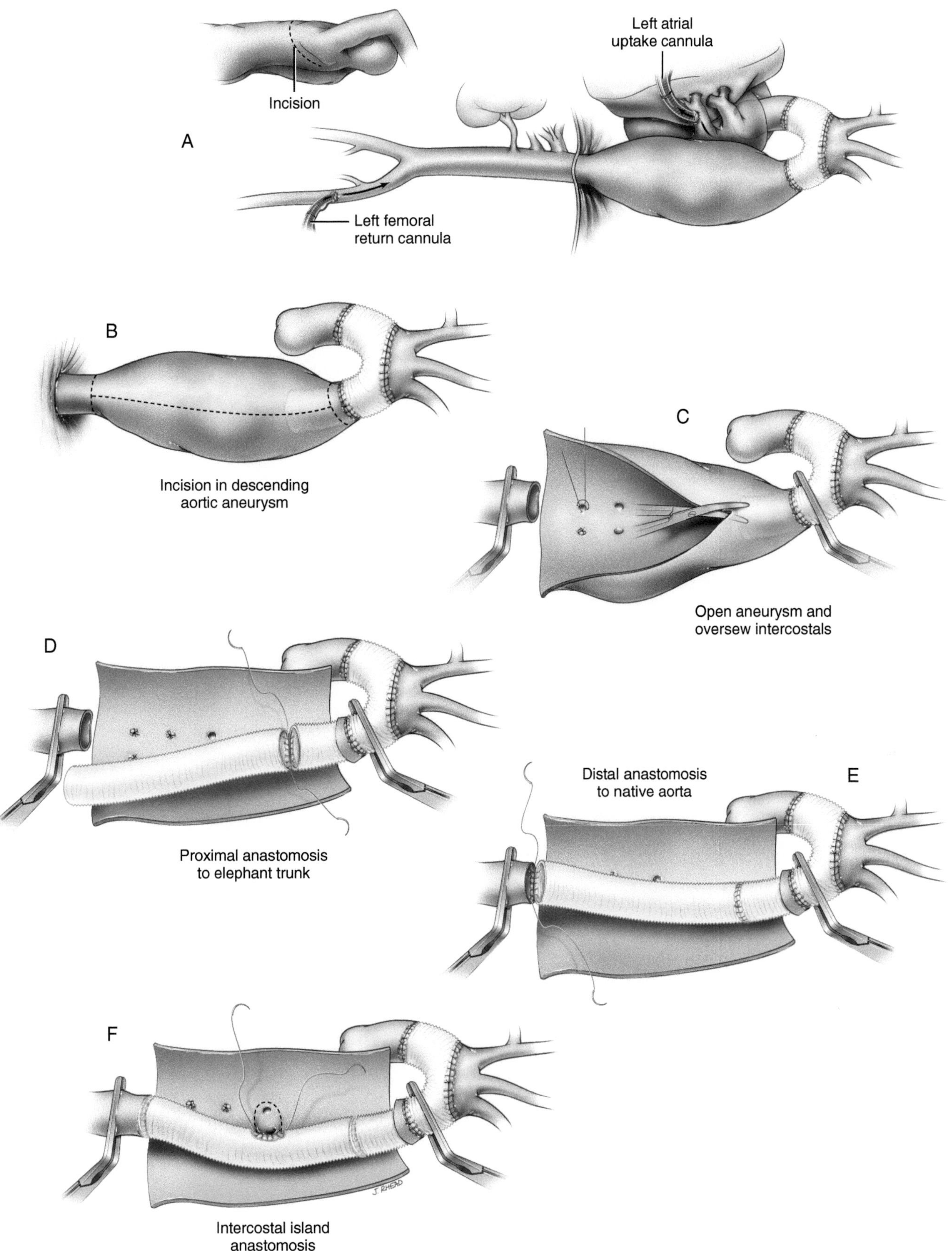
Left atrial uptake cannula
Incision
A
Left femoral return cannula
B
Incision in descending aortic aneurysm
C
Open aneurysm and oversew intercostals
D
Proximal anastomosis to elephant trunk
Distal anastomosis to native aorta
E
F
J. RHEAD
Intercostal island anastomosis

Figure 38-19 (continued)

G An alternative technique for the second-stage repair is to use an endovascular approach. The previous prosthetic arch graft is used for the proximal landing zone for the endovascular graft. Guidewires and a pigtail imaging catheter are placed into the aortic arch, and an aortogram is performed. The distal end of the elephant trunk graft is identified and measured for endovascular graft selection.

H The delivery catheter is placed into the aortic arch, and the endovascular graft is partially deployed in the elephant trunk graft. The endovascular graft is gradually pulled down into position, placing the proximal end at the distal margin of the origin of the left subclavian artery.

I The endovascular graft is fully deployed through the elephant trunk and into the descending thoracic aorta. Additional endovascular grafts are placed as indicated, and a final aortogram is performed to assess the completed repair.

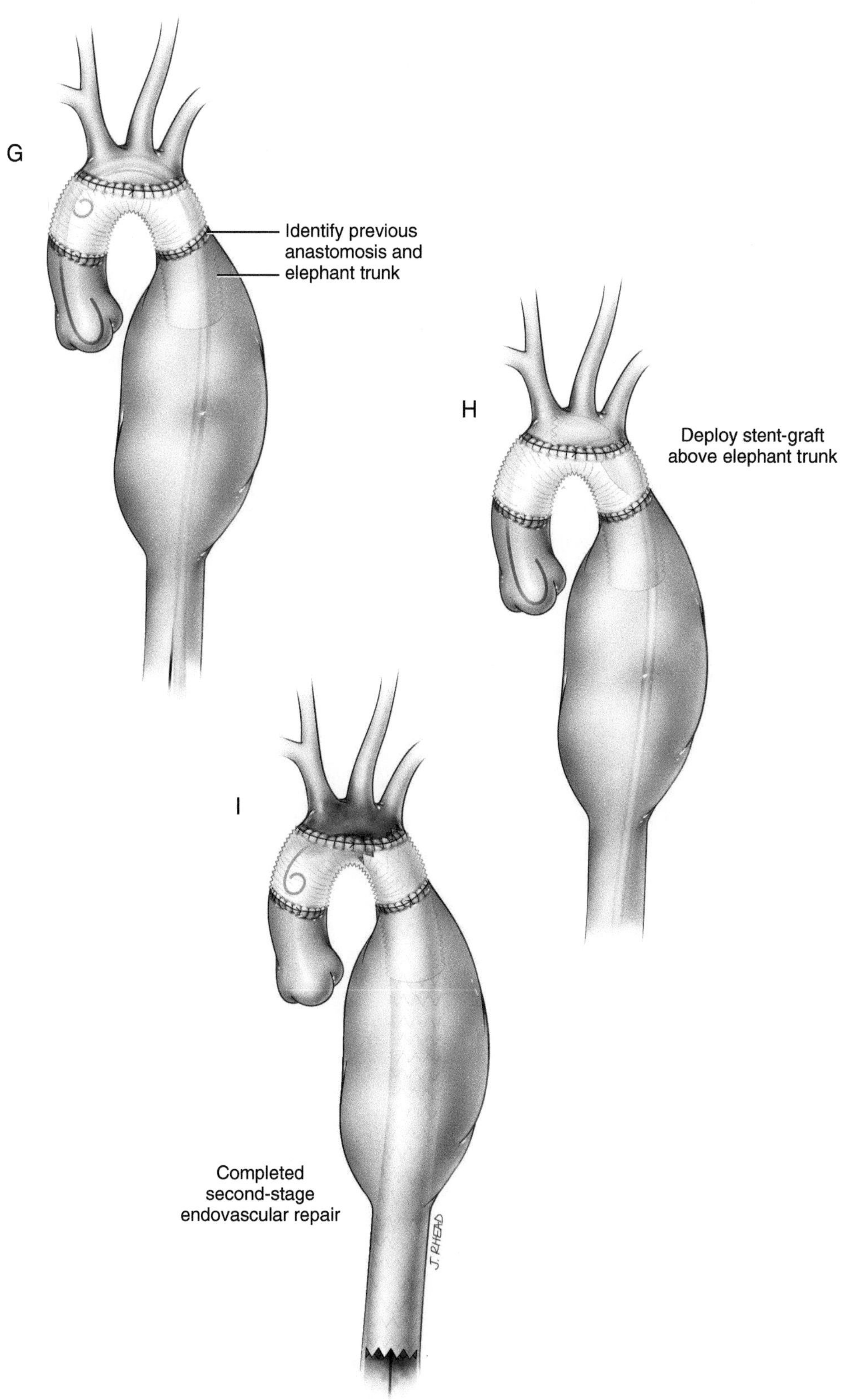
G
Identify previous anastomosis and elephant trunk
H
Deploy stent-graft above elephant trunk
I
Completed second-stage endovascular repair
J. RHEAD

"Frozen Elephant Trunk" Repair

Combined open replacement of the aortic arch and endovascular repair of the proximal descending thoracic aorta can be performed in a single operation. Termed the "frozen elephant trunk" repair, this operation involves deployment of an endovascular graft in the open descending thoracic aorta, followed by attachment of a standard surgical graft for reconstruction of the aortic arch.

Figure 38-20

A After the institution of cardiopulmonary bypass via the axillary artery, either hypothermic circulatory arrest or selective antegrade head vessel perfusion is used to resect the aortic arch and prepare the proximal descending thoracic aorta. An endovascular graft is inserted directly down the open descending thoracic aorta and deployed in a retrograde fashion.

B A small length of the endovascular graft is now outside the proximal descending thoracic aorta, with the remainder of the graft fixed inside the descending thoracic aorta ("frozen elephant trunk").

C A prosthetic graft is attached to the end of the endovascular graft using continuous stitches of 4/0 polypropylene. Care is taken not to dislodge the endovascular graft. The suture line is reinforced with BioGlue.

D The arch vessels are reimplanted onto the prosthetic graft either as an island or by the individual attachment of each vessel using continuous stitiches of 5/0 polypropylene.

E The repair is completed by trimming the graft to length and attaching it to the ascending aorta in an end-to-end fashion using continuous stitches of 4/0 polypropylene. All anastomoses are sealed with BioGlue.

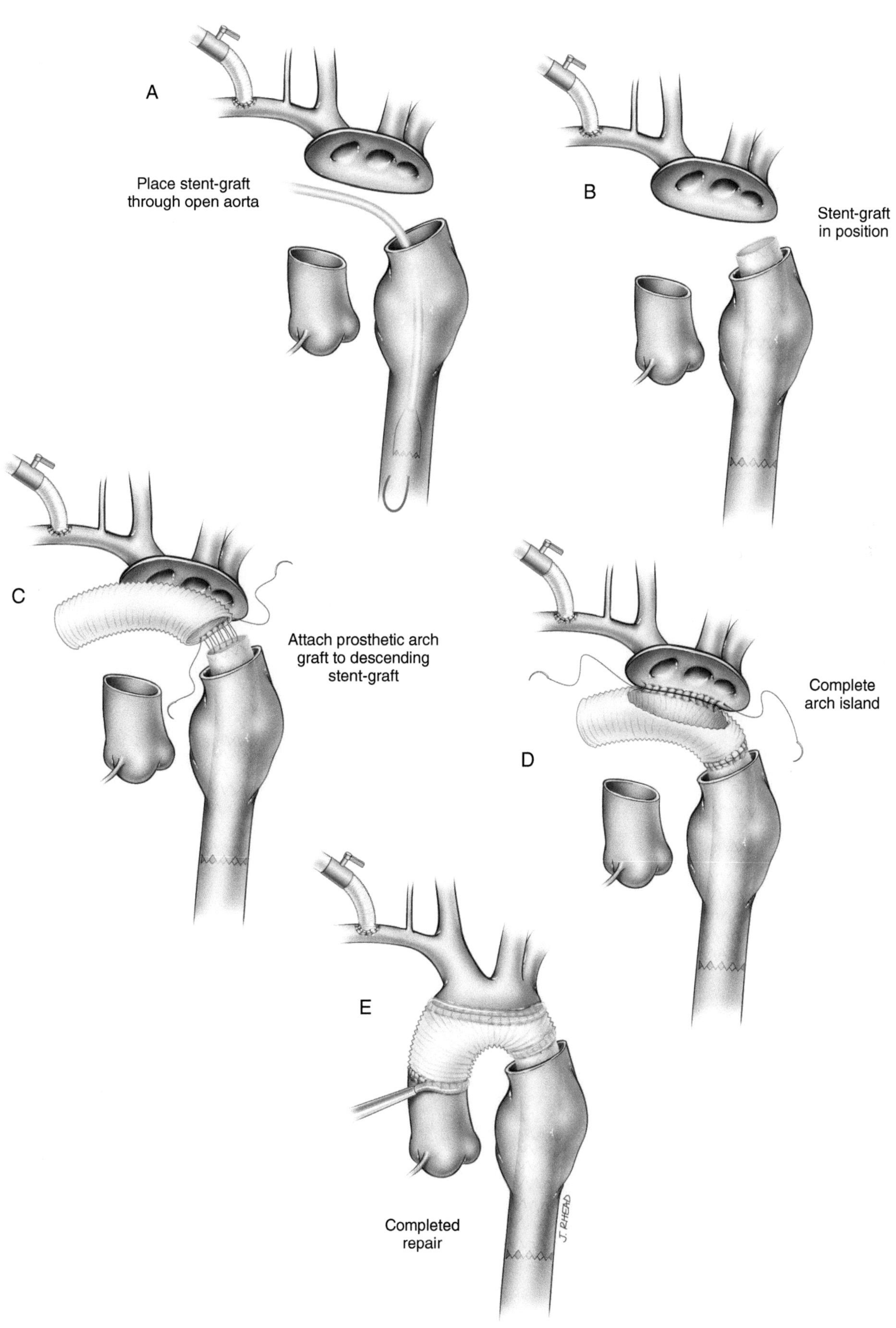
A
Place stent-graft through open aorta
B
Stent-graft in position
C
Attach prosthetic arch graft to descending stent-graft
D
Complete arch island
E
Completed repair
J. RHEAD

Thoracoabdominal Debranching

Reconstruction of the arterial supply to the abdominal vessels combined with endovascular repair of the thoracoabdominal aorta is an alternative solution for extensive aneurysmal disease. Thoracoabdominal debranching combines revascularization to the abdominal and renal arteries with endovascular repair, avoiding cardiopulmonary bypass.

Figure 38-21

A Thorough preoperative evaluation and planning are crucial to adequately revascularize the abdominal vasculature and to ensure proper endovascular graft selection. Computed tomography with three-dimensional reconstruction can identify concomitant peripheral vascular and abdominal vascular disease.

B A midline abdominal incision is used for exposure of the abdominal aorta. Extension of the incision into the chest may be necessary for the proximal anastomosis of the prosthetic graft to the distal descending thoracic aorta. The origins of the celiac, superior mesenteric, and renal arteries are mobilized and divided. Each stump is oversewn with 4/0 polypropylene suture. After completion of the proximal anastomosis, separate anastomoses are constructed to each abdominal vessel using continuous stitches of 5/0 polypropylene.

C Alternatively, separate bypass grafts can be attached to the iliac arteries using continuous stitches of 5/0 polypropylene. A sequential graft is then constructed on the right side to supply the right renal artery, the superior mesenteric artery, and the celiac artery. A separate graft on the left side supplies the left renal artery. A prefabricated arch graft as shown in Fig. 38-14, *M* could also be used to revascularize the abdominal viscera.

D After completion of the abdominal revascularization, endovascular grafts are used to repair the thoracoabdominal aorta. This may require additional endovascular grafting into the descending thoracic aorta or the iliac arteries.

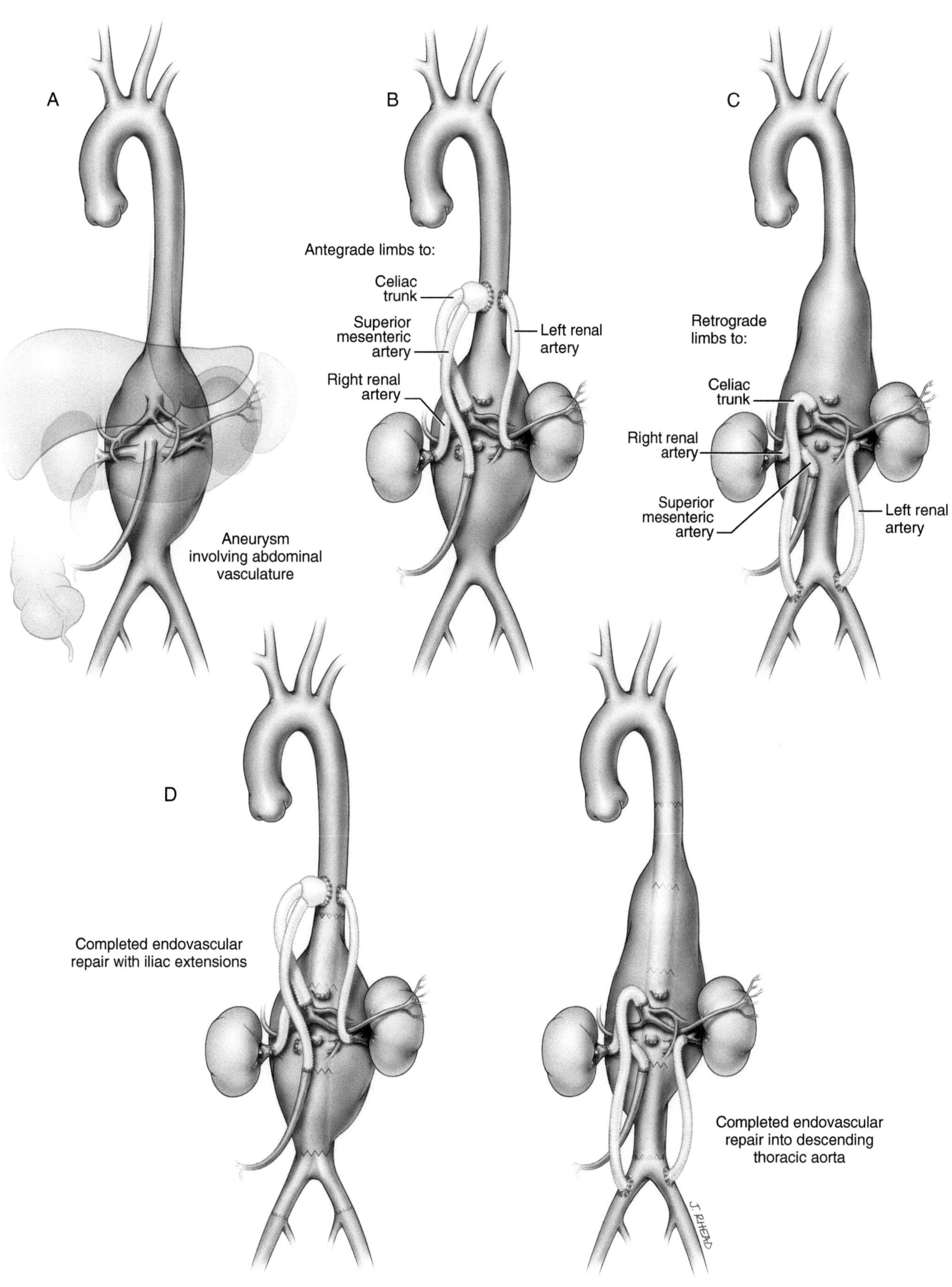
A
B
C
Antegrade limbs to:
Celiac trunk
Superior mesenteric artery
Right renal artery
Left renal artery
Retrograde limbs to:
Celiac trunk
Right renal artery
Superior mesenteric artery
Left renal artery
Aneurysm involving abdominal vasculature
D
Completed endovascular repair with iliac extensions
Completed endovascular repair into descending thoracic aorta
J. RHEAD

chapter 39 BYPASS OF SUPERIOR VENA CAVA

Composite Spiral Vein Graft

Benign and malignant conditions causing obstruction of the superior vena cava may result in severe superior vena cava syndrome. Some of the so-called benign causes of superior vena cava obstruction are severe and relentless fibrotic processes that result in recurrent and extensive obstruction. Clot propagation within the venous system proximal to the primary site of caval obstruction may present as progression of superior vena cava syndrome in patients with a benign etiology. Some patients with obstruction of the superior vena cava never develop adequate collateral circulation, even though the causative process is stabilized or arrested. Most patients with malignant tumors in the thorax causing superior vena cava obstruction are treated by radiation or chemotherapy. In some cases of malignant disease, the superior vena cava syndrome is so severe that it is life threatening and may require immediate intervention. Incapacitating symptoms and signs of superior vena cava syndrome may be relieved by bypass of the caval obstruction. Conduits constructed from autogenous vein are immediately beneficial and associated with long-term patency.

Morphology

Figure 39-1

A Operative photograph of superior vena cava obstruction by malignant tumor, anterior view. Obstruction may be the result of direct tumor invasion, as in this case, or it may occur when the inflammatory reaction in the tissues around the tumor results in thrombosis of the vena cava.

B Operative photographs of construction of a composite spiral saphenous vein graft. The greater saphenous vein has been removed from the thigh, opened longitudinally, and wrapped around a catheter in spiral fashion. The lower photograph shows the completed graft after the edges of the vein have been sewn together with 7/0 polypropylene suture.

C Operative photograph of superior vena cava bypass graft, anterior view. Bypass of the obstructed superior vena cava lowers venous pressure sufficiently to reduce tissue edema and relieve the signs and symptoms of superior vena cava syndrome. Adequate decompression of the upper compartment venous system can generally be accomplished by drainage through a single jugular vein, usually the left innominate vein, because of the connected venous sinuses in the skull. The bypass graft shown here is a composite spiral saphenous vein graft anastomosed to the left innominate vein and to the right atrial appendage.

D Operative photograph of a bifurcated composite spiral saphenous vein graft, completed. In some cases, bypass of an obstruction to both sides of the upper compartment is desirable. A bifurcated bypass graft is used in these cases.

E Operative photograph of superior vena cava bypass with a bifurcated composite spiral saphenous vein graft, anterior view. The long limb of the graft is anastomosed to the left internal jugular vein (not shown). The graft is brought into the thorax through an externally reinforced polytetrafluoroethylene (PTFE) tubular graft to prevent compression at the thoracic inlet. The short limb is anastomosed to the patent remnant of a previously placed spiral saphenous vein graft. The distal end of the graft is anastomosed to the right atrium.

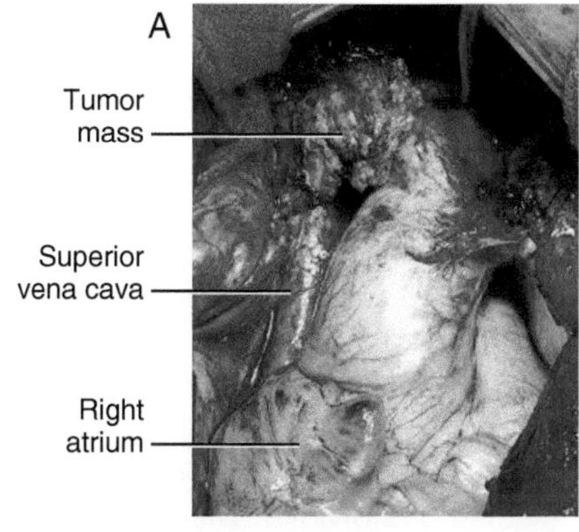

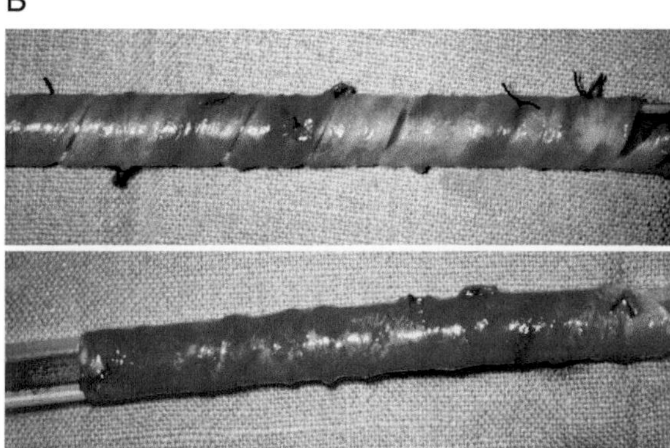

Construction of spiral saphenous vein graft

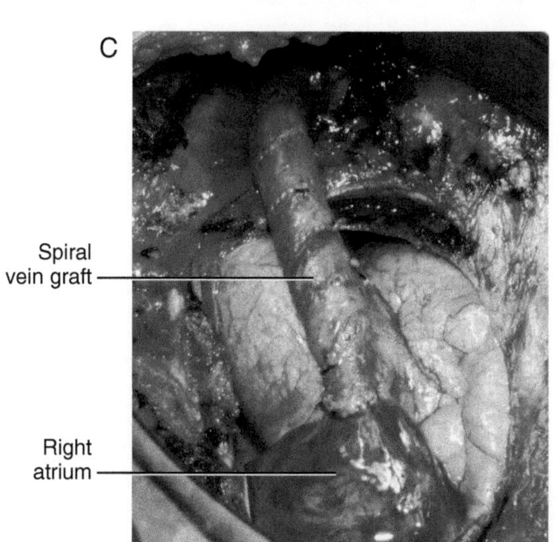

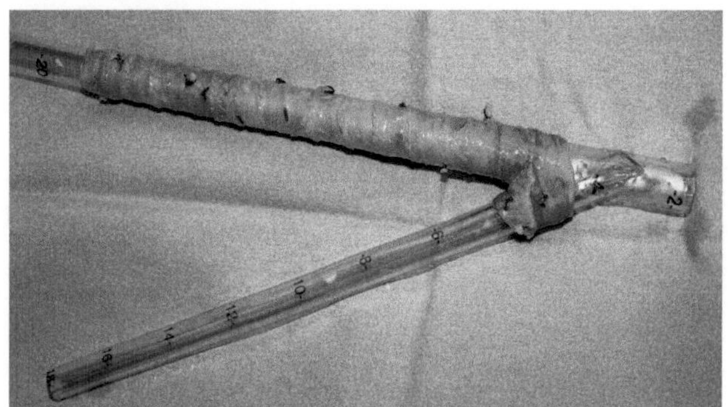

Bifurcated spiral saphenous vein graft

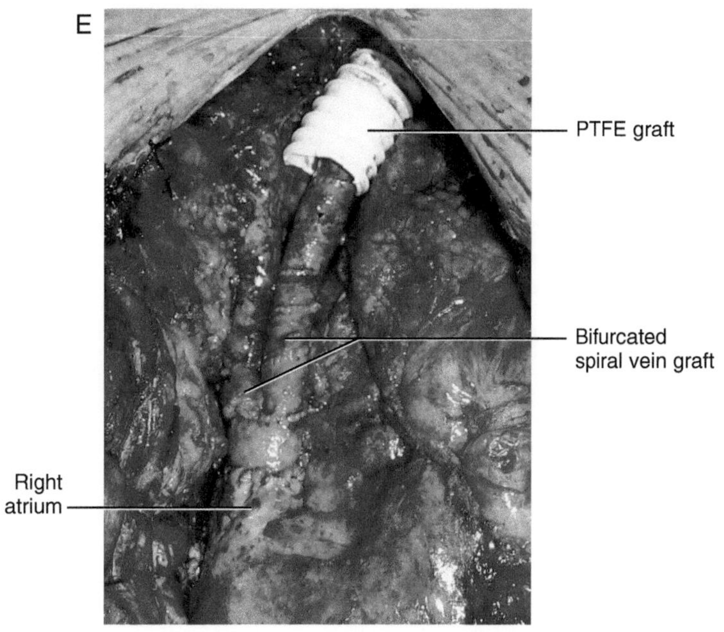

Figure 39-2

A A midsternal incision is made. A partial upper-half sternotomy is usually sufficient for this operation. The incision can be extended into the left or right side of the neck if necessary to expose the internal jugular vein. A secondary cervical incision can also be made, with the incisions communicating at the thoracic inlet. Chest wall collateral circulation may be extensive, but it is controlled by compression and electrocautery. A cell-saving system is helpful to reduce blood replacement requirements. A biopsy of the obstructing process in the mediastinum is performed. The pericardium is opened to expose the right atrial appendage. The thymic remnant is removed, and the innominate vein is completely mobilized. Once the feasibility of bypass has been established by assessing innominate or internal jugular vein patency, the length of the proposed bypass graft is measured by stretching a silk suture between the inflow vein and the right atrial appendage.

B The greater saphenous vein is exposed by making an incision in the thigh from the groin to the knee. The diameter of the innominate or jugular vein is measured and compared with the average diameter of the saphenous vein, and a ratio is determined. This ratio multiplied by the length of the proposed bypass graft determines the length of saphenous vein required to construct a composite spiral vein graft of the same diameter as the inflow vein and of sufficient length to reach the right atrial appendage. For example, if the diameter of the innominate vein is 12 mm and the average diameter of the saphenous vein is 4 mm, three times the length of saphenous vein will be required to bridge the distance between the innominate vein and the right atrial appendage. As a practical matter, excision of the saphenous vein from groin to knee is usually sufficient. The side branches of the saphenous vein are ligated and divided. The vein is excised from the leg and gently distended using heparinized electrolyte solution. Unligated branches of the vein are controlled. The vein is opened longitudinally through its entire length. A catheter of the same diameter as the inflow vein is used as a stent over which the composite spiral graft is constructed. The saphenous vein is wrapped around the stent in spiral fashion, placing the endothelium against the stent. The graft edges at the first complete wrap are secured by suture, allowing some tension to be maintained on the saphenous vein to achieve maximal length as it is spiraled around the catheter. Securing the edges at the last complete wrap maintains the configuration. The edges of the saphenous vein are then approximated by continuous stitches using 7/0 polypropylene. Gentle traction on the suture elevates the vein slightly from the catheter stent, allowing the needle to pass easily from edge to edge. Optical magnification (2.5×) is used to ensure the accuracy of the anastomosis. About 30 minutes is required to prepare the graft. A bifurcated graft is constructed over a stent made from two catheters of an appropriate size. One of the catheters is inserted into the side of the other catheter at a 30-degree angle. More length of saphenous vein is obviously required. The saphenous vein is wrapped around one limb of the stent past the point of bifurcation. The vein is brought through the angle of bifurcation and continued on the other limb of the stent. The edges of the vein graft are approximated by continuous stitches using 7/0 polypropylene.

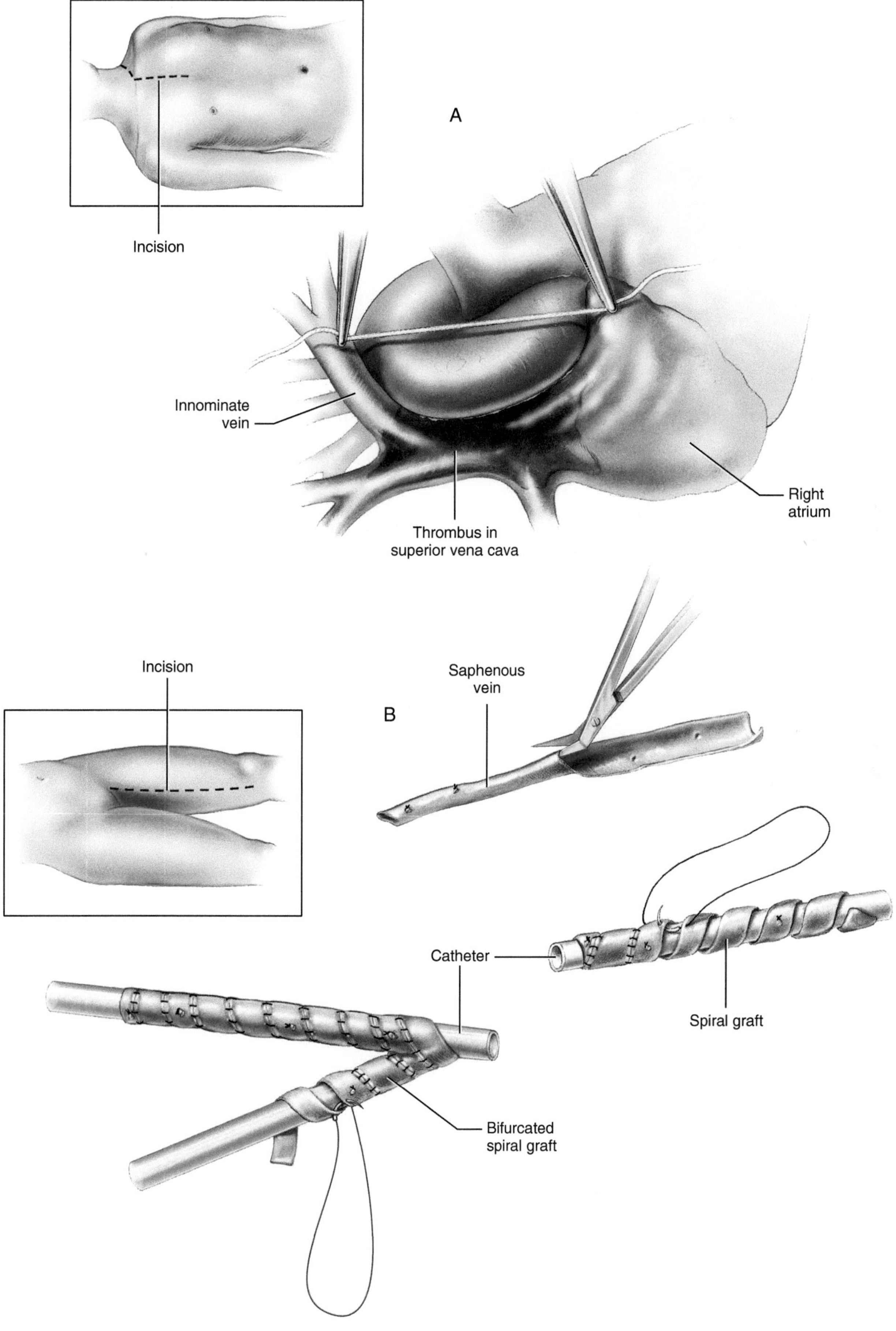
A
Incision
Innominate vein
Thrombus in superior vena cava
Right atrium
B
Incision
Saphenous vein
Catheter
Spiral graft
Catheter
Bifurcated spiral graft

Figure 39-2 (continued)

C Heparin 100 U/kg is administered intravenously to the patient. The innominate vein is ligated as close to the superior vena cava as possible. A soft-jaw vascular clamp (Fogarty) is applied at the jugular-subclavian confluence on the left side, and the innominate vein is divided, preserving as much length as possible. The intima of the vein is inspected to ensure that it is normal and that all organized thrombus has been removed. The end of the composite spiral vein graft is trimmed to ensure a uniform circumference, and then the graft is pushed off the end of the stent slightly. An end-to-end anastomosis of the graft to the innominate vein is constructed using continuous stitches of 6/0 or 7/0 polypropylene. Several suture loops can be placed in the back row for convenience and accuracy before pulling up the suture and approximating the graft to the innominate vein. The front row of the anastomosis can then be completed. The stent is removed, and the graft is allowed to be free in the mediastinum, anterior to the aorta.

D The right atrial appendage is excluded by a vascular clamp. The tip of the appendage is excised, and all trabeculae within the appendage are removed to ensure an unrestricted passageway into the atrium. An end-to-end anastomosis of the vein graft to the right atrial appendage is made with 5/0 polypropylene suture. Prior planning of the graft's orientation allows use of its naturally occurring bevel for correct approximation to the atrial appendage.

E The vascular clamps are removed, protamine is administered, and the graft is packed for a few minutes to achieve hemostasis. Correct measurement of graft length is essential. Excessive length has no advantage because hemostasis will not be satisfactory, and any angles in the graft are likely to be detrimental to patency. The pericardium is left open, the mediastinum is drained with a single tube, and wound closure is routine.

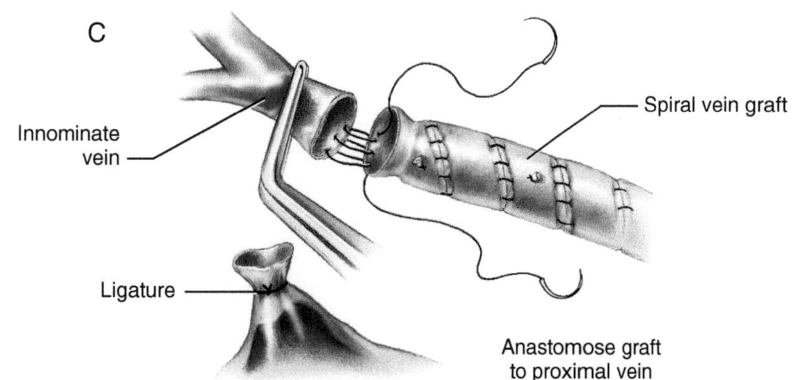
C
Innominate vein
Spiral vein graft
Ligature
Anastomose graft to proximal vein

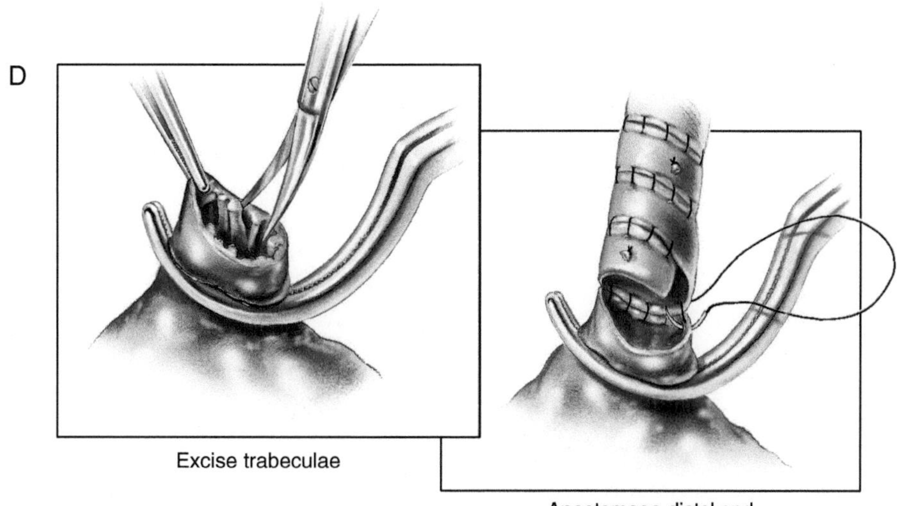
D
Excise trabeculae
Anastomose distal end of graft to right atrium

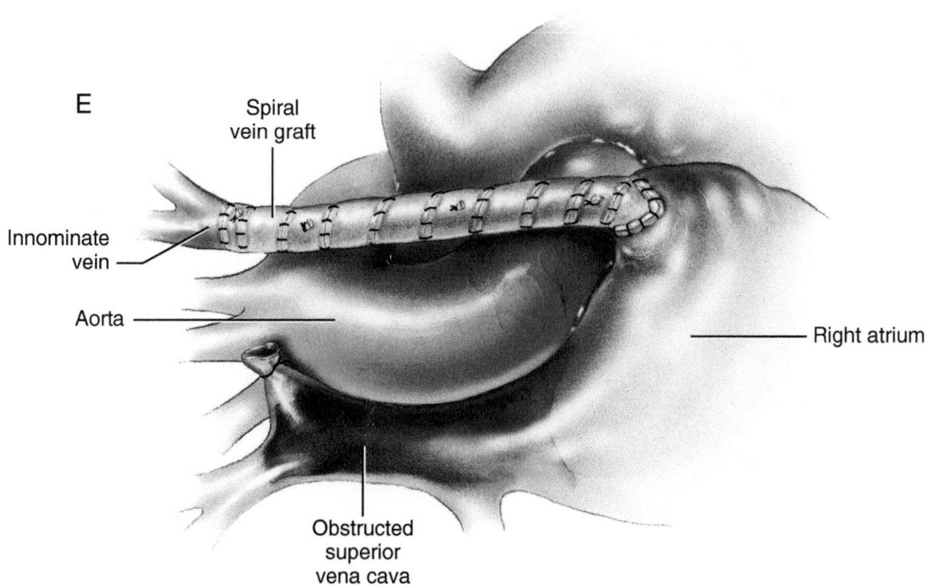
E
Spiral vein graft
Innominate vein
Aorta
Right atrium
Obstructed superior vena cava

part XII

Special Operations

chapter 40 CARDIAC TRANSPLANTATION

Improved means of controlling tissue rejection have made transplantation of the human heart a useful clinical procedure that is widely applied in cardiovascular centers throughout the world. Cooperative organizations for the sharing of facilities and long-distance transportation of cryopreserved tissue for transplantation have made this procedure available to many individuals who otherwise might have died of congestive cardiac failure. All these organizational and immunological advances make possible a procedure that is remarkable to observe in total perspective and offers its own technical challenges.

Morphology

Two human beings are involved. One donates the heart (having died from brain injury), and the other receives it after having his or her own heart removed and discarded. The donor heart is carefully evaluated to verify its normal performance. Its size should be normal and should match within 20% of the expected size of the recipient's heart, predicted by his or her body weight. The heart of the recipient is always considerably enlarged due to dilation from congestive cardiac failure.

Figure 40-1

A Recipient heart and donor heart after excision. The significant size disparity is obvious and must be accounted for during implantation of the donor heart.

B In addition to the size discrepancy, the surgeon must account for the absence of great vessels resulting from the prior operations to excise the hearts from both the donor and the recipient. The heart is separated from the donor by dividing pulmonary veins, venae cavae, aorta, and pulmonary artery and/or branch pulmonary arteries at the pericardial reflection, preserving as much vessel length as possible. The heart of the recipient is removed by incising the atria along the atrioventricular groove and dividing the aorta and pulmonary arteries just above the sinuses of Valsalva.

A

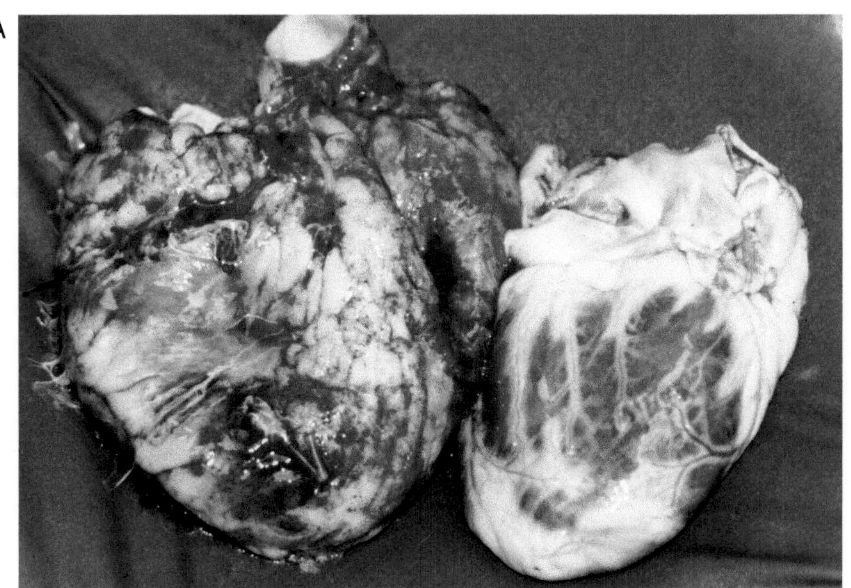

Recipient heart Donor heart

B

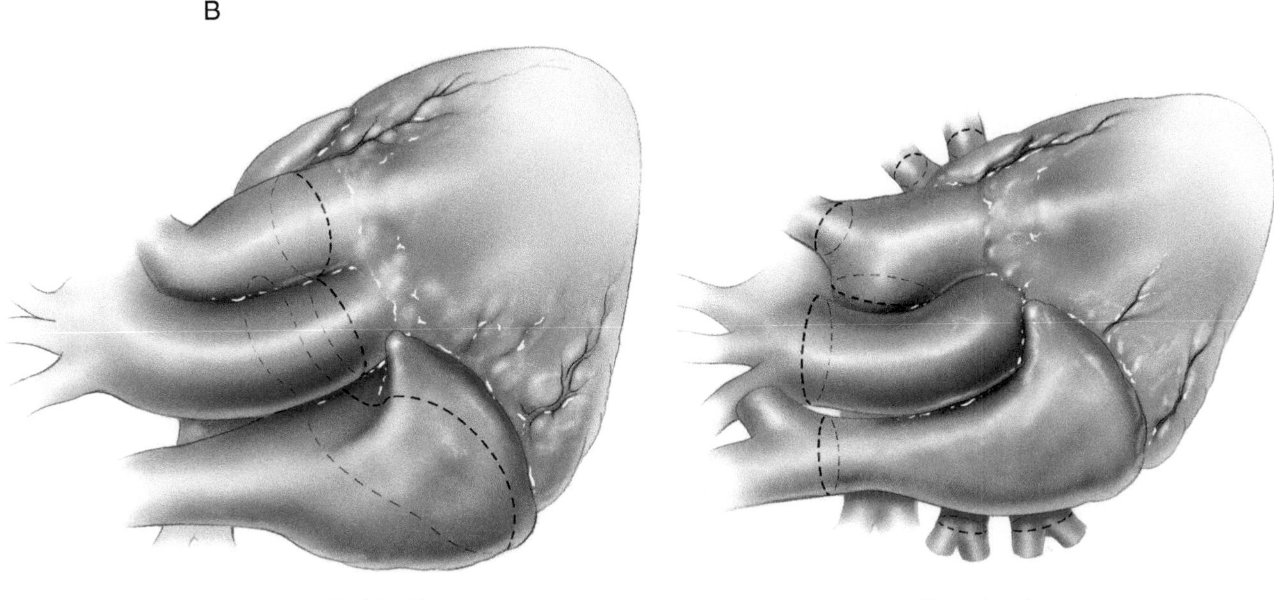

Areas of excision for cardiectomy

Donor Cardiectomy

Operation on the donor is performed after verifying proper donor identification, consent, blood type, and normal cardiac function. After inspection of the heart, the donor's surgeon informs the recipient's surgeon of the findings and estimates the operating time and transport time to establish an estimated time of arrival of the donor heart.

Figure 40-2

A Removal of the donor heart is performed through a midsternal incision. Pericardial retraction stitches are placed for exposure. The pericardium is mobilized off the superior vena cava, and a ligature is placed around the vessel. A needle catheter is placed in the ascending aorta and secured by tourniquet for the administration of cold cardioplegic solution. Heparin is administered systemically. The superior vena cava is ligated. The inferior vena cava is divided at the diaphragm. After a few heartbeats, the left ventricle empties, and cardiac ejection ceases. An occlusion clamp is placed on the ascending aorta at the pericardial reflection. The right superior pulmonary vein is incised to further empty the left side of the heart. Cold cardioplegic solution is administered through the aortic root to cool the heart and ensure electromechanical arrest. Cold isotonic solution poured into the pericardial sac hastens the process of myocardial cooling. Coronary sinus effluent is allowed to escape to the pericardial sac through the open inferior vena cava. Cardiectomy proceeds by dividing the right pulmonary veins at the pericardial reflection. The heart is retracted superiorly and to the right to expose the left pulmonary veins. These vessels are divided at the pericardial reflection.

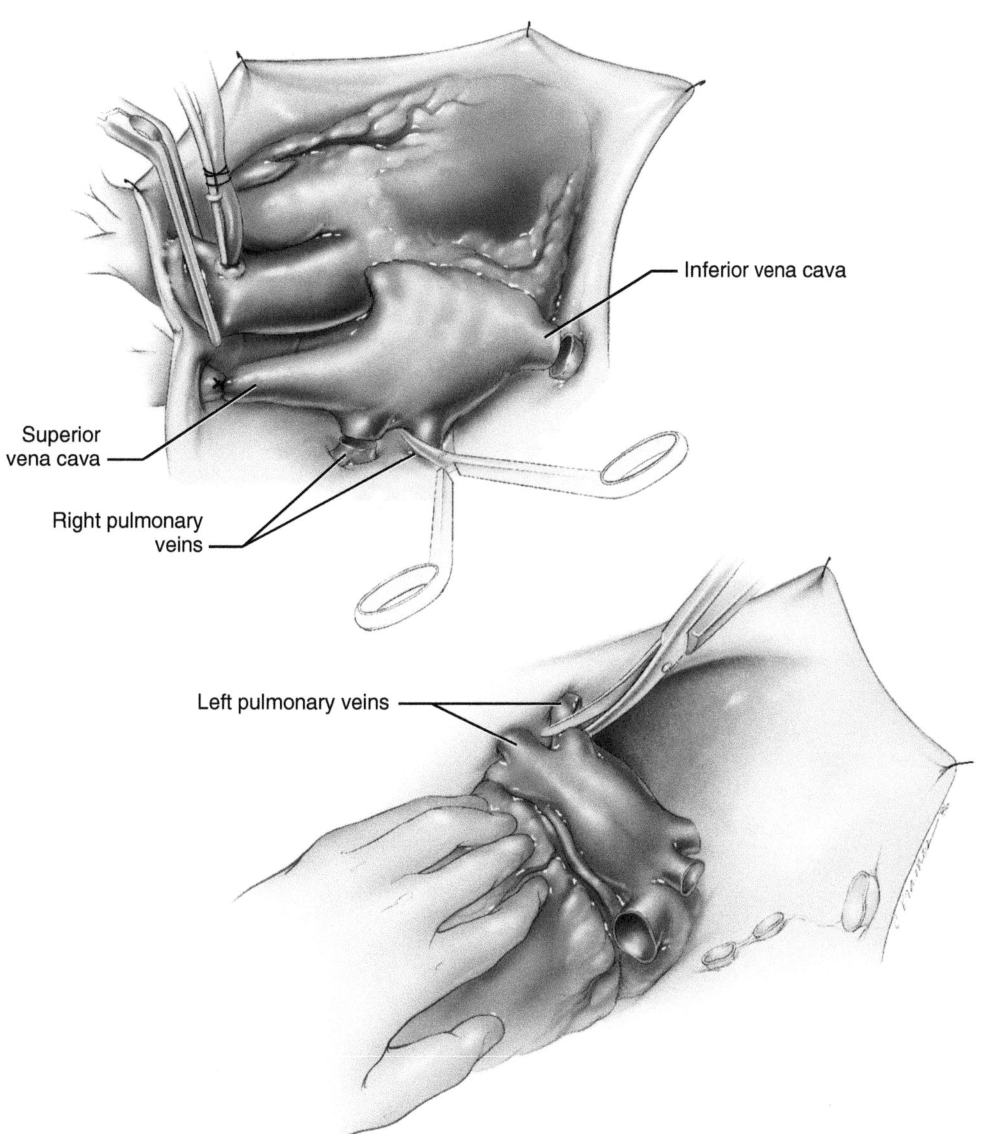
A
Inferior vena cava
Superior vena cava
Right pulmonary veins
Left pulmonary veins

Figure 40-2 (continued)

B Downward traction alongside the aorta and pulmonary artery exposes the maximal length of these vessels. The aorta is divided at the origin of the right brachiocephalic artery. The left pulmonary artery is divided at the pericardial reflection. The superior vena cava is divided at the pericardial reflection above the previously placed ligature, and the right pulmonary artery is divided behind the superior vena cava. All that remains to be divided is the connective tissue behind the left atrium at the pericardial reflection and the lymphatic tissue that lies between the left atrium and the tracheal bifurcation.

C The heart is removed from the body and taken to a back table, where it is immersed in cold isotonic solution. A few minutes are spent trimming the heart and preparing it for implantation. The right pulmonary veins are joined by incision. The left pulmonary veins are treated similarly. The left atrium is opened posteriorly between the pulmonary veins. This provides the maximal available length for the left atrial suture line. The right atrium is opened by incision from the inferior vena cava toward the right atrial appendage. This places the suture line on the right atrium, well away from the sinoatrial node and the intraatrial conduction pathways. The aorta is separated from the pulmonary artery. The pulmonary artery is opened at the bifurcation to preserve the maximal circumference, which may be needed to match the dilated recipient vessel. The cardiac chambers are thoroughly irrigated with cold isotonic solution and inspected to verify the absence of a patent foramen ovale, any other anomaly or abnormality, and any retained debris. The organ is placed in triple sterile plastic bags and transferred to an ice chest for transport.

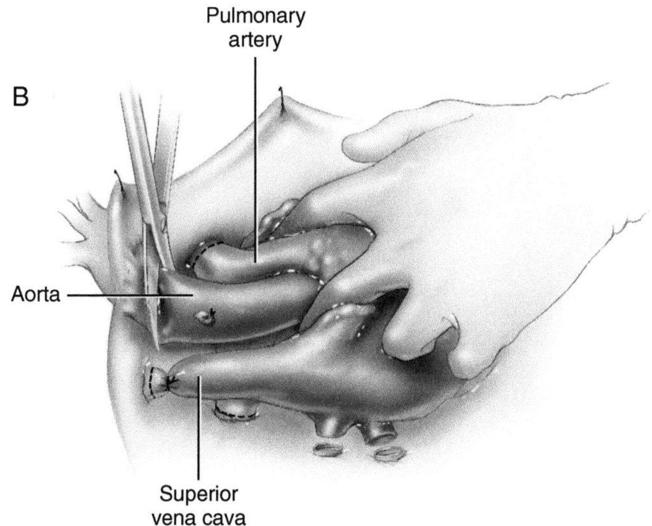
B
Pulmonary
artery
Aorta
Superior
vena cava

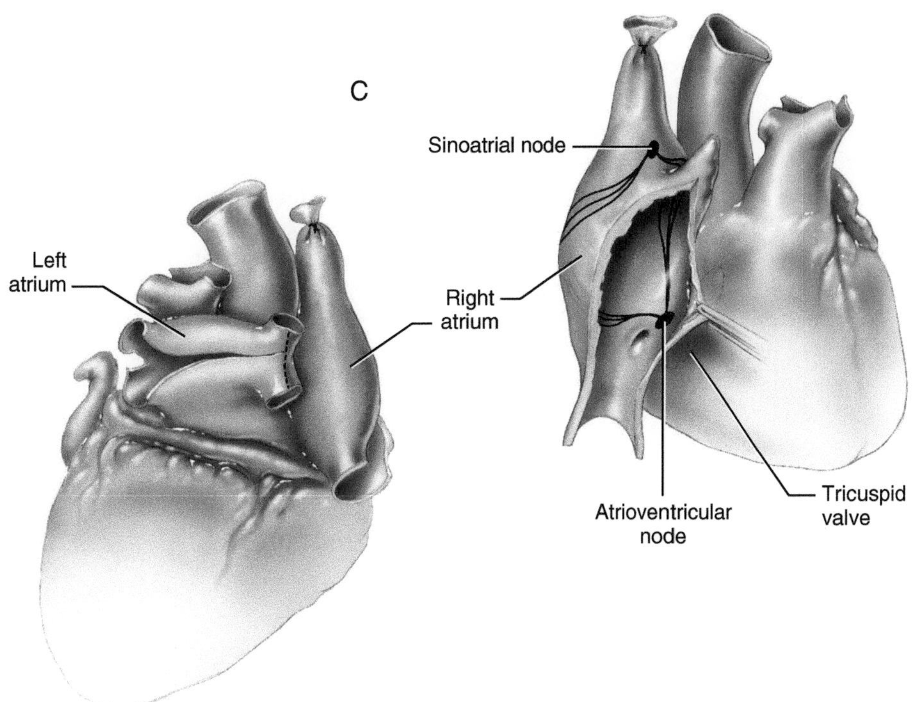
C
Left
atrium
Right
atrium
Sinoatrial node
Atrioventricular
node
Tricuspid
valve

Recipient Operation

The recipient operation is started sufficiently in advance of the arrival of the donor heart to minimize its ischemic time. Recipient cardiectomy usually awaits the arrival of the donor heart in the operating room.

Figure 40-3

Recipient Cardiectomy

A Cardiopulmonary bypass is established using two cannulae for venous drainage, with oxygenated blood returned to the ascending aorta. The venous cannulae are placed through incisions within purse-string stitches located well posteriorly on the right atrium and passed into the venae cavae. Right-angled cannulae may be used, and the superior vena cava may be cannulated directly. The cavae are closed around the cannulae with tourniquets. The aorta is occluded proximal to the perfusion cannula. The right atrium is incised parallel to the atrioventricular groove. This incision is extended superiorly toward the left atrium and inferiorly to a convenient place medial to the inferior vena cava. The incision must stay close to the atrioventricular groove at the inferior vena cava junction to preserve as much tissue as possible in this area.

B The heart is retracted superiorly to expose the left atrium. The left atrium is opened, and the blood is allowed to escape. At this point, with the heart completely empty, cardiectomy becomes much easier. The left atrial incision is extended to the right until it approaches the incision previously made in the right atrium. The septum lies between these two incisions. The incisions are joined, and the septum is partially incised. The left atrial incision is then extended to the left and superiorly, in front of the left pulmonary veins and behind the left atrial appendage.

C The aorta is divided just above the sinus rim. The pulmonary artery is also divided above the sinus rim. The proximal ends of the aorta and pulmonary artery are retracted inferiorly to expose the superior aspect of the left atrium. The right atrial incision is extended across the atrial septum into the left atrium.

D At this point, the septum can be easily visualized and incised. All that remains to be divided is a short segment of the superior aspect of the left atrium so that the heart can be removed. The distal aorta and pulmonary artery are separated by incision of the connective tissue between them.

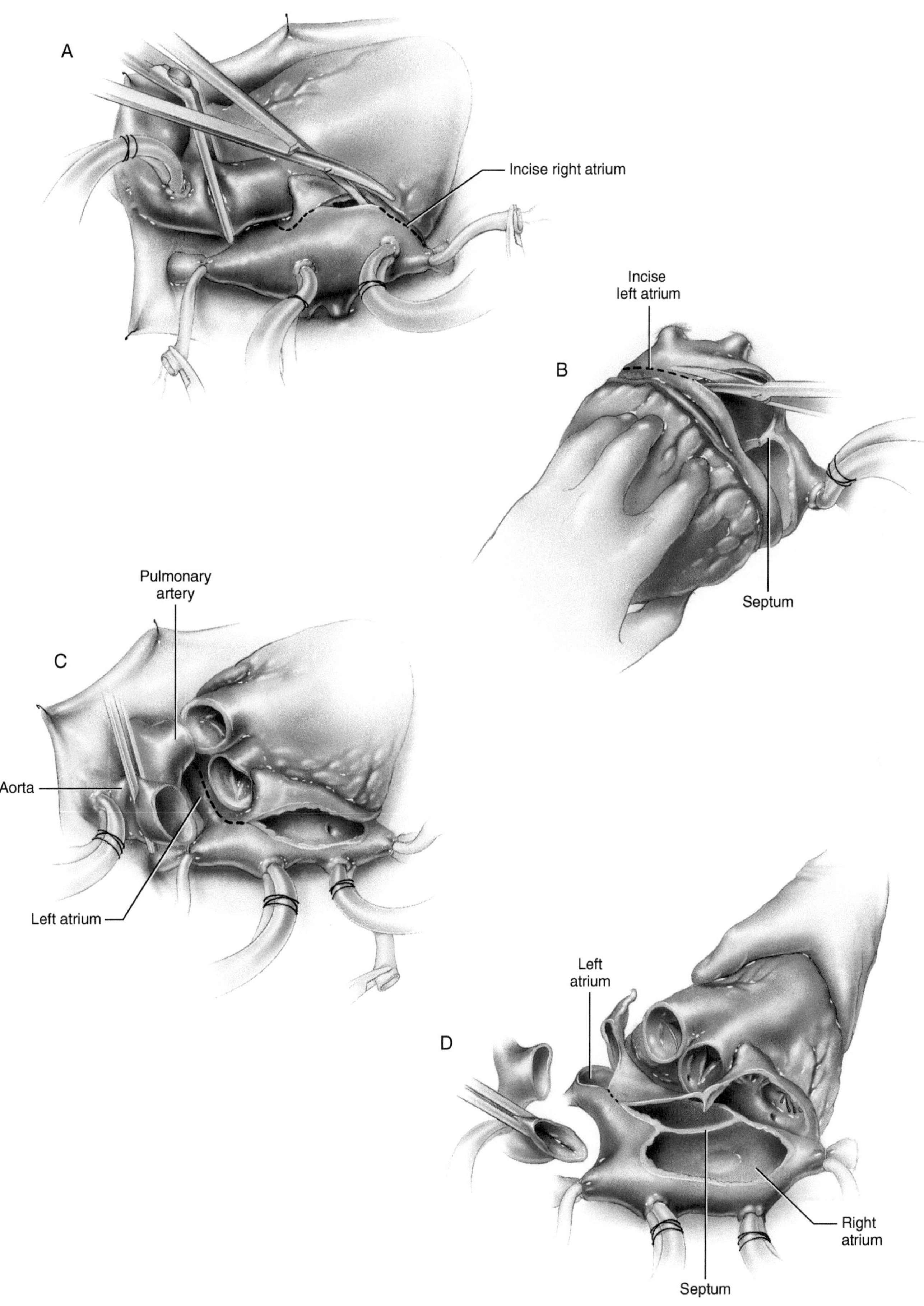
A
Incise right atrium
Incise
left atrium
B
Septum
Pulmonary
artery
C
Aorta
Left atrium
Left
atrium
D
Right
atrium
Septum

Figure 40-3 (continued)

Implantation of the Donor Heart

The donor heart is brought into the operating field. A final check of the trimming of the suture lines is performed, and the cardiac chambers are reexamined.

E Stay ligatures are placed through the recipient left atrium, at its junction with the septum superiorly and inferiorly. This maneuver helps straighten the cut edge of the recipient left atrium and makes it easier to approximate the tissues, especially inferiorly. Long suture (54 inch) with needles at both ends is used. Suture material of 3/0 polypropylene is preferred. The donor heart is oriented so that the left atrial appendage is clearly identified. The suture line joining the left atria is started from the endocardial surface of the donor left atrium below the left atrial appendage. The needle is passed from outside the left atrium of the recipient into the chamber just above the left superior pulmonary vein. Three or four suture loops are placed between the donor and recipient left atria, proceeding inferiorly, before pulling up the suture and bringing the donor heart into the pericardial sac. The suture line proceeds from the endocardial surface of the donor heart inferiorly and to the right, to the junction of the left atrium and the atrial septum. The opposite needle is already on the inside of the donor heart so that it can be passed from inside the recipient left atrium when performing the anastomosis superiorly.

F The anastomosis of the left atria is completed by bringing the suture line across from the left atrium onto the atrial septum. The recipient left atrium along the area of the right pulmonary veins is attached to the atrial septum.

G The anastomosis of the right atria commences with the septal closure. The posterior edge of the right atriotomy of the donor heart is approximated to the atrial septum. It should be noted that the left atrium has already been anastomosed to the septum, so the right atrium is approximated by oversewing the previously placed suture line. At the superior end of the septum, the right atrial suture line is deviated away from the septum onto the recipient right atrium.

H The suture line is continued around the right atrium below the superior vena cava. The inferior portion of the suture line around the inferior vena cava may be difficult to complete unless care was taken to keep the line of atrial excision close to the atrioventricular groove. Assuming this precaution has been taken, the suture line is completed around the inferior vena cava by gaining exposure through retraction of the inferior venous uptake cannula. The right atrial anastomosis is completed laterally.

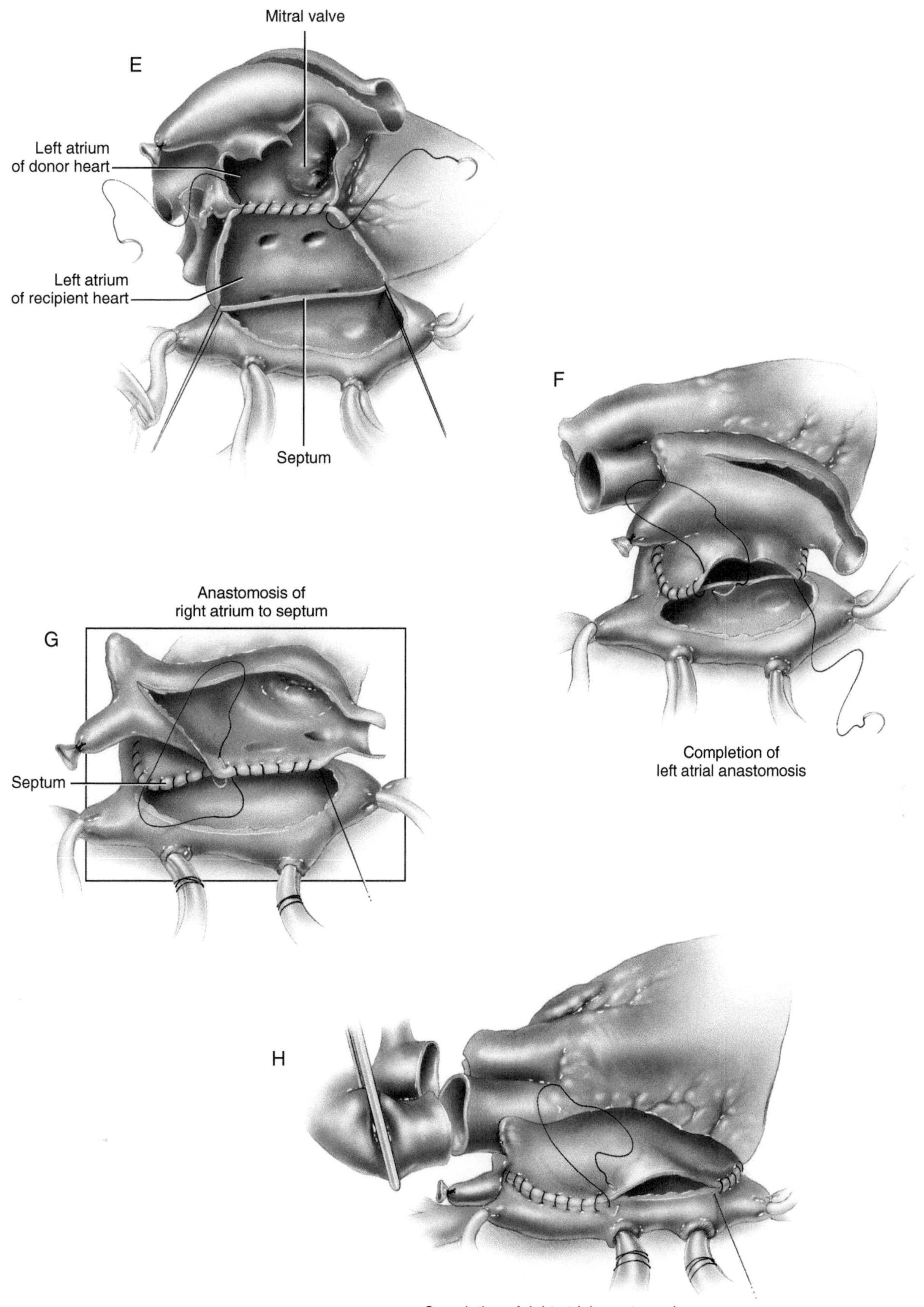

Completion of left atrial anastomosis

Completion of right atrial anastomosis

Figure 40-3 (continued)

I Anastomosis of the donor and recipient pulmonary arteries is performed after tailoring the donor artery to an appropriate circumference. While the anastomosis is being performed, visibility in the operating field is enhanced by aspirating blood from the distal pulmonary artery and occasionally massaging the heart gently to expel blood from the aorta. A continuous stitch technique with 4/0 polypropylene and double needles is used. The initial stitch is placed from outside to inside the recipient pulmonary artery at the left lateral aspect of the vessel. The needle is then passed from inside to outside the donor pulmonary artery on the lateral aspect of the vessel. The needle is returned to the inside of the recipient vessel, setting up a situation whereby the sutures can be placed from inside the donor vessel in continuous fashion, working toward the operator. The anastomosis is interrupted once the suture line reaches a convenient point on the anteromedial aspect of the pulmonary arteries. The suture line is then continued with the opposite needle, working from outside the donor vessel and proceeding toward the surgeon. The anastomosis is completed anteriorly, but the suture is left untied until later to allow the removal of air from the right cardiac chambers.

J The anastomosis of the donor aorta and recipient aorta proceeds in exactly the same fashion as for the pulmonary arteries. Before final closure of the aorta and pulmonary artery, blood is allowed to reenter the heart, which is gently massaged to expel air. The anastomoses are then secured, a vent needle is placed in the aorta, and the heart is reperfused by removal of the aortic clamp.

I

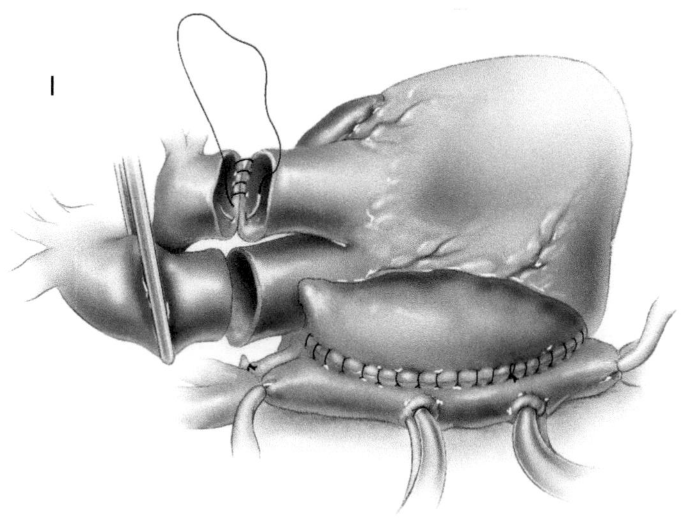

Anastomosis of pulmonary artery

J

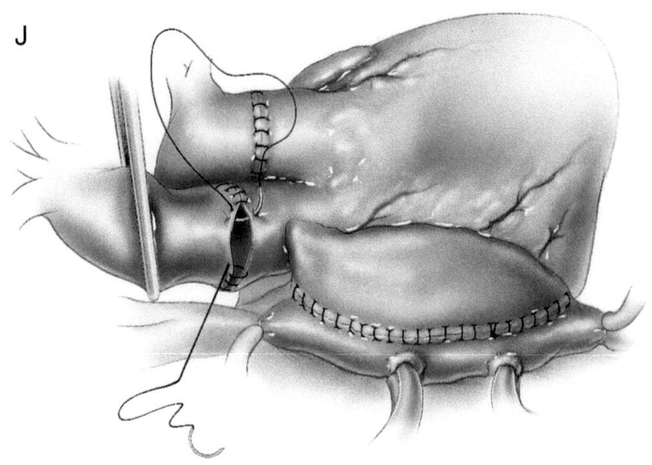

Anastomosis of aorta

Bicaval Anastomosis Technique

Standard techniques of heart transplantation retain the right and left atria of both donor and recipient. The resultant increased volume of the atria may predispose to atrial arrhythmia and incompetence of the tricuspid valve. Direct bicaval venous anastomosis achieves a more anatomic position of the donor heart in the thorax. There is less tricuspid valve incompetence and better hemodynamic performance of the donor heart when this implantation technique is used.

Figure 40-4

A The donor heart is prepared by retaining as much superior vena cava as possible. There is usually quite a large opening into the right atrium at the inferior vena cava because of the requirements for liver transplantation in multiorgan removal procedures. The left atrium is opened through the middle of the posterior wall. The atrial septum is checked for defects, and any deficiency is repaired.

B Recipient cardiectomy proceeds as usual, with excision of the atria near the atrioventricular groove. The *dashed lines* in this illustration show the line of cardiac excision. Venous uptake cannulae are placed directly in the superior vena cava at the pericardial reflection and in the inferior vena cava through the right atrium as low as possible, near the diaphragm.

C To complete the cardiac excision, the aorta and pulmonary artery are divided above the sinus rim. The left atrium is removed except for a bridge posteriorly, which joins the right and left pulmonary veins. The superior vena cava is divided at a comfortable length below the uptake cannula. A generous rim of right atrium is retained inferiorly above the uptake cannula for ease of anastomosis. Removal of too much atrium at the lower end makes anastomosis very difficult.

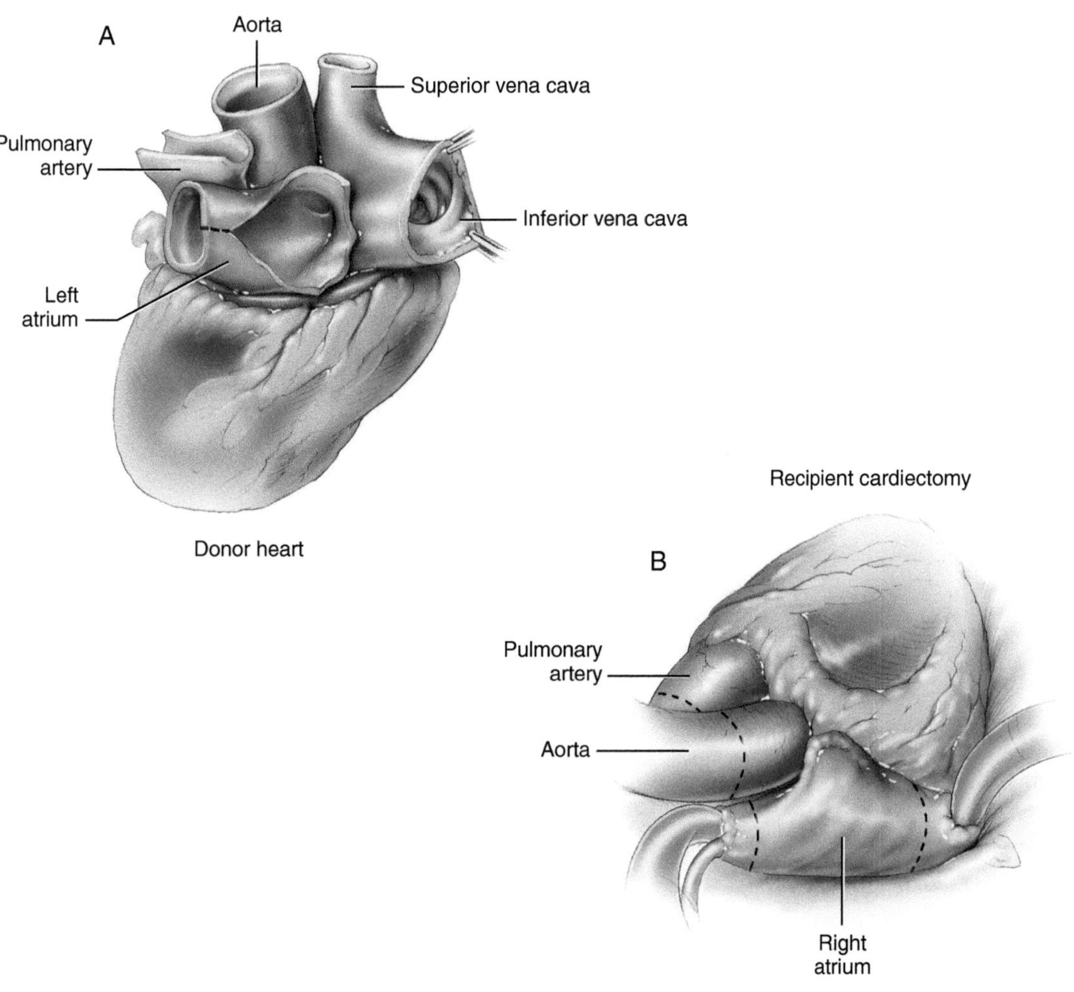

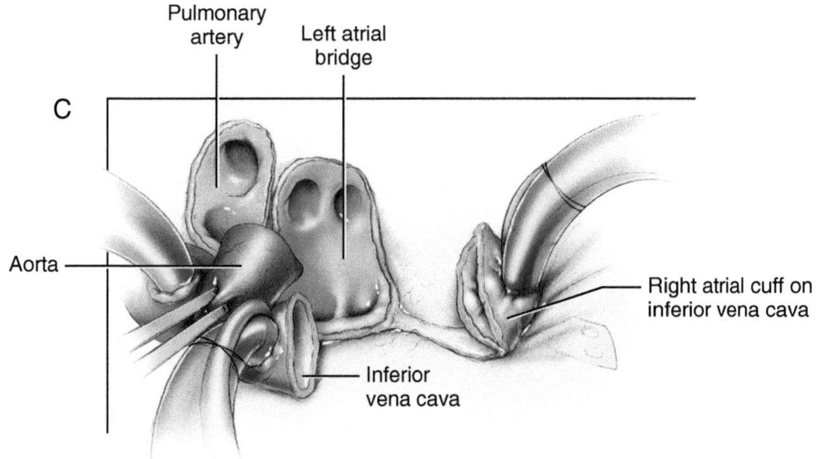

Completed cardiectomy

Figure 40-4 (continued)

D The left atria are anastomosed using continuous stitches of 3/0 polypropylene. The reduced perimeter of the recipient left atrium makes this anastomosis easier than in the "classic" technique.

E The anastomosis of the left atria is completed laterally over the right pulmonary veins. The septum of the donor is intact, so the double suture line for septal reconstruction used in a standard repair is not necessary.

F The anastomosis of the inferior venae cavae is performed. This is the most fixed point in the atrial anastomosis and has the least possibility for adjustment in location. Continuous stitches of 3/0 polypropylene are appropriate for this anastomosis. The use of a small half-circle needle is helpful.

G An end-to-end anastomosis of the superior venae cavae is performed using continuous stitches of 5/0 polypropylene. The donor superior vena cava is shortened to exactly the right length. There is no advantage in leaving excess length on the superior vena cava to reduce tension. In fact, extra length may cause the vena cava to kink, predisposing to thrombosis or making passage of a bioptome more difficult later.

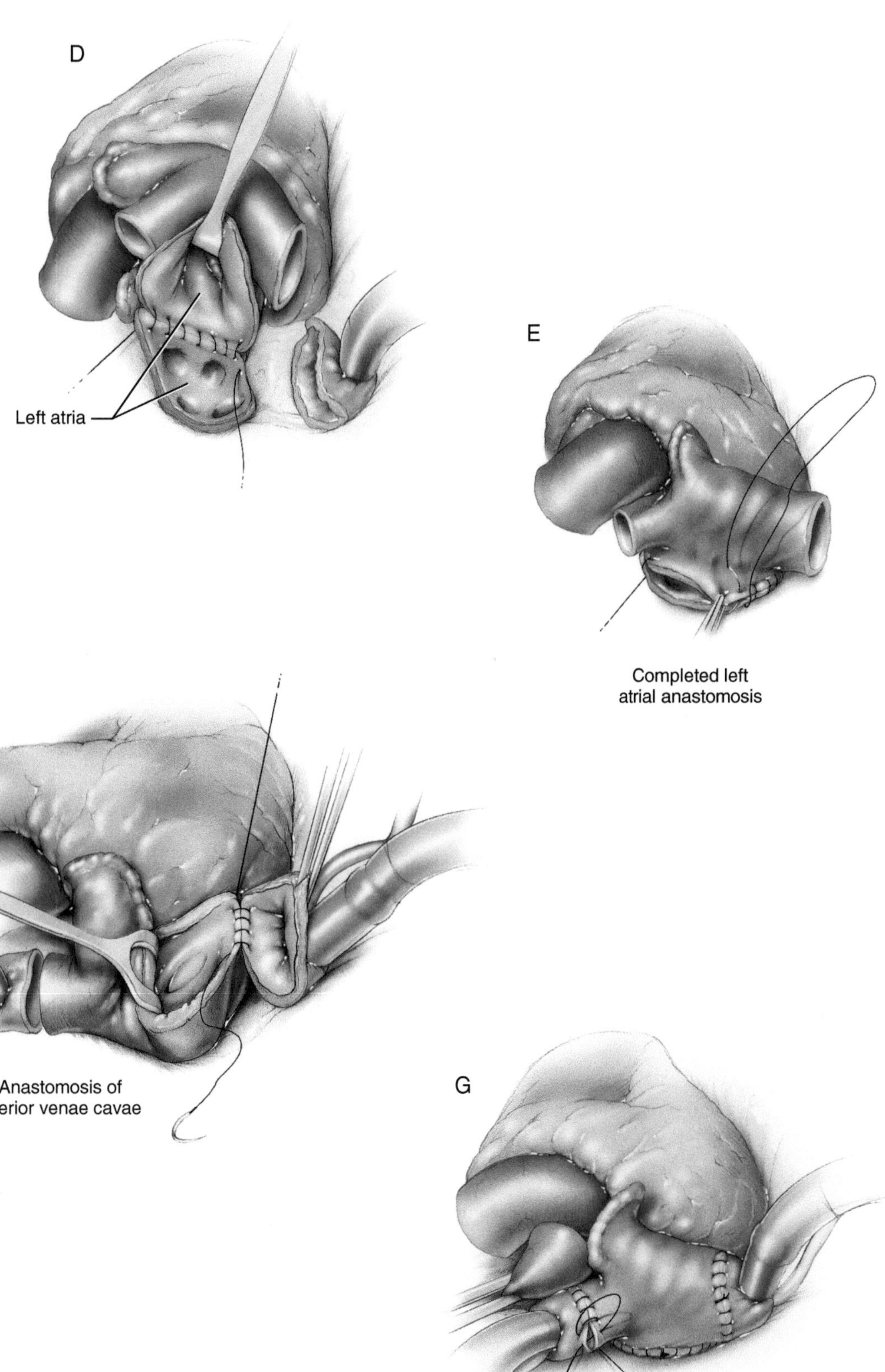
D
Left atria
E
Completed left
atrial anastomosis
F
Anastomosis of
inferior venae cavae
G
Anastomosis of
superior venae cavae

chapter 41 SPECIAL PROCEDURES IN CARDIAC TRANSPLANTATION

Left Thoracotomy

In contemporary practice, cardiac transplantation is occasionally undertaken in patients who have undergone previous cardiac procedures that render reentry by midsternal incision impractical or inadvisable. Prior sternal wound infection is an obvious case in which a midline incision is best avoided. In these patients, cardiac transplantation can be performed through a left anterior thoracotomy. The procedure is technically more demanding than a midline approach, but it is certainly feasible and may be preferable to a dangerous reentry.

Figure 41-1

A Cardiopulmonary bypass is established by cannulation of the right ventricle with a single venous uptake cannula, with oxygenated blood returned to the descending thoracic aorta. The venous cannula is simple to insert in the dilated right ventricle through a purse-string stitch for retention. The aortic return site is conveniently located at the posterior margin of the exposure.

B The body temperature is reduced to 20°C by the usual core-cooling technique. The circulation from the bypass pump is temporarily stopped, and the venous cannula is removed. The heart is excised, and the great vessels are divided. The lateral wall of the right atrium is easily exposed once the enlarged heart is out of the chest. Purse-string stitches are placed in the wall of the right atrium and the superior vena cava. Venous uptake cannulae are inserted, passing them into the superior and inferior venae cavae. Caval tourniquets are secured, and bypass flow is restored. Circulatory arrest is required for about 10 to 15 minutes during this part of the procedure.

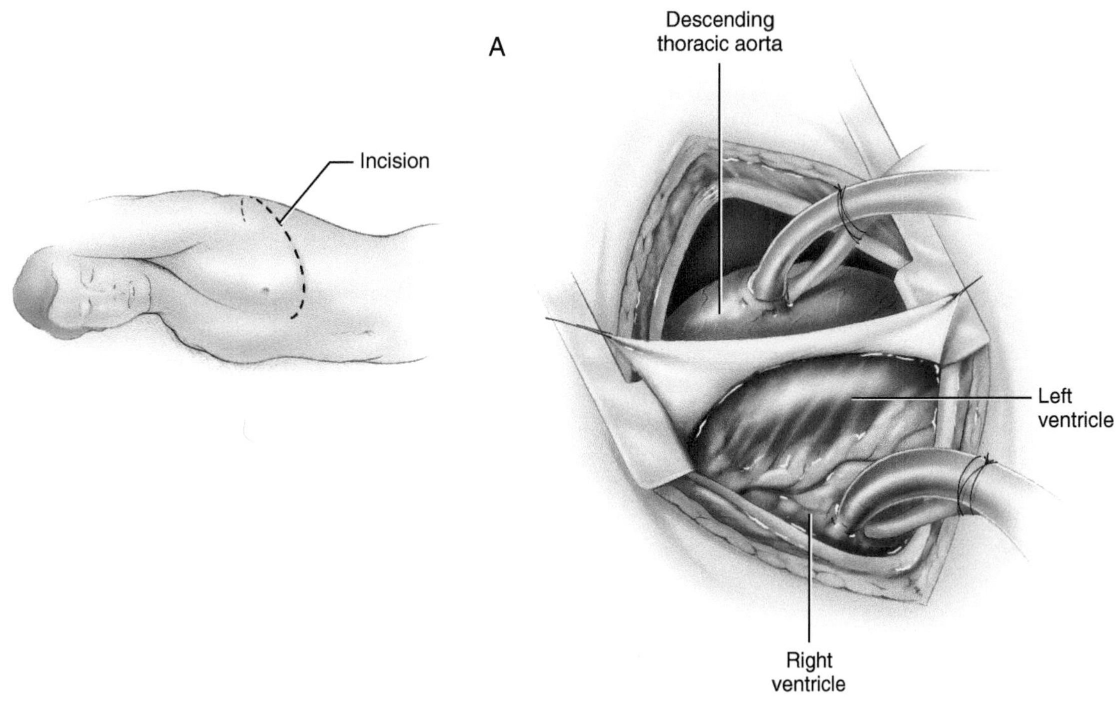
A
Descending thoracic aorta
Incision
Left ventricle
Right ventricle

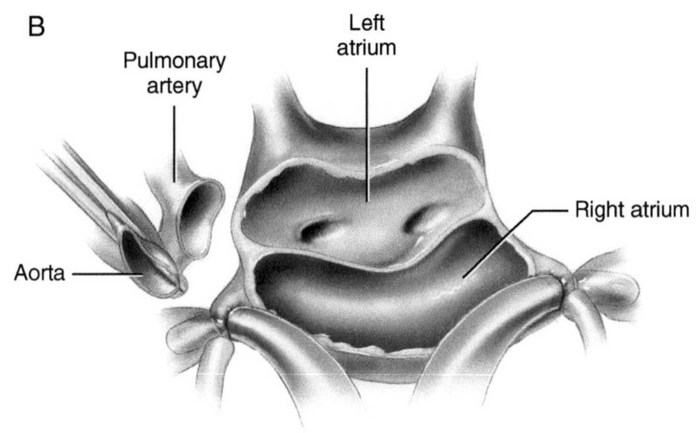
B
Left atrium
Pulmonary artery
Right atrium
Aorta

Figure 41-1 (continued)

C One would imagine that the exposure for implantation of the donor heart would be difficult. Actually, the orientation is simply rotated 90 degrees anteriorly, and the arrangement of the atria is such that the operation proceeds exactly as it would for a midline anastomosis of the atria. The only difficult part is that the heart must be held anteriorly rather than allowing it to lie back in the pericardium, as is the practice when working through a midsternal incision. The suturing begins in the left atrium near the appendage and proceeds inferiorly to the atrial septum, then superiorly to complete the joining of the left atria.

D As in usual transplant operations, a double septal suture line is placed as the posterior edge of the right atriotomy of the donor heart is folded back to the septum of the recipient. The right atrial anastomosis is completed anteriorly.

E The great vessel anastomoses overlie each other more in the left approach than they do in the midline operation. The aortic anastomosis is performed in an end-to-end fashion. Attention to detail during suture placement is especially important because the anastomosis will be covered by the pulmonary artery. The pulmonary artery anastomosis is the final step of the operation.

F Decannulation of the atrium may provoke some anxiety because the stab incisions in the right atrium and superior vena cava are relatively inaccessible. They can be reached, however, if necessary. Normally, once the transplant is complete, the apex of the heart is oriented anteriorly into the thoracotomy wound. When the patient is placed supine, the transplant settles into its natural position.

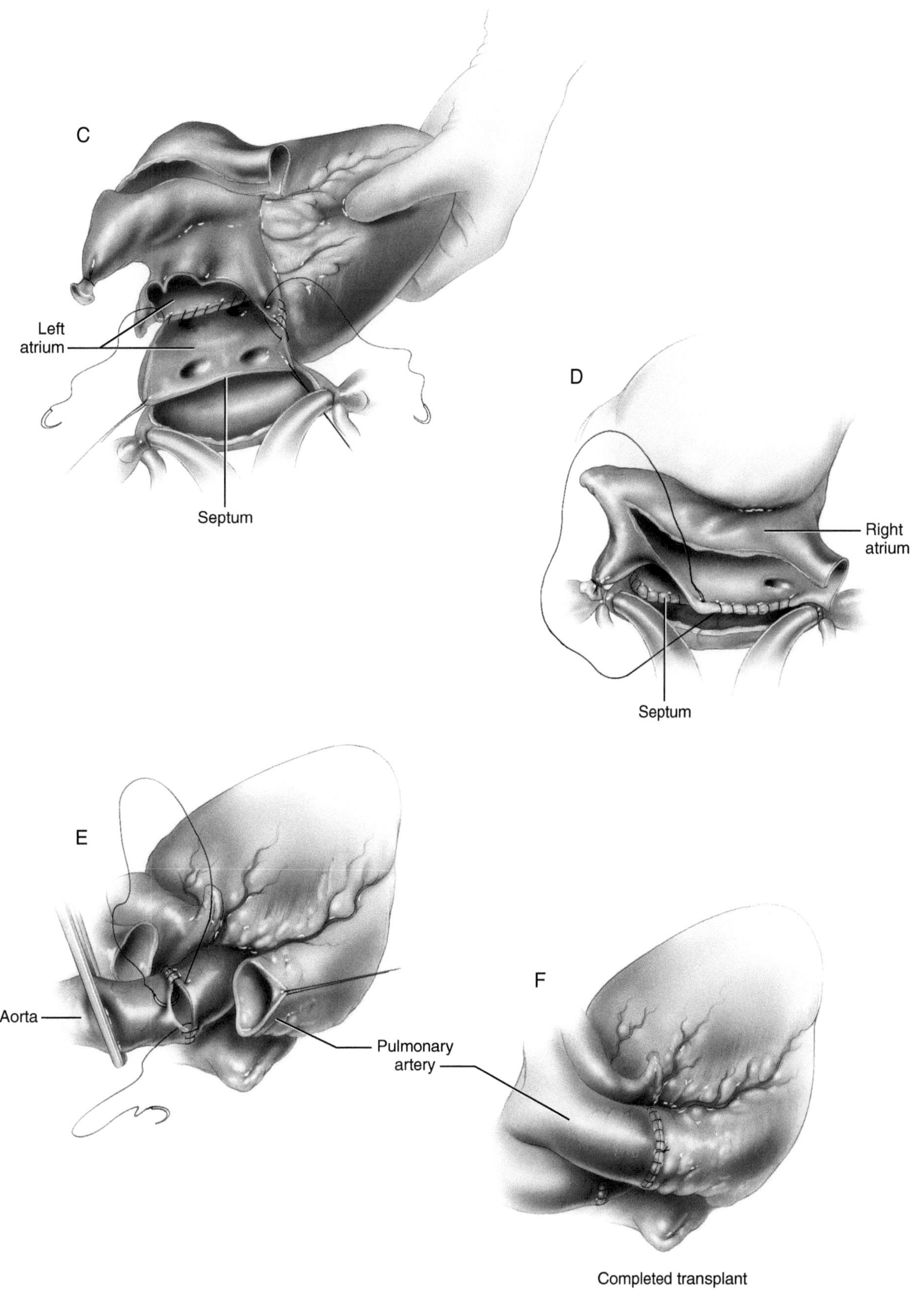
C
Left atrium
Septum
D
Right atrium
Septum
E
Aorta
Pulmonary artery
F
Completed transplant

Transposition of the Great Arteries

Many congenital cardiac anomalies that eventually require cardiac transplantation, especially those with single ventricles, may include transposition of the great arteries. The abnormal position of the great arteries might suggest that cardiac transplantation would be extraordinarily difficult. Actually, it is not difficult at all to directly anastomose the great arteries, and no prosthetic material is required.

Figure 41-2

A The heart is cannulated and excised in the usual manner, retaining as much of the aorta as possible.

B Knowledge of the location of the great vessels at the pericardial reflection is key to understanding the simplicity of heart transplantation when there is transposition of the great arteries. The location of the venae cavae and pulmonary veins is normal, and the left atrium is always a midline structure. Thus, anastomosis of the atria proceeds as usual. The pulmonary artery bifurcation is essentially a midline structure, regardless of the orientation of the great arteries at their origin from the ventricles of the heart. Similarly, the aorta assumes a position anterior and to the right of the pulmonary artery at the pericardial reflection, regardless of whether the great arteries are normally related or transposed.

C The keys to performing heart transplantation when there is transposition of the great arteries are thorough mobilization of the aorta up to the pericardial reflection and separation of the aorta from the pulmonary artery. Retaining adequate length on both recipient and donor aortae allows the transposed recipient aorta to be shifted to a normal position and normal relationship with the normally related donor aorta.

D End-to-end anastomosis of the great arteries is possible after mobilization and shifting of the recipient aorta. The pulmonary arteries usually match up nicely, although it may be necessary to excise the recipient pulmonary artery up to the bifurcation or perhaps extend an incision to the right or left to accommodate the donor heart. The donor aortic arch should be retained so that tailoring the ends of the donor and recipient aortae allows good approximation.

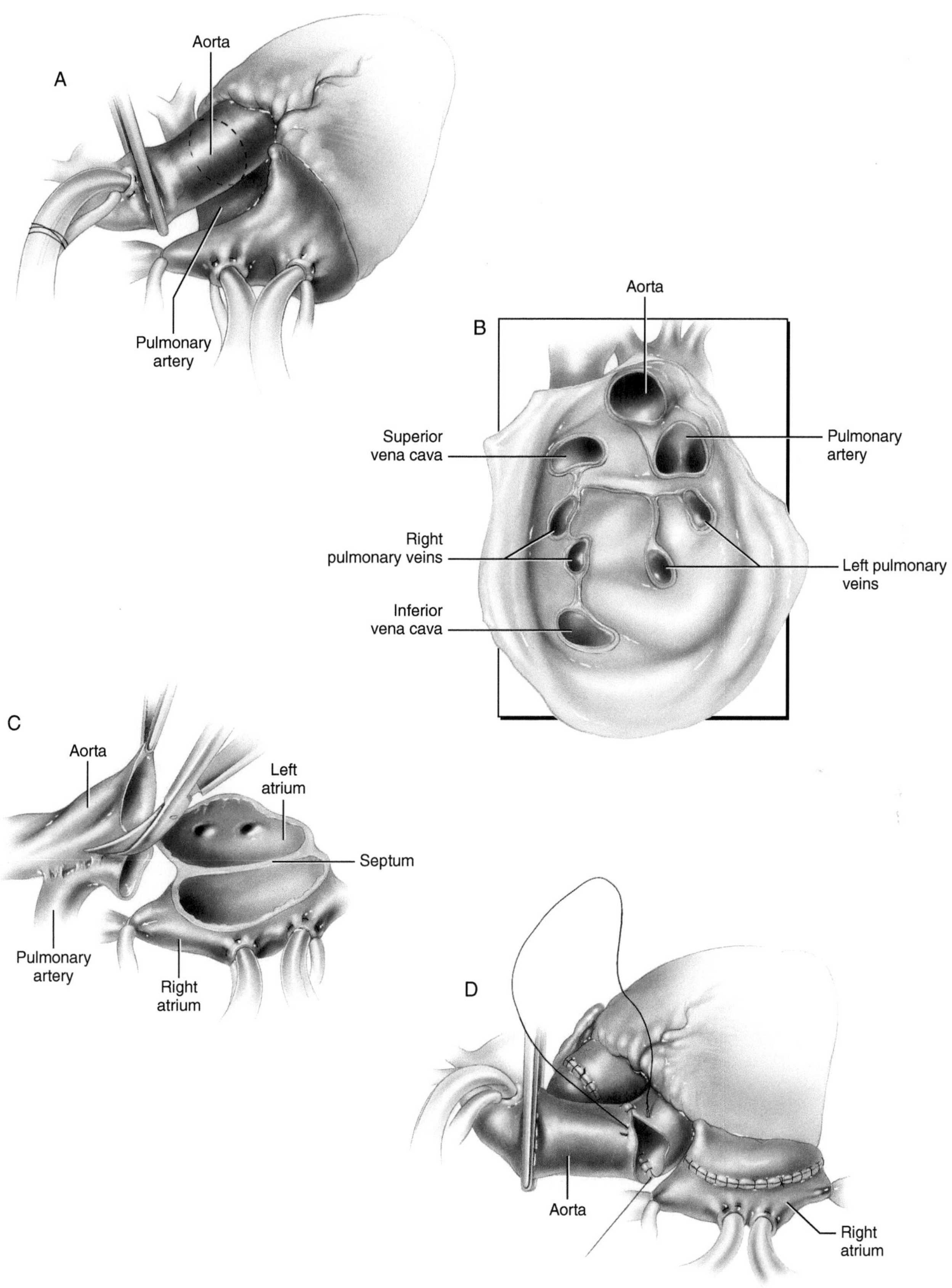
A
Aorta
Pulmonary artery
B
Aorta
Superior vena cava
Pulmonary artery
Right pulmonary veins
Left pulmonary veins
Inferior vena cava
C
Aorta
Left atrium
Septum
Pulmonary artery
Right atrium
D
Aorta
Right atrium

Situs Inversus

Cardiac transplantation in a patient with situs inversus is a significant technical challenge. The complete reversal of the anatomic position of the systemic venous return to the heart does not permit a simple operation. A systemic venous passageway to provide direct access to the right ventricle of the transplanted heart is essential to allow biopsy to monitor for immunological rejection patterns. The bioptome requires a nearly straight pathway to the right ventricle, and circuitous pathways are almost impossible to negotiate. Even in cases of situs inversus, some constants remain: the aorta is nearly always anterior and to the right of the pulmonary artery at the pericardial reflection; the pulmonary bifurcation is essentially midline, even in the most complex anomalies; and the left atrium is a midline structure that receives the pulmonary veins from the right and left sides. Thus, it is the systemic venous structures in a patient with situs inversus that must be mated to a donor heart with a normal situs (solitus). Systemic venous reconstruction is the key to the operation.

Figure 41-3

A Illustrated is a complex congenital anomaly that might be encountered in a patient presenting for cardiac transplantation. There is a single ventricle and transposition of the great arteries, with accompanying situs inversus of the viscera and atria and discordant positions of the atria and ventricles. The apex of the single ventricle presents to the right. The cavae enter the right atrium (RA) to the left side. When the heart is excised, as much length of the aorta (Ao) and pulmonary artery (PA) as possible should be preserved. The superior vena cava (SVC) must be excised for translocation to the right. IVC, inferior vena cava; LA, left atrium; LV, left ventricle; RV, right ventricle.

B Cannulation for cardiopulmonary bypass is performed with two cannulae for venous drainage. Venous drainage of the upper compartment is via a cannula passed into the left internal jugular–innominate vein junction. The inferior vena cava is cannulated at the diaphragm on the left side. Oxygenated blood is returned to the ascending aorta. The patient is perfused with cold blood to reduce body temperature in preparation for temporary circulatory arrest. The heart is excised during the cooling period. The empty pericardium is visualized with the right atrium anterior and to the left side. The left atrium is somewhat to the left but related to the midline. The superior vena cava is excised, and the ends are oversewn.

C The excised segment of the superior vena cava is translocated to the right side, where an end-to-side anastomosis is made to the innominate vein directly below the right internal jugular vein. This provides a passageway to the right side of the transplanted heart for biopsy. The innominate vein is higher than one might imagine on the right side, and the new superior vena cava will be much longer than anticipated.

D The right atrium is separated from the atrial septum and mobilized completely away from the left atrium, without disrupting the attachment to the inferior vena cava. The right atrial remnant will form the extension of the inferior vena cava to the right side. Removal of the right atrium will also provide the opening required for the donor apex to lie in its natural position to the left.

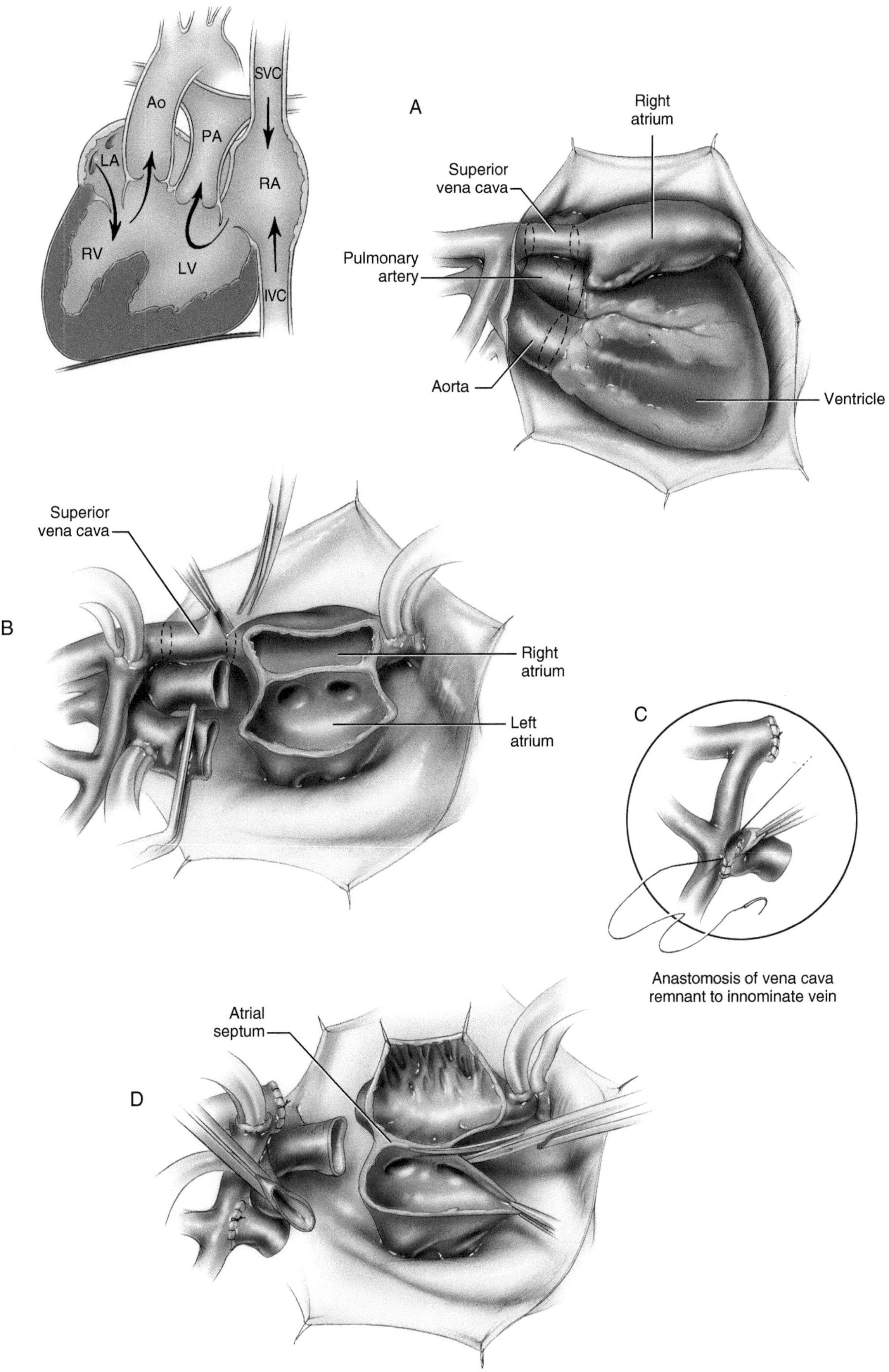

Ao
SVC
PA
LA
RA
RV
LV
IVC
A
Right atrium
Superior vena cava
Pulmonary artery
Aorta
Ventricle
Superior vena cava
B
Right atrium
Left atrium
C
Anastomosis of vena cava remnant to innominate vein
Atrial septum
D

Figure 41-3 (continued)

E The pericardium is incised on the left side back to the phrenic nerve, and the left pleural space is opened widely to accommodate the apex of the ventricle of the donor heart to the left side. Reconstruction of the inferior vena cava proceeds under circulatory arrest so that the inferior vena cava cannula can be removed for accurate visualization of the caval orifice. A composite passageway to the right side is created using the remnant of the right atrium and the pericardium over the diaphragm. The inferior vena cava is carefully cut back medially to the level of the diaphragm. Continuous stitches of 3/0 or 4/0 polypropylene are used to anastomose the caval orifice to the pericardium of the diaphragm.

F Double-ended needles are used to continue the suture lines in two parallel rows, attaching the right atrial remnant as the roof of a tunnel created on the pericardium of the diaphragm. A tunnel is required to divert the inferior vena cava to the right side to the point where it would naturally enter the pericardial sac. Some tailoring of the right atrial remnant is required to achieve a tunnel of the appropriate dimensions and configuration. The operation up to this point should be completed before arrival of the donor heart. This requires some coordination because at least an hour of cardiopulmonary bypass time will be consumed to complete this stage of the operation.

G The donor heart is excised, preserving as much systemic vein as possible. The entire inferior and superior venae cavae and the innominate vein are required. Maximal length of the aorta and pulmonary artery is also required. Preservation of the entire aortic arch is desirable to ensure sufficient length to compensate for transposition of the great arteries in the recipient.

H Anastomosis of the left atria proceeds as usual, except that the left portion of the recipient left atrium is actually the atrial septum.

I Anastomosis of the great vessels is the next step, leaving the systemic venous anastomoses for last. The pulmonary artery of the donor is anastomosed to the recipient pulmonary artery. Care must be taken to shorten these arteries appropriately. Too much length in the pulmonary arteries can result in kinking and obstruction.

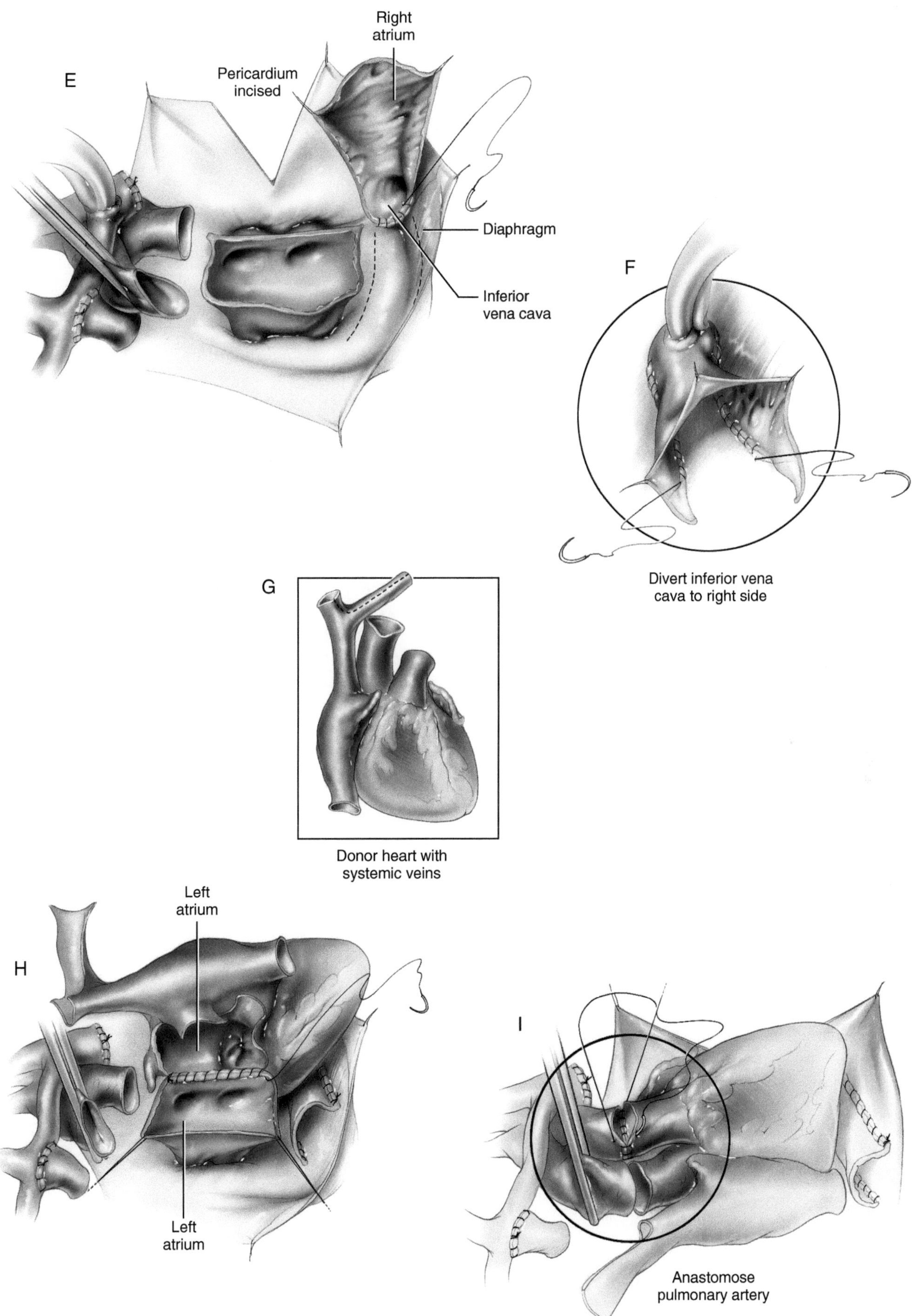
E
Right atrium
Pericardium incised
Diaphragm
Inferior vena cava
F
Divert inferior vena cava to right side
G
Donor heart with systemic veins
H
Left atrium
Left atrium
I
Anastomose pulmonary artery

Figure 41-3 (continued)

J The aortic anastomosis proceeds in end-to-end fashion. The aortic arch of the donor may be required for sufficient length. Complete mobilization of the recipient aorta is essential to allow the aortic anastomosis to assume a natural position anterior and to the right of the pulmonary artery.

K The inferior vena cava of the donor heart is anastomosed to the tunnel extension of the inferior vena cava of the recipient. The lateral aspect of the donor caval opening is anastomosed to the pericardium over the diaphragm at the end of the tunnel passageway.

The anastomosis of the inferior vena cava is completed by joining the medial aspect of the recipient caval opening to the right atrial remnant portion of the tunnel.

L The superior vena cava is reconstructed by creating a composite tunnel. The distance from the innominate vein to the right atrium of the donor heart is too great to bridge by simply joining the translocated superior vena cava to the superior vena cava of the donor heart. In addition, the diameter of the innominate vein is insufficient to serve as an extension of the vena cava. Thus, a composite conduit consisting of the pericardium posteriorly in situ and the opened innominate vein is created. The donor innominate vein is incised longitudinally on the posterior aspect to the caval junction. This incision includes the right internal jugular junction. The translocated recipient superior vena cava is anastomosed to the pericardium along its posterior one third. The left aspect of the innominate vein of the donor is anastomosed to the pericardium.

M The right aspect of the innominate vein is anastomosed to the pericardium. Care should be taken not to separate the parallel suture lines excessively in the hope of creating a larger passageway because a slit-like, obstructed conduit will result. The repair is completed by anastomosing the donor innominate vein to the translocated recipient vena cava anteriorly. The reconstructed composite superior vena cava is very long but provides a nearly straight route from the right internal jugular vein to the right ventricle of the donor heart for a bioptome.

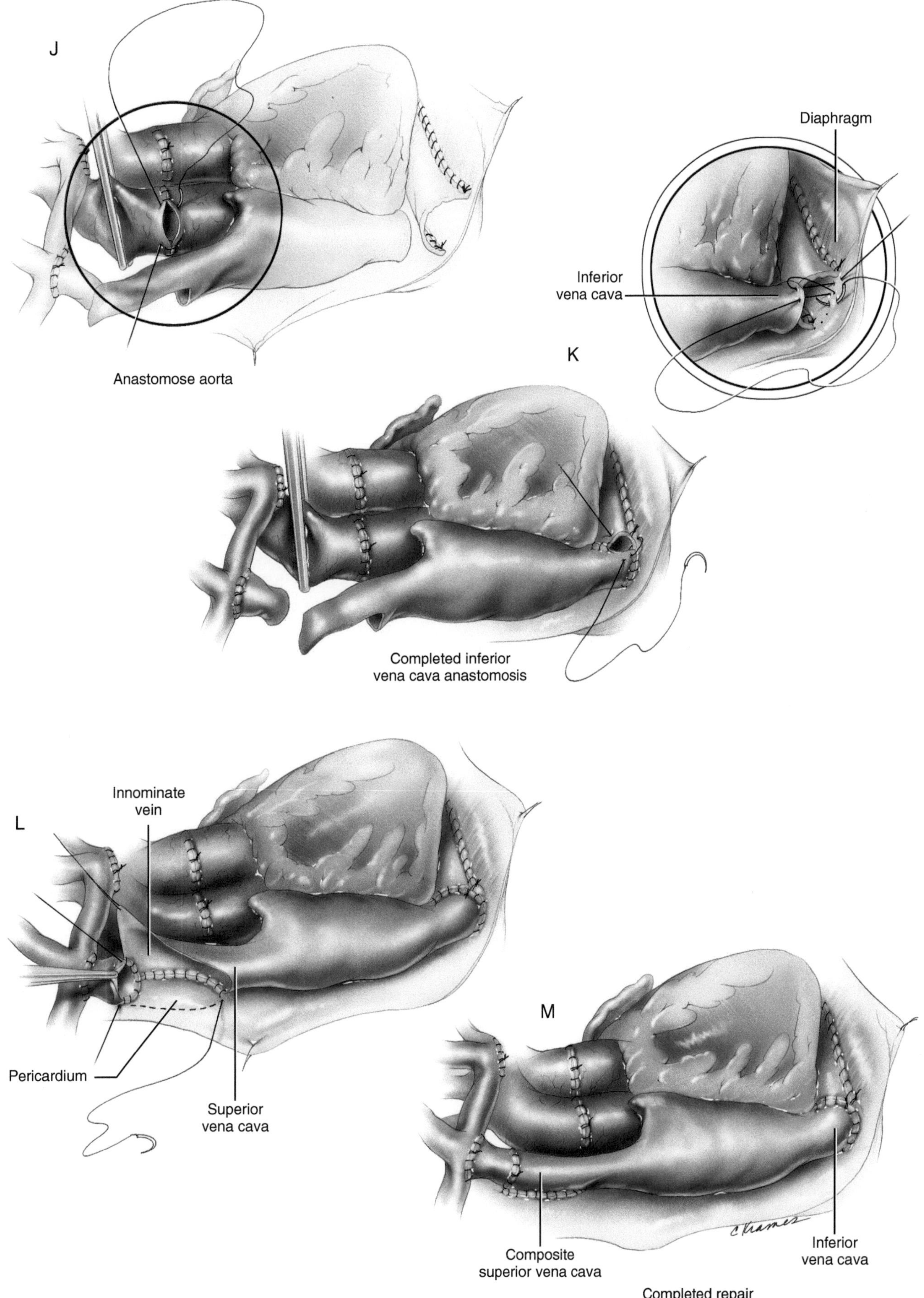
J
Anastomose aorta
Diaphragm
Inferior
vena cava
K
Completed inferior
vena cava anastomosis
L
Innominate
vein
Pericardium
Superior
vena cava
M
Composite
superior vena cava
Inferior
vena cava
Completed repair

Hypoplastic Left Heart Syndrome

Cardiac transplantation in patients with hypoplastic left heart syndrome has become accepted treatment and may be preferable to staged palliative operations. The lack of availability of donor hearts is the major obstacle to more widespread application of this treatment.

Figure 41-4

A Patients presenting with hypoplastic left heart syndrome may have a spectrum of anomalies. Common to all, however, is hypoplasia of the left ventricle and ascending aorta. The aortic arch is usually small as well. There may be associated coarctation of the aorta (Ao). The right ventricle (RV) and pulmonary artery (PA) are usually large, and the ductus arteriosus continues to the descending aorta. The ductus arteriosus must be identified relative to the left pulmonary artery (LPA). The right atrium (RA) may be enlarged due to high pressure and flow through a patent foramen ovale. The superior vena cava (SVC) and inferior vena cava connect normally to the heart.

B The operation is performed with the patient on cardiopulmonary bypass. The superior vena cava is cannulated directly at the pericardial reflection. The inferior vena cava is cannulated through the right atrium (RA) at the diaphragm. Arterial return is to the ductus arteriosus. The pulmonary artery is occluded proximal to the perfusion cannula to prevent flooding of the lungs. The perfusate is cooled to lower the body temperature to 18°C. Excision of the heart is commenced during the cooling phase. The heart is excised in the usual fashion near the atrioventricular groove, retaining most of the atria. When the body temperature reaches the target, cardiopulmonary bypass is discontinued, and much of the operation is accomplished during circulatory arrest. The pulmonary artery is divided at the bifurcation. The aorta is divided near the innominate artery, and the ascending aorta remnant is removed with the heart. The aortic arch is opened through the inferior aspect, and the incision is extended past the ductus arteriosus into the upper portion of the descending thoracic aorta to encompass any coarctated segment. The ductus arteriosus is removed completely, and the pulmonary end is oversewn with 6/0 polypropylene suture. LA, left atrium; RPA, right pulmonary artery.

C The donor heart is excised, along with the entire aortic arch and some of the descending thoracic aorta. The aortic arch of the donor heart is tailored to fit the recipient aortic arch. The left atria are anastomosed using the standard method of cardiac transplantation. This anastomosis fixes the position of the heart so that the lengths of the great vessels on the donor heart can be accurately determined. Continuous stitches of 4/0 polypropylene or polydioxanone are used. Direct caval anastomoses are avoided to prevent subsequent caval stenoses. The donor right atrium is cut back from the inferior vena cava in the usual fashion.

D The donor aortic arch is anastomosed to the recipient aortic arch by continuous stitches of 6/0 or 7/0 polypropylene or polydioxanone, depending on the thickness of the tissues. The most difficult portion of the repair is anastomosis of the distal donor aortic arch to the apex of the aortotomy in the upper portion of the recipient descending thoracic aorta. This repair should be done with complete accuracy because bleeding from this point can be difficult to control. Several suture loops are placed at the apex of the aortotomy before bringing the tissues together. The rest of the arch repair is routine. On completion of the anastomosis of the aortic arch, cardiopulmonary bypass can be reestablished via a perfusion cannula in the ascending aorta of the donor.

Rewarming of the patient is accomplished during the remainder of the transplant procedure. The right atria are anastomosed in standard fashion by continuous suture technique. An end-to-end anastomosis of the pulmonary arteries is performed. LV, left ventricle.

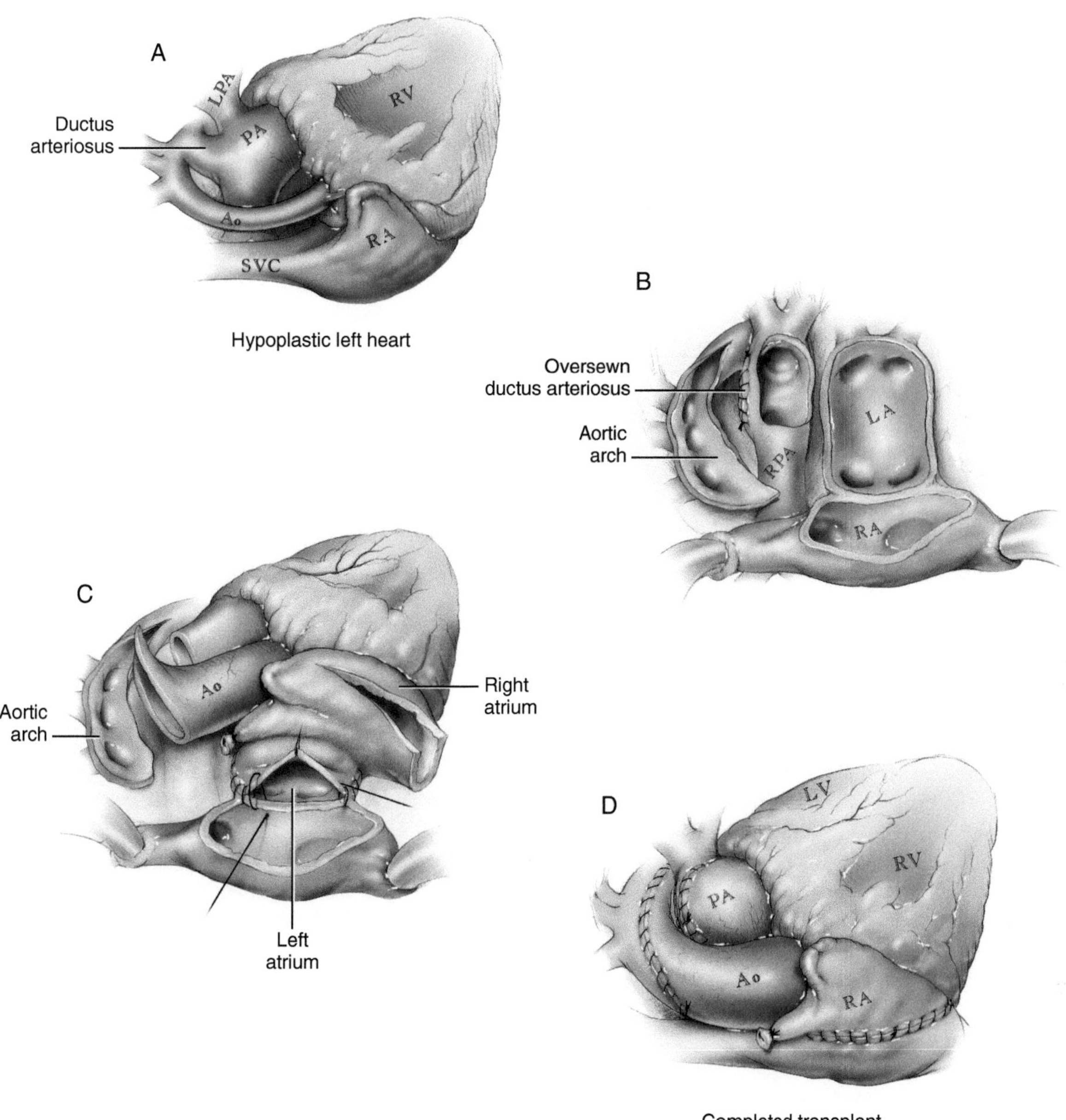
A
LPA
RV
Ductus arteriosus
PA
Ao
RA
SVC
Hypoplastic left heart
B
Oversewn ductus arteriosus
LA
Aortic arch
RPA
RA
C
Ao
Right atrium
Aortic arch
Left atrium
D
LV
RV
PA
Ao
RA
Completed transplant

Cardiac Transplantation After the Fontan Operation

A previous Fontan operation presents significant technical challenges to cardiac transplantation. The general principle in this situation is to excise all tissues that were previously treated surgically and replace them with donor tissue.

Figure 41-5

A This heart has undergone a previous Fontan procedure with bicaval anastomosis. The cardiac transplantation operation is performed with the patient on cardiopulmonary bypass. Venous uptake is via cannulae placed in the inferior vena cava through the right atrium at the diaphragm and in the innominate vein (not shown). Oxygenated blood is returned via a cannula in the ascending aorta or the common femoral artery. The *dashed lines* show where the heart and great vessels are divided to remove all previous suture lines. Direct caval anastomoses are planned for the transplanted heart because these patients are usually older and not at high risk for caval stenoses. The superior vena cava is divided above the bicaval anastomoses, and the right pulmonary artery is divided distal to the previous caval anastomoses. The left pulmonary artery is divided at the bifurcation. The ascending aorta is divided at about the midpoint. The right atrium is separated as a cuff above the inferior vena cava uptake cannula.

B The remnant recipient tissues are shown. Only a bridge of the left atrium between the right and left pulmonary veins is retained. The venae cavae, pulmonary arteries, and aorta are fashioned for direct anastomoses to the donor heart and great vessels.

C The donor heart and great vessels are completely retained. The superior vena cava, innominate vein, and pulmonary arteries are totally retained.

D The donor left atrium is anastomosed posteriorly to a bridge of left atrium that connects the recipient pulmonary veins. The right atrium at the inferior vena cava of the donor heart is anastomosed to the recipient right atrial cuff. The donor superior vena cava is tailored for direct end-to-end anastomosis to the recipient superior vena cava. The right and left pulmonary arteries are anastomosed in end-to-end fashion. An end-to-end anastomosis of the aortae is performed. The great vessel anastomoses are performed using continuous stitches of 4/0 to 6/0 polypropylene, depending on the thickness of the tissues.

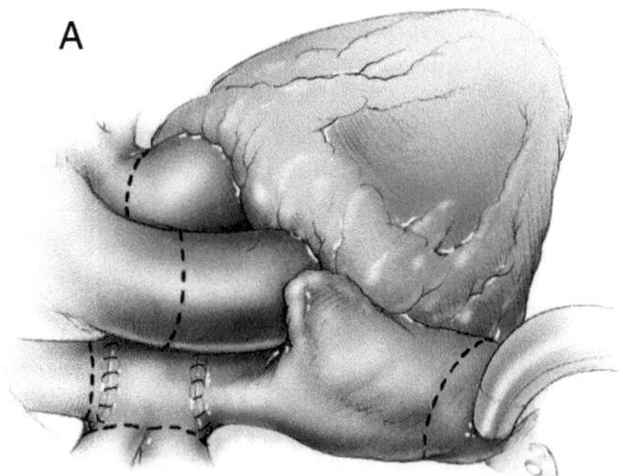

Donor cardiectomy

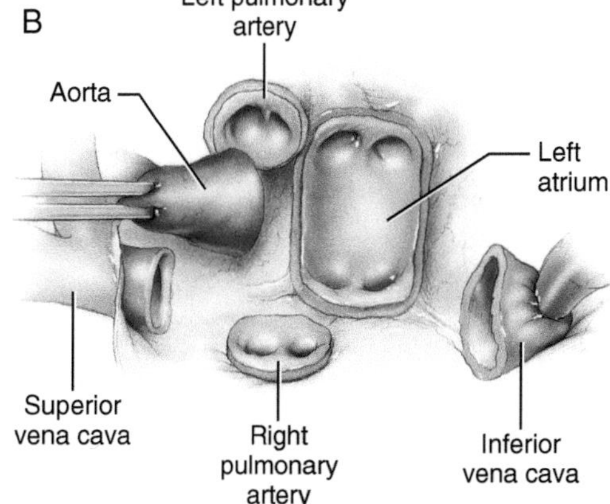

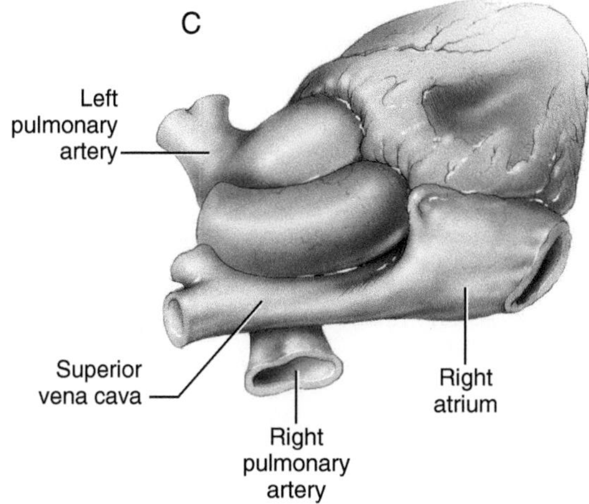

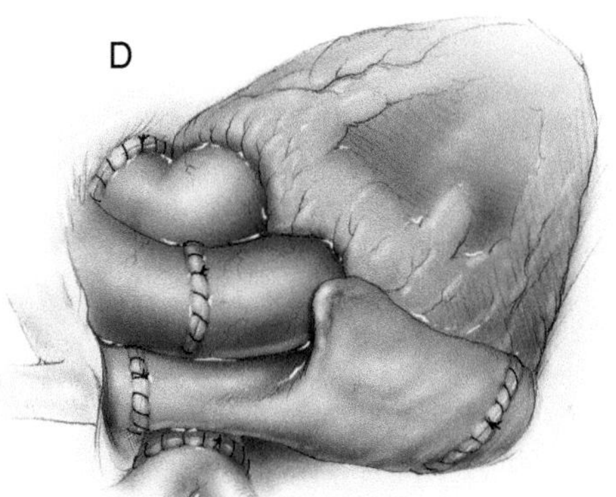

Completed transplant

chapter 42 HEART-LUNG TRANSPLANTATION

Transplantation of the heart and lung may be performed in selected patients with cardiac defects and heart failure in association with pulmonary hypertension.

Donor Selection and Operation

The lungs in a brain-dead patient deteriorate rapidly, and either pulmonary edema or infection develops. The donor should have a normal chest x-ray. Tracheal aspirate should consist of clear mucus without any purulence. Blood gas analysis should reveal PaO_2 greater than 100 mm Hg with FIO_2 0.4, and peak inspiratory pressures on the respirator should be less than 30 mm Hg. Donor and recipient body weight and chest x-ray configuration should be compatible; ideally, the donor should be 10% to 20% smaller than the recipient.

Figure 42-1

A A midline sternotomy incision is made. Because the abdominal organs are usually harvested as well, the midline incision is typically extended to the pubis. The pleura is opened anteriorly to expose the lungs. The pericardium is excised completely back to the hilum of the lungs, removing both phrenic nerves in the process. The pericardial excision is extended over the great arteries superiorly and to the diaphragm inferiorly. The inferior pulmonary ligament is mobilized.

B The innominate vein is ligated and divided to gain access to the trachea. The aorta is retracted medially, and the superior vena cava is retracted laterally to expose the trachea. The pericardium is opened, and the trachea is mobilized as high as possible, retaining at least five or six rings above the bifurcation.

C Perfusion catheters are placed in the aorta and pulmonary artery. The aorta is occluded. The superior vena cava is ligated and divided. The inferior vena cava is divided to empty the heart and allow the egress of cold cardioplegia solution, which is administered to the aortic root. The tip of the left atrial appendage is removed to allow the escape of cold modified Collins solution, which is infused to the main pulmonary artery. Ventilation of the lungs is continued during this phase.

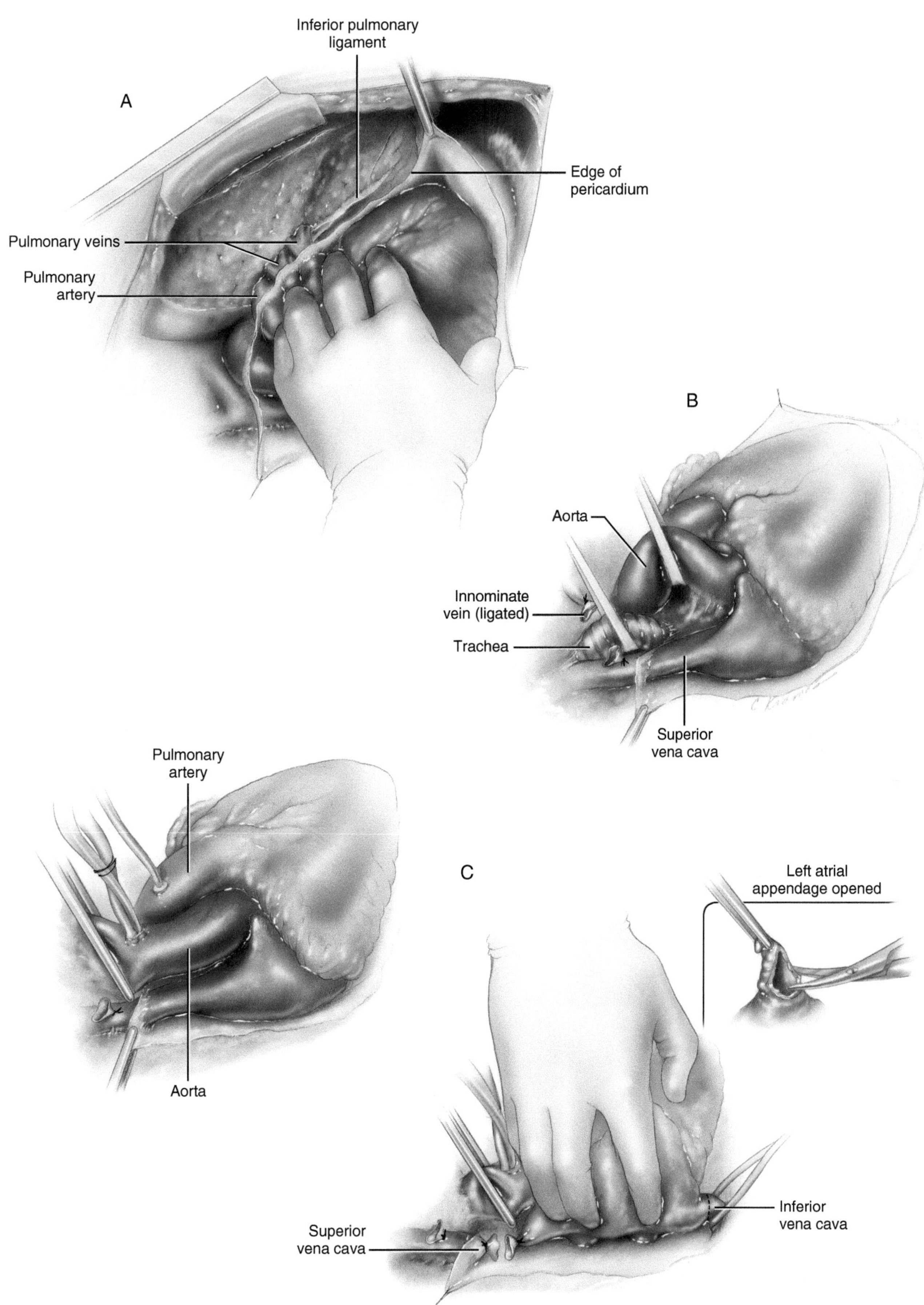
A
Inferior pulmonary ligament
Edge of pericardium
Pulmonary veins
Pulmonary artery
B
Aorta
Innominate vein (ligated)
Trachea
Superior vena cava
Pulmonary artery
Aorta
C
Left atrial appendage opened
Inferior vena cava
Superior vena cava

Figure 42-1 (continued)

D The heart is retracted to expose the pericardium posterior to it. The pericardium is opened posteriorly, near the diaphragm and over the esophagus. Upward retraction on the pericardium provides access to the tissue plane in front of the esophagus. The space anterior to the esophagus is cleared up to the inferior pulmonary veins and in back of the left atrium.

E The left lung is gently retracted superiorly and to the right to expose its posterior surface. The pleural incision from the inferior pulmonary ligament is extended posterior to the hilum of the left lung.

F The pleural incision is continued over the aorta anteriorly to join with the point of pericardial excision over the aorta.

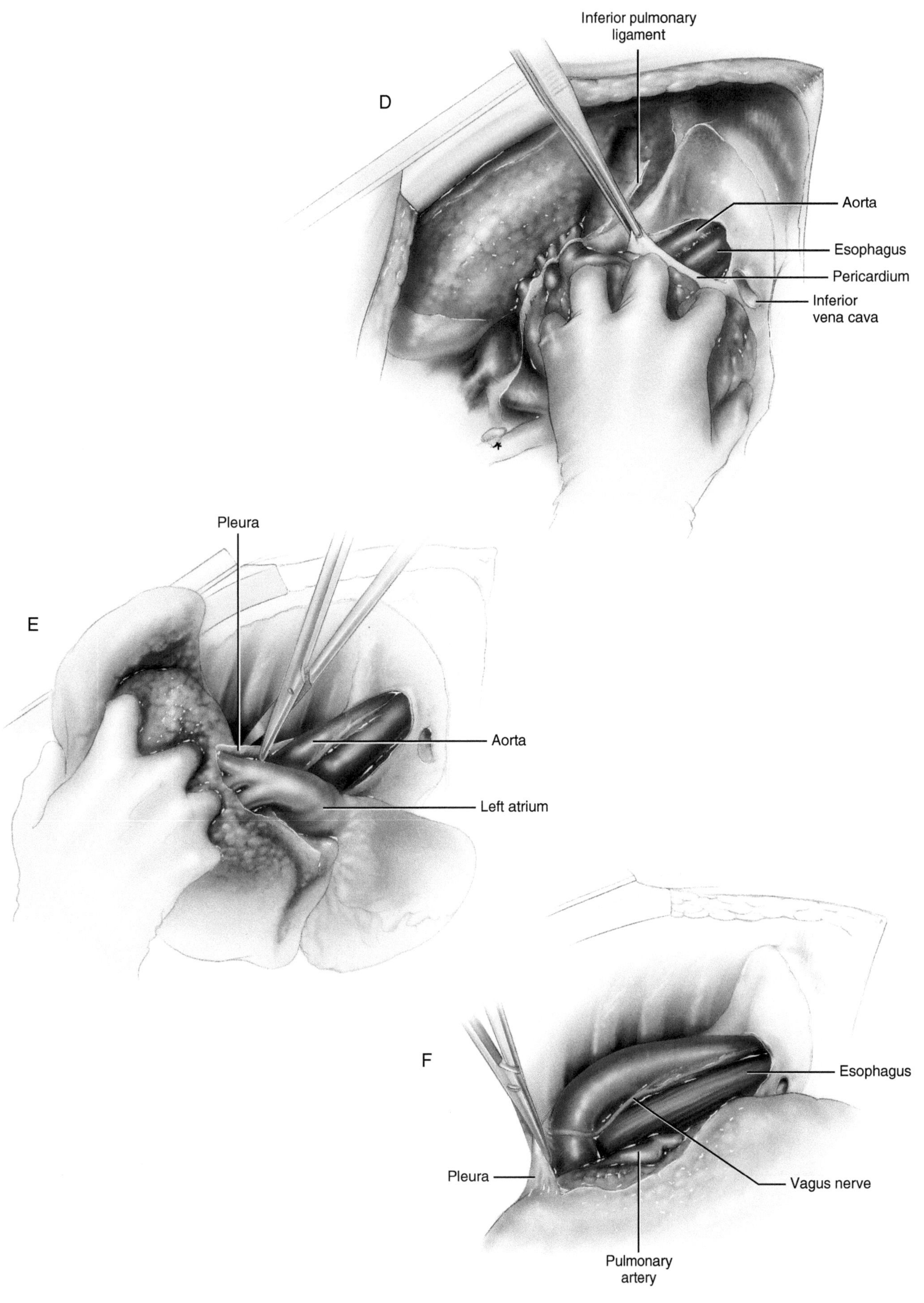
D
Inferior pulmonary ligament
Aorta
Esophagus
Pericardium
Inferior vena cava
E
Pleura
Aorta
Left atrium
F
Esophagus
Pleura
Vagus nerve
Pulmonary artery

Figure 42-1 (continued)

G The right lung is retracted anteriorly. The inferior pulmonary ligament is divided up to the inferior pulmonary veins. The pleural incision is extended along the surface of the esophagus over the posterior aspect of the pulmonary hilum. The azygos vein is ligated and divided. The pleural incision is extended anteriorly to join with the point of pericardial excision anterior to the superior vena cava.

H The limits of the pleuropericardial excision are shown. The incision begins at the diaphragm, includes the inferior pulmonary ligament, passes behind the pulmonary hilum and in front of the esophagus and aorta, and finally crosses the ascending aorta at the arch.

I The aorta is divided just below the innominate artery. The cardioplegia administration site is closed by purse-string suture. The lungs are ventilated until the trachea is occluded and are kept about two-thirds inflated. The trachea is clamped about five rings above the bifurcation and divided. Anterior mobilization of the trachea frees the heart-lung block from the mediastinum.

J The complete heart-lung block is removed from the thorax and immersed in iced saline solution. The pulmonary perfusion site is closed by purse-string suture. The right atrium is opened by an incision extending from the inferior vena cava toward the appendage. The interior of the heart is irrigated with chilled saline solution. The graft is now ready to be transplanted in the recipient.

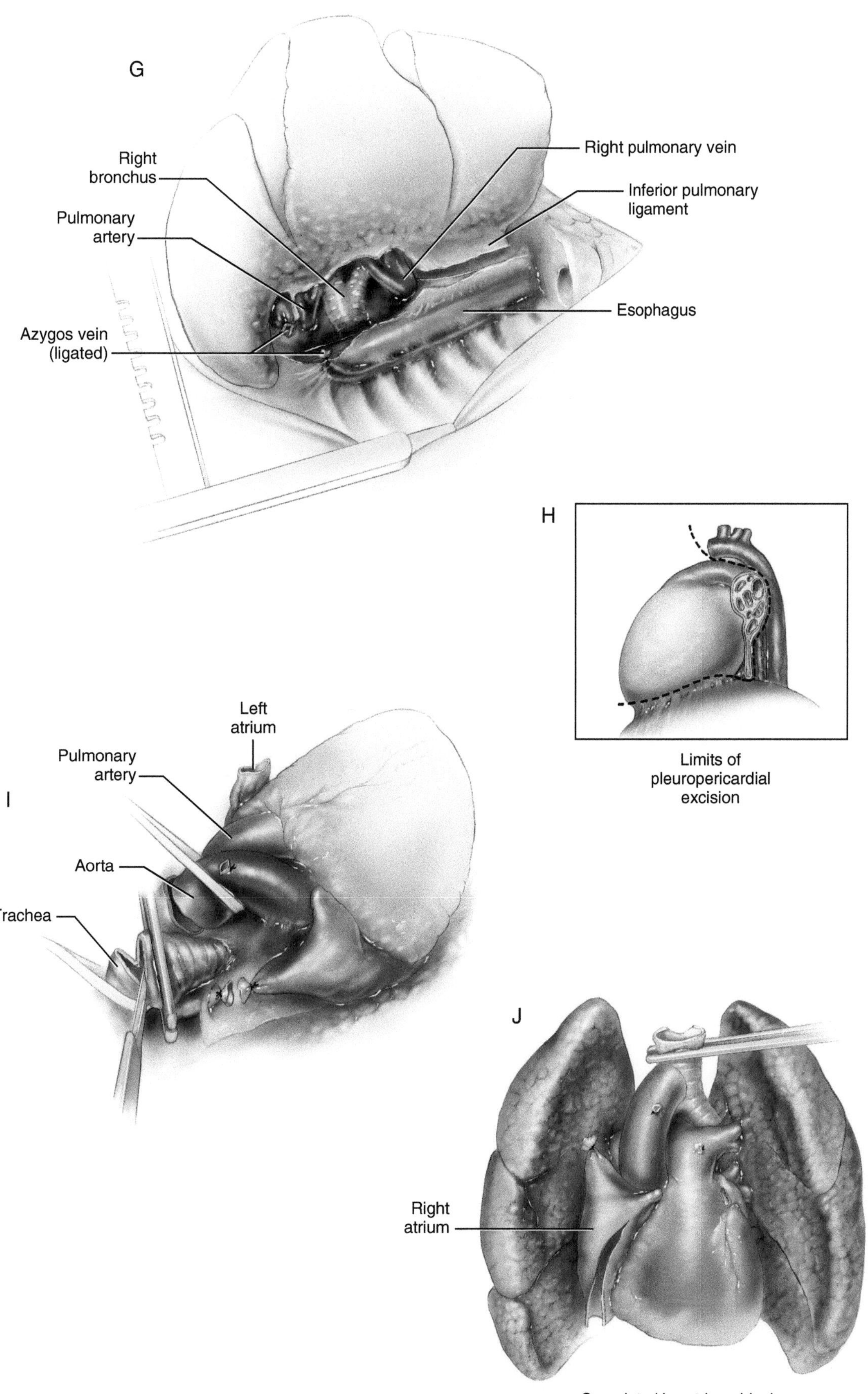

Limits of pleuropericardial excision

Completed heart-lung block

Recipient Operation

The recipient operation includes excision of the heart and lungs and implantation of the donor heart-lung block.

Figure 42-2

A The most difficult aspect of the heart-lung transplant operation is excision of the recipient heart and lungs. Function of the phrenic and vagus nerves (recurrent branch) must be preserved. Hemostasis must be meticulous in the mediastinum because the graft will cover this area when the operation is complete.

A midsternal incision is made. The pericardium is opened in the midline, and both pleural spaces are opened widely. Retraction stitches are placed on the pericardial edge. Some of the dissection can be done before the institution of cardiopulmonary bypass, but eventually it is necessary to establish bypass using two venous uptake cannulae, with oxygenated blood returned to the ascending aorta. Cardiectomy is performed exactly as described for cardiac transplantation. An incision is made in the pericardium just anterior to the left pulmonary veins and well behind the phrenic nerve. Dissection extends anterior to the pulmonary veins until the pleural space is entered. The incision is extended superiorly and inferiorly for a few centimeters, leaving the phrenic nerve anterior on the pleuropericardial flap. The left atrium is divided through the oblique sinus between the left and right pulmonary veins. The pericardial reflection on the posterosuperior aspect of the left atrium is divided to free the two halves of the left atrium.

B Dissection continues posteriorly on the surface of the left pulmonary veins. The left atrial remnant may be pushed through beneath the phrenic nerve. The left bronchus and left pulmonary artery are exposed. The pulmonary artery is divided proximal to the first branch.

C The inferior pulmonary ligament on the left side is divided up to the inferior pulmonary veins. The left lung is retracted anteriorly so that the pleural incision can be continued on the posterior aspect of the hilum in front of the aorta. Bronchial arteries are identified, ligated with hemoclips, and divided.

D The left bronchus is closed by staples. The bronchus is divided distal to the staple line, and the left lung is removed.

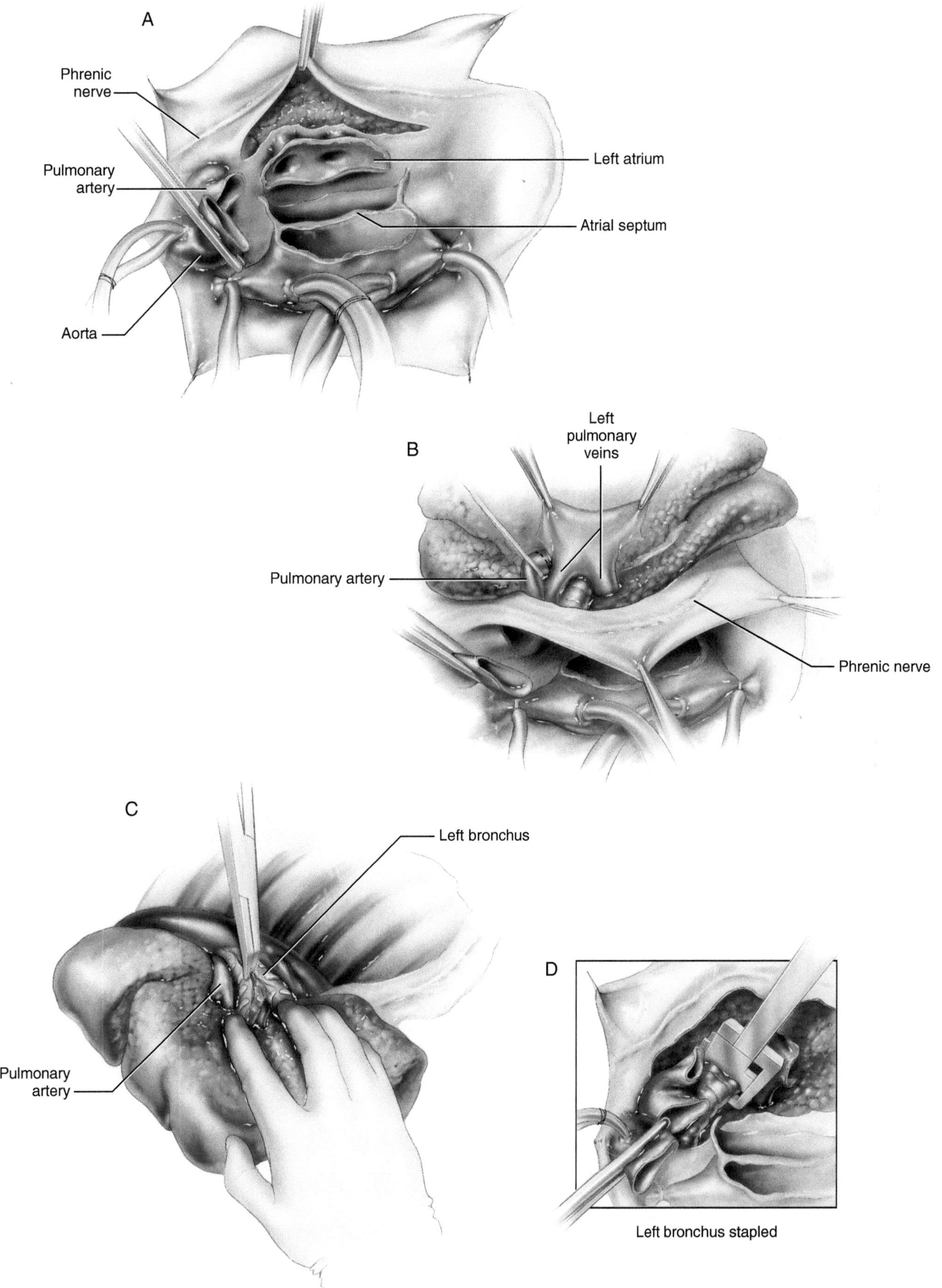
A
Phrenic nerve
Pulmonary artery
Aorta
Left atrium
Atrial septum
B
Left pulmonary veins
Pulmonary artery
Phrenic nerve
C
Left bronchus
Pulmonary artery
D
Left bronchus stapled

Figure 42-2 (continued)

E The right lung is resected next. An incision in the pericardium, anterior to the right pulmonary veins, is made into the right pleural space so that the right phrenic nerve remains intact on the pleuro-pericardial flap. The left atrium is incised posterior to the interatrial groove on the right side to allow the pulmonary veins to separate from the cardiac remnant.

F The remainder of the left atrium is resected from the atrial septum, working anteriorly from the left side of the septum. This leaves only the rim of atrial septum continuous with the right atrium near the atrioventricular groove for anastomosis to the transplant graft.

G The right inferior pulmonary ligament is divided, and the lung is mobilized posterior and anterior to the hilum as described for the left side. As the right pulmonary veins are mobilized to the right, the right pulmonary artery comes into view. It is divided. All that remains is the underlying right bronchus. It is dissected free of surrounding mediastinal tissues. The bronchial arteries are ligated with hemoclips. The right bronchus is closed by staples. The bronchus is divided distal to the staple line, and the right lung is removed from the chest. The mediastinum is carefully inspected, and all bleeding points are meticulously controlled.

H The trachea is divided just above the bifurcation. It is prepared for anastomosis by careful inspection of mediastinal surfaces posterior to it. Excess remnants of the right and left pulmonary arteries are removed, leaving the pulmonary artery bifurcation in place so as not to dissect the ligamentum arteriosum and the recurrent branch of the left vagus nerve.

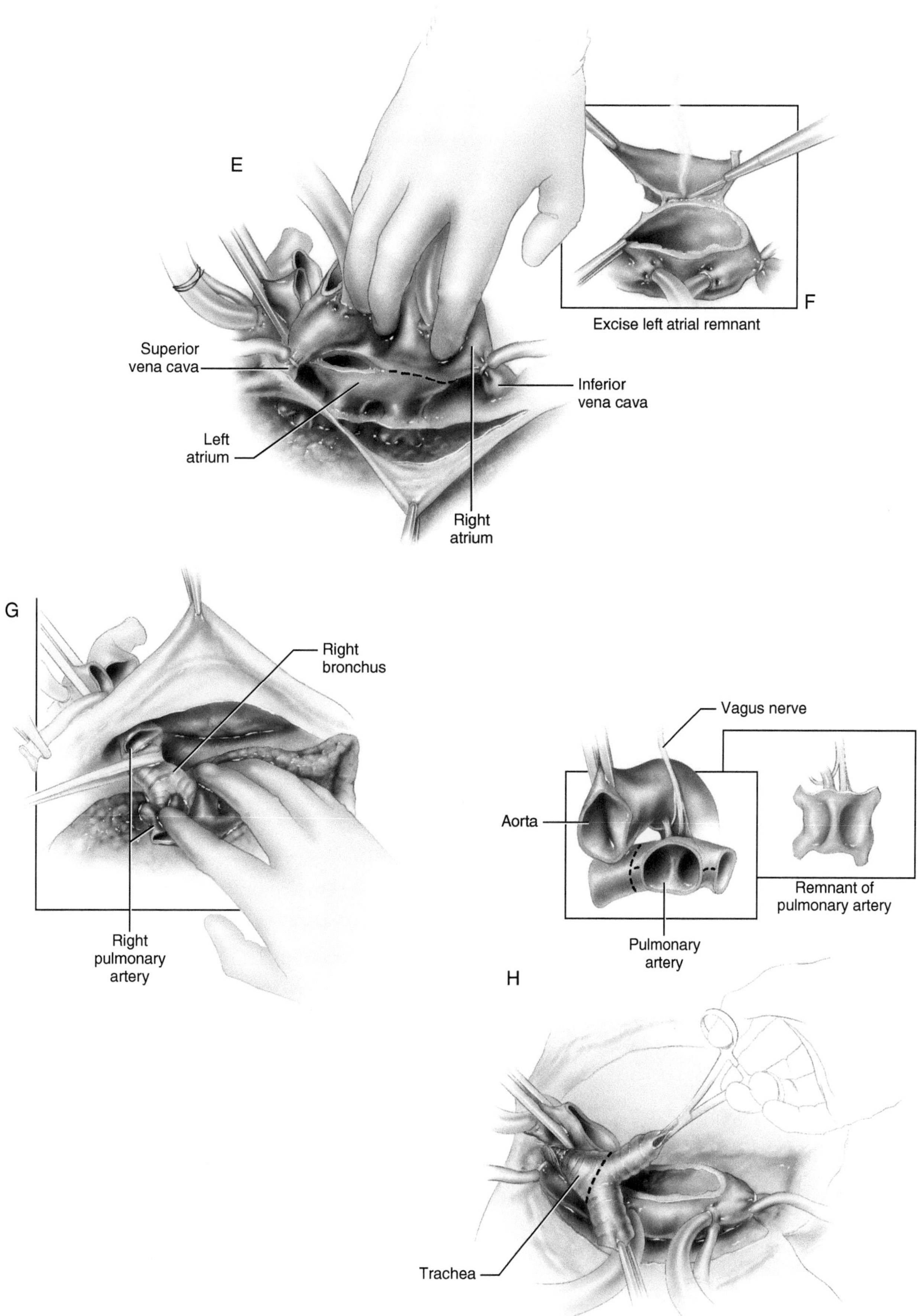
E
Superior vena cava
Left atrium
Inferior vena cava
Right atrium
F
Excise left atrial remnant
G
Right bronchus
Right pulmonary artery
Vagus nerve
Aorta
Remnant of pulmonary artery
Pulmonary artery
H
Trachea

Figure 42-2 (continued)

I The heart-lung block is placed into the recipient thorax. The right lung is passed behind the right atrium and venae cavae of the recipient. The left lung is passed behind the pleuropericardial flap into the left hemithorax. The tracheae, aortae, and right atria are aligned for anastomosis.

J An end-to-end anastomosis of the tracheae is constructed by continuous stitches of 3/0 polypropylene. The stitch is brought from outside the recipient trachea so that the suture line on the membranous portion posteriorly is from inside the donor trachea. The anastomosis must be meticulous and accurate, with the ends abutting precisely without buckling. Attention to detail is extremely important to prevent leakage at this critical anastomosis.

K The right atria are anastomosed by continuous stitches of 3/0 polypropylene. The donor right atrial opening is adjusted to the size of the recipient right atrium by modifying the length of the incision into the right atrium. The suture line is started inferiorly, continued around the inferior vena cava and superiorly along the septal remnant, and completed laterally on the surface of the right atrium.

L The graft aorta is anastomosed to the recipient aorta using continuous stitches of 4/0 polypropylene. The suture line is started from the outside medial surface of the recipient aorta so that the stitches can be placed from inside the donor aorta on the posterior aspect of the anastomosis. The suture line is completed anteriorly. Before final closure of the suture line, air is removed from cardiac chambers on the left side through the untied suture line. The left atrial appendage must be ligated. Following completion of the repair, the heart is reperfused to restore cardiac contraction, and ventilation is reestablished to the transplanted lungs.

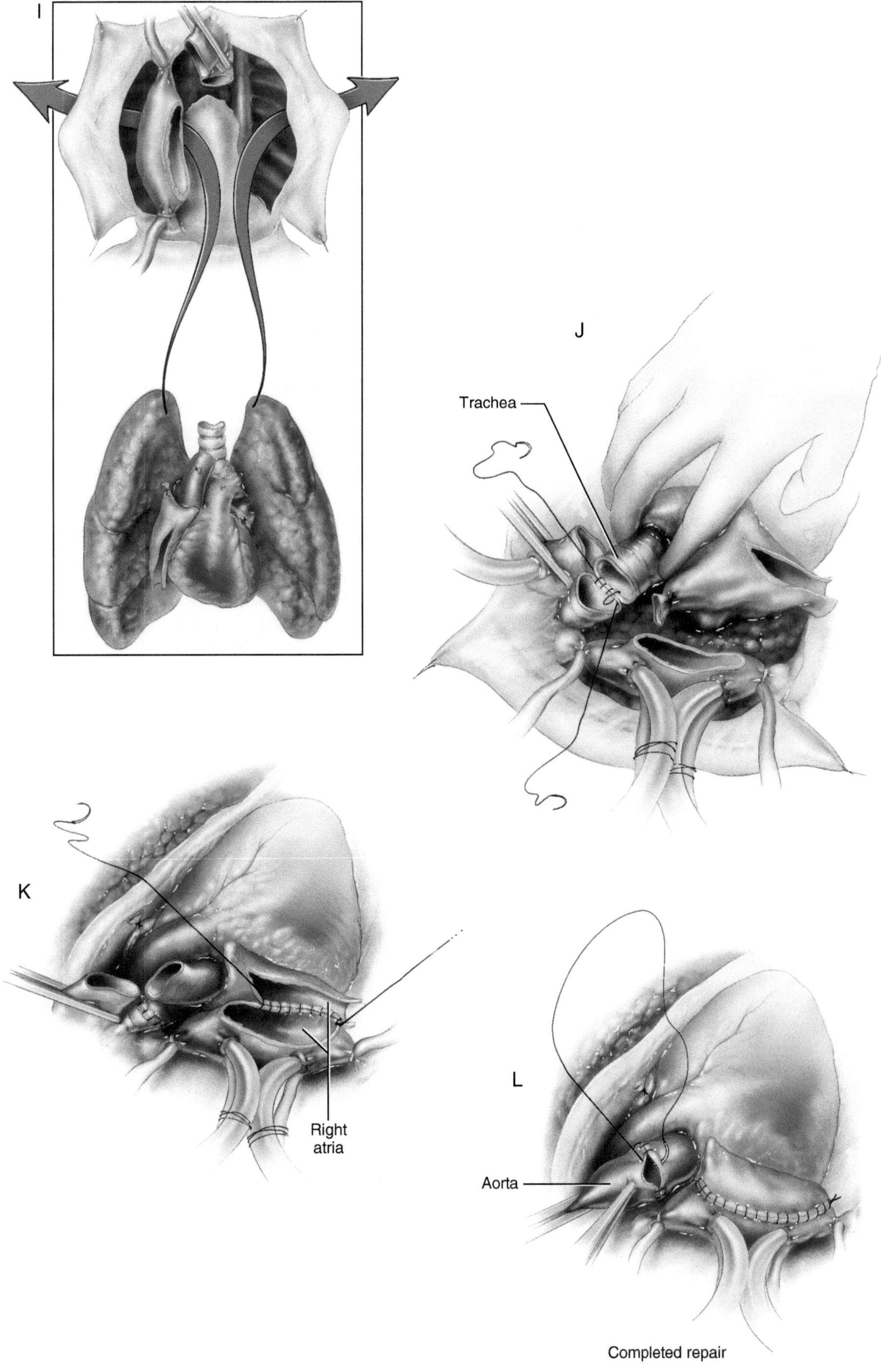
I
J
Trachea
K
Right
atria
L
Aorta
Completed repair

chapter 43 # LUNG TRANSPLANTATION

Double-Lung Transplantation

Transplantation of both lungs to a recipient may be indicated for patients with pulmonary hypertension or cystic fibrosis in whom both lungs have been destroyed but the heart remains healthy.

Figure 43-1

A The donor operation is exactly as described for heart-lung transplantation. After the heart-lung block is removed, the heart is separated by making an incision in the left atrium just outside the pulmonary venous ostia to leave an adequate cuff of left atrium on the lungs and an adequate cuff of left atrium on the heart. The pulmonary artery is divided slightly above the sinus rim, preserving the bifurcation with the lungs and preserving the valve with the heart. The heart is used in another patient for heart transplantation.

The recipient operation proceeds similarly to the heart-lung transplantation operation, except that the heart is not removed. The pericardium is opened in the midline, and both pleural spaces are opened anteriorly. An incision is made in the pericardium just anterior to the pulmonary veins, allowing dissection into the hilum posterior to the phrenic nerve. The nerve is preserved with the anterior pericardial flap. The pulmonary veins are ligated and divided. The pulmonary artery is divided at the bifurcation. The bronchi are mobilized by dissection through the posterior pericardium and in the hilum. The right and left bronchi are divided between staples in the hilum, allowing the lungs to be removed separately.

B This posterior view of the left atrium and hilum demonstrates ligation and separation of the pulmonary veins and the point of division of the pulmonary arteries. The bronchi are divided in the hilum to remove the lungs, and the trachea is later divided above the bifurcation.

C The recipient heart is arrested with cold cardioplegic solution after occlusion of the ascending aorta. The heart is retracted superiorly and to the right to allow the donor double-lung block to be positioned in the thorax. The lungs are passed individually behind the phrenic nerves into the pleural spaces. Note that the right lung must also pass posterior to the inferior vena cava. The pleural spaces are partly filled with cold saline solution to keep the lungs cool. An incision is made in the posterior wall of the left atrium between the pulmonary veins and extending to the base of the left atrial appendage.

D The left atrial anastomosis is constructed using continuous stitches of 3/0 polypropylene. Attention is given to proper orientation and planning of the suture line so that the relationship of the left atrium and the lung block will be appropriate when the heart is in its natural position.

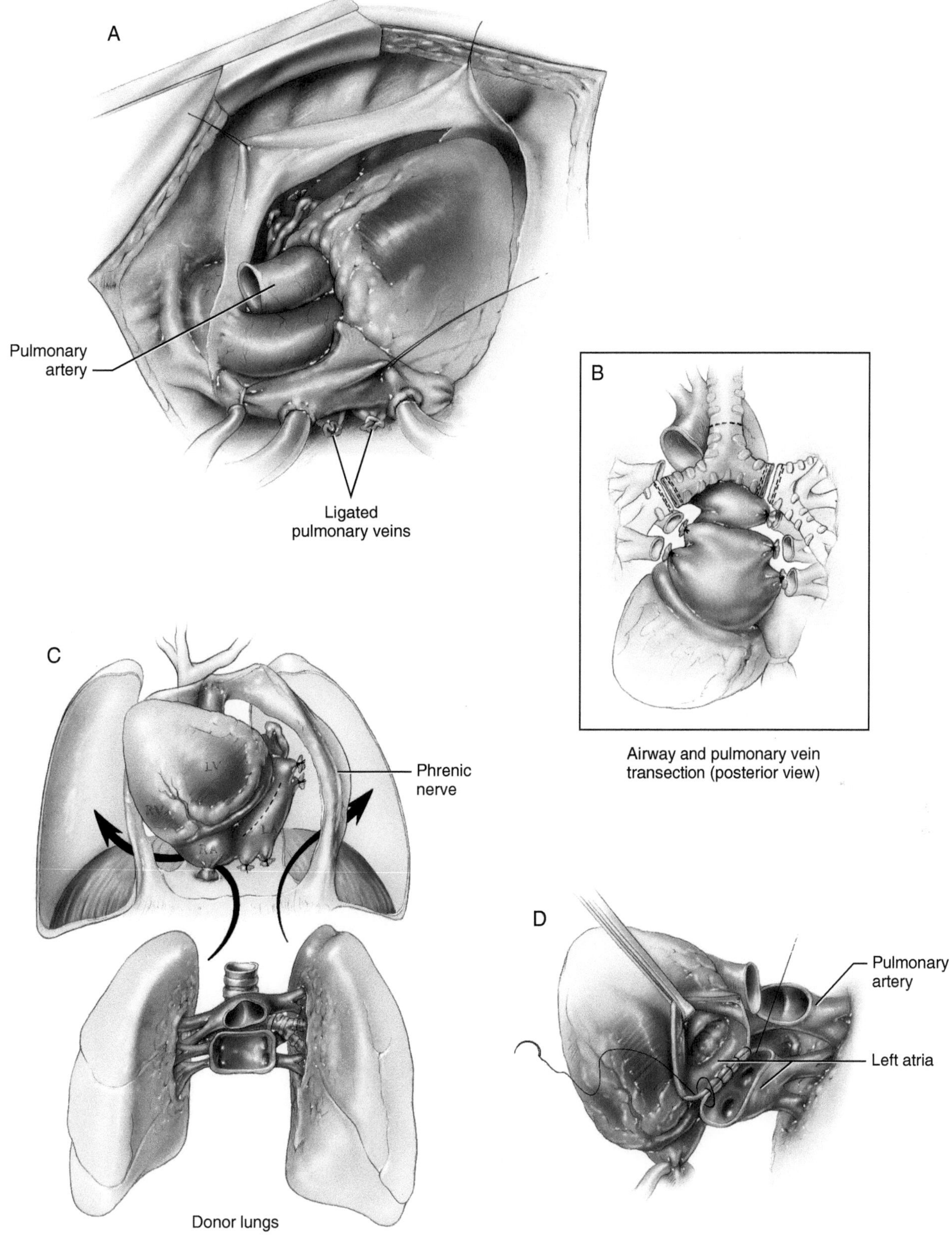
A
Pulmonary artery
Ligated pulmonary veins
B
Airway and pulmonary vein transection (posterior view)
C
Phrenic nerve
LV
RV
RA
Donor lungs
D
Pulmonary artery
Left atria

Figure 43-1 (continued)

E An end-to-end anastomosis of the pulmonary arteries is constructed. The recipient pulmonary artery is shortened appropriately, with care taken to leave no excess that could kink and obstruct the outflow from the heart. Continuous suture technique with 4/0 polypropylene is employed. It is easiest to begin from the outside of the donor pulmonary artery so that stitches are placed from inside the recipient pulmonary artery on the posterior wall of the anastomosis. The heart is reperfused after the anastomosis is completed.

F The trachea is exposed between the aorta and the superior vena cava through the posterior pericardium. The recipient trachea is divided above the bifurcation, and the remaining right and left bronchi are removed, with care taken to control the bronchial arteries. The donor trachea is shortened to an appropriate length above the bifurcation. Blood and fluid are kept out of the airway. Cultures are taken from the donor and recipient tracheae. An end-to-end anastomosis of the tracheae is constructed with continuous stitches of 3/0 polypropylene. Sutures are placed first in the posterior wall of the anastomosis and then in the anterior wall, as for great vessel anastomosis. The omentum is brought up from the peritoneal cavity through an incision in the pericardium just above the esophageal hiatus. The peritoneum may be opened anteriorly in the midline to facilitate dissection of the omentum. The omentum is wrapped around the tracheal anastomosis and secured to the peritracheal tissues and pericardial edges with fine sutures.

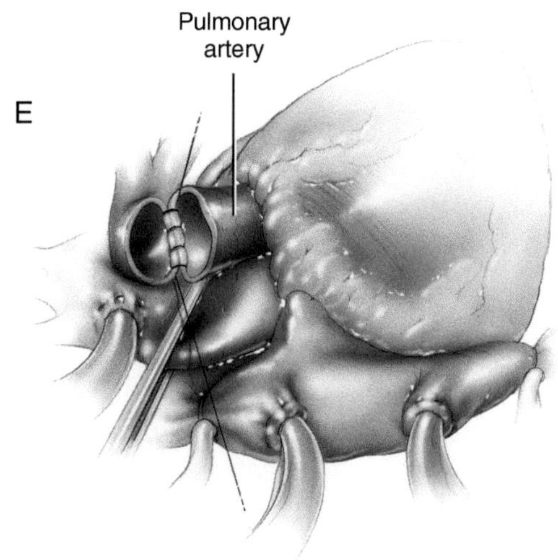
E
Pulmonary
artery

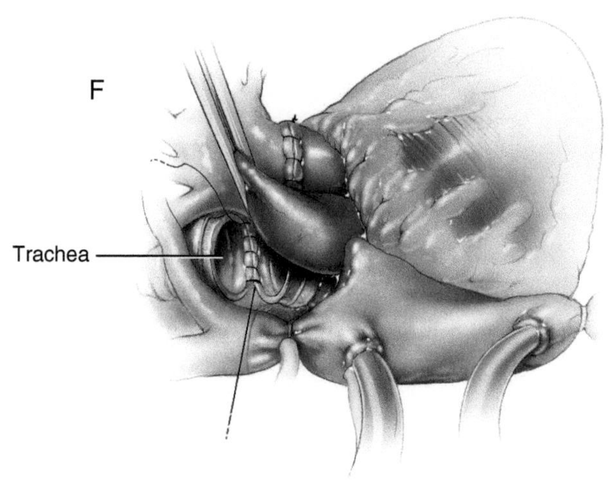
F
Trachea

Single-Lung Transplantation

Single-lung transplantation has become the standard whenever lung transplantation is necessary. A single lung often suffices for patients with pulmonary hypertension. In cases in which double-lung transplantation is required, the operation can be performed as sequential single-lung transplants. The operation is usually performed without cardiopulmonary bypass support unless there is an associated intracardiac defect that requires simultaneous correction or oxygenation is inadequate on single-lung ventilation.

Figure 43-2

A Shown here is single-lung transplantation on the right side. Similar principles apply to single-lung transplantation on the left side. The azygos vein is ligated and divided. A pneumonectomy is performed, preserving the right mainstem bronchus, most of the pulmonary artery, and a cuff of the left atrium. The pulmonary veins are cut back to the left atrium so that a single anastomosis can include both pulmonary veins of the donor.

B The donor pneumonectomy should leave the donor lung with a generous portion of the mainstem bronchus, the pulmonary artery to the bifurcation, and a good-sized cuff of left atrium encompassing both pulmonary veins. The pericardium is left attached to the hilum of the lung.

C An end-to-end anastomosis of the mainstem bronchi is constructed using continuous stitches of 3/0 polypropylene. A telescoping anastomosis has been recommended. Accuracy of the bronchial anastomosis is probably the most important determinant of its success. The left atrial cuff of the graft is anastomosed to the recipient left atrium. Continuous stitches of 3/0 polypropylene are employed.

D An end-to-end anastomosis of the pulmonary arteries is constructed using continuous stitches of 4/0 or 5/0 polypropylene, depending on the thickness of the tissues.

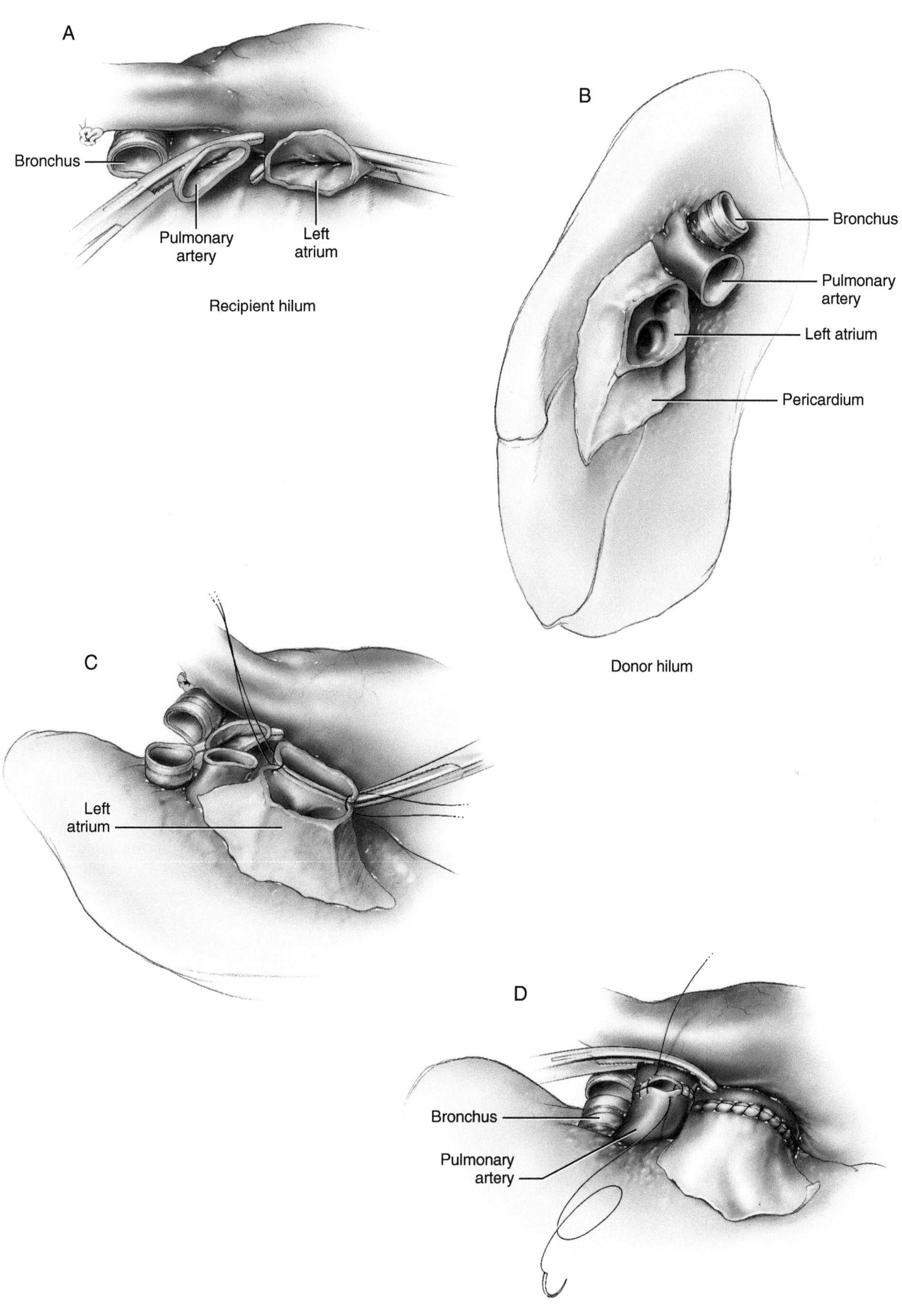
A
Bronchus
Pulmonary artery
Left atrium
Recipient hilum
B
Bronchus
Pulmonary artery
Left atrium
Pericardium
Donor hilum
C
Left atrium
D
Bronchus
Pulmonary artery

chapter 44 CARDIAC ARRHYTHMIA

Pacemaker Insertion

Permanent pacing systems require the implantation of pacing electrodes in contact with the myocardium and the placement of a pulse generator in the body. There are a number of options for accomplishing these tasks. In certain circumstances it may be advisable to implant permanent myocardial electrodes on the surface of the heart at the time of open cardiac surgery. Endocardial contact with the electrode, however, appears to be more satisfactory in achieving long-term, low-threshold function of the electrode. The availability of small-diameter, flexible electrode catheters and small pulse generators makes electrode implantation via the subclavian vein and placement of the pulse generator in the chest wall possible and preferable in nearly every case in both adults and children.

Figure 44-1

A An incision is made on the anterior chest wall below the clavicle. An incision placed on either the right or left side of the chest can be used with equal ease; the choice is based on surgeon preference or patient handedness. Local anesthesia is used. A pocket is formed by separating the subcutaneous tissues from the fascia of the pectoralis major muscle. Hemostasis in the pocket must be meticulous. In children and in some adults with insufficient subcutaneous tissues, the pocket for the pulse generator can be formed beneath the pectoralis major muscle to protect the pulse generator from trauma. General anesthesia is required in these cases.

B The superior edge of the incision is retracted to provide access to the first rib–clavicle passageway, beneath which lies the subclavian vein. A needle with a syringe attached is used to locate and penetrate the vein. A flexible J-tip guidewire is passed through the needle into the superior vena cava. The position of the guidewire is confirmed by fluoroscopy.

C The needle is withdrawn and replaced with a peel-away catheter sheath. The pacing electrode is passed with ease through the sheath into the superior vena cava. The sheath is then peeled away from the electrode catheter. The electrode is manipulated under fluoroscopic guidance into the right atrial appendage or the apex of the right ventricle, depending on the desired location of cardiac stimulation. When two electrodes are required for atrioventricular sequential pacing, it is usually easier to make separate entry into the subclavian vein rather than attempting to simultaneously place two electrodes through a single catheter sheath. Based on individual patient conditions, a number of tricks for shaping and manipulating the electrode catheter guidewires may be required to reach the desired point in the right heart. A gentle curve anteriorly usually guides the electrode into the right ventricle and out the pulmonary artery. Withdrawal of the electrode allows it to drop into the apex of the right ventricle, where it can be firmly seated with a straight guidewire. A full J-shaped curve of the guidewire allows the electrode to be pulled back into the right atrial appendage. The tines near the tip of the electrode catch in right heart trabeculations to hold its position; generally, however, more secure fixation is desired and is accomplished using a screw-in electrode.

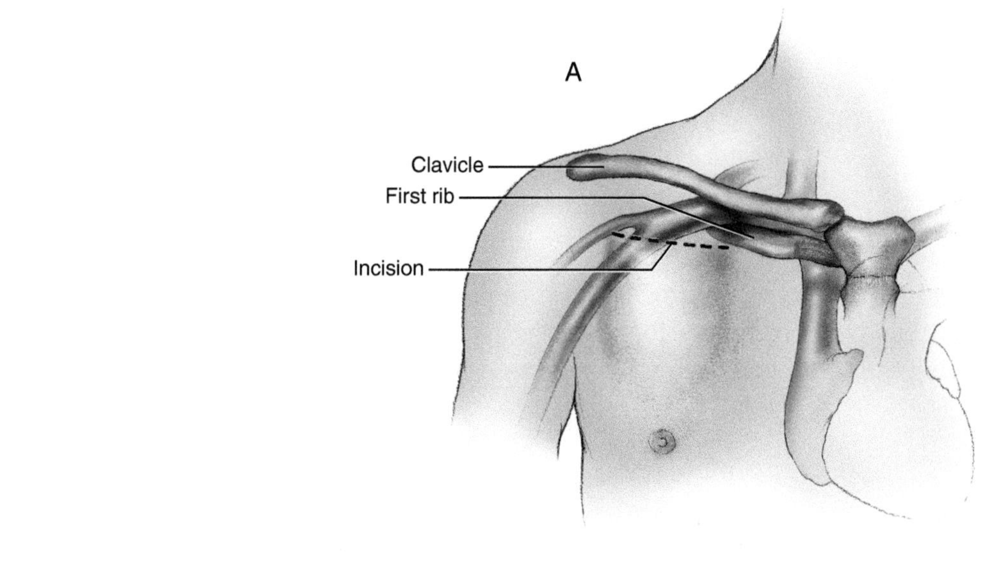
A
Clavicle
First rib
Incision

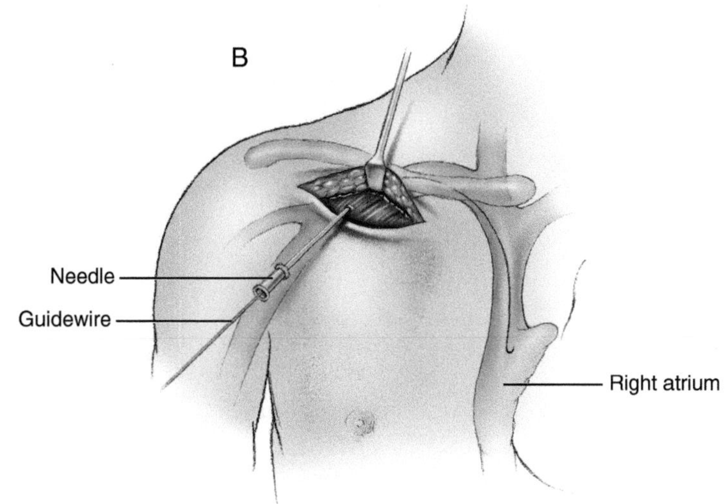
B
Needle
Guidewire
Right atrium

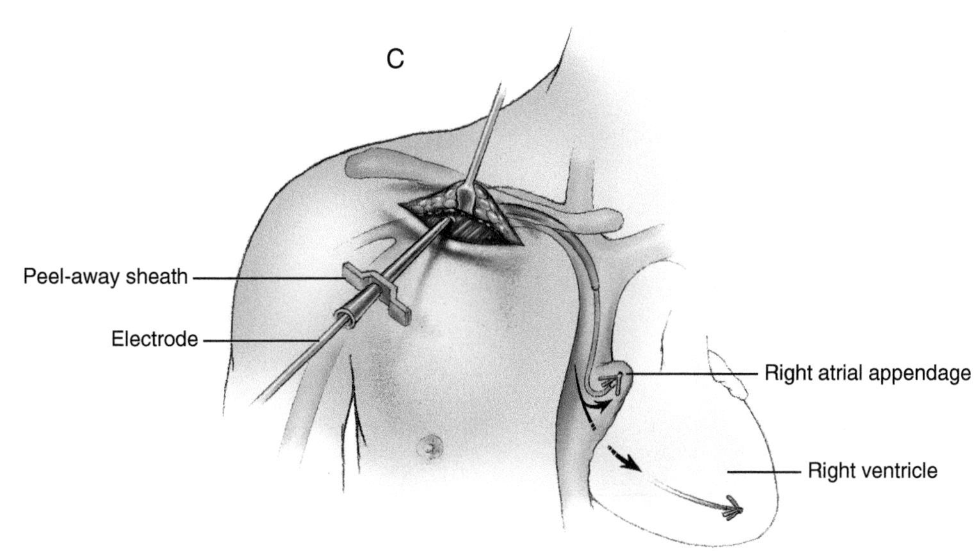
C
Peel-away sheath
Electrode
Right atrial appendage
Right ventricle

Automatic Internal Cardioverter Defibrillator Insertion

Insertion of an automatic internal cardioverter defibrillator (AICD) is also accomplished by electrode implantation using a transvenous technique and subcutaneous implantation of the AICD generator.

Figure 44-2

A An incision is made below the clavicle on the side of the nondominant hand (usually the left side). A subcutaneous pouch may be created if there is sufficient fat to cover the device adequately. Otherwise, the device is implanted beneath the pectoralis major muscle.

B The electrodes are implanted via the veins using a needle-catheter technique. The subclavian vein is punctured by a needle, and a guidewire is passed through the needle into the vein.

C A catheter sheath is passed over a dilator and the guidewire. The ventricular electrode is passed through the sheath and positioned at the apex of the right ventricle with fluoroscopic guidance.

D The simplest AICD configuration uses the ventricular electrode and the generator container as the two electrodes between which the mass of the ventricle is placed to effect cardioversion. In most cases the defibrillation threshold is satisfactory with this simple electrical setup.

E Another commonly used configuration employs a second transvenously placed electrode in the superior vena cava.

F For patients with previously placed epicardial patch electrodes that are still functional, it may be desirable to use one of these patches in the electrical circuit.

B

Incision

A

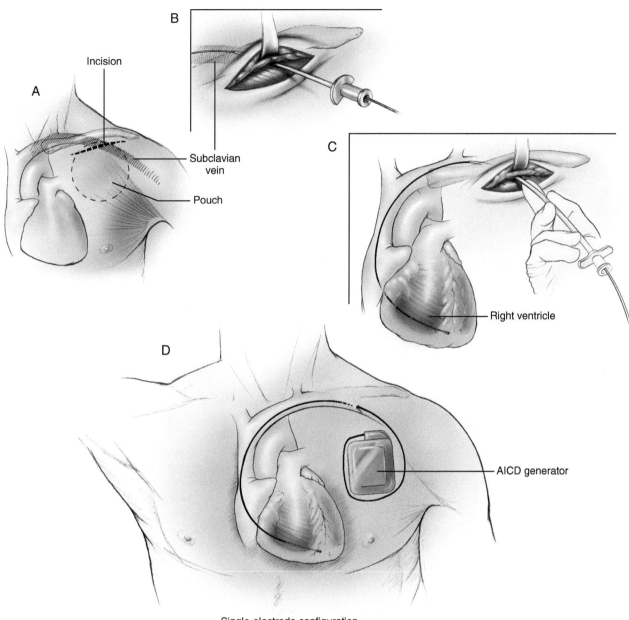

Subclavian vein

Pouch

C

Right ventricle

D

AICD generator

Single-electrode configuration

Double-electrode configuration

E

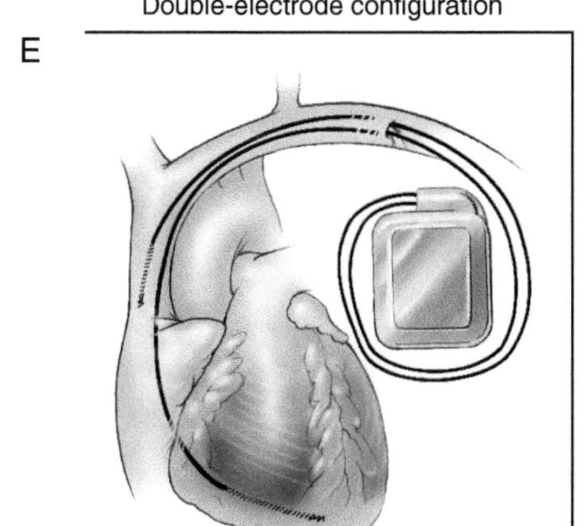

Transvenous and patch configuration

F

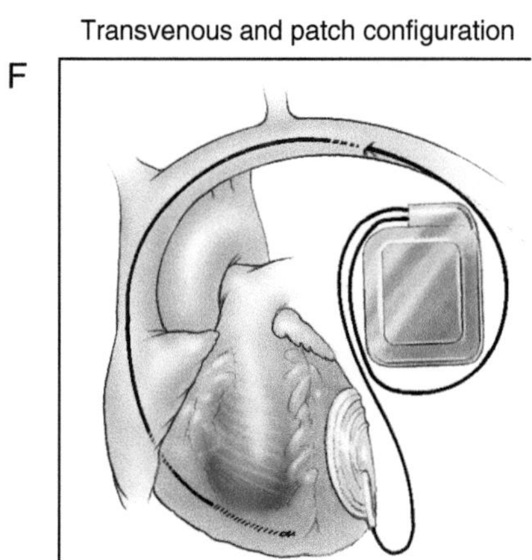

Ventricular Tachyarrhythmia

Catheter techniques for the localization and characterization of cardiac arrhythmia precede operation. Most rhythm disturbances can be controlled with properly selected medications. A large number of drugs are available, and new ones are continuously being developed. Should the arrhythmia prove refractory to medical therapy, radiofrequency ablation by intravascular catheter techniques may be indicated. In some cases operation may be indicated when less invasive techniques have failed or in conjunction with other intracardiac operations such as coronary artery bypass, resection of ventricular aneurysm, or cardiac valve reconstruction or replacement.

Figure 44-3

A At operation, the arrhythmia is characterized and localized by a combination of epicardial and endocardial mapping. Epicardial mapping is performed by systematically moving an electrode over the surface of the heart while recording electrocardiograms. A grid is developed from the various electrograms. This technique is essential during operation for Wolff-Parkinson-White syndrome. Only electrograms obtained from the ventricular surface near the atrioventricular groove (shown in larger typeface in the illustration) are important in this syndrome. These electrograms detect early entry of depolarization on the ventricle. Devices that contain multiple electrodes in a net or sock have been developed so that electrograms from multiple points can be obtained simultaneously. The information is analyzed by computer to simplify the process of localizing the focus of the arrhythmia.

Endocardial mapping can be performed through a ventriculotomy using either the probe or an electrode placed on a ring. Again, the systematic acquisition of surface electrograms and the development of a grid aid in localizing the focus of the rhythm disturbance.

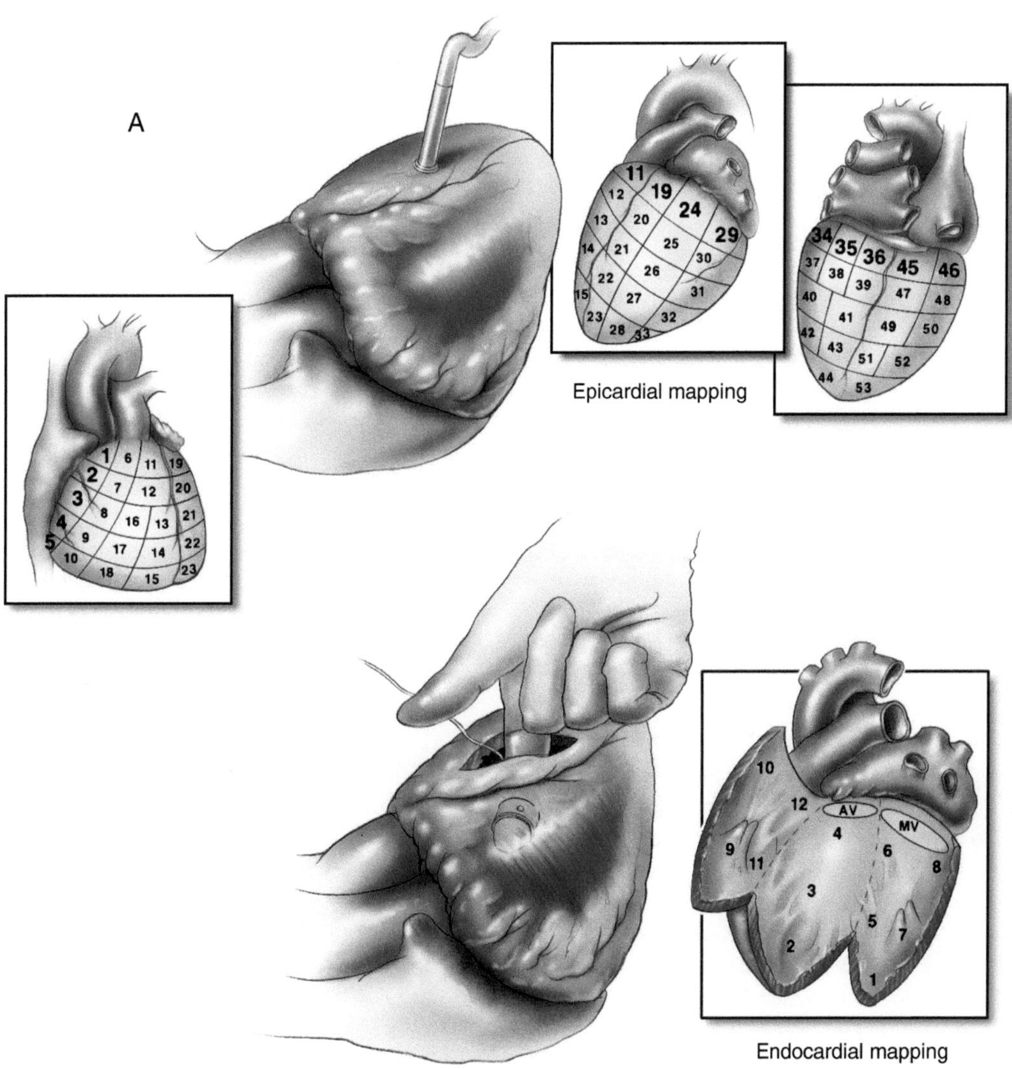
A
Epicardial mapping
Endocardial mapping
AV
MV

Figure 44-3 (continued)

B Operation may be indicated for ventricular tachyarrhythmia refractory to medical therapy or catheter ablation. The location of the irritable myocardium responsible for initiating the rhythm disturbance is usually well known prior to operation because these patients have had multiple catheter studies and multiple attempts to induce and control the problem medically or to ablate the focus of the arrhythmia. Further operative mapping using the surface electrograms directs the surgeon to the areas of the heart most likely to respond to operative intervention. Arrhythmogenic myocardium is usually located at the margin of a myocardial scar, the result of ischemic damage to the heart. Two approaches are commonly used to treat the affected myocardium. The irritable myocardium may be resected by removing a peel of the endocardium, or it may be isolated by an encircling incision on the endocardial surface of the ventricle.

C When the focus of the rhythm disturbance is located at the margin of a scar on the anterolateral surface of the left ventricle near the apex, an incision is made into the scar to gain access to the ventricle. Localized endocardial resection of the arrhythmogenic focus is accomplished by dissecting a partial thickness of the ventricular wall. The dissection is started at the margin of the scar and proceeds in a well-developed subendocardial plane of partial scar to normal myocardium. Removal of this portion of the myocardium should eliminate the irritable focus causing the rhythm disturbance.

D When the focus of the rhythm disturbance is located on the posterior wall of the left ventricle, a combination of techniques is required to isolate the area. The most complex lesions are those located in proximity to the mitral valve and the posterior papillary muscle. An incision is made through the surface myocardial scar.

E The myocardium near the posterior papillary muscle can be isolated by a combination of encircling ventriculotomy and cryoablation. An incision is made in the endocardium and part way through the ventricle wall, around the base of the papillary muscle, and continued to a point near the annulus of the mitral valve. A cryoprobe is used to destroy the myocardium near the mitral annulus. Cryoablation of myocardium is safer and more effective than incision near the mitral annulus and the aortic valve.

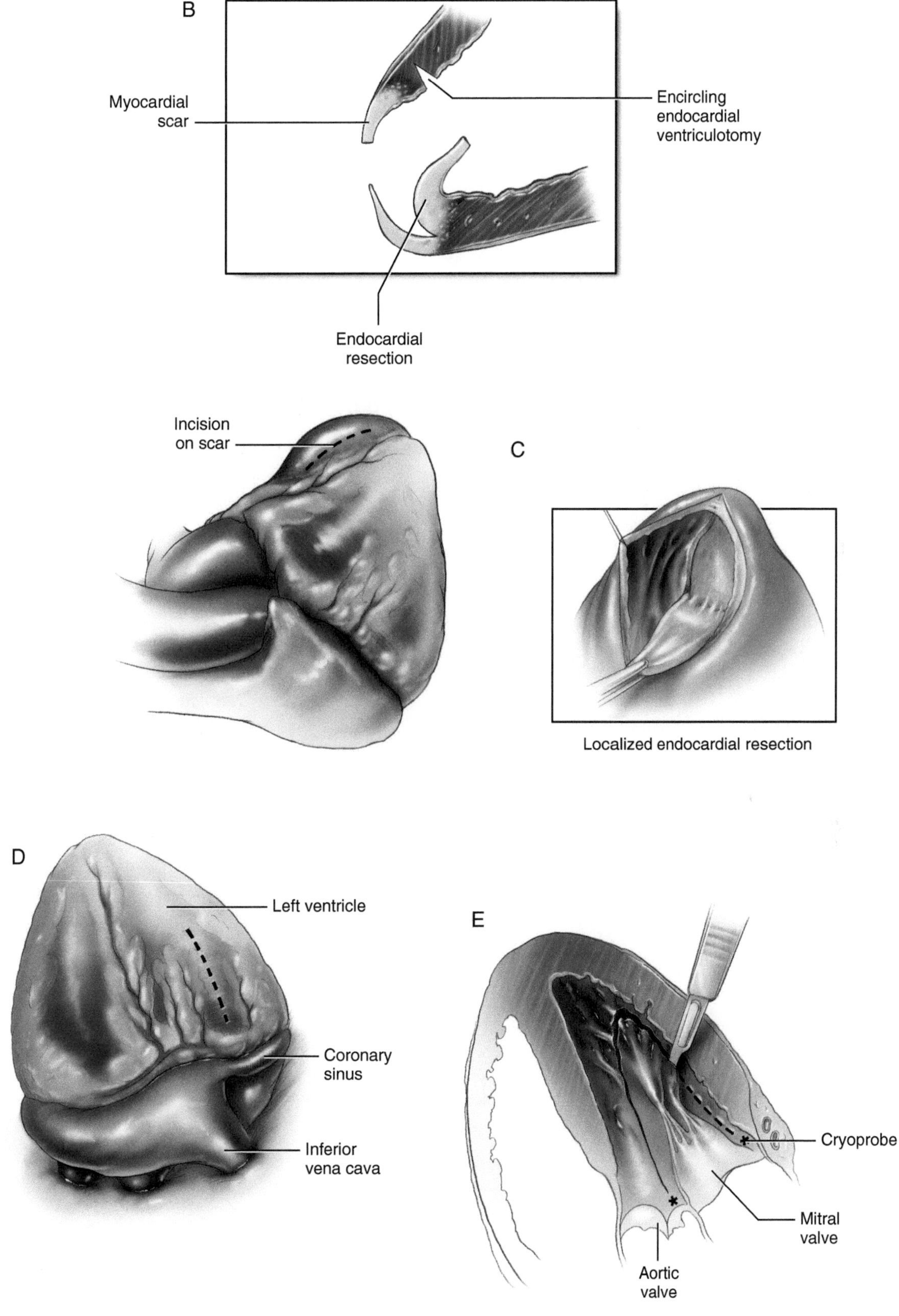
B
Myocardial scar
Encircling endocardial ventriculotomy
Endocardial resection
Incision on scar
C
Localized endocardial resection
D
Left ventricle
Coronary sinus
Inferior vena cava
E
Cryoprobe
Mitral valve
Aortic valve

Wolff-Parkinson-White Syndrome: Right Free Wall Type

Wolff-Parkinson-White syndrome may be associated with life-threatening or disabling cardiac arrhythmias caused by preexcitation or early depolarization of the ventricles through anomalous conduction tissue connections between the atrium and the ventricle (Kent's bundles). These anomalous conduction pathways, which course from the right atrium to the anterior free wall of the right ventricle, can be divided through either an epicardial or an endocardial approach. The former can be accomplished as a closed heart procedure; the latter requires cardiopulmonary bypass.

Figure 44-4

A The epicardial approach is performed through an incision in the epicardium near the atrioventricular groove. The fat of the groove is dissected from the surface of the right atrium and the right ventricle to the tricuspid valve annulus. This dissection should divide any accessory pathway between the right atrium and right ventricle, except those that course within the wall of the atrium to the ventricle. Although this approach may be easier than the endocardial approach, there is a small chance that some pathways could be missed.

B The endocardial approach is accomplished with the patient on cardiopulmonary bypass. An incision is made in the atrium anterior to the tricuspid annulus. The dissection is taken into the fat of the atrioventricular groove over the surface of the right ventricle. This should divide every possible accessory pathway from atrium to ventricle. The incision is repaired from within the right atrium.

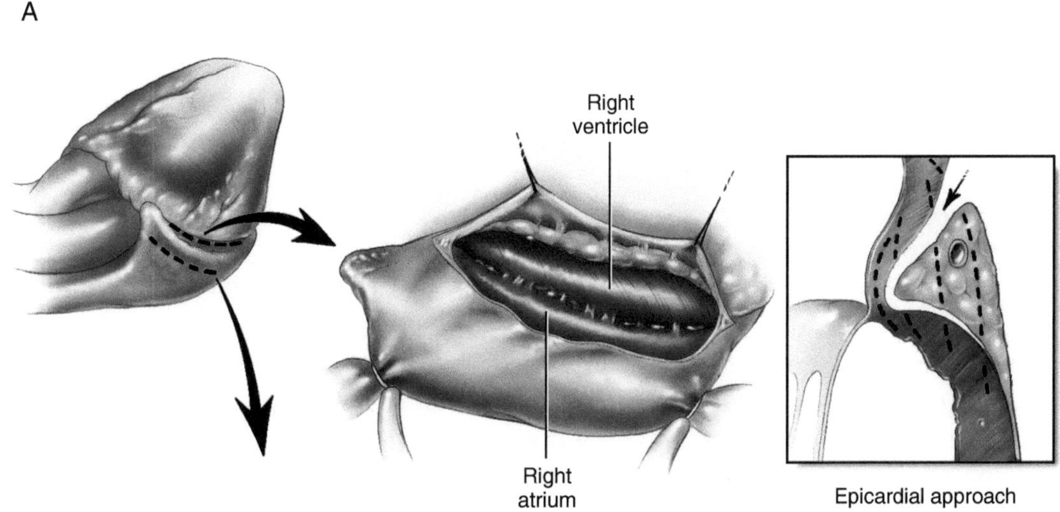
A
Right ventricle
Right atrium
Epicardial approach

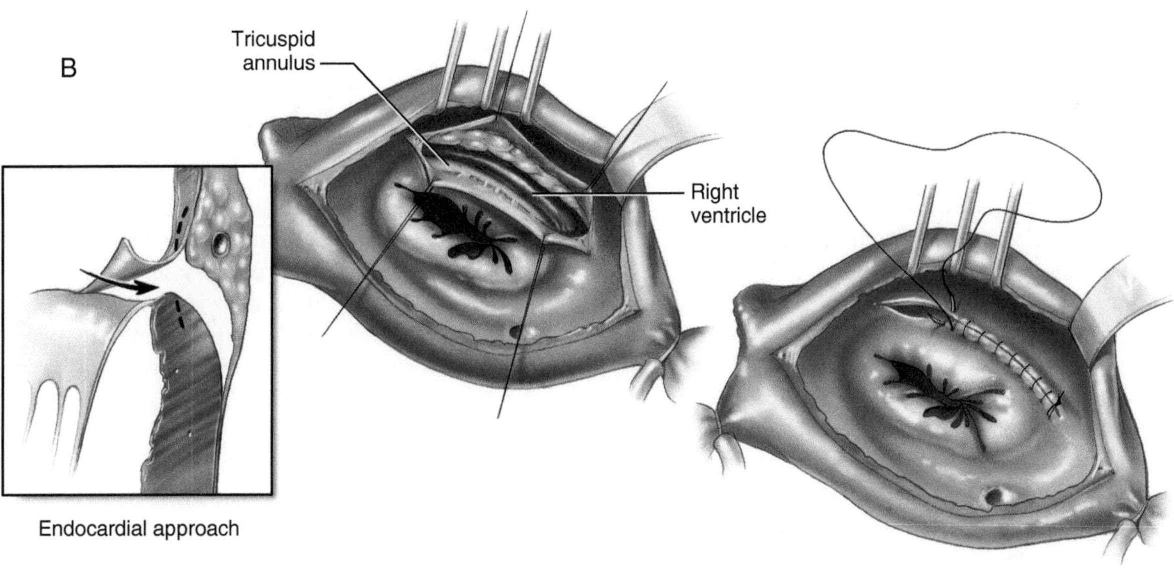
B
Tricuspid annulus
Right ventricle
Endocardial approach

Wolff-Parkinson-White Syndrome: Left Free Wall and Posterior Type

A left atrial endocardial approach is preferred for patients with accessory pathways localized at the atrioventricular groove of the left ventricle. Although closed heart procedures to divide or cryoablate accessory pathways in the left atrioventricular groove have been described, the risks of cardiac manipulation and associated exposure problems outweigh the benefits derived from avoiding cardiopulmonary bypass.

Figure 44-5

A As for mitral valve operations, a left atriotomy is made on the right side posterior to the intraatrial groove. An incision is made in the atrium near the posterior mitral valve annulus. Most of the dissection is over the shoulder of the left ventricle beneath the epicardium. The coronary artery and vein are mobilized away from the surface of the ventricle. The dissection extends to the mitral annulus and on the surface of the atrium to ensure that all accessory bundles have been divided. The incision in the left atrium is repaired from within the atrium.

B Accessory preexcitation pathways located posterior to either the right or left ventricle near the septum are approached through a right atriotomy. An incision is made near the annulus of the tricuspid valve, posterior to the bundle of His. The incision may proceed into the triangle of Koch, as long as it is close to the tricuspid annulus and avoids the area of the atrioventricular node.

C Dissection proceeds into the fat of the atrioventricular groove at the crux of the heart. The dissection should expose the myocardium of both the right and left ventricles in the area of the septum. The mitral valve annulus is exposed, as well as the annulus of the tricuspid valve. The coronary sinus and right coronary artery are mobilized away from the ventricular surfaces, with care taken to preserve the blood supply to the atrioventricular node. Any accessory pathways located in this area should be divided by this dissection.

D Although the epicardial approach is not recommended because division of the coronary veins is required, this approach is shown for completeness and to clarify the area of dissection. The surfaces of both right and left ventricles may be exposed to the septum.

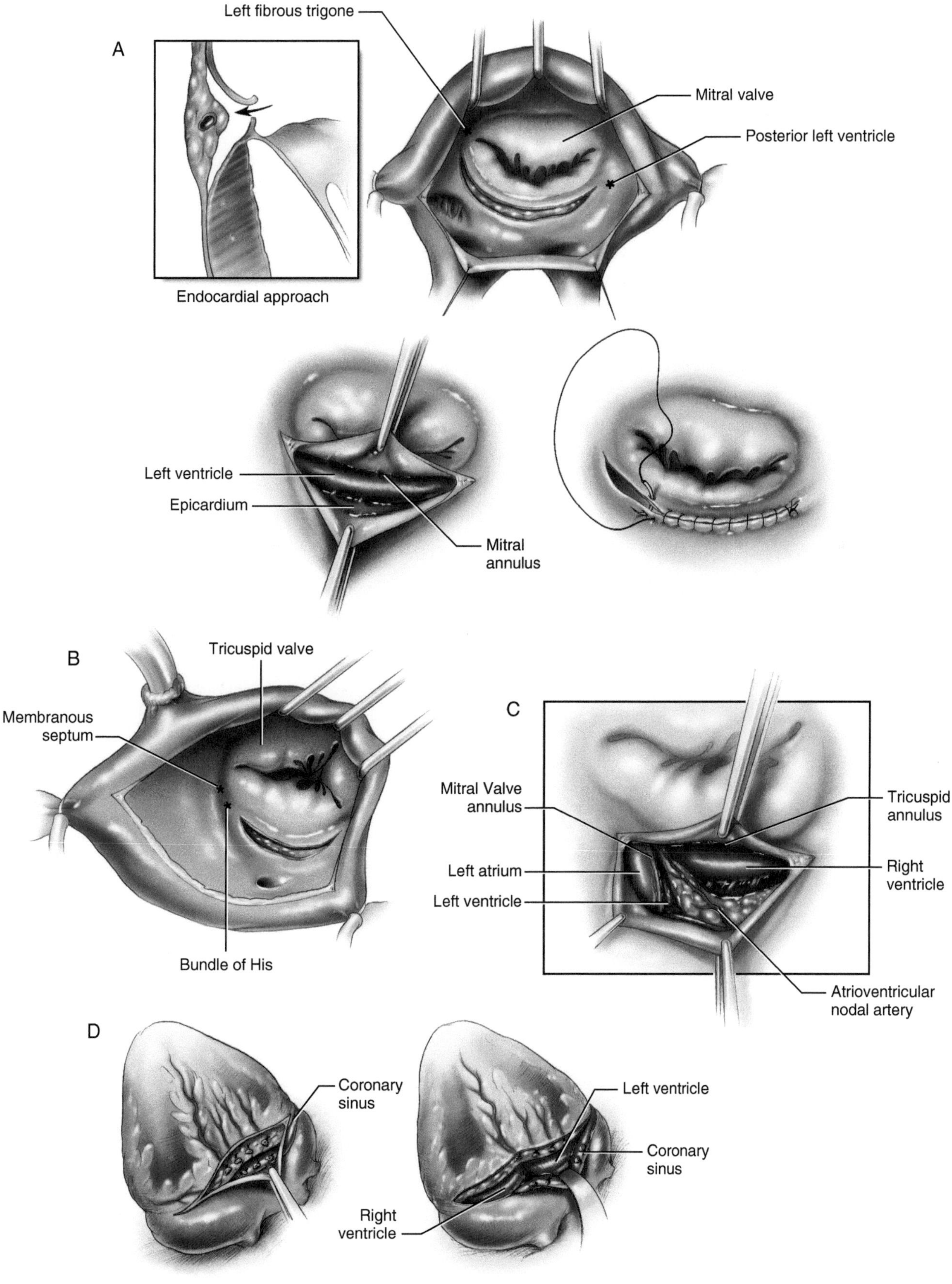
A
Left fibrous trigone
Mitral valve
Posterior left ventricle
Endocardial approach
Left ventricle
Epicardium
Mitral annulus
B
Tricuspid valve
Membranous septum
Bundle of His
C
Mitral Valve annulus
Left atrium
Left ventricle
Tricuspid annulus
Right ventricle
Atrioventricular nodal artery
D
Coronary sinus
Left ventricle
Coronary sinus
Right ventricle

Maze III Procedure

The Maze III procedure is performed for patients with chronic atrial fibrillation who have tachyarrhythmia that is resistant to medical treatment. Selected patients with mitral valve disease may have the Maze III procedure in conjunction with operation on the mitral valve. The operation was devised by Cox and follows his technique with minor modifications. Incisions are made in the right and left atria, producing an orderly passage of the electrical impulse from the sinoatrial node to the atrioventricular node. Blind passageways are created that suppress reentry cycles.

Figure 44-6

A Bicaval cannulation is required. A right-angled cannula is inserted directly into the superior vena cava (SVC). The inferior vena cava (IVC) is cannulated through the right atrium (RA) as close as possible to the diaphragm. Perfusion is at normothermia to maintain the heartbeat during the initial phases of the operation on the right atrium. The right atrial appendage is excised, removing all trabeculations attached to it. An incision is made in the lateral aspect of the right atrial opening, extending toward the midpoint of the right atrium.

B A longitudinal incision is made in the lateral wall of the right atrium just anterior to the interatrial groove. This incision extends onto the superior vena cava above and the inferior vena cava below.

C The lower end of the incision is immediately closed by continuous stitches of 4/0 polypropylene to a point about 2 cm cephalad to the inferior vena cava cannula.

D At this point a vertical incision is made, extending anteriorly.

E The inside of the right atrium is exposed so that an intraatrial incision can be extended to the tricuspid valve annulus at about the midpoint of the posterior leaflet. The inset shows the placement of a cryolesion (*asterisk*) at approximately the 2 o'clock position on the tricuspid annulus.

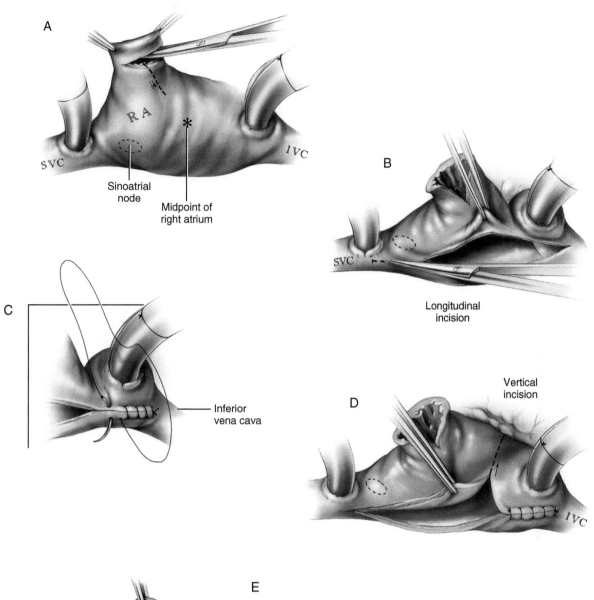

A

RA

SVC

IVC

Sinoatrial node

Midpoint of right atrium

B

SVC

Longitudinal incision

C

Inferior vena cava

D

Vertical incision

IVC

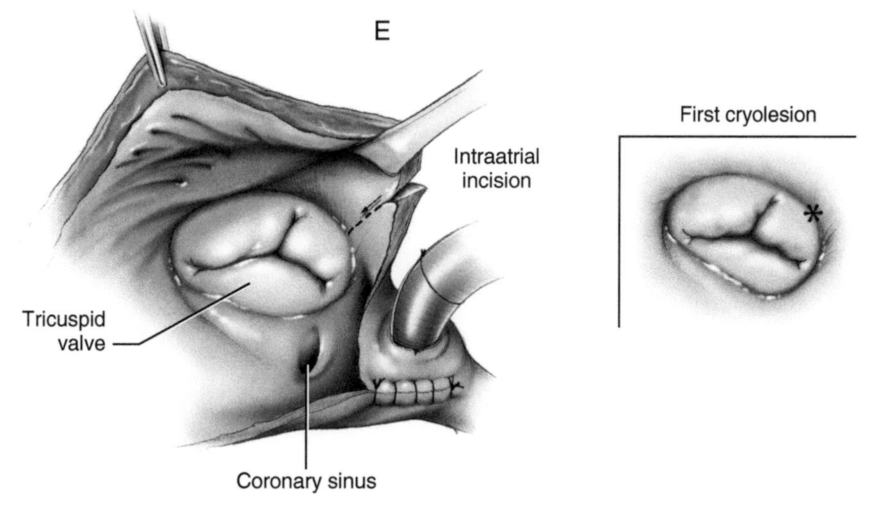

Figure 44-6 (continued)

F All muscle fibers of the right atrial wall are divided, exposing the fat of the atrioventricular groove and occasionally the right coronary artery. A 3-mm cryolesion is placed at the tricuspid annulus for 2 minutes at –70°C.

G The atrial incision is closed from the annulus of the tricuspid valve to the free wall of the right atrium by continuous stitches of 4/0 polypropylene.

H An incision is made on the medial aspect of the remnant of the appendage.

I This incision extends to the tricuspid valve annulus at the midpoint of the anterior leaflet, or to approximately the 10 o'clock position.

J Another 3-mm cryolesion (*asterisk*) is placed at the tricuspid annulus for 2 minutes at –70°C. Systemic cooling is started during this maneuver. The aorta is occluded in preparation for the left atrial portion of the operation. Cold cardioplegic solution is administered to the heart via retrograde perfusion of the coronary sinus through an appropriate cannula (not shown).

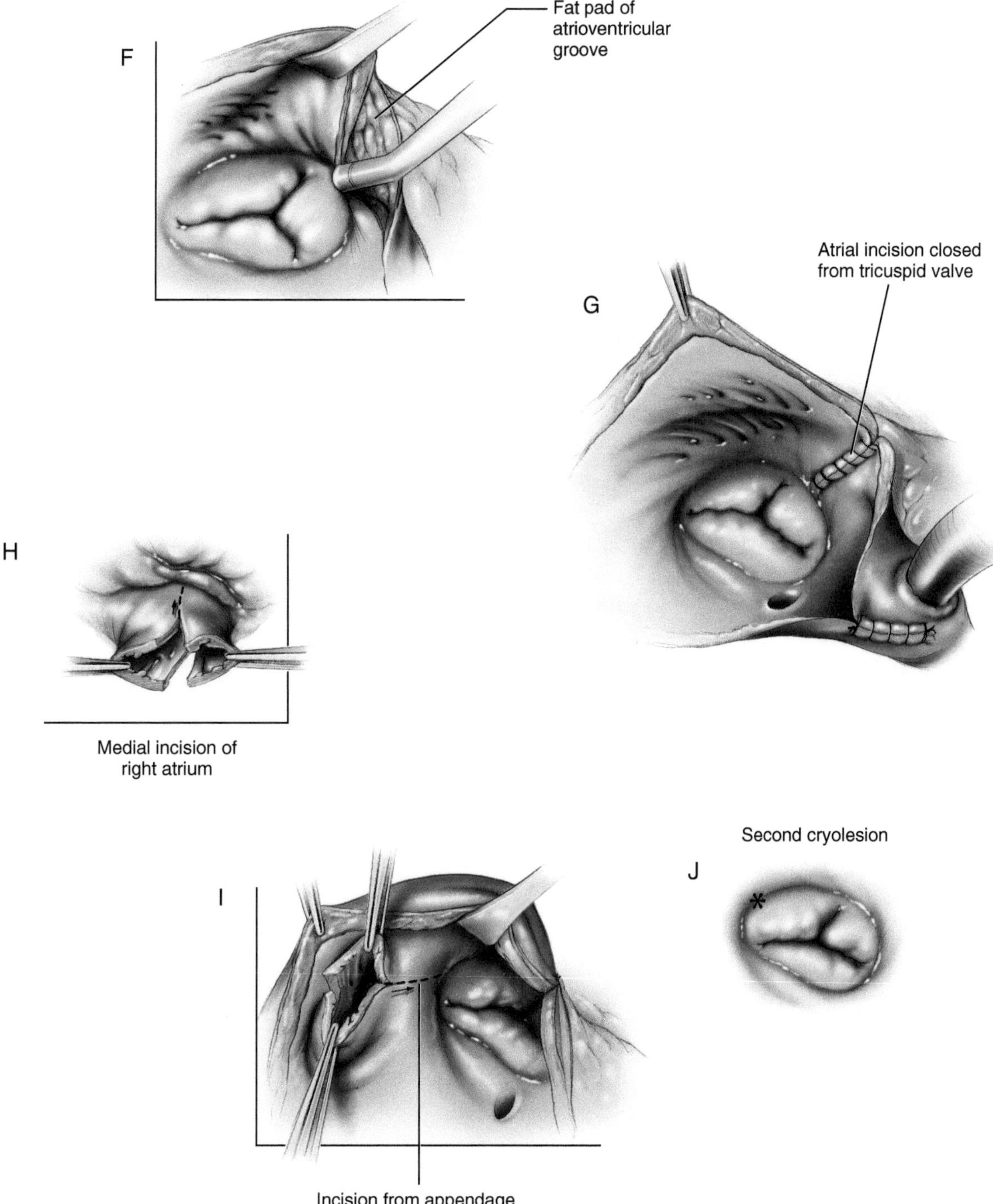
F
Fat pad of
atrioventricular
groove
G
Atrial incision closed
from tricuspid valve
H
Medial incision of
right atrium
Second cryolesion
J
*
I
Incision from appendage
to tricuspid valve annulua

Figure 44-6 (continued)

K The left atrium is opened by an incision just posterior to the interatrial groove near the orifices of the right pulmonary veins. RA, right atrium.

L The incision is extended onto the left atrium (LA), around the superior and inferior pulmonary veins. The incision is continued across the left atrium toward the left pulmonary veins to isolate and encircle the veins.

M The atrial septum is incised above the fossa ovalis. The incision is curved across the limbus of the fossa ovalis and across the membrane of the fossa to its inferior margin near but not into the tendon of Todaro.

N The pulmonary vein-encircling incision is continued. Retention stitches of 3/0 polypropylene are placed near the left superior and inferior pulmonary veins prior to completing the left side of the encircling incision. These stitches maintain the proper orientation of the atrial structures for later reconstruction.

O The heart is retracted to the right to expose the left atrial appendage. The left atrial appendage is excised at its base.

P The appendage is incised in a cephalad direction near the atrioventricular groove, across its base, and back into the left atrium. This incision is closed with continuous stitches of 3/0 polypropylene. The suture is passed from the outside into the left atrium and retrieved from within the atrium. PA, pulmonary artery.

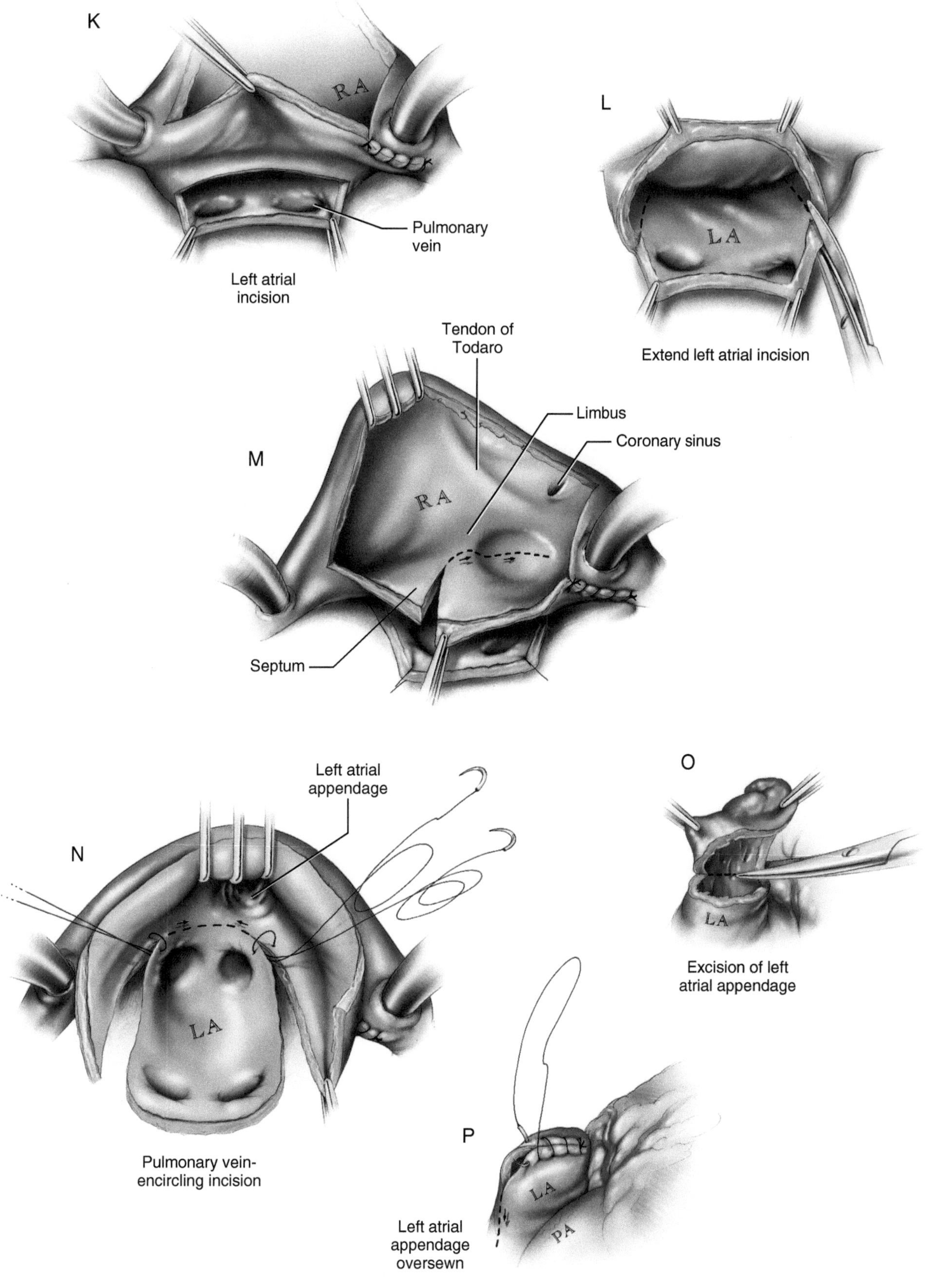
K
RA
Pulmonary vein
Left atrial incision
L
LA
Extend left atrial incision
Tendon of Todaro
Limbus
Coronary sinus
M
RA
Septum
Left atrial appendage
N
LA
Pulmonary vein-encircling incision
O
LA
Excision of left atrial appendage
P
LA
PA
Left atrial appendage oversewn

Figure 44-6 (continued)

Q The incision in the left atrial appendage is joined to the pulmonary vein–encircling incision from inside the left atrium at a point near the left superior pulmonary vein retention stitch.

R With the previously placed suture, the incision in the base of the left atrial appendage is closed back to the encircling incision. The encircling incision is closed beginning with the inferior pulmonary vein retention suture and continuing cephalad.

S The closure continues around the superior aspect of the encircling incision to the midpoint. The encircling incision is closed inferiorly to the midpoint. An incision is made across the floor of the left atrium to the midpoint of the posterior mitral valve annulus.

T This incision is carefully opened by sharp dissection. The coronary sinus is exposed by the incision in the fat of the atrioventricular groove. The circumflex coronary artery may also be visualized in the incision. A 15-mm cryoprobe at –60°C is placed posteriorly on the coronary sinus for 3 minutes. After 1 minute of freezing, a 3-mm cryoprobe is placed at the mitral valve annulus at –70°C for 2 minutes. The timing of freezing with the twp probes is coordinated so that thawing occurs simultaneously.

U The incision in the floor of the left atrium is closed by continuous stitches of 4/0 polypropylene, beginning at the mitral annulus and continuing to the encircling incision. The sutures are joined and continued to close the encircling incision over to the right pulmonary veins.

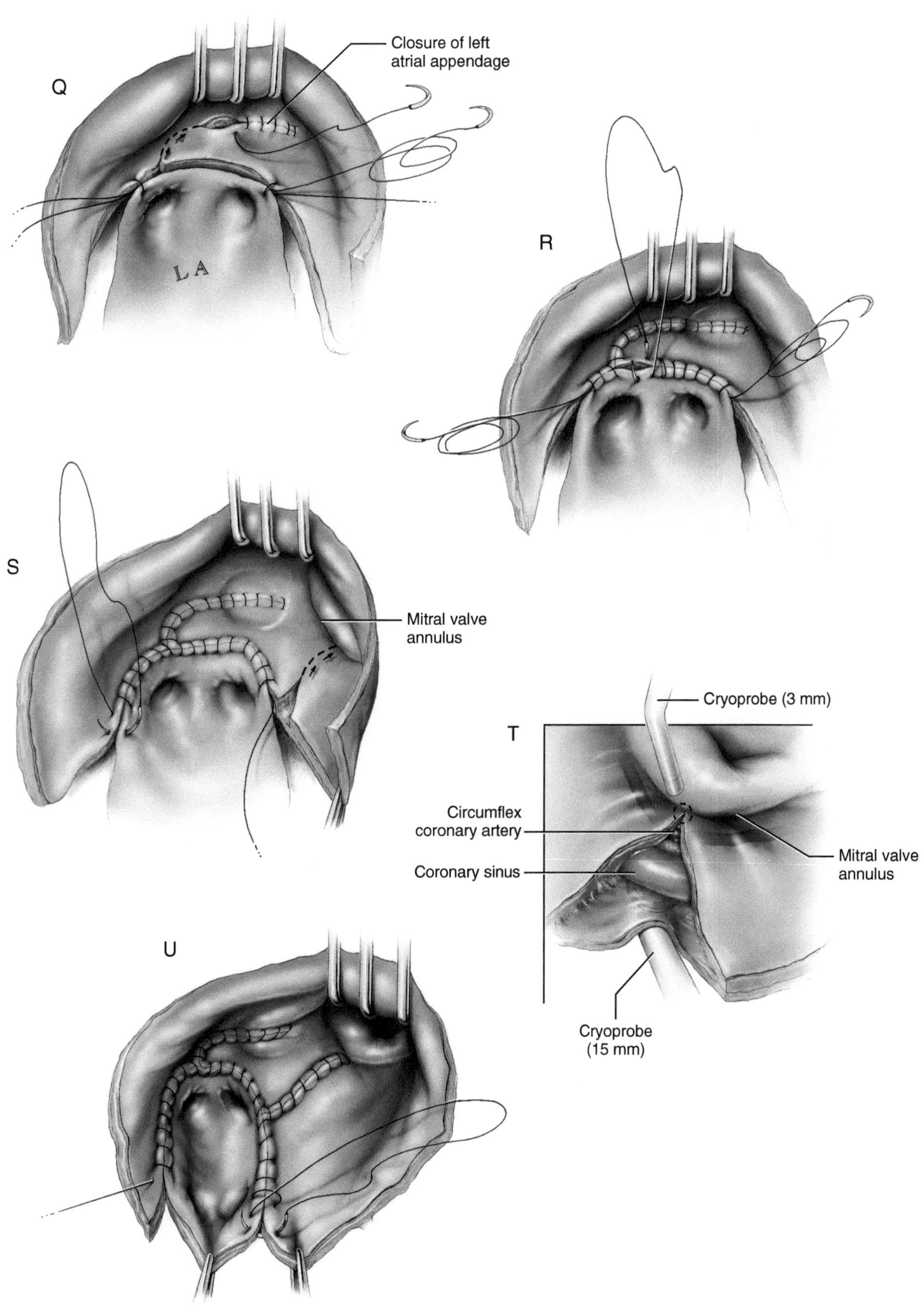
Q
Closure of left
atrial appendage
LA
R
S
Mitral valve
annulus
T
Cryoprobe (3 mm)
Circumflex
coronary artery
Mitral valve
annulus
Coronary sinus
Cryoprobe
(15 mm)
U

Figure 44-6 (continued)

V The atrial septum is a thin membrane within the fossa ovalis. The limbus is muscular and thicker. There are discrete layers of the right and left atria that represent infolding of the atria at the interatrial groove rather than the true septum. These layers should be closed separately.

W Septal closure begins at the inferior border of the fossa ovalis using continuous stitches of 4/0 polypropylene. The suturing continues across the limbus and along the left atrial fold to the free margin.

X A second layer of closure starts at the limbus and continues along the right atrial fold to the junction with the longitudinal incision in the right atrium. The remainder of the pulmonary vein–encircling incision is closed and joined to the left atrial septal closure. A vent catheter is inserted via the left superior pulmonary vein. Air is evacuated from the left cardiac chambers and aorta, and the aortic occlusion clamp is removed. The heart is reperfused and may be defibrillated.

Y The longitudinal incision in the right atrium is closed beginning at the superior vena cava and working inferiorly. The suture is joined to the right atrial septal closure, then continued to the vertical right atrial incision. The vertical incision is closed.

Z The operation is completed by closure of the right atrial appendage opening, with the suture line beginning at the midpoint of the right atrium and continuing through the appendage incision.

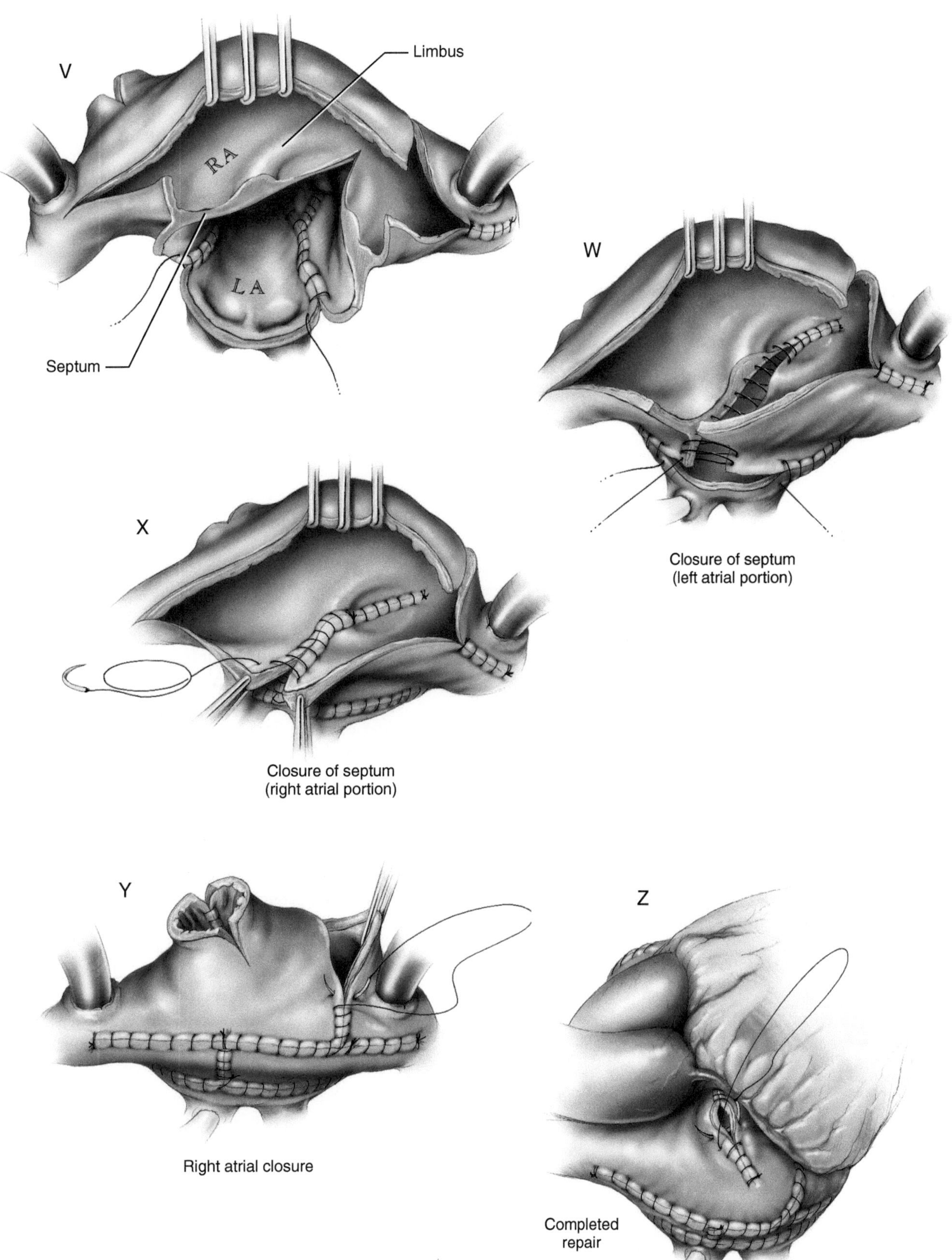
V
Limbus
RA
LA
Septum
W
Closure of septum
(left atrial portion)
X
Closure of septum
(right atrial portion)
Y
Right atrial closure
Z
Completed
repair

Modified Maze III Procedure Using Irrigated Radiofrequency

The Maze III procedure is a long, complex operation even when performed by the most technically adept surgeons. Less than 10% of surgeons used it. Adapting techniques of radiofrequency ablation utilized by cardiologists in the cardiac catheterization laboratory, surgeons began simulating the Maze III lesion pattern using various energies to create scarring in segments of the atria and control atrial fibrillation. Irrigated radiofrequency applied through a monopolar electrode provides reproducible deep injury to the atrial myocardium and is simple to perform.

Figure 44-7

A An incision is made through the right atrial appendage. An incision made in the lateral wall of the right atrium curves from the fat of the atrioventricular groove toward the right superior pulmonary vein, crossing the crista terminalis. The left-side surgical incisions to amputate the left atrial appendage and enter the left atrium on the right side behind the interatrial groove are also shown, but these incisions are actually made later.

B Working through the primary incision in the lateral wall of the right atrium, linear radiofrequency ablation lesions are created to extend the primary incision posteriorly into the superior vena cava and then cephalad to the caval tourniquet. The primary incision is also extended by an ablation line directed posteriorly into the inferior vena cava to the caval tourniquet. An inferior isthmus ablation is performed to control atrial flutter by extending the inferior vena cava ablation line across the inferior isthmus to the tricuspid valve annulus at the posterior leaflet. The primary incision is not extended by an ablation line to the annulus of the tricuspid valve in order to allow depolarization of the inferior isthmus. The appendage incision is extended to the tricuspid valve annulus. An occlusion clamp is placed on the ascending aorta, and cold cardioplegic solution is infused by a catheter in the coronary sinus. The left atrial appendage is amputated at the base. Working through the base of the appendage, an ablation line is created anterior to the left pulmonary veins and joined to the base of the appendage. The appendage is closed by suture.

C Working through the primary incision posterior to the interatrial groove into the left atrium, the left pulmonary vein–encircling ablation line is completed posterior to the veins. This encircling ablation line is extended to the annulus of the mitral valve. The right pulmonary vein–encircling incision is completed by using radiofrequency ablation to extend the primary incision around the right pulmonary veins. The encircling ablation lines are connected by tissue ablation. A coronary sinus ablation line extends from the mitral annulus line along the course of the coronary sinus. The thickness of the atrial septal tissues and the presence of a fat layer between the right and left atrial portions of the septum make full-thickness ablation by radiofrequency energy unreliable. In other areas where radiofrequency is employed, such as around the atrioventricular valves, in the cavae, around the pulmonary veins, and over the coronary sinus, the atrial tissues are thin and smooth, making full-thickness tissue penetration by ablation energy easier and more reliable.

D The atrial septum is therefore ablated both on the left atrial endocardial surface from the fossa ovalis to the primary left atrial incision and on the right atrial endocardium from the fossa ovalis and over the limbus to the primary incision in the right atrium.

E Surgical incisions are closed in the usual fashion to complete the modified Maze III procedure.

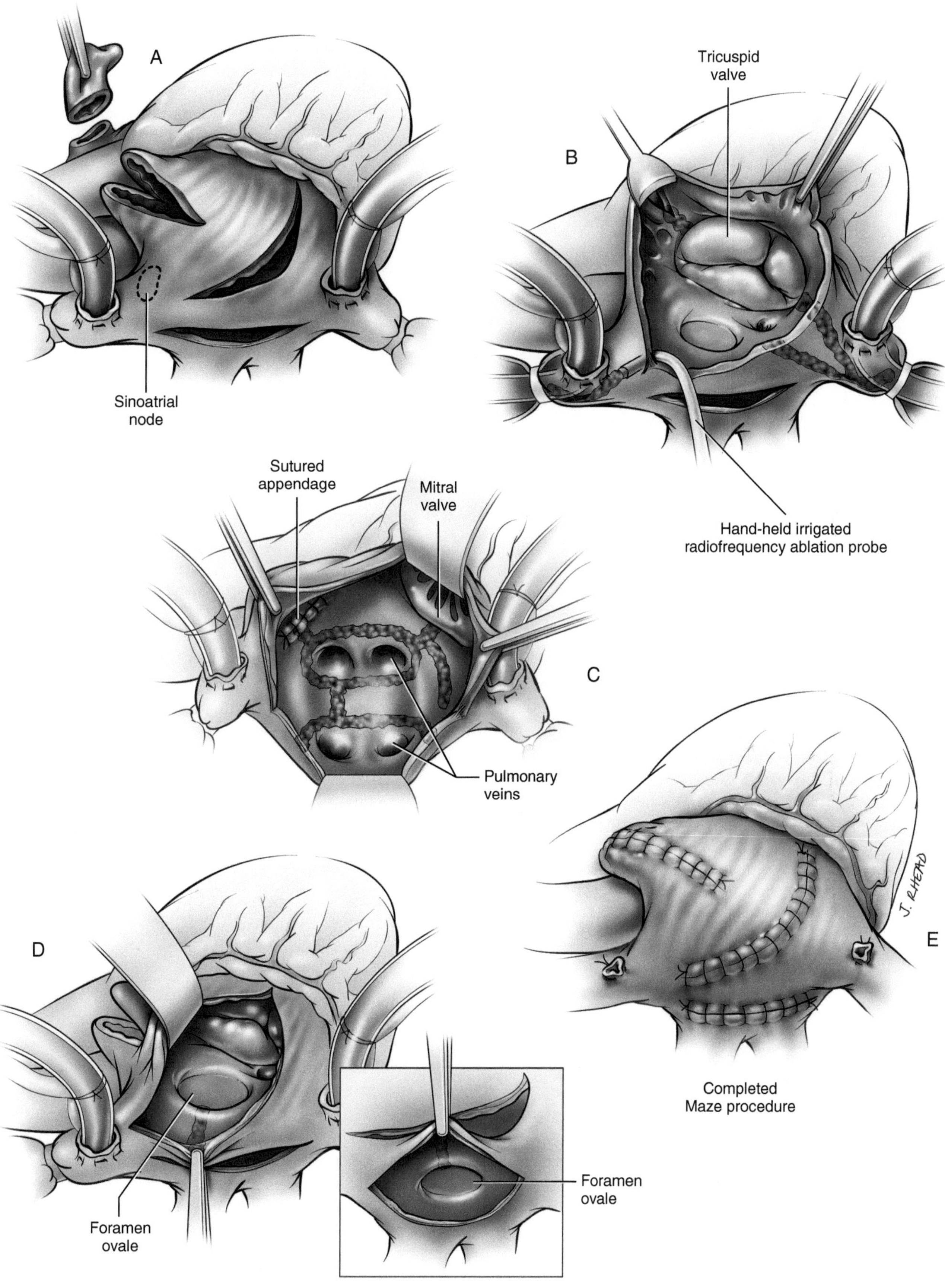
A
Sinoatrial
node
B
Tricuspid
valve
Hand-held irrigated
radiofrequency ablation probe
Sutured
appendage
Mitral
valve
C
Pulmonary
veins
D
Foramen
ovale
Foramen
ovale
E
J. RHEAD
Completed
Maze procedure

Modified Maze Operation Using Cardioblate BP System

The Cardioblate BP (bipolar) surgical ablation system (Medtronic, Minneapolis, MN) combines saline-irrigated radiofrequency with an ergonomic design and an electrode head with pitch and rotation control, as well as malleable electrodes for ease of use. The Cardioblate BP device can be used for a modified Maze procedure in which both right and left atrial ablation lesions are employed.

Figure 44-8

A A midline sternotomy incision is made. Cardiopulmonary bypass is established using active suction through two cannulae for venous drainage. A 24 F thin-walled percutaneous venous cannula is placed directly into the superior vena cava at the pericardial reflection. A second cannula is placed through the right atrial wall into the inferior vena cava at a position somewhat higher on the atrium than usual for dual venous cannulation. Oxygenated blood is returned to a cannula in the ascending aorta. The atria are defibrillated to check sinoatrial node function. Tourniquets are secured around the caval cannulae. The tip of the right atrial appendage is incised. The primary incision in the right atrium extends transversely across the free wall of the right atrium from the atrioventricular groove to the crista terminalis. Suction drainage is placed in the coronary sinus.

Right Atrial Ablation

B One electrode blade of the Cardioblate BP device is placed through the right atrial appendage onto the endocardial surface. The other blade is placed on the epicardial surface of the right atrium, leaving a 3- to 4-cm bridge of intact atrial wall between the ends of the blades and the primary atrial incision. The blades are closed and locked into position to create the ablation lesion. An audible signal alerts the surgeon when transmural ablation is complete. The blades are opened and reapplied on the wall of the right atrium through the appendage, toward the annulus of the tricuspid valve up to the atrioventricular groove. An ablation lesion is created in this position.

C The blades of the Cardioblate BP device are shaped with a curve to the right. The blades are inserted through the posterior aspect of the primary incision and advanced to the superior vena cava. The blades are closed posterior to the sinoatrial node on the posterolateral wall of the superior vena cava, up to the level of the venous uptake cannula, and an ablation lesion is created. The blades are then replaced through the posterior aspect of the primary incision into the inferior vena cava (inset). Positioning of the blades is made easier by rotating the head of the device three clicks to the right (90 degrees). An ablation lesion is created on the posterolateral wall of the inferior vena cava up to the venous uptake cannula. The blades are withdrawn, and the head is returned to the neutral position.

D Next, a small opening is made in the right atrium medial to the inferior vena cava. One blade of the Cardioblate BP device is placed inside the right atrium on the endocardium behind the caval uptake cannula. The other blade is placed on the epicardial surface and directed laterally, toward the inferior vena cava ablation line. Loosening the purse-string stitch on the inferior vena cava venous uptake cannula makes this maneuver easier. An ablation lesion is created across the inferior isthmus, joining the inferior vena cava ablation lesion. The blades of the device are withdrawn and replaced in a medial direction toward the tricuspid valve annulus (inset). This maneuver is made easier by adjusting the blade pitch to 90 degrees. An ablation lesion is created up to the atrioventricular groove.

E The monopolar Cardioblate pen device is used to extend both this ablation line and the atrial appendage ablation line to the tricuspid annulus. This completes the right atrial portion of the Maze procedure.

A retrograde perfusion cannula is placed in a coronary sinus. The aorta is occluded, and the ascending aorta is vented by a needle. A 12 F pediatric vent catheter is placed through the right superior pulmonary vein into the left atrium. Cold cardioplegic solution is administered through the coronary sinus to achieve total electromechanical arrest of the heart.

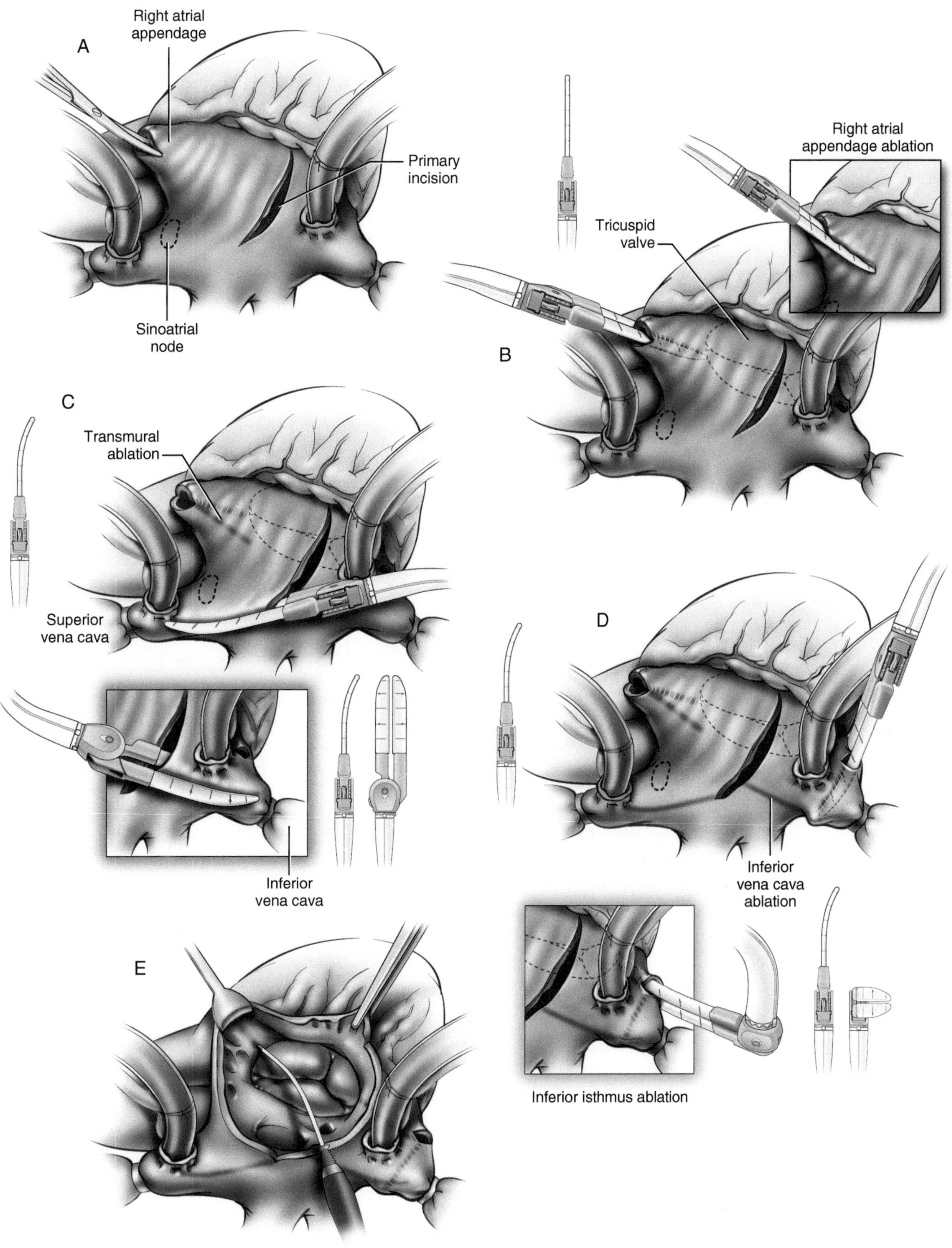
A
Right atrial appendage
Primary incision
Sinoatrial node
B
Tricuspid valve
Right atrial appendage ablation
C
Transmural ablation
Superior vena cava
Inferior vena cava
D
Inferior vena cava ablation
Inferior isthmus ablation
E
Monopolar ablation to tricuspid annulus

Figure 44-8 (continued)

Left Atrial Ablation

F The heart is retracted anteriorly and to the right to expose the left pulmonary veins. The pericardial reflection over the posterior aspect of the left pulmonary veins is opened to allow passage of a right-angled clamp behind the veins. The blades of the Cardioblate BP device are rotated one click to the left. The pitch remains at 90 degrees. One blade is passed behind the pulmonary veins from below, and the other is placed in front of the veins. The blades are closed on the left atrium to create the left pulmonary vein isolation lesion. The blades are opened, the device is removed from the pulmonary veins, and the head is returned to the neutral position.

G The left atrial appendage is excised at the base, removing all trabecular tissue. The blades of the Cardioblate BP device are inserted through the base of the appendage into the left superior pulmonary vein. An ablation lesion is created at this position, joining the appendage to the left pulmonary vein isolation lesion. The base of the appendage is closed by continuous suture in two layers using 4/0 polypropylene.

H The heart is returned to its normal position in the pericardial sac. The pericardial reflection behind the right pulmonary veins is opened to allow a right-angled clamp to be passed behind the veins. An incision is made on the right side of the left atrium in the interatrial groove. One blade of the Cardioblate BP device is passed from above, posterior to the right pulmonary veins; the other blade is placed on the endocardial surface of the left atrium. An ablation lesion is created in this position to complete the right pulmonary vein isolation. The blades are withdrawn and reshaped with a curve to the left.

I The blades are placed across the posterior wall of the left atrium and into the left inferior pulmonary vein from the inferior aspect of the primary incision, below the right inferior pulmonary vein. An ablation lesion is created to join the right and left pulmonary vein isolation lesions. The monopolar pen is used to join the left pulmonary vein isolation lesion to the midpoint of the posterior mitral valve annulus (inset).

Septal Ablation

J The monopolar pen is used to ablate the left atrial aspect of the interatrial septum from the fossa ovalis to the primary incision in the left atrium. The pen is then used to ablate the interatrial septum on the right side from the fossa ovalis, across the limbus, to the primary incision in the right atrium. The left atriotomy is closed by continuous stitches of 3/0 polypropylene. The right atrial incisions are closed with 4/0 polypropylene suture.

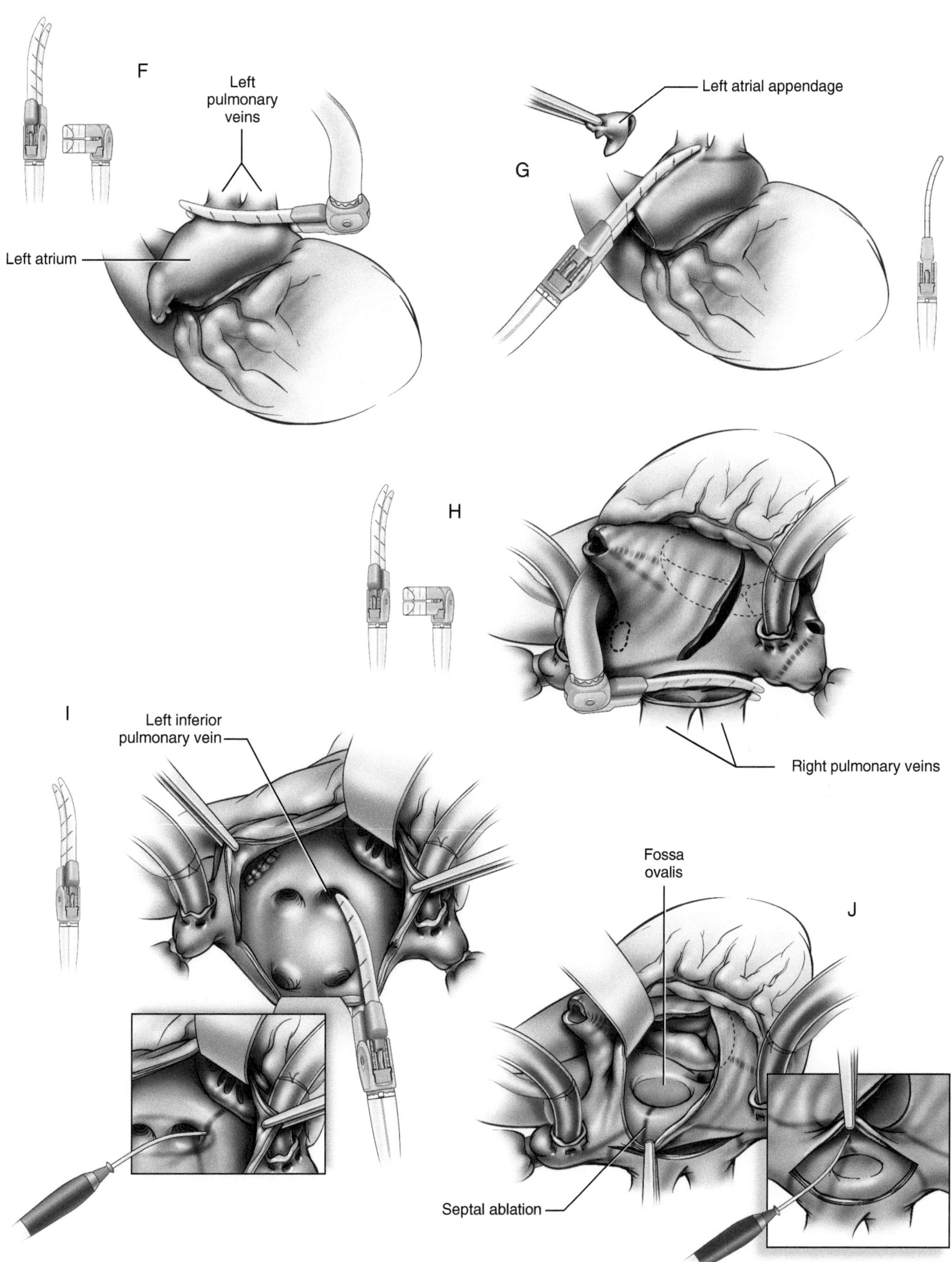
F
Left pulmonary veins
Left atrium
Left atrial appendage
G
H
Right pulmonary veins
I
Left inferior pulmonary vein
Fossa ovalis
J
Septal ablation

Pulmonary Vein Isolation (Bilateral Vertical Approach)

Pulmonary vein isolation, either as a stand-alone operation or as part of the full Maze III lesion set, is indicated for any patient with atrial fibrillation. Bilateral pulmonary vein isolation is performed with radiofrequency ablation, isolating the right and left pulmonary veins independently.

Figure 44-9

A Blunt dissection is used to develop a space behind the left atrium near the confluence of the left pulmonary veins. One jaw of the bipolar radiofrequency clamp is passed behind the veins, and the other jaw is placed in front of the veins. The clamp is angled so that the convexity places the jaws well up onto the left atrial wall. This avoids creating a lesion on the pulmonary veins, which can result in pulmonary vein stenosis.

The left atrial appendage is divided near its base, and one jaw of the clamp is placed inside the left atrium, forming a connecting lesion into the left superior pulmonary vein. The stump of the left atrial appendage is then oversewn with continuous suture.

B In a similar fashion, blunt dissection is used to develop a space behind the left atrium near the confluence of the right pulmonary veins. One jaw of the bipolar radiofrequency clamp is passed behind the veins, and the other jaw is placed in front of the veins to create the right pulmonary vein isolation lesion. Care is taken to ensure that the jaws are placed well up onto the left atrial wall.

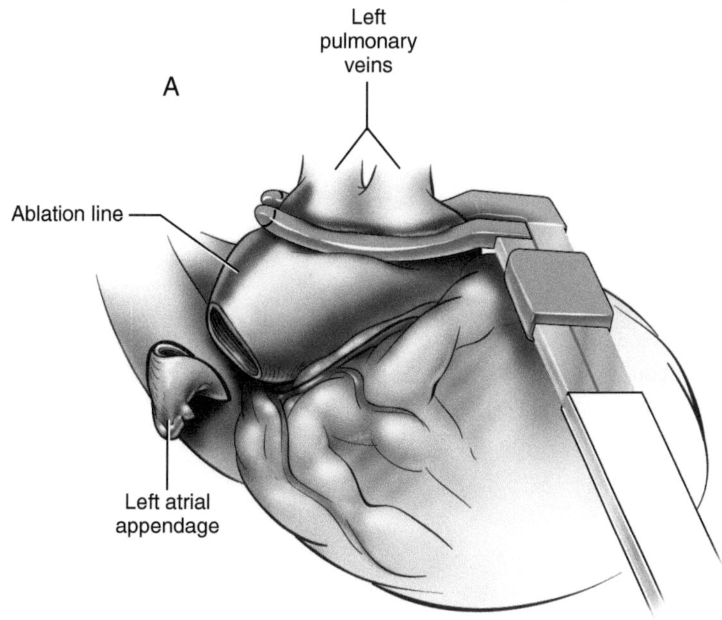
A
Left pulmonary veins
Ablation line
Left atrial appendage

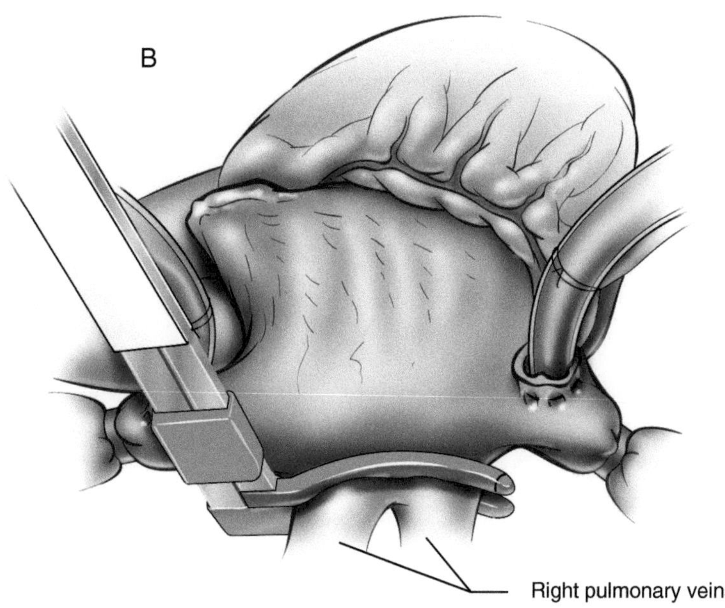
B
Right pulmonary veins

GALAXY Procedure (Gemini Ablation and Left Atrial Appendage Excision)

Patients with isolated atrial fibrillation are suitable candidates for less invasive operations to ablate atrial tissue. Such procedures are performed on the beating heart without cardiopulmonary bypass, utilizing either small bilateral thoracotomies or video-assisted thoracoscopy.

Figure 44-10

A The patient is placed in a supine position with inflatable thyroid pillows on each side of the spine. The arms are tucked laterally; alternatively, they may be extended out 90 degrees. Double-lumen intubation is required to allow selective single-lung ventilation.

A small thoracotomy is performed in the right fourth interspace centered below the nipple, and the right lung is deflated. The thyroid pillow is inflated behind the right chest, and the operating table is tilted to the left to improve exposure. An 8-mm port is placed in the sixth or seventh interspace, and a 30-degree thoracoscope is inserted. A No. 0 silk suture is placed in the central tendon of the right hemidiaphragm and pulled through the incision next to the port to retract the diaphragm inferiorly.

B The pericardium is opened longitudinally, well above the phrenic nerve, and retraction sutures are placed to expose the heart. A lighted, flexible dissector is used to open the oblique sinus between the right inferior pulmonary vein and the inferior vena cava, and a guide is passed through to the left side of the pericardial space. The dissector is used to dissect behind the superior vena cava and above the roof of the left atrium to enter the transverse sinus. A second guide is passed through the transverse sinus into the left side of the pericardial space.

C The right-sided autonomic ganglia are mapped by placing the tip of the irrigated probe in a sequential, logical pattern, beginning on the medial and superior aspect of the right pulmonary veins and ending on the lateral and inferior aspect of the veins. High-frequency stimulation is performed at each of the ten points in the grid. Monopolar ablation is performed at any grid point where there is positive autonomic activity. Following ablation, the point is retested to ensure destruction of that area.

D A small thoracotomy is performed in the left third or fourth interspace in a more posterior location to allow access to the left atrial appendage. The right lung is reinflated, and the left lung is deflated. The thyroid pillow is deflated behind the right chest and inflated behind the left chest, and the table is tilted toward the right to improve exposure. A 15-mm port is placed in the seventh or eight interspace, and a 30-degree thoracoscope is inserted. The pericardium is opened longitudinally, well below the phrenic nerve, and retention sutures are placed to expose the heart. The guides are retrieved and brought out through the thoracotomy.

E Mapping of the left-sided autonomic ganglia is performed in a similar manner, with stimulation, ablation, and retesting. The ligament of Marshall represents an important focus of autonomic activity and lies between the left pulmonary artery and the left superior pulmonary vein. This structure should routinely be ablated as part of the procedure.

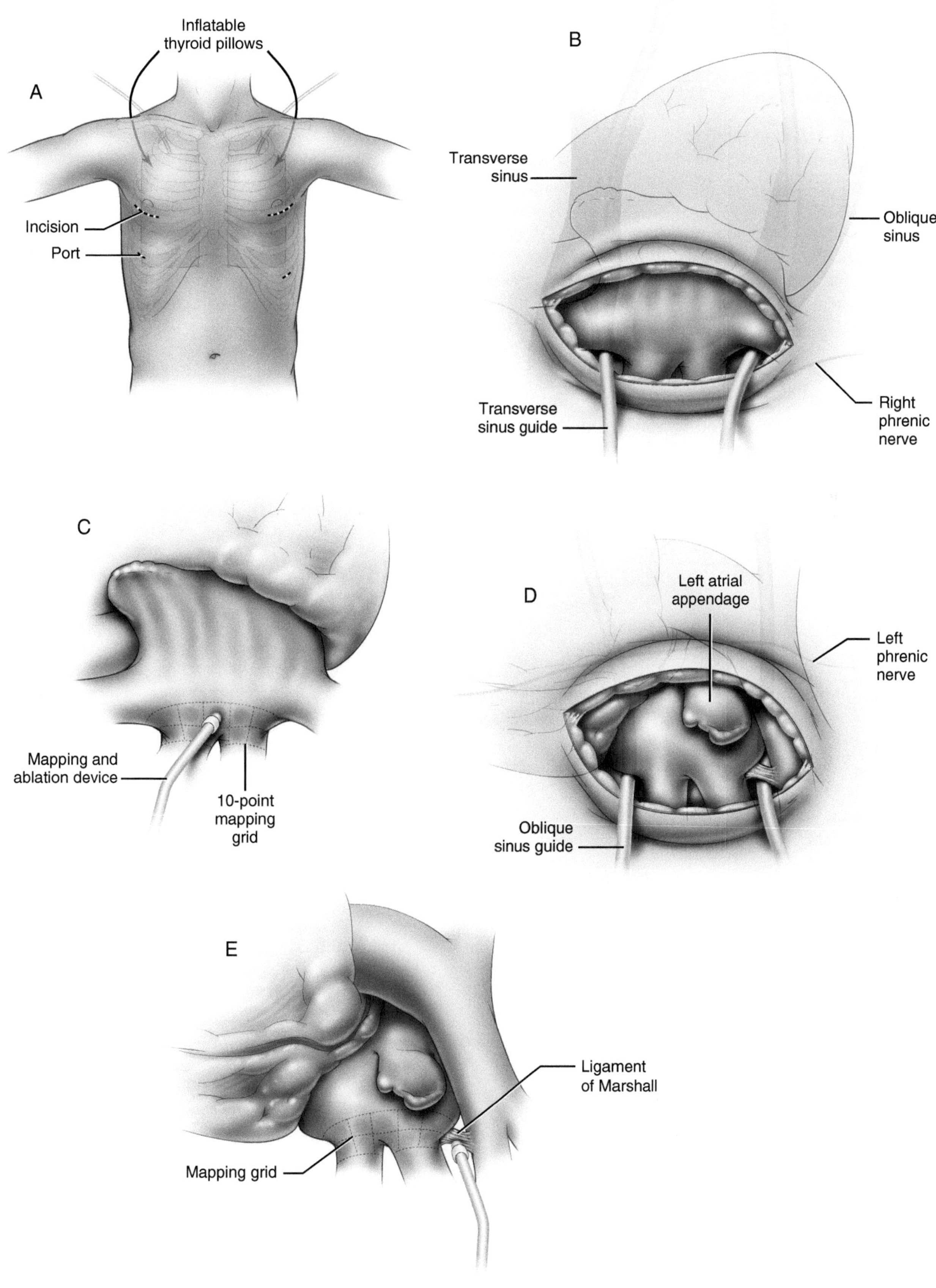
A
Inflatable
thyroid pillows
Incision
Port
B
Transverse
sinus
Oblique
sinus
Transverse
sinus guide
Right
phrenic
nerve
C
Mapping and
ablation device
10-point
mapping
grid
D
Left atrial
appendage
Left
phrenic
nerve
Oblique
sinus guide
E
Ligament
of Marshall
Mapping grid

Figure 44-10 (continued)

F The irrigated bipolar ablation device is attached to the guides and smoothly drawn into the chest, placing the jaws across the left pulmonary veins and across the back of the left atrium. Three ablations are performed, withdrawing the jaws 2 cm after each ablation. The bipolar device is then removed, and the guides are secured.

G The left lung is reinflated, and the right lung is deflated. The bipolar device is attached to the guides on the right side and smoothly drawn into the chest, placing the jaws across the right pulmonary veins and across the back of the left atrium. Three ablations are performed, withdrawing the jaws 2 cm after each ablation. This completes the box or oval lesion encircling all four pulmonary veins. The bipolar device is removed.

H The irrigated probe is used to confirm entrance and exit block at all four pulmonary veins and the atrium. If the pulmonary vein isolation is incomplete, additional ablation with either the irrigated probe for autonomic ganglia or the bipolar device for the pulmonary veins should be performed.

I The right lung is reinflated, and the left lung is deflated. A 60-mm thoracoscopic stapler is inserted into the left port and advanced up to the left atrial appendage. Gentle traction is used to guide the left atrial appendage into the stapler. The appendage is completely stapled and transected, leaving a smooth staple line with minimal residual appendage tissue to avoid thrombus formation. The stapler is withdrawn, and the thoracoscope is reintroduced.

An alternative method is to ligate the left atrial appendage using an endo-loop. The loop is positioned around the appendage at the base. The loop is tightened under echocardiographic control until no blood is seen entering the appendage. The loop is then secured with a hemoclip. This has the advantage of nothing penetrating the appendage that could cause bleeding.

The pericardial incisions are closed with interrupted suture, and a small chest tube is placed in each pleural space. A single figure-eight 1 Vicryl suture is used to reapproximate the ribs, and the wounds are closed in standard multiple-layer fashion.

If the patient remains in atrial fibrillation at the conclusion of the operation, cardioversion should be attempted while the patient is still under anesthesia to restore sinus rhythm.

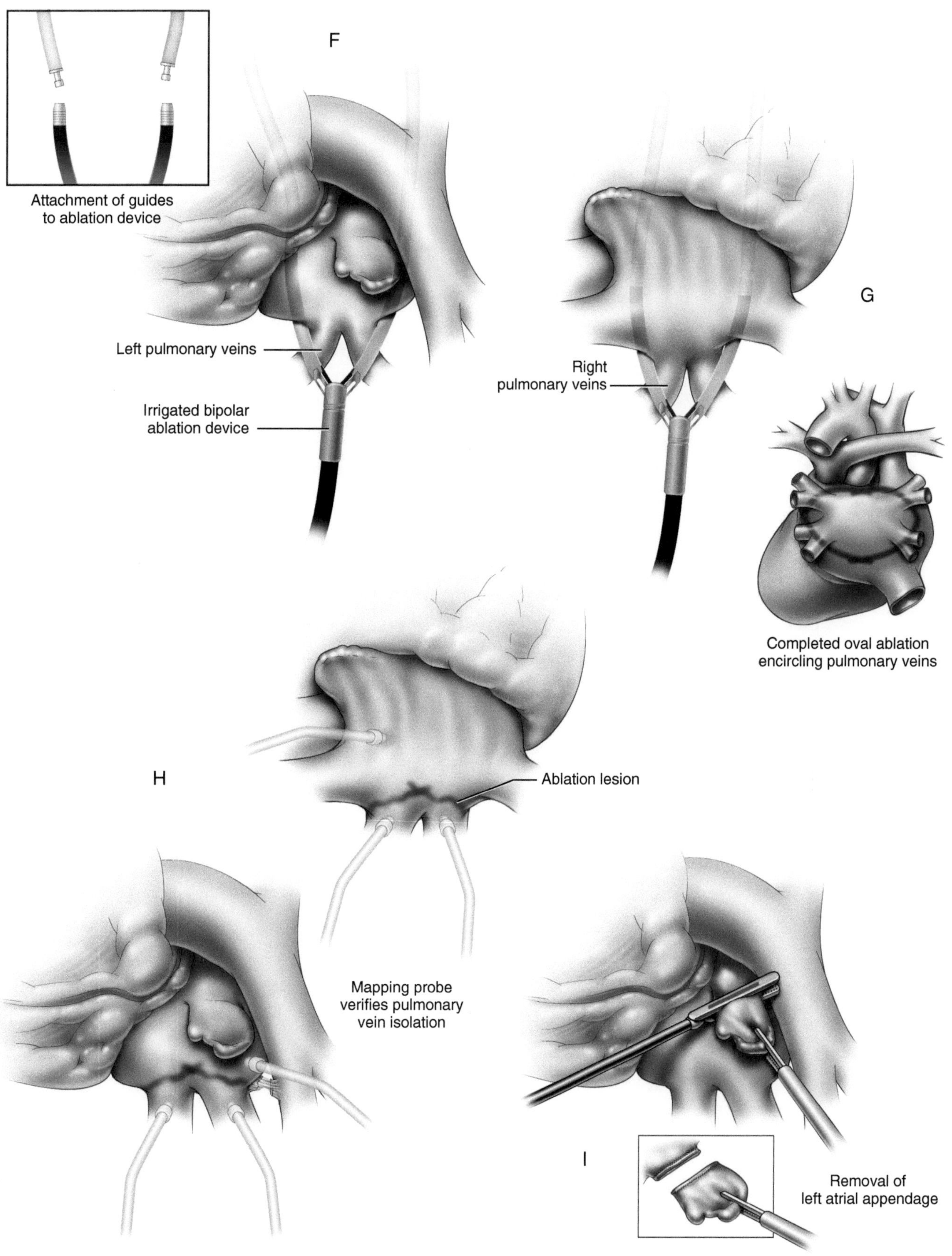
F
Attachment of guides
to ablation device
Left pulmonary veins
Irrigated bipolar
ablation device
Right
pulmonary veins
G
Completed oval ablation
encircling pulmonary veins
H
Ablation lesion
Mapping probe
verifies pulmonary
vein isolation
I
Removal of
left atrial appendage

Figure 44-10 (continued)

Thoracoscopic Approach

J The ablation system can also be used with a closed-chest thoracoscopic approach. Patient positioning is identical to that for the small, bilateral thoracotomy approach.

Two 10-mm ports are placed in the third and seventh interspaces on the right side. A 15-mm port is placed in the fifth interspace for the thoracoscope and the guides. Thoracoscopic instruments are used for all dissection and for the placement of retention sutures. After opening the transverse and oblique sinuses, the guides are passed through to the left side of the pericardial space. Mapping and autonomic ablation are performed as described earlier.

Three ports are placed on the left side: two 10-mm ports in the third and seventh interspaces, and one 15-mm port in the fifth interspace for the thoracoscope and the guides. Thoracoscopic instruments are used for dissection, guide retrieval, and mapping and ablation. The thoracoscopic stapler is inserted through the fifth interspace or through an additional incision in the eighth interspace. Alternatively, an endo-loop may be used to ligate the appendage.

The guides are passed through the 15 mm port in the fifth interspace on each side. Alternatively, the port can be removed and the bipolar device can be passed with the guides directly through the skin incision. Bipolar ablation and confirmation of exit and entrance block are performed as described in Figure 44-10, *H*.

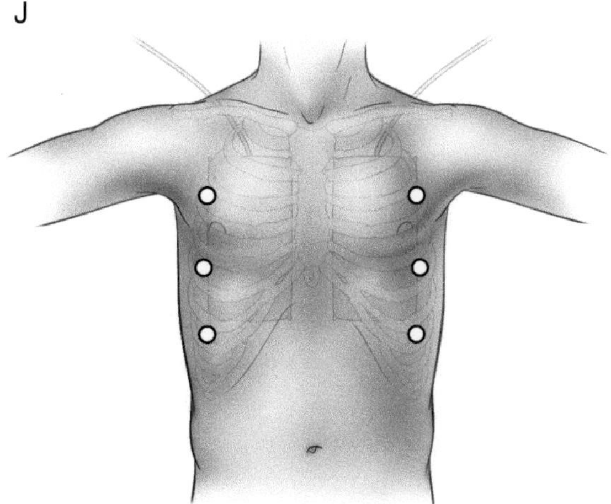

Port sites for thoracoscopic approach

chapter 45 CARDIAC TUMORS

Left Atrial Myxoma

The most common tumor of the heart is benign myxoma. It is usually located within the left atrium. The tumor tissue is friable and prone to break away and embolize. The tumor may obstruct the mitral valve and left ventricular inlet. Echocardiography is diagnostic and is usually the only test required. The point of tumor attachment can often be demonstrated on echocardiography. Operation is performed urgently after the diagnosis is established.

Figure 45-1

A The lesion is approached through an incision in the right atrium. The atrial septum is incised at the fossa ovalis. A flap of the atrial septum is developed, making sure it is free of tumor attachment.

B The flap of atrial septum is further developed until the point of attachment of the tumor stalk is clearly defined. The attachment point is frequently on the atrial septum, allowing the tumor's complete removal with a substantial margin of normal atrial septal tissue. When the tumor is attached to the left atrial wall or the mitral valve, the extent of resection of normal tissue must be evaluated on an individual basis.

C Small retractors are used to widen the opening in the atrial septum to allow the tumor to be removed from the left atrium. Some patience is required to deliver a large tumor intact. The tumor can be fragmented, but this is less desirable than removing the whole tumor intact.

D The defect in the atrial septum is repaired by suturing a pericardial patch to the rim of the defect with 4/0 polypropylene.

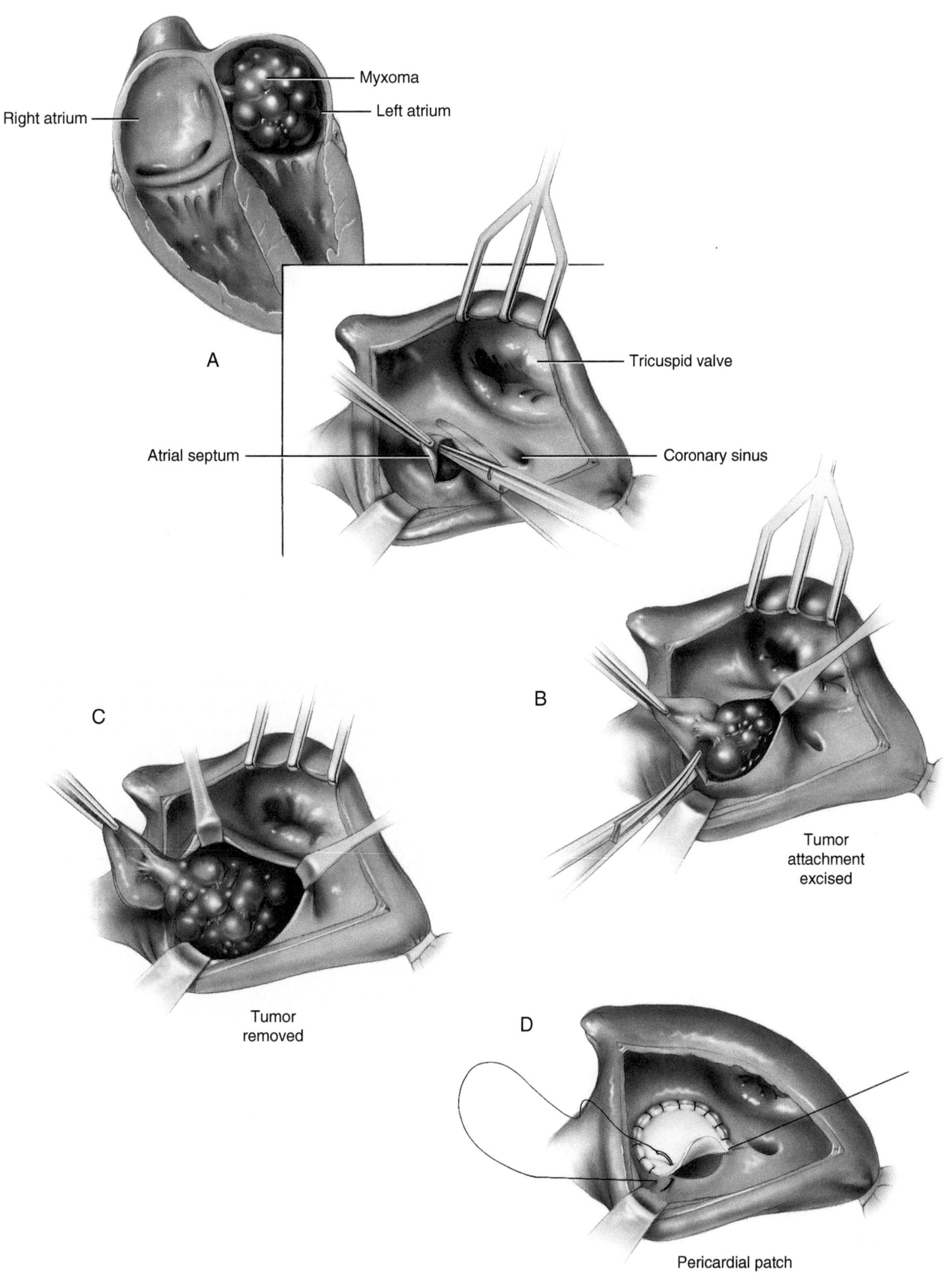
Myxoma
Right atrium
Left atrium
A
Tricuspid valve
Atrial septum
Coronary sinus
B
C
Tumor attachment excised
Tumor removed
D
Pericardial patch

Sarcoma and Other Malignant Tumors in the Left Atrium

Patients with malignant tumors in the left atrium are usually incapacitated by obstruction of blood flow from the pulmonary veins. Presence of tumor in the bloodstream predisposes to early metastasis. Resection of a tumor in the left atrium is a technical challenge. Because the tumor is located behind and covered by the cardiac mass, access is difficult. Furthermore, resection of the wall of the atrium to excise the tumor necessitates reconstruction of the left atrium to provide sufficient reservoir capacity. Operative treatment of malignant tumors of the left atrium has been accomplished by cardiac explantation to gain access. After resection of the tumor, the left atrium is reconstructed using autologous or bovine pericardium. The heart is then reimplanted.

Figure 45-2

A A primary median sternotomy is made. Cardiopulmonary bypass is established using two venous uptake cannulae; one is placed high in the superior vena cava, and the other is passed through the right atrium into the inferior vena cava. Oxygenated blood is returned through a cannula placed in the ascending aorta. An occlusion clamp is placed on the ascending aorta, and the aortic root is perfused with cold cardioplegic solution without blood cells. The superior vena cava is divided above the tumor mass, the ascending aorta is divided, the pulmonary artery is divided at the bifurcation, and the inferior vena cava is divided on the right atrium. The heart is elevated anteriorly and superiorly to expose the left atrium. (In the case illustrated here, a bulky tumor in the right superior pulmonary vein extended across the roof of the left atrium. The tumor was very close to but did not extend into the orifices of the right inferior and left pulmonary veins.) The left atrium is opened just above the atrioventricular groove, and the incision is extended in front of the tumor in the left atrium, preserving the left atrial wall not involved with tumor. The pulmonary veins are divided individually, leaving no atrium attached. (In this case, the right superior pulmonary vein was removed with the tumor.) The left atrial incision is extended superiorly around the left atrial appendage and the aorta, leaving a small cuff of atrium attached to the aorta. (The superior vena cava, right pulmonary vein, and atrial septum were firmly attached to the tumor in this case, so a portion of the right atrium and the septum were left attached to the tumor as the incision was extended. The right pulmonary artery was divided near the bifurcation and at the hilum, leaving the major part of the artery attached to the tumor.) The heart is then separated from the patient and placed in an ice-saline bath for cold preservation. With the heart removed, it is possible to remove the tumor and any attached pericardium posteriorly, leaving the orifices of the uninvolved pulmonary veins cut flush with the pericardial sac. En bloc pulmonary resection can also be performed if required to excise the tumor. The illustration shows the remnant of the pericardial sac and the cut ends of the great vessels (minus the right superior pulmonary vein) after removal of the heart and the tumor mass.

B Reconstruction of the left atrium is accomplished by attaching the orifices of the pulmonary veins securely to the remaining posterior pericardium by continuous stitches of 4/0 polypropylene.

C The posterior cut edge of the pericardium between the pulmonary veins is attached to a free patch of autogenous pericardium obtained from the sac anteriorly and fixed for 3 minutes in glutaraldehyde solution. This achieves continuity between the pericardial sac posteriorly and the pulmonary veins draining into the reconstructed sac.

D The heart is reimplanted. The remaining left atrial cuff on the heart is attached to the pericardial sac, forming a ridge of the in situ pericardium below and around the pulmonary veins.

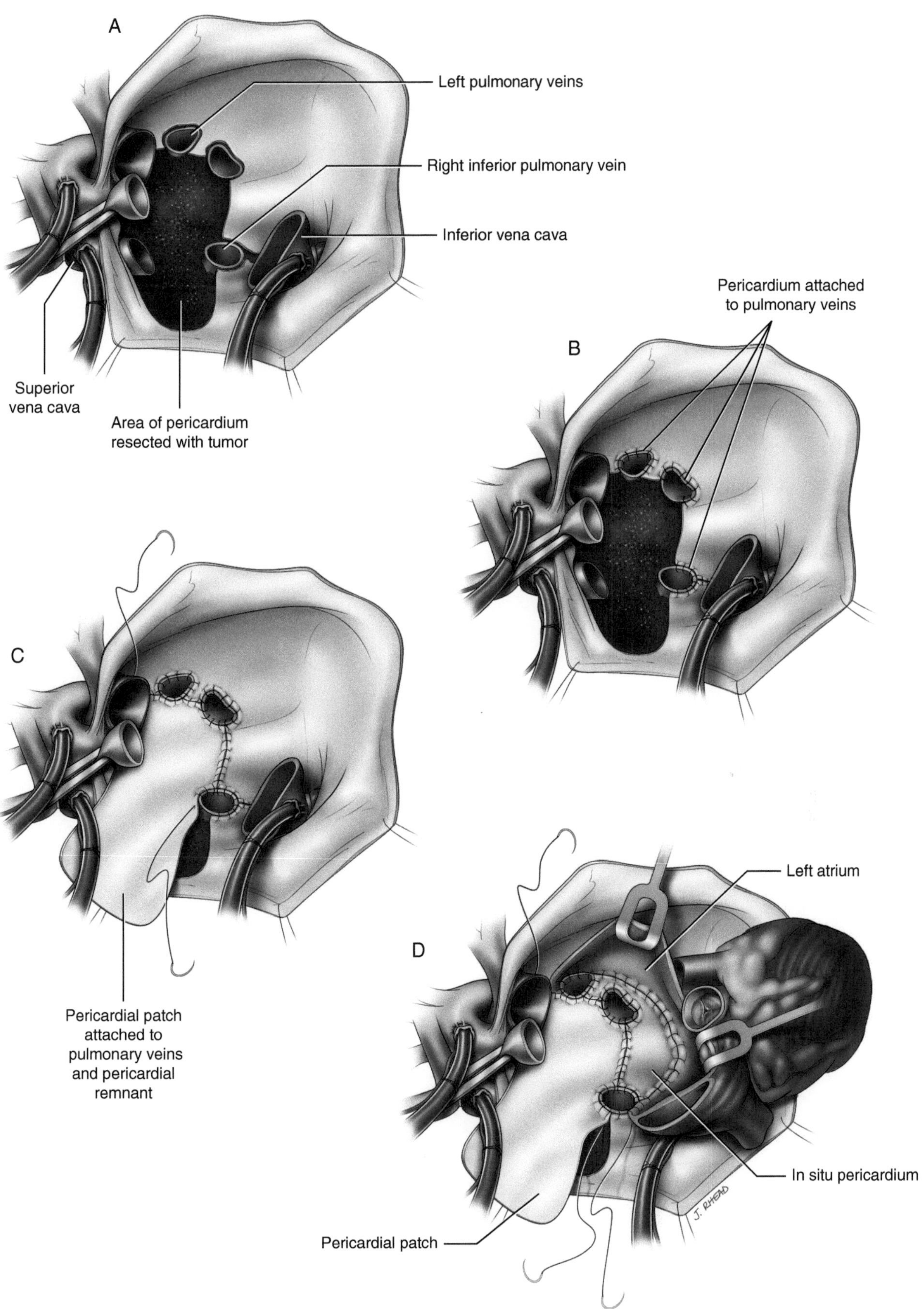
A
Left pulmonary veins
Right inferior pulmonary vein
Inferior vena cava
Superior vena cava
Area of pericardium resected with tumor
B
Pericardium attached to pulmonary veins
C
Pericardial patch attached to pulmonary veins and pericardial remnant
D
Left atrium
In situ pericardium
Pericardial patch
J. RHEAD

Figure 45-2 (continued)

E Superiorly, the free pericardial patch is shortened and tailored to form the dome of the reconstructed left atrium. Continuous stitches of 4/0 polypropylene are used for the repair.

F The completed left atrial reconstruction has good capacity.

G The inferior vena cava is reanastomosed to the right atrium. The right pulmonary artery is reconstructed using an 8 mm externally reinforced polytetrafluoroethylene (PTFE) graft to create a bridge from the bifurcation to the right pulmonary artery at the hilum. The main pulmonary artery is reanastomosed separately (inset).

H The tip of the right atrial appendage is excised. The large opening that remains in the right atrium as a consequence of resection is extended to allow rotation of the appendage superiorly for anastomosis to the superior vena cava. The right atrium is closed, and the septum is repaired in a single suture line. The operation is completed by anastomosis of the aorta.

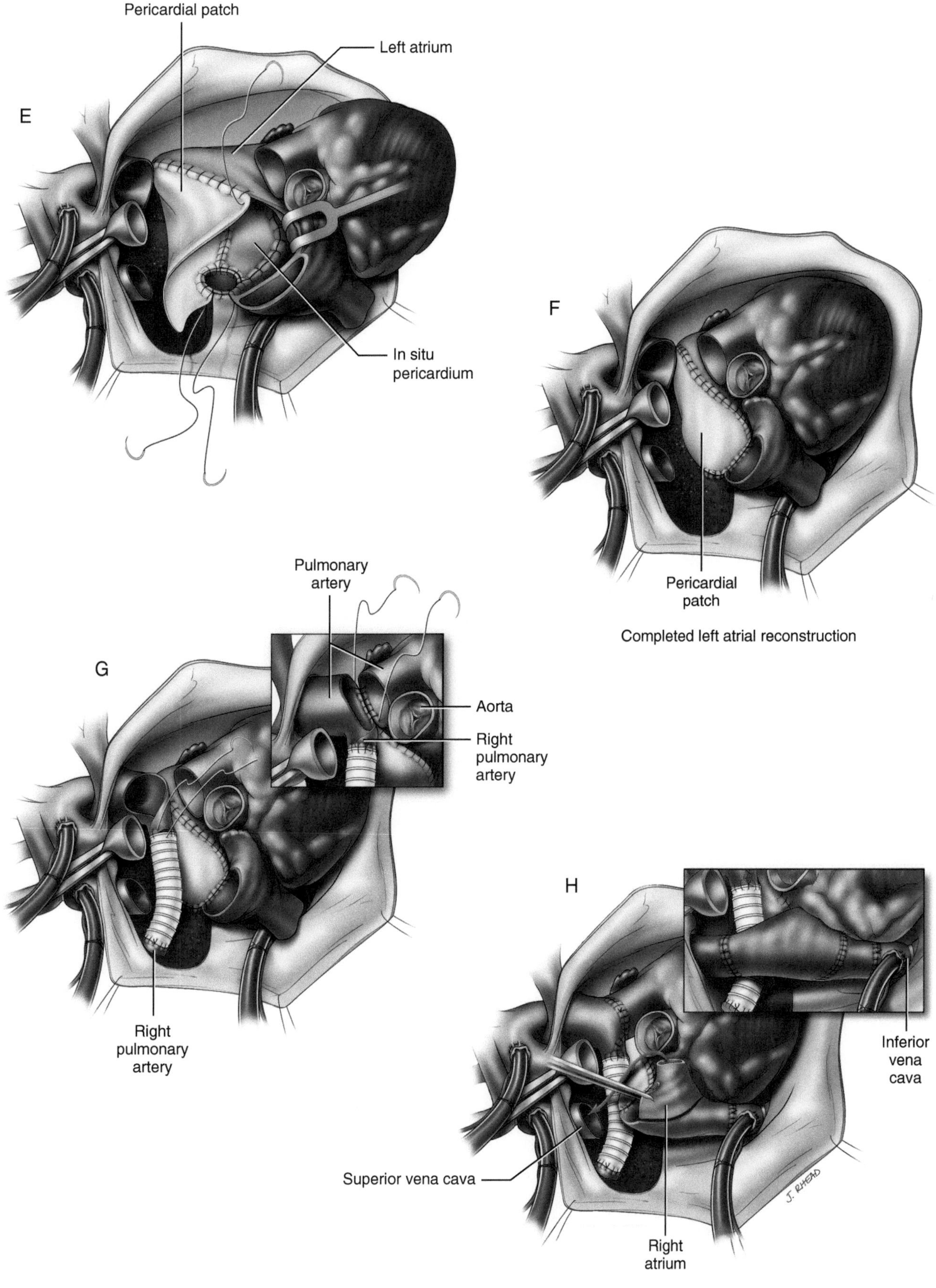

Completed left atrial reconstruction

INDEX

Note: Page numbers followed by *f, t,* and *b* refer to figures, tables, and boxes.

E

F

G

H

M

R

S

T

U

V